ANEURYSM

Edited by **Yasuo Murai**

Aneurysm
http://dx.doi.org/10.5772/3152
Edited by Yasuo Murai

Contributors

Simona Celi, Sergio Berti, Katarzyna Socha, Maria H. Borawska, Ivanilson Alves de Oliveira, Krzysztof Siemianowicz, Guillermo Vilalta, Félix Nieto, Enrique San Norberto, María Ángeles Pérez, José A. Vilalta, Carlos Vaquero, Ana Mladenovic, Zeljko Markovic, Sandra Grujicic-Sipetic, Hideki Hyodoh, Ahmad Alsheikhly, Efstratios Georgakarakos, Antonios Xenakis, George S. Georgiadis, Konstantinos C. Kapoulas, Evagelos Nikolopoulos, Miltos Lazarides, Ionel Droc, Dieter Raithel, Blanca Calinescu, Julia Mikhal, Cornelis H. Slump, Bernard J. Geurts, Yiyi Wei, Stéphane Cotin, Jérémie Dequidt, Christian Duriez, Jérémie Allard, Erwan Kerrien, Ivan Vulev, Andrej Klepanec, Xu Gao, Guobiao Liang, Igor Lima Maldonado, Alain Bonafé, Yasuo Murai, Akira Teramoto, Václav Procházka, Michaela Vávrová, Tomáš Jonszta, Daniel Czerný, Jan Krajča, Tomáš Hrbáč, G. Kang, K. Kang, Tomasz Szmuda, Pawel Sloniewski, Vishal N. Patel, Owen B. Samuels, Igor Banzić, Lazar Davidović, Oliver Radmili, Igor Končar, Nikola Ilić, Miroslav Marković, Miguel Angel Ramirez-Marrero, Beatriz Perez-Villardon, Ricardo Vivancos-Delgado, Manuel de Mora-Martin, Ivica Maleta, Božidar Vujičić, Iva Mesaroš Devčić, Sanjin Rački, Soh Hosoba, Tohru Asai, Tomoaki Suzuki

Published by InTech

Janeza Trdine 9, 51000 Rijeka, Croatia

Publishing Process Manager Dragana Manestar
Technical Editor InTech Prepress, Novi Sad
Cover InTech Design team

Additional hard copies can be obtained from orders@intechopen.com

Aneurysm, Edited by Yasuo Murai
p. cm.
ISBN 978-953-51-0730-9

For EU product safety concerns:
IN TECH d.o.o., Prolaz Marije Krucifikse Kozulić 3, 51000 Rijeka, Croatia,
info@intechopen.com or visit our website at intechopen.com.

Meet the editor

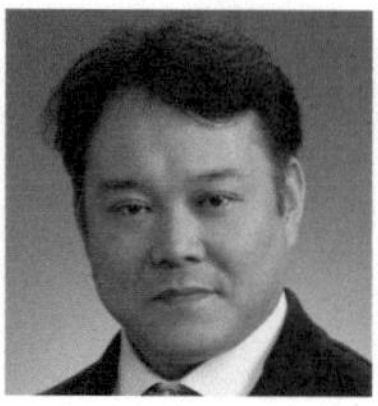

Dr Yasuo Murai MD, PhD who graduated from Nippon Medical School in 1993, trained at the Department of Neurosurgery, Nippon Medical School and specialized in Neurovascular surgery and skull base surgery at the Nippon Medical School hospital. His areas of expertise include neurovascular surgery, vascular reconstructive surgery and skull base neurosurgery both within Japan and abroad. A highly respected surgeon, teacher and researcher, he is one of the leading authorities on advanced vascular reconstructive surgery in Japan. He is the author of many peer-reviewed articles on these topics. He has been serving as acting head of the Nippon Medical School of neurovascular surgery and is an internationally recognized authority in vascular reconstructive surgery. He is currently clinical Assistant Professor of the Department of Neurosurgery at the Nippon Medical School hospital. He has received numerous scientific awards for his contributions to neurovascular surgery within Japan.

Contents

Preface XI

Section 1 Basic Research of Aneurysm 1

Chapter 1 **Biomechanics and FE Modelling of Aneurysm: Review and Advances in Computational Models 3**
Simona Celi and Sergio Berti

Chapter 2 **Mineral Components in Aneurysms 27**
Katarzyna Socha and Maria H. Borawska

Chapter 3 **Main Models of Experimental Saccular Aneurysm in Animals 43**
Ivanilson Alves de Oliveira

Chapter 4 **The Role of Metalloproteinases in the Development of Aneurysm 65**
Krzysztof Siemianowicz

Section 2 Abdominal Aneurysm 75

Chapter 5 **Biomechanical Approach to Improve the Abdominal Aortic Aneurysm (AAA) Rupture Risk Prediction 77**
Guillermo Vilalta, Félix Nieto, Enrique San Norberto, María Ángeles Pérez, José A. Vilalta and Carlos Vaquero

Chapter 6 **Abdominal Aortic Aneurysm in Different Races Epidemiologic Features and Morphologic-Clinical Implications Evaluated by CT Aortography 109**
Ana Mladenovic, Zeljko Markovic, Sandra Grujicic-Sipetic and Hideki Hyodoh

Chapter 7 **Splenic Artery Aneurysms 135**
Ahmad Alsheikhly

Chapter 8 **Studying the Flow Dynamics Within Endografts in Abdominal Aortic Aneurysms 151**
Efstratios Georgakarakos, Antonios Xenakis, George S. Georgiadis, Konstantinos C. Kapoulas, Evagelos Nikolopoulos and Miltos Lazarides

Chapter 9 **Abdominal Aortic Aneurysms – Actual Therapeutic Strategies 169**
Ionel Droc, Dieter Raithel and Blanca Calinescu

Section 3 Cerebral Aneurysm 197

Chapter 10 **Simulation of Pulsatile Flow in Cerebral Aneurysms: From Medical Images to Flow and Forces 199**
Julia Mikhal, Cornelis H. Slump and Bernard J. Geurts

Chapter 11 **A (Near) Real-Time Simulation Method of Aneurysm Coil Embolization 223**
Yiyi Wei, Stéphane Cotin, Jérémie Dequidt, Christian Duriez, Jérémie Allard and Erwan Kerrien

Chapter 12 **Endovascular Treatment of Internal Carotid and Vertebral Artery Aneurysms Using Covered Stents 249**
Ivan Vulev and Andrej Klepanec

Chapter 13 **Complications and Adverse Events Associated with Stent-Assisted Coiling of Wide-Neck Intracranial Aneurysms 269**
Xu Gao and Guobiao Liang

Chapter 14 **Stent-Assisted Techniques for Intracranial Aneurysms 291**
Igor Lima Maldonado and Alain Bonafé

Chapter 15 **Retroperitoneal Haemorrhage as a Dangerous Complication of Endovascular Cerebral Aneurysmal Coiling 313**
Yasuo Murai and Akira Teramoto

Chapter 16 **Intracranial and Extracranial Infectious Pseudoaneurysms 327**
Václav Procházka, Michaela Vávrová, Tomáš Jonszta, Daniel Czerný, Jan Krajča and Tomáš Hrbáč

Chapter 17 **Saphenous Vein Graft Aneurysms 343**
G. Kang and K. Kang

Chapter 18 **Giant Intracranial Aneurysms – Surgical Treatment, Accessory Techniques and Outcome 351**
Tomasz Szmuda and Pawel Sloniewski

Chapter 19 **The Critical Care Management of Aneurysmal Subarachnoid Hemorrhage 383**
Vishal N. Patel and Owen B. Samuels

Section 4 Special Case 403

Chapter 20 **False Aneurysms 405**
Igor Banzić, Lazar Davidović, Oliver Radmili, Igor Končar, Nikola Ilić and Miroslav Marković

Chapter 21 **Marfan Syndrome – Advances in Diagnosis and Management 427**
Miguel Angel Ramirez-Marrero, Beatriz Perez-Villardon, Ricardo Vivancos-Delgado and Manuel de Mora-Martin

Chapter 22 **Vascular Access for Hemodialysis 453**
Ivica Maleta, Božidar Vujičić, Iva Mesaroš Devčić and Sanjin Rački

Chapter 23 **Atrial Septal Aneurysm 471**
Soh Hosoba, Tohru Asai and Tomoaki Suzuki

Preface

This book focus is on diagnosis and treatment of intracranial aneurysm, abdominal and thoracic aortic aneurysms. It addresses neurosurgical, vascular and cardiothoracic surgeons and interventional radiologists, but also anyone engaged in vascular medicine. The book presents an effort to collect an up-to-date account of existing knowledge, involving recent development in this field. Various experts described details of established knowledge or newly recognized advances associated with diagnosis, treatment, perioperative management and mechanisms. The chapters are written by recognized vascular surgeons and scientists from around the world, collecting the work of internationally acknowledged experts sharing their opinions about the important topics of the current vascular surgery practice and research. The chapters selected for this book bring scientific input from authors who come from different specialities, countries, and sometimes even cultures, which has facilitated a comprehensive and interesting approach to the problem of aneurysm treatment. The book chapters include epidemiology, symptoms and signs, clinical, radiological imaging, medications, direct open surgery, intravascular surgeries and ultrastructural pathological diagnosis, therapeutic approaches and outcome of the whole body aneurys. Surgical procedures in this area have received increasing attention in the last few years and have been subjected to several modifications, especially the progress of interventional radiological endovascular techniques that reduce the invasive nature of surgery as well as complication rates led to rapid advancements. This book looks at current basic knowledge on aneurysm and some of the developments in research which have the potential to change the prognosis. This is the first book that deals with the whole body aneurysm, such as cerebral aneurysm, abdominal aneurysm, and splenial aneurysm and to learn the latest research in other fields is always very useful. I hope this book will be used worldwide by vascular surgeons and interventionalists enhancing their knowledge and stimulating the advancement of this field.

Yasuo Murai
Nippon Medical School, Tokyo,
Japan

Section 1

Basic Research of Aneurysm

Chapter 1

Biomechanics and FE Modelling of Aneurysm: Review and Advances in Computational Models

Simona Celi and Sergio Berti

Additional information is available at the end of the chapter

http://dx.doi.org/10.5772/46030

1. Introduction

Abdominal aortic aneurysm (AAA) disease is the 18th most common cause of death in all individuals and the 15th most common in individuals aged over 65 [48]. Clinical treatment for this disorder can consist of open surgical repair or, more recently, of minimally invasive endovascular repair procedures [71]. However, both clinical treatments present significant risks and, consequently, require specific patient selection. Given the risks of current repair techniques, during the course of an aneurysm it is important to determine when the risk of rupture justifies the risk of repair. In this scenario, how to determine the rupture risk of an aneurysm is still an open question. Currently, the trend in determining the severity of an AAA is to use the maximum diameter criterion. Unfortunately, this criterion is only a general rule and not a reliable indicator since small aneurysms can also rupture, as reported in autopsy studies, while many aneurysms can become very large without rupturing [16]. The maximum diameter criterion, in fact, is based on the law of Laplace that establish a linear relationship between diameter and wall stress. However, the law of Laplace is simply based on cylindrical geometries, where only one radius of curvature is involved, whereas aneurysms are complex structures, and therefore the law fails to predict realistic wall stresses. From a biomechanical point of view, rupture events occur when acting wall stresses exceed the tensile strength of the degenerated aortic abdominal (AA) wall. Biomechanics relates the function of a physiological system to its structure and its objective is to deduce the function of a system from its geometry, material properties and boundary conditions based on the balance laws of mechanics (e.g. conservation of mass, momentum and energy). Consequently, from a more general and extensive perspective, the stress state in a body is determined by several factors such as geometry, material properties, load and boundary conditions. In order to understand the capability to estimate the potential rupture risk, it is fundamental to capture the mechanical response of the aortic tissue and its changes during aneurysmal formation. In fact, while, to date, the precise pathogenesis of AAA is poorly understood, it is well known that this change significantly impact on the structure of the aortic wall and on its mechanical behavior.

This chapter will review the state of literature on the mechanical properties and modelling of AAA tissue and will present advanced computational models. The first part (Sec. 2) includes a description of the mechanical test currently used (2.1), the aortic mechanical properties (2.2) and a review of the literature on material constitutive equations (2.3) and geometrical models (2.4). To stress out the morphological complexity of the aortic segment, in Sec 3 the regional variations of material properties and wall thickness reported in literature form experimental investigations are reported. The second part (Sec. 4) describes our original contribution with a description of our Finite Element (FE) models and our probabilistic approach implemented into FE simulations to perform sensitivity analysis (Sec. 4.1). The main results are reported in Sec. 4.2 and discussed in detail in Sec. 5.

2. Review

In order to understand the biomechanical issues in the etiology and treatment of abdominal aortic aneurysms, it is important to understand the structures of the aortic wall and how they affect the mechanical response. Biological tissues are subject to the same balance laws of conservation of mass, momentum and energy of the classical engineering material. What distinguish biological tissues from materials of the field of classical engineering mechanics is their unique structure. Soft biological tissues, in fact, have a very complex structure that can be regarded as either *active* and *passive*. The active components arise from the activation of the smooth muscle cells while the passive response is governed primarily by the elastin and collagen fibres [15]. The distribution and the arrangement of the collagen fibres, in particular, have a significant influence on the mechanical properties due to they attribute anisotropic properties [49] to the tissue. Different studies have shown that this structural arrangement is very complex and varies according to the aortic segment (thoracic or abdominal) [20]. As well as being anisotropic, the material response of soft biological tissue is also highly non-linear.

2.1. Experimental test

To determine mechanical properties of AAA, studies have used both *in-vivo* "tests" and *ex-vivo/in-vitro* testing. As reported by Raghavan and da Silva [53], both of them offer advantages and disadvantages. In particular, in the first case the main difficult is to accurately determine the true force and the displacement distribution ascertaining stress-free configuration of the biological entity. On the other side, isolating samples may introduce as yet unknown changes to their behavior affecting the results of such tests. In vivo measurement are often performed by using imaging modality. By using ultrasound phase-locked echo-tracking, Lanne et al. [43] reported that the pressure-strain elastic modulus (E_p), Eq. 1, was higher on average and more widely dispersed in aneurysmal abdominal aorta compared to the non-aneurysmal aorta group. The E_p modulus was calculated based on the diameter (D_s,D_d) and pressure (P_s, P_d) at the systolic and diastolic values as follow:

$$E_p = D_p \frac{P_s - P_d}{D_s - D_d} \tag{1}$$

Using similar consideration, MacSweeney et al. [44] founded that E_p was higher in aneurysmal abdominal aorta compared to controls.

More recently, van't Veer et al. [75] estimated the compliance and distensibility of the AAA by means of simultaneous instantaneous pressure and volume measurements obtained with the magnetic resonance imaging (MRI). By using time resolved ECG-gated CT imaging data from 67 patients, Ganten et al. [27] found that the compliance of AAA did not differ between small and large lesions. In 2011 Molacek and co-authors [47] did not find any correlation between aneurysm diameter and distensibility of AAA wall and of normal aorta. However it is worth to notice that all these studies do not provide intrinsic mechanical properties of the tissue but more general extrinsic AAA behavior. As far as the *ex-vivo* testing, there are several types of mechanical tests that can be carried out on materials to obtain information on their mechanical behavior. Such tests include simple tension test, biaxial tension, conducted on thin samples of material, and extension/inflation test of thin-walled tubes.

Uniaxial test. Uniaxial extension testing is the simplest and most common of *ex-vivo* testing methods. Here, a rectangular planar sample is subjected to extension along its length at a constant displacement (or load) rate while the force (or the displacement) is recorded during extension. Under the assumption of incompressibility (zero changes of volume during the tensile test, Eq. 2) the recorded force-extension data are converted to stress/strain:

$$A_0 L_0 = AL \tag{2}$$

where A_0 and L_0 are the initial cross sectional area and the initial length while A and L are the values in the current configuration. Interested reader can refer to Di Puccio et al. [19] for a recent review on the incompressibility assumption on soft biological tissue.

Biaxial test. Due to the presence of the collagen fibers, the uniaxial testing is not sufficient for highlighting the aorta tissue and the stress distribution does not fully conform to physiological conditions. Therefore, biaxial tension tests should be performed. During biaxial test, an initial square thin sheet of material is stress normally to both edges. Even if, theoretically, the biaxial test are not sufficient to fully characterized anisotropic materials, [40, 50] they are able to capture additional information regarding the mechanical behavior of the specimens with respect to uniaxial one. By contrast, biaxial tests provides a complete characterization of the material properties for isotropic material. To some extent soft biological tissues can be considered as isotropic within certain limitation, however, in their general formulation, they respond anisotropically under loads. Figure 1 depicts as example the mechanical test and response of a soft tissue under uniaxial (a) and biaxial (b) test.

As we can observe, a distinctive mechanical characteristic of soft tissue in tension tests is its initial flat response and relatively large extensions followed by an increased stiffening at higher extension. As it is well known, this behavior is the result of collagen fibres recruitment as proposed by Roach and Burton [61]. The non-linear stress strain curve arises from the phenomenon of the fibres recruitment. As the material is stretched, the fibres gradually become uncrimped and become more aligned with the direction of applied load.

The results of uniaxial and biaxial tests are used to characterize the mechanical behavior of soft tissue under investigation. Due to the large deformation that characterizes this type of tissue, from a mathematical point of view, a Strain Energy Function (SEF) denoted by W is introduced. The Cauchy stress tensor ($\boldsymbol{\sigma}$) is calculated as:

$$\boldsymbol{\sigma} = J^{-1}\mathbf{F}\frac{\partial W}{\partial \mathbf{F}} \tag{3}$$

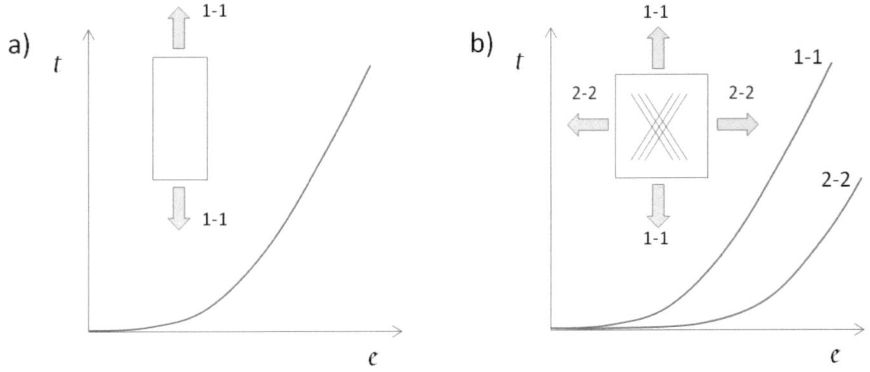

Figure 1. Schematic of uniaxial (a) and biaxial (b) test and curves. The t value is a rappresentative tension value and e a typical extension dimension.

where $\mathbf{F}$ is the deformation gradient tensor, defined as $\mathbf{F} = \partial\mathbf{x}/\partial\mathbf{X}$, i.e. the derivative of the current position $\mathbf{x}$ as regards to the initial position $\mathbf{X}$ during a deformation process and J is the determinant of $\mathbf{F}$. Under the assumption of incompressibility (J=1), the SEF is split in a volumetric (W_{vol}) and isochoric (W_{isoch}) component. In case of uniaxial test we have:

$$\sigma_{11} = \lambda_{11}\frac{\partial W_{isoch}}{\partial \lambda_{11}} \tag{4}$$

where λ_{11} is the stretch in the 1-1 direction (see Fig. 1 (a)). For biaxial test both components can be calculated:

$$\sigma_{\theta\theta} = \lambda_{\theta\theta}\frac{\partial W_{isoch}}{\partial \lambda_{\theta\theta}} \tag{5}$$

$$\sigma_{zz} = \lambda_{zz}\frac{\partial W_{isoch}}{\partial \lambda_{zz}} \tag{6}$$

Equations 5-6 represent the stress components used in the follow sections. With respect to Fig. 1 direction 1-1 and 2-2 are now defined as the circumferential $\sigma_{\theta\theta}$ and the axial σ_{zz} ones, respectively.

2.2. Mechanical properties of healthy and pathological aortic tissue

AAA development is multifactorial phenomenon. A mechanism postulated for AAA formation focuses on inflammatory processes where macrophages recruitment leads to MMP production and elastase release. The biomechanical change associated with enzymatic degradation of structural proteins suggests that AAA expansion is primarily related to elastolysis [21]: a decreasing quadratic relationship was found between elastin concentration and diameter for normal aortas and for pathological increasing diameter [65]. Despite universal recognition of the importance of wall mechanics in the natural history of AAAs [2, 38, 81], there are few detailed studies of the mechanical properties.

Early studies focused on simple uniaxial tests. He and Roach [32] obtained rectangular specimen strips during surgical resection of eight AAA patients and subjected them to uniaxial extension tests up to a pre-defined maximum load rather than until failure. They showed that the stress-strain behavior of AAA tissue was non-linear. Later, in two reports,

Vorp et al. [82] and Raghavan et al. [57] reported on uniaxial extension testing of strips harvested from the anterior midsection of 69 AAA. The specimens were extended until failure. In most cases, the rectangular specimens' length was in the axial orientation, but in a small population, they were oriented circumferentially. Results have found that aneurysmal tissue is substantially weaker and stiffer than normal aorta [18, 57, 70].

To date, the most complete data on both the biaxial mechanical behavior of aorta and AAAs comes from Vande Geest et al. [76, 77]. The source of these specimens becomes from AAA ventral tissue available during the open surgical repair of unruptured lesions. They reported biaxial mechanical data for AAA (26 samples) and normal human AA as a function of age: less than 30, between 30 and 60 and over 60 years of age. In particular Vande Geest and co-workers confirmed that the aortic tissue becomes less compliant with age and that AAA tissue is significantly stiffer than normal abdominal aortic tissue, Figure 2.

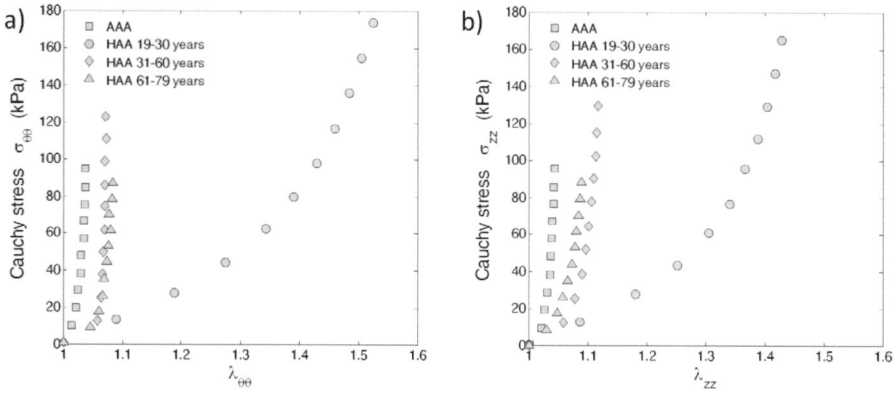

Figure 2. Stress-stretch plot comparing the equibiaxial response for AAA and HAA for four patient groups, for circumferential direction (a) and axial direction (b). Modified from [22].

The specimen was subjected to force-controlled testing with varying prescribed forces between the two orthogonal directions. A CCD camera was used to track the displacement of markers forming a 5x5 mm square placed on the specimen. It is worth to stress out that the use of optical extensometer (markers tracking with CCD camera) is fundamental to measure the deformation during test avoiding the potential tissue slippage from the clamps. Figure 3 depicts a representative biaxial stress-stretch data for healthy (a-b) and pathological (c-d) samples considering three different tension ratios ($T_\theta : T_z$) equal to 1:1 , 0.75:1 and 1:0.75.

2.3. Material models

Equations that characterize a material and its response to applied loads are called constitutive relations since they describe the gross behavior resulting from the internal constitution of a material. Constitutive modelling of vascular tissue is an active field of research and numerous descriptions have been reported. Constitutive models for biological tissues can be established following a so-called phenomenological or structural approach. The first type of formulation [14, 26, 36, 73] does not take into account any histological constituents and attempt to describe the global mechanical behavior of the tissue without referring to its underlying microstructure. The phenomenological approach is commonly used but has led to a number of difficulties in describing the mechanical behavior of tissues. Among phenomenological

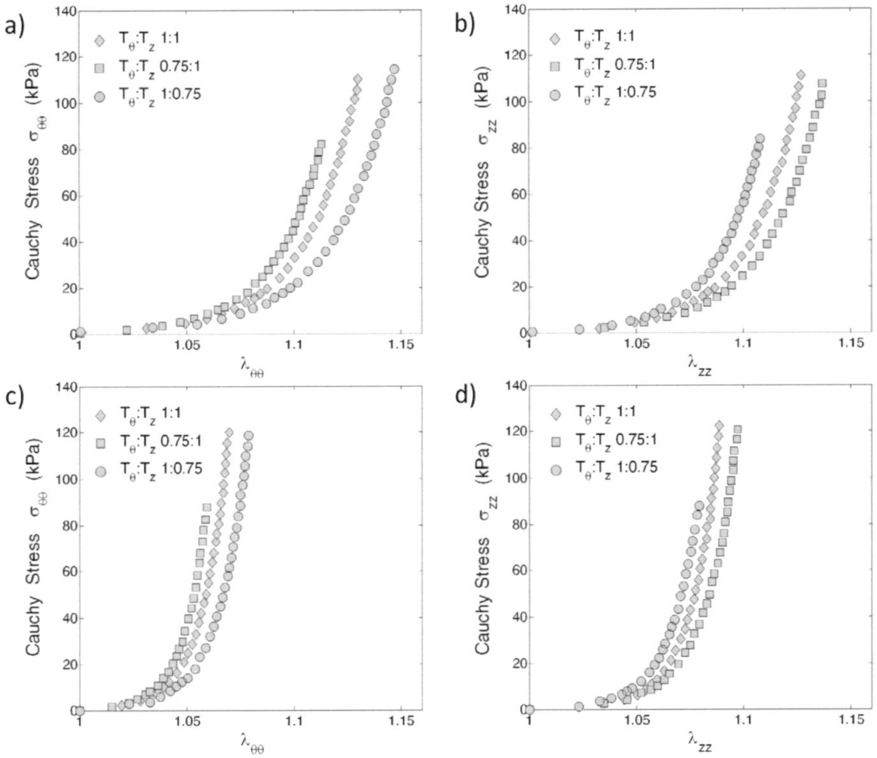

Figure 3. Experimental biaxial data for both healthy (a-b) and pathological (c-d) samples with different tension ratio. Open diamonds, 1 : 1; open squares, 0.75 : 1 and open circles, 1 : 0.75. Modified from [9].

SEFs, Vande Geest and co-authors [77] found that a constitutive functional form used earlier by Choi and Vito [12], Equation 7, would best suit their experimental data:

$$W_{isoch} = b_0 \left(e^{\frac{1}{2}b_1 E_{\theta\theta}^2} + e^{\frac{1}{2}b_2 E_{zz}^2} + e^{\frac{1}{2}b_3 E_{\theta\theta} E_{zz}} - 3 \right) \tag{7}$$

where b_0, b_1, b_2 and b_3 are the material parameters and $E_{\theta\theta}$ and E_{zz} are the components of the Green-strain tensor (Eq. 8) defined as follows:

$$\mathbf{E} = \frac{1}{2}\left(\mathbf{C} - \mathbf{I}\right) = \frac{1}{2}\left(\mathbf{F}\mathbf{F}^T - \mathbf{I}\right) \tag{8}$$

where **I** is the identity matrix and **C** is the right Cauchy-Green strain tensor.

Alternatively, structural constitutive descriptions [5, 28, 34, 35] overcome this limitation and integrate histological and mechanical information of the arterial wall. In particular, the contributions of constitutive cells, fibers and networks of elements are added together to depict the whole tissue behavior. The structural-based approach has become common with the advent of microstructural imaging methods [64, 80]. In fact, soft biological tissues have a very complex microstructure, consisting of many different components and including elastin fibres, collagen fibres, smooth muscle cells and extracellular matrix.

The same experimental data obtained by vande Geest et al. [77] were then fitted by using an invariant based constitutive equation with two fibre families (2FF) by Basciano et al. [5], Eq.

9, and Rodriguez et al. [62, 63], Eq. 10.

$$W_{isoch} = \alpha \left(\bar{I}_1 - 3\right)^2 + \beta \left(\bar{I}_4 - 1\right)^6 + \gamma \left(\bar{I}_6 - 1\right)^6 \tag{9}$$

$$W_{isoch} = C_1 \left(\bar{I}_1 - 3\right) + \sum_{i=3}^{4} \frac{k_1^i}{2k_2^i} \left(e^{k_2^i\left((1-\rho)\left(\bar{I}_1-3\right)^2+\rho\left(\bar{I}_4-I_0\right)^2\right)} - 1\right) \tag{10}$$

where $\bar{I}_1$ is the first invariant of the isochoric portion of the right Cauchy-Green stretch tensor (Eq. 11) and $\bar{I}_4$ and $\bar{I}_6$ are mixed invariants of the isochoric portion of the right Cauchy-Green deformation tensor (Eq. 12-13), introduced from embedded fibers [6, 33, 69].

$$\bar{I}_1 = tr\bar{\mathbf{C}} \tag{11}$$

$$\bar{I}_4 = \mathbf{a}_0 \cdot \bar{\mathbf{C}}\,\mathbf{a}_0 \tag{12}$$

$$\bar{I}_6 = \mathbf{b}_0 \cdot \bar{\mathbf{C}}\,\mathbf{b}_0 \tag{13}$$

where $\mathbf{a}_0$, $\mathbf{b}_0$ are the direction of the fibers as reported in Figure 4(a-b). In Eq. 9, α is the coefficients for the isotropic part while β and γ for the anisotropic component. In the same manner, in Eq. 10, C_1 is a stress-like material parameter for the purely elastin contribute, and k_j^i are material parameters corresponding to the fibers ($k_1^3 = k_1^4$ and $k_2^3 = k_2^4$). The parameter $\rho \in [0;1]$ is a (dimensionless) measure of anisotropy, $I_0 > 1$ is dimensionless parameters regarded as the initial crimping of the fibers (Fig. 4(b)).

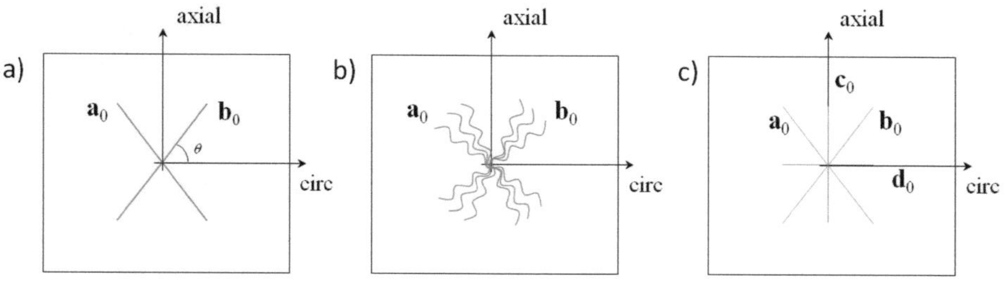

Figure 4. Collagen fiber orientation ($\mathbf{a}_0$, $\mathbf{b}_0$) in a square specimen of tissue for the 2FF model (a), the 2FF model with dispersion (b) and for the 4FF model (c). Note the crimp and fibres dispersion in case (b) and the two additional fibre family ($\mathbf{c}_0$, $\mathbf{d}_0$) in (c).

A constitutive relation based on four fibres family (4FF) (Fig. 4(c)) was proposed by Baek et al. [4], including two additionally fibres family (in longitudinal and circumferential direction, [86]), Equation 14:

$$W_{isoch} = \frac{c}{2} \left(\bar{I}_1 - 3\right) + \sum_{i=1}^{4} \frac{c_1^i}{4c_2^i} \left(e^{c_2^i\left(\bar{I}_4^i-1\right)^2} - 1\right) \tag{14}$$

where c, c_1^i and c_2^i are material parameters for this specific SEF. Ferruzzi et al. [22] assumed that diagonal families of collagen were regarded as mechanically equivalent, hence $c_1^3 = c_1^4$, $c_2^3 = c_2^4$. By fitting the biaxial data, the model parameter associated with the isotropic term decreased with increasing age for AA specimens and decreased markedly for AAA specimens [22, 31]. These finding are in good agreement with histopathological results of reduced elastin in ageing [30, 51] and AAAs, e.g. [32, 60].

For all models, the diagonal fibres are accounted for by $\mathbf{a}_0 = -\mathbf{b}_0$; in the 4FF model, axial ($\mathbf{c}_0$) and circumferential ($\mathbf{d}_0$) fibres are fixed at 90° and 0°, respectively.

Among the variety of constitutive equations reported in literature, the most significant difference in structural formulation were included by Holzapfel group [62] and by Baek and co-authors [4]. For a more detailed analysis on the effect of this assumption and a comparison between the two constitutive model, interested reader can refer to [17]. It is worth to stress out that, as observed by Zeinali-Davarani and co-authors [87], in parameter estimation, the larger number of parameters for a model provides more flexibility and generally gives better fitting, i.e., decreases the residual error. A common assumption in all previous models is to assume the same fibers distribution and mechanical response throughout the thickness. More recently Schriefl et al. [66] has observed that in the case of the intima layer, due to the higher fibers dispersion, the number of fiber families varying from two to four. However, not all intimas investigated had more than two fiber families while two prominent fibers families were always visible. The number of fiber families equal to two was previously reported by Haskett et al. [31] by analyzing 207 aortic samples.

Finally, it is worth to notice that it is fundamental to define a constitutive model and its material constants over some specific range, from experiments that replicate conditions (physiological or pathological), [17], in order to provide more accurate response. In fact all constitutive formulation are based on specific assumptions and hypotheses. The complexities of the artery wall poses several new conceptual and methodological challenges in the cardiovascular biomechanics. There exist several recent frameworks, in fact, to develop theories of arterial growth and remodeling (G&R) of soft tissues. Interested reader can refer to a more complete and detailed review by Humphrey and Rajagopal [38, 39] and in [41]. However, in this study, we restrict our attention to structural based formulations to emphasize their particular effects.

2.4. Geometrical model

By using Finite Element analyses, Fillinger et al. [23] showed that peak wall stress is a more reliable parameter than maximum transverse diameter in predicting potential rupture event. These findings appear to be supported by the results obtained by Venkatasubramaniam et al. [79], who indicated that the location of the maximum wall stress correlates well with the site of rupture and, additionally, by the observation that AAA formation is accompanied by an increase in wall stress [55, 83], and a decrease in wall strength [84]. Simulation on 3D patient-specific models are aimed to analyze the distribution of the wall stress to estimate the rupture risk during the evolution of the pathology [23], the effect of the thrombus [29, 85] or calcification [42, 45, 68] on the peak stress. Integration of geometry data with solid modelling is used for estimation of vessel wall distension, strain and stress patterns. Studies, to date, have typically used 3D geometries usually obtained from computer tomography (CT) [52] or MRI [7] scans or have used simplified morphologies [17, 62]. Figure 5 reports as example the phases from a CT reconstruction. However, both approaches present some limitations. In particular, it is worth pointing out that 3D simulations are not fully patient-specific models but only based on 3D patient-specific geometries while the material properties are assumed as mean population values due to the difficulty of assessing *in-vivo* material properties. Consequently, to date, no fully patient-specific model has been performed. Additionally, due to the complexity of the structure and the high computational cost required by patient-specific models, sensitivity analyses have not been performed on 3D real geometries, and only univariate investigations have been performed on idealized shapes, to estimate the influence of a single parameter on the whole stress map [63].

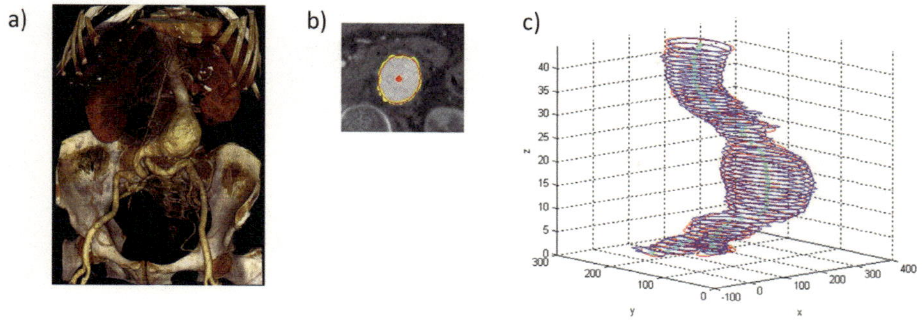

Figure 5. Example of AAA (a), segmentation of a CT cross section (b) and 3D reconstruction of a AAA (c), from [10].

3. Regional variations in wall thickness and material properties

As reported in previous section, starting from the observation that most AAAs are characterized by a complex not axisymmetric geometries a growing amount of literature has been published on the influence of the geometrical features. However one limitation in all the studies published so far is a constant wall thickness and homogeneous material assumed in the FE models.

Wall thickness. While the segmentation of the arterial lumen is a well established technique and has been performed with different modalities in living subjects, the segmentation of the wall and its connective components is not a feasible process due to the low contrast between the wall and the surrounding tissues. The conventional imaging techniques, in fact, do not provide sufficient spatial resolution to assess the wall thickness measurement and variant *in-vivo*.

During the AAA formation the artery wall is subjected to the remodelling process [77] and, as a consequence, the ratio between AA and AAA wall thickness changes. Di Martino et al. [18] noted a significant difference in wall thickness between ruptured and elective AAAs (3.6±0.3 mm vs 2.5±0.1 mm, respectively). By comparing the wall thickness between healthy and pathological samples, Vande Geest et al. [77] reported that the mean measured thickness values were 1.49±0.11 and 1.32±0.08 mm for the AA and AAA specimens, respectively. In all these studies, samples were measured only in the anterior area and consequently no information regarding regional variation between ventral and dorsal was reported. Thubrikar et al. [70] obtained five whole unruptured AAA specimens during surgical resection. Raghavan et al. [54] performed similar measures on three unruptured and one ruptured AAA, harvested as a whole during necropsy. More recently Celi et al. [10] performed measurements on 12 harvested unrupture ascending segments. In Table 1, the main results of these experimental measures are reported for both anterior and posterior region (mean±sd).

It is worth to notice that the thickness distribution seems to be opposite of that in the normal abdominal aorta where the wall is thicker than the posterior wall in 64% of cases [74].

From the computational point of view, in literature only few authors have investigated the effect on wall thickness reduction. Scotti et al. [67] used a non uniform wall thickness in an

N. of samples	District	$Thk_{anterior}$ (mm)	$Thk_{posterior}$ (mm)	Ref
5	AAA	2.09±0.51	2.73±0.46	[70]
4	AAA	2.25±0.37	2.34±0.48	[54]
12	aTAA	1.63±0.48	2.18±0.35	[10]

Table 1. Wall thickness measurements, reported in literature, categorized by circumferential location as anterior and posterior

idealized isotropic model to performed FSI simulations. Their results show that the models with a non uniform wall thickness have a maximum wall stress nearly four times that of a uniform one. Starting from experimental measurement on 12 human harvested ascending aortic samples, Celi et al. [10] developed structural 3D models of ascending AAA by including wall thickness regional variation between dorsal and ventral areas.

Material properties. As far as the material properties, to date, different behavior has funded between healthy (HAA) and pathological samples. However, due to the lack of sufficient biaxial data, a full characterization in regional variations are not provided (in circumferential direction in particular), and mechanical tests have been performed mainly in the ventral area where the bulge was formed. As well as the material properties change during the AAA progression, also the wall strength value changes. This aspect plays a fundamental role in the rupture phenomenon. In fact, the concept is that AAA rupture follows the basic principles of material failure; i.e., an aneurysm ruptures when the mural stresses or deformation meets an appropriate failure criterion. In the filed of the classical mechanics, this concept is defined by means of the potential rupture risk (RPI) parameter and quantify as the ratio of local wall stress to local wall strength:

$$RPI = \frac{local\,stress}{local\,strength} \tag{15}$$

In the same manner the safety factor (SF) can be used as the inverse of the RPI.

Thubrikar et al. [70] performed uniaxial tensile tests in both longitudinal and circumferential direction, on samples from five aneurysms. To study the regional variation they obtained samples from anterior, lateral (without distinction between left and right side) and posterior regions. In this study, however, authors did not perform tests until failure and they recorded the yield stress to define the initial point of a permanent damage. Thubrikar et al. observed that in both directions, the yield stress was greater in the lateral region with respect to the anterior and the posterior region, Figure 6(a). Experimental values regarding ultimate stress were reported by Raghavan et al. [54], Figure 6(b). They cut multiple longitudinally oriented rectangular specimen strips at various locations from three unruptured AAA and one ruptured AAA for a total of 48 strips. Samples were tested uniaxially until failure. They observed that the failure tension (ultimate) of specimen strips varied regionally from 55 kPa (near the rupture site) to 423 kPa at the undilated neck. However they report that there was no perceptible pattern in failure properties along the circumference.

Using multiple linear regression, Vande Geest et al. [78] proposed a mathematical model to estimate the wall strength by including several mixed parameters such as the gender, the presence of the intraluminal thrombus (ILT) and the family history. The final statistical model for local Cauchy wall strength (Eq. 16, dimension in kPa) was given by:

$$\sigma_u = 719 - 379\left(ILT^{\frac{1}{2}} - 0.81\right) - 156\,(D_{NORM} - 2.46) - 213\,HIST + 193\,SEX \tag{16}$$

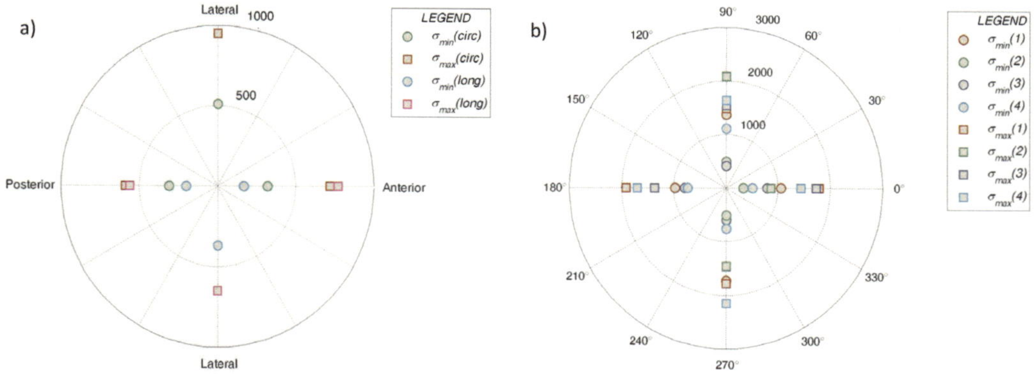

Figure 6. Yield stress in circumferential (upper side) and longitudinal (lower side) direction from [70] (a). Failure stress by circumferential location as anterior (0°), left (90°), posterior (180°) and right (270°) regions from [54] (b).

where $ILT^{\frac{1}{2}}$ is the square root of the ILT thickness whose units, D_{NORM} is a dimensionless parameter for local normalized diameter, HIST is a dimensionless binary variable (1/2 for positive family history, -1/2 for no family history), and SEX is a dimensionless binary variable for gender (1/2 for males, -1/2 for females). Table 2 depicts some examples of the effect of the coefficients of Eq. 16 by varing the gender and the ILT thickness.

Case	ILT (cm)	D_{NORM}	$HIST$	SEX	σ_u (kPa)
1	0	3.9	0.5	0.5	917.71
2	0	3.9	0.5	-0.5	598.35
3	1	3.9	0.5	-0.5	219.35

Table 2. Effect of the gender (case 1 vs. case 2) and of ILT thickness (case 2 vs. case 3) on the wall strength by using Eq. 16.

As we can notice the presence of the ILT decreases significantly the σ_u of about 63%. However, it is worth to notice that Eq. 16 describes local variation of the wall strength only in terms of normalized diameter and ILT thickness. Indeed Fillinger et al. [24] report that aneurysms likely rupture at stresses of 450 kPa or lower.

4. Finite element analyses

In order to get some indications on how regional variation of wall thickness and material properties affect the wall stress, two different FE models were developed. The first case describes a simplified model where an isotropic SEF has been adopted [56]. The tissue was described as homogeneous and consequently no distinction between healthy and pathological tissues was modeled. The second model introduces anisotropy and material regional variation to obtain more realistic simulations. For this last model, three different regions were considered and characterized with specific anisotropic SEFs: healthy material for the necks (HAA), pathological for the anterior bulge (AAA) and pathological for the posterior (AHA). Due to no data were available for the posterior region, a simple data manipulation was applied to define the new AHA pathological dataset starting from AAA experimental data as previously described in [9]. Figure 7 depicts the anisotropic dataset for the three rappresentative materials. As we can observe, the AHA dataset is able to reproduce an intermediate mechanical behavior between full healthy and pathological material.

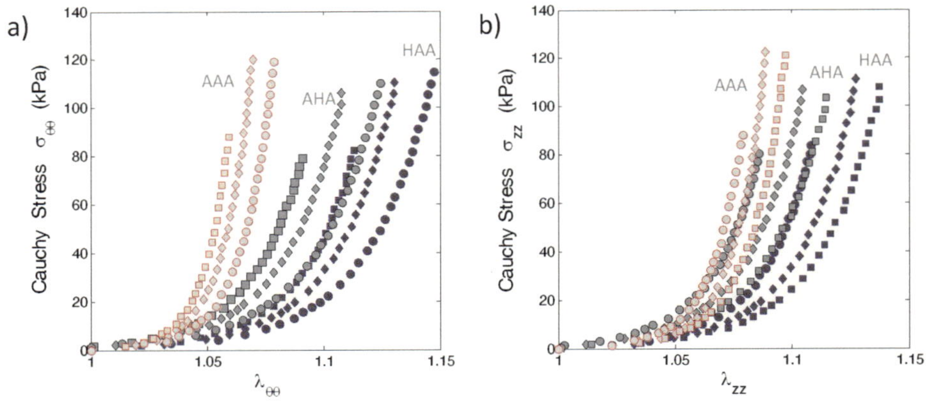

Figure 7. Example of HAA and AAA material models and virtual dataset (AHA) adopted for the transition region.

Both FE models are characterized by a wall thickness reduction in longitudinal and circumferential direction. For the necks, a wall thickness value equal to 1.8 mm was used while reduction of 30% and 50% was applied for the ventral area and of 20% for the dorsal one. Aneurysm shapes were defined as idealized 3D geometries with circular cross sections. Meridian lines describing the interior surface were based on a SZ-shaped function reported in Equation 17:

$$z(r) = \begin{cases} R_0 & 0 \le z \le a \\ 2(R_{AAA} - R_0)\left(\frac{z-a}{b-a}\right)^2 + R_0 & a < z \le \frac{a+b}{2} \\ (R_{AAA} - R_0) - 2\left(\frac{z-b}{b-a}\right)^2 + R_0 & \frac{a+b}{2} < z \le b \\ R_{AAA} & b < z \le \frac{L}{2} \end{cases} \quad (17)$$

where the parameter a and b locate the extremes of the slope portion of the curve. Due to symmetry only one-half of the profile is reported. Geometrical profiles are reported in Fig. 8.

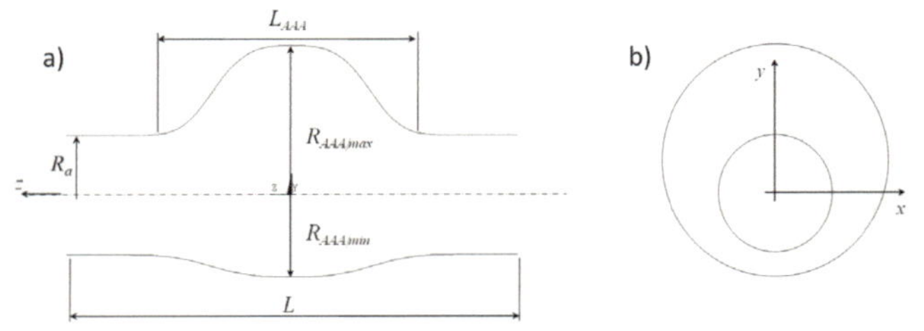

Figure 8. Lateral (a) and frontal (b) view of an asymmetrical aneurysmatic shape.

where where R_a is the radius of the healthy artery, $R_{AAA|max}$ is the maximum radius of the aneurysm in the ventral region, $R_{AAA|min}$ is the maximum radius of the aneurysm in the dorsal site. L (equal to 80 mm) defines the length of the abdominal vessel and L_{AAA} is the length of the aneurysmatic area. Figure 9(a) depicts an example of meshed asymmetric aneurysm with indication of the three anisotropic materials (in accordance with Fig. 7, while in Figure 9(b)) transversal cross section at the maximum diameter is reported with indication of circumferential wall thickness reduction.

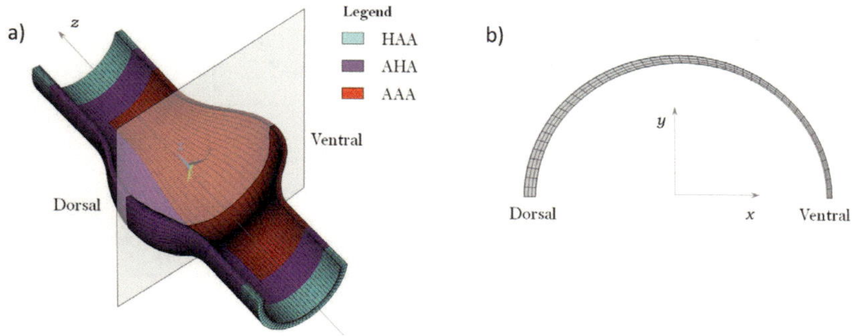

Figure 9. Example of asymmetric aneurysm and assignment of local material properties (a) and transversal cross section (b) with a wall thickness reduction of 50% and 20% in the ventral and dorsal region respectively.

For the constitutive equations for both healthy and pathological tissue, an invariant-based anisotropic polynomial SEF was chosen, as reported in Eq. 18. The material coefficients were calculated by using a specific weighted non-linear regression procedure implemented in Matlab and based on the Levenberg-Marquardt algorithm.

$$W_{isoch} = \sum_{i=1}^{3} a_i \left(\bar{I}_1 - 3\right)^i + 2\sum_{j=2}^{6} b_j \left(\bar{I}_4 - 1\right)^j \qquad (18)$$

Aneurysms were inflated applying a uniform inner pressure of 16 kPa, corresponding to the nominal value of peak systolic pressure. The ends of the vessels were left free to move in the radial direction.

4.1. Sensitivity analysis

To evaluate the sensitivity of the maximum stress state with respect to geometrical features, sensitivity and multivariate analyzes were also carried out by means of ANSYS Probabilistic Design Toolbox. This type of investigation presents two main advantages: the spread of the response of the output variables can be found, and it is possible to define the parameters that mainly influence the response of the system, for further details see [3, 46, 58]. Correlation coefficients are used as a measure of the strength of the relationship between input parameter and output measure.

In this study, analyzes were performed using the Monte Carlo method, in which the correlations between input and output variables are defined in a completely statistical way. In order to reduce the number of samples, the Latin Hypercube technique, instead of a direct sampling, was adopted. The effectiveness of these procedures was previously tested by Celi [8] and Celi et al. [11]. In order to study the effect of the AAA geometry on the distribution of the wall stresses, we introduced three dimensionless geometrical parameters:

$$F_R = \frac{R_{AAA}}{R_a}; \quad F_L = \frac{L_{AAA}}{R_{AAA}}; \quad F_{sym} = \frac{R_{AAA|min} - R_a}{R_{AAA|max} - R_a}; \quad F_{thk} = \frac{thk_0 - thk_{min}}{thk_0} 100 \qquad (19)$$

The parameter F_R defines the ratio between the maximum AAA radius and the healthy arterial radius, F_L defines the ratio between the length of the aneurysm and the maximum AAA radius, while $F_{sym} \in [0,1]$ is a measure of the aneurysmal eccentricity. The extreme cases F_{sym}=1 and F_{sym}=0 define the symmetrical situation and the most asymmetric geometry, respectively. Table 3 summarizes the FE analyses performed in this study.

Parameter	Definition	Distribution	Range
F_R	Dilatation ratio	uniform	1.5-3
F_L	Shape factor	uniform	1.5-4
F_{sym}	Symmetry factor	uniform	0-1
F_{thk}	Thickness ratio	uniform	0-50

Table 3. Range of the geometric parameters defining the aneurysmal shape.

Model	Thk	N. of materials	Type of Material	Type of Analysis
Iso_1	variable	1 (AAA)	Iso	Det./Prob.
$Aniso_1$	variable	1 (AAA)	Aniso	Det.
$Aniso_3$	variable	3 (AAA, AHA, HAA)	Aniso	Det.

Table 4. Scheme of the simulations performed in this study.

4.2. Results

Fitting procedure. The results of the best fit procedures for the anisotropic SEFs are reported in Figure 10. For all models very good results were obtained and, as a metric of the goodness of fit, the root mean square of the fitting error were computed: R^2=0.992, R^2=0.992 and R^2=0.983 from healthy to pathological tissue, respectively.

Table 5 lists the parameters values for the HAA, AHA and AAA models. The angle θ represents the embedded fiber orientations, as illustrated in Fig. 4(a).

Model	a_1	a_3	a_3	b_4	b_5	b_6	θ	R^2
HAA	2.503	1.641	896.714	3.467	1.564	102.677	45.510	0.992
AHA	12.194	40.869	2166.994	2.483	41.883	64.650	52.199	0.992
AAA	1.5	0.1	4966.781	54.381	3856.291	4997.367	45.989	0.983

Table 5. Coefficients for the models for the three SEFs. Vales in kPa

Thus, the new models adequately reproduce the experimental data sets for HAA, AHA and AAA tissues using only one SEF with six parameters per model. Figure 10(c-f-i) points out the changes in the anisotropic effect by increasing the pathological response of a tissue from healthy to aneurysmatic state.

FE simulations. Distributions of the circumferential stresses for the isotropic and anisotropic models for three different values of F_{thk} are shown in Fig. 11. It can be observed that for all models and geometries, the maximum stress is localized in the interior wall surface and in the proximity of the minor radius of curvature, due to the geometrical effect of the curvature itself, and that there exists a stress gradient through the aneurysm wall thickness. As expected, the isotropic model underestimates the peak stress value of about 40%, 38%, 42% with respect to the 2FF homogeneous anisotropic model, Fig. 11(d-e-f), of about 44%, 40%, 43% with respect to the 2FF heterogeneous model, Fig. 11(g-h-i). By focusing our attention on the anisotropic

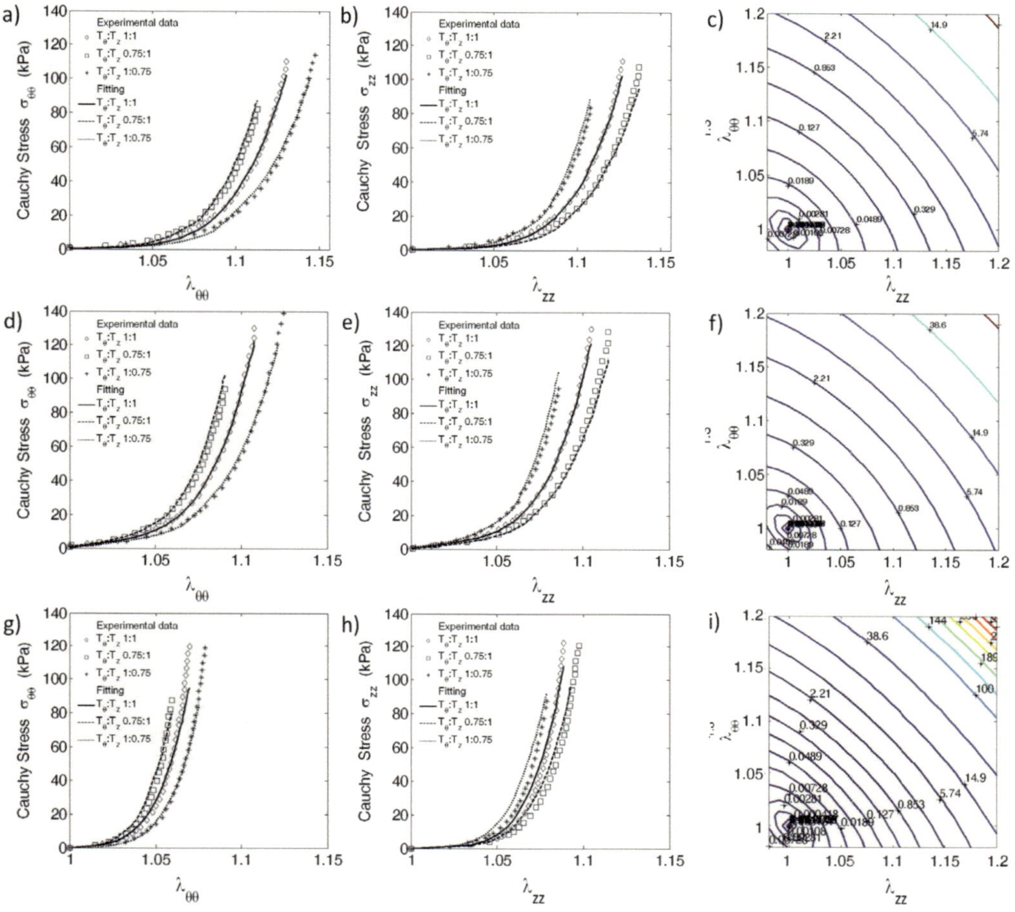

Figure 10. Representative stress-stretch data and fitting results for an HAA (a-b), AHA (d-e) and AAA (g-h) in circumferential and axial direction, see Fig. 7. The isolines of the SEFs for all models are reported in (c), (f) and (i).

models, as we can observe, the 2FF heterogeneous models present the highest maximum stress values due to the presence of the additional two material (HAA and AHA). The effect of these materials is to increase deformation in both radial and axial directions of the ventral and dorsal regions by changing, as a consequence, the local curvature.

As far as the stress gradient, Figure 12 depicts the transmural circumferential stress for model $Aniso_1$ and $Aniso_3$ for the two extreme cases of constant wall thickness and of maximum reduction. In the bulge area, Fig. 12(a), models $Aniso_1$ and $Aniso_3$ present the same stress gradient behavior due to the use of the same material (AAA). The effect of the wall thickness reduction is an increase of about 30% in the bulge region where the maximum diameter is reached. In the dorsal region, Fig. 12(b) the wall thickness reduction increases the maximum stress of about 8% for both models, while, the combined effect of the wall thickness reduction and different material produces an increase of about 21%. As far as the multivariate analysis, under the assumption of a constant wall thickness, the peak stress, is primarily affected by F_R, while if the wall thickness reduction in the bulge (F_{thk}) is considered, F_{thk} plays the main role.

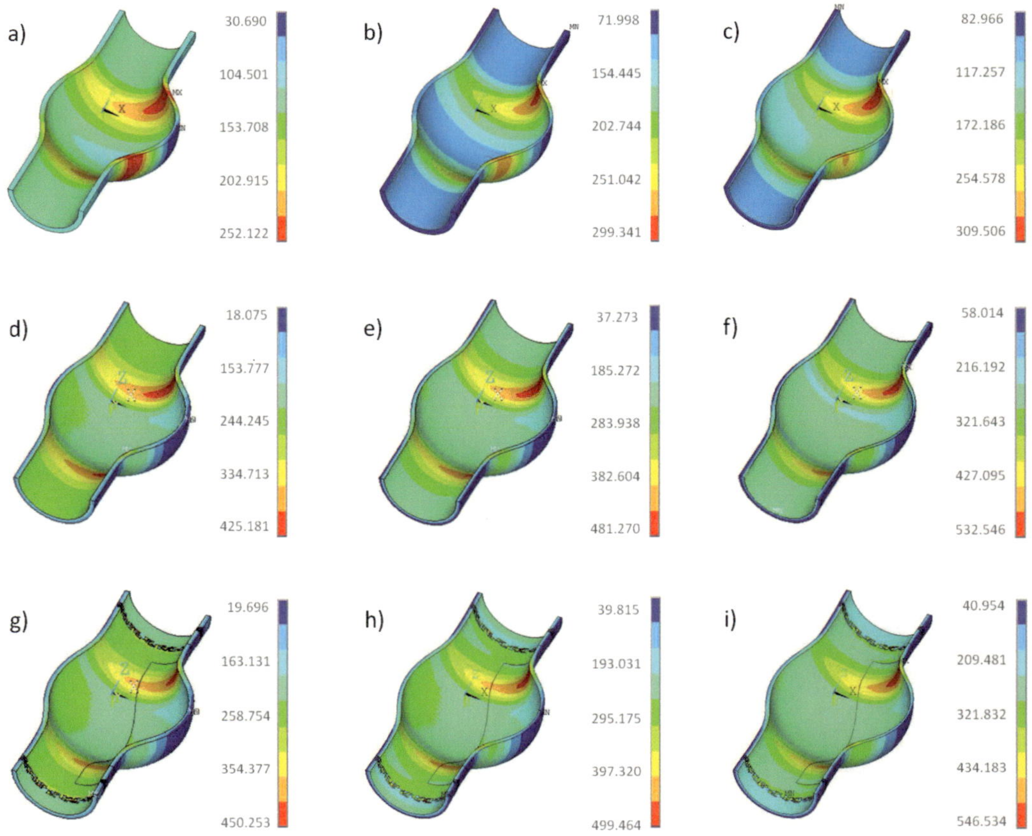

Figure 11. Contour plots of the circumferential stress for model Iso_1 (a-c), $Aniso_1$ (d-f) and $Aniso_3$ (g-i) with progressive wall thickness reduction. Constant wall *thk* (a,d,g), reduction of 30% and 20% (b,e,h) and reduction of 50% and 20% (c,f,i) in ventral and dorsal area. Stress in kPa.

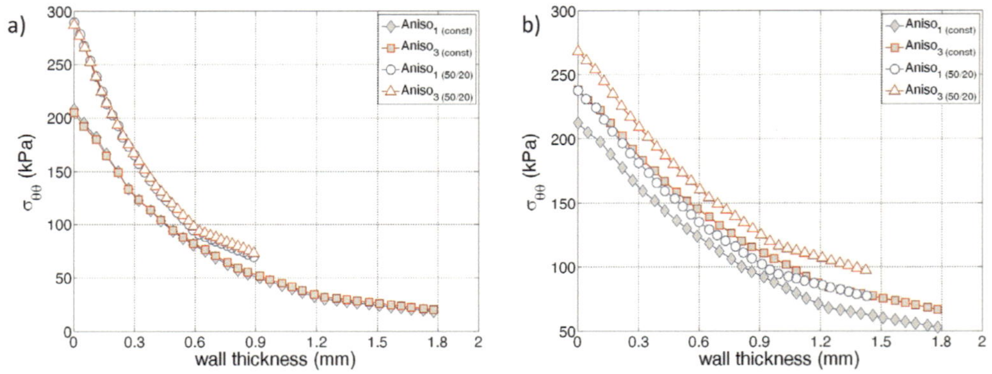

Figure 12. Stress gradient (kPa) in the ventral (a) and dorsal (b) area for the anisotropic models by considering constant wall thickness and the reduction of 50% and 20% in ventral and dorsal area.

Moreover, the same stress value is obtained both in fusiform aneurysm with critical dimension ($F_{thk} \simeq 2.5$) and in saccular with $F_{thk} \simeq 2$, see Figure 13(a). Including the wall thickness variation in the multivariate analyses points out the importance of these parameters. Figure 13(b) depicts the correlation coefficients (C.C.) for each input variable: the stresses increase as the diameter increases, but decrease as the thickness increases. Additionally, shorter models had higher wall stress.

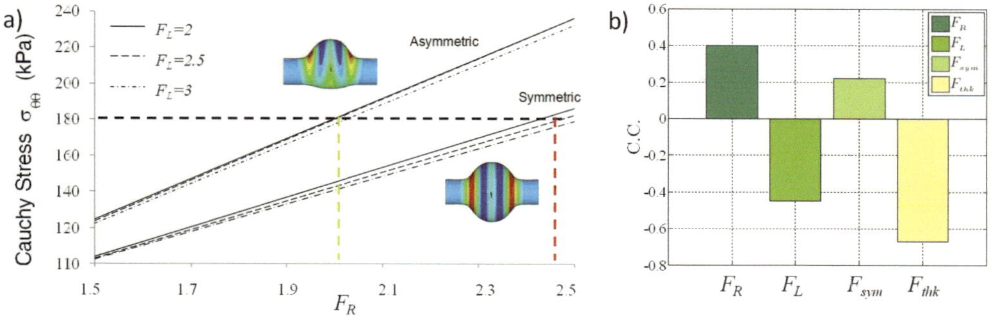

Figure 13. Maximum circumferential stresses as a function of F_R and F_L parameters (a) and correlation coefficients (C.C.) for each geometrical parameters (b).

5. Discussion and conclusion

In the first part of this work a literature survey on AAA biomechanics is reported by including several aspects from experimental test to constitutive model formulations. In the second part our FE models are presented, aimed at simulating and enhancing the computational study of the aneurismatic pathology. With respect to previous works, a more realistic type of AAA, even if idealized, was considered defined by means of regional variation of wall thickness and material properties. Notwithstanding many important findings from prior finite element stress analyses, all models are limited by the assumption of material homogeneity and constant wall thickness, e.g. [17, 55, 59, 62, 63]. Starting from the principle that intramural cells seek to remodel the arterial wall in order to maintain and to restore stresses towards homeostatic values, the material and geometrical properties must vary from region to region. This concept is the base of the remodeling phenomena as suggest by Humphrey [37]. In order to include material regional variation, in this work, we have introduced a simplified form of the stored energy function (Equation 18), motivated directly by microstructural information on two collagen fiber families [66]. This constitutive form fits well (e.g. mean R^2 of about 0.9) healthy and pathological available human biaxial data without complexity. Our SEF, in fact, is able to cope the progressive decrease in the elastin contribute (associated with the isotropic contribution attributed to an elastin-dominated amorphous matrix [34]) and increase in the anisotropic effects (associated with the predominant families of collagen fibers). The decrease of the elastin from heathy to pathological state as well as the increase of anisotropy are reported in Figure 14 where the isotropic (W_{iso}) and anisotropic (W_{aniso}) components of the SEF for HAA and AAA models are reported.

The present nonlinear regression focused not only on the estimating global best-fit values of model parameters suitable for performing stress analyses, but also on their effect in terms of energy behavior and changes from heathy to pathological tissue (Figure 10(c-i)). In

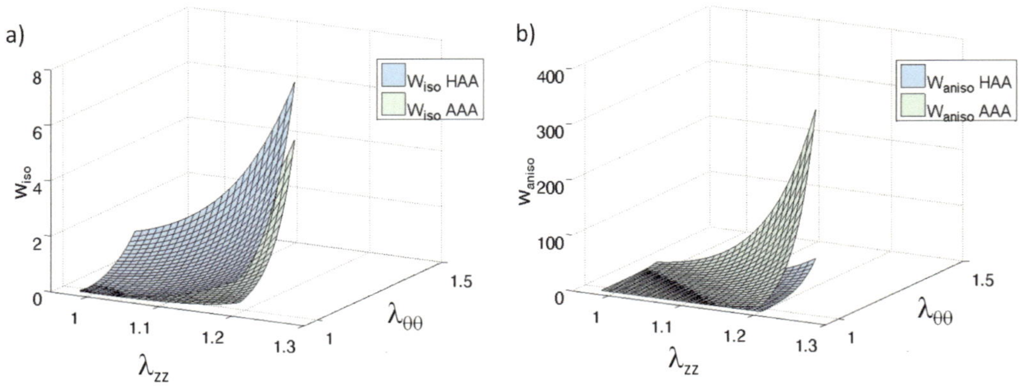

Figure 14. Isotopic (a) and anisotropic (b) component of the SEF reported in Eq. 18 for healthy (HAA) and pathological (AAA) tissue.

parallel to the marked decrease in the isotropic stored energy for AAA tissues (as describe above), we can observed an increase of stiffness capturing the observed biaxial reduction in extensibility/distensibility in particular in the circumferential direction (see Fig. 10(g)). As mention in Sec. 1, in current clinical practise, the aortic diameter is the main feature that is used to predict the risk of rupture. The more reliable quantification of the rupture risk is provided by the RPI parameter of Eq. 15 (and similar), however, which stress (principal stress, circumferential stress or von Mises stress) and strength is still matter of controversy. Gaining an understanding of the mechanical properties of the AAA tissue therefore is of clinical significance. Due to the difficult to reliably predict abdominal aortic aneurysm expansion and rupture in individuals several clinical trials have been performed [25, 72]. At the same time, from the computational point of view, literature systematically reports the evidence to support the role of patient-specific biomechanical profiles in the management of patients with AAA both from imaging and FE approach [1, 13, 81]. In order to accurately predict the risk of rupture of AAA, is necessary to predict the AAA wall strength distribution and the material properties non-invasively. With regard to our work, our specific FE simulations (both deterministic and probabilistic), reveal the importance to define a more realistic geometrical shape by including also wall thickness regional variation. Several previous studies were devoted to the definition of the geometrical parameters that mainly influence the wall stress (Vorp et al. [83] and more recently Rodríguez et al. [62] found that wall stress is substantially increased by an asymmetric bulge in AAAs, just to cite but a few), but, to the best of our knowledge, this is the first structural study in which also the wall thickness is considered as variable. Figure 15 depicts results from two deterministic simulations extracted by the multivariate analysis: aneurysm with a large diameter and constant wall thickness (a) and FE model small diameter and a wall thickness reduction of 50% in the ventral area. The stress contour plot points out how the wall thickness reduction influence the maximum stress value and its localization.

To conclude, there is, therefore, a pressing need to include patient specific regional variations to identify regions within AAAs that have the highest ratio of stress to strength. Future studies on patient-specific geometries of AAAs should consider the actual wall thickness. Moreover, the understanding the mechanical properties of the AAA wall will enhance our ability to design implants that can stay in place and/or protect the aneurysm wall from blood pressure.

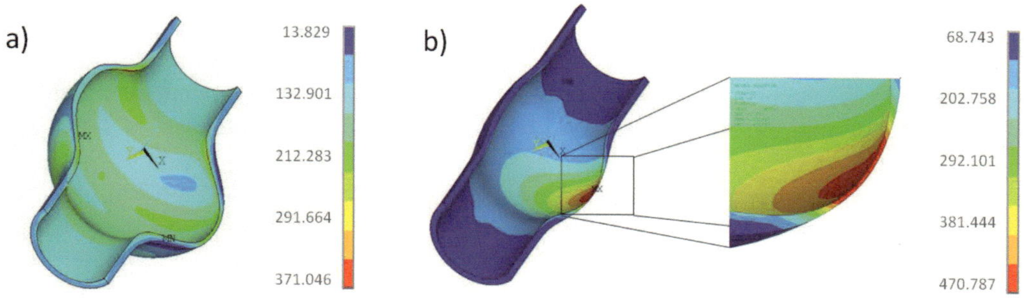

Figure 15. Stress contour plot of aneurysm with a large diameter and constant wall thickness (a) and a FE model small diameter and a wall thickness reduction of 50% in the ventral area.

Author details

Simona Celi
Institute of Clinical Physiology National Research Council IFC-CNR, Massa
Fondazione Toscana CNR "G. Monasterio", Heart Hospital, Massa, Italy

Sergio Berti
Fondazione Toscana CNR "G. Monasterio", Heart Hospital, Massa, Italy

6. References

[1] Abbas, A., Attia, R., Smith, A. & M.Waltham [2011]. Can we predict abdominal aortic aneurysm (aaa) progression and rupture by non-invasive imaging?-a systematic review, *International Journal of Clinical Medicine* 2: 484–499.

[2] Alexander, J. J. [2004]. The pathobiology of aortic aneurysms, *Journal of Surgical Research* 117: 163–175.

[3] Ang, A. S. & Tang, W. H. [1984]. *Probabilistic concepts in engineering planning and design, Decision, risk and reliability*, John Wiley & Sons Inc.

[4] Baek, S., Gleason, R., Rajagopal, K. & Humphrey, J. [2007]. Theory of small on large: Potential utility in computations of fluidŰsolid interactions in arteries, *Computer Methods in Applied Mechanics and Engineering* 196: 3070–3078.

[5] Basciano, C. A. & Kleinstreuer, C. [2009]. Invariant-based anisotropic constitutive models of the healthy and aneurysmal abdominal aortic wall, *Journal of Biomechanical Engineering* 131(2): 021009 (11 pages).

[6] Boehler, J. P. [1987]. *Introduction to the Invariant Formulation of Anisotropic Constitutive Equations*, Springer-Verlag, Wien,, chapter Applications of Tensor Functions in Solid Mechanics, CISM Courses and Lectures No., 292, pp. 13–30.

[7] Borghi, A., Wood, N., Mohiaddin, R. & Xu, X. [2006]. 3d geometric reconstruction of thoracic aortic aneurysms, *BioMedical Engineering OnLine* 5(59): 1–13.

[8] Celi, S. [2012]. Numerical and experimental simulations of surgical procedures, *PhD Thesis*, University of Pisa.

[9] Celi, S. & Berti, S. [2012]. FE simulations on the effect of regional variations of material properties and wall thickness on AAA, *GNB congress*, ISBN: 978 88 555 3182-5.

[10] Celi, S., Berti, S., Mariani, M., Di Puccio, F. & Forte, P. [2010]. Investigation on the effect of the wall thickness in rupture risk estimation of aaa by a probabilistic finite element approach, *European Heart Journal* 31 (Supp)(1): 284.

[11] Celi, S., Di Puccio, F. & Forte, P. [2011]. Advances in finite element simulations of elastosonography for breast lesion detection, *Journal of Biomechanical Engineering* 133: 081006–13.

[12] Choi, H. S. & Vito, R. P. [1990]. Two-dimensional stress-strain relationship for canine pericardium, *Journal of Biomechanical Engineering* 112(2): 153–159.

[13] Choke, E., Cockerill, G., Wilson, W., Sayed, S., Dawson, J., Loftus, I. & Thompson, M. [2005]. A review of biological factors implicated in abdominal aortic aneurysm rupture, *European Journal of Vascular and Endovascular Surgery* 30(3): 227–244.

[14] Chuong, C. J. & Fung, Y. C. [1983]. Three-dimensional stress distribution in arteries, *Journal of Biomechanical Engineering* 105(3): 268–274.

[15] Cox, R. [1978]. Regional variation of series elasticity in canine arterial smooth muscles., *American Journal of Physiology* 234(5): H542–51.

[16] Darling, R., Messina, C., Brewster, D. & Ottinger, L. [1977]. Autopsy study of unoperated abdominal aortic aneurysms, *Circulation* 56: 161–164.

[17] Di Achille, P., Celi, S., Di Puccio, F. & Forte, P. [2011]. Anisotropic aaa: computational comparison between four and two fiber family material models, *Journal of Biomechanics* 44(13): 2418–26.

[18] Di Martino, E., Bohra, A., Geest, J. V., Gupta, N. & Vorp, M. M. D. [2006]. Biomechanical properties of ruptured versus electively repaired abdominal aortic aneurysm wall tissue, *Journal of Vascular Surgery* 43(3): 570–576.

[19] Di Puccio, F., Celi, S. & Forte, P. [2012]. Review of experimental investigations on compressibility of arteries and the introduction of a new apparatus, *Experimental Mechanics* 52(7): 1–8, DOI: 10.1007/s11340-012-9614-4.

[20] Dingemans, K., Teeling, P., Lagendijk, J. & Becker, A. [2000]. Extracellular matrix of the human aortic media: an ultrastructural histochemical and immunohistochemical study of the adult aortic media, *The Anatomical Record* 258(1): 1–14.

[21] Dobrin, P. [1989]. Pathophysiology and pathogenesis of aortic aneurysms. current concepts, *Surgical Clinics of North America Journal* 69(4): 687–703.

[22] Ferruzzi, J., Vorp, D. A. & Humphrey, J. D. [2011]. On constitutive descriptors of the biaxial mechanical behaviour of human abdominal aorta and aneurysms, *Journal of the Royal Society Interface* 8: 435–450.

[23] Fillinger, M. F., Marra, S. P., Raghavan, M. L. & Kennedy, F. E. [2003]. Prediction of rupture risk in abdominal aortic aneurysm during observation: wall stress versus diameter, *Journal of Vascular Surgery* 37: 724–732.

[24] Fillinger, M. F., Raghavan, M. L., Marra, S. P., C., J. L. & Kennedy, F. E. [2002]. In vivo analysis of mechanical wall stress and abdominal aortic aneurysm rupture risk, *Journal of Vascular Surgery* 36(3): 589–597.

[25] Fleming, C., Whitlock, E. P., Beil, T. L. & Lederle, F. A. [2005]. Screening for abdominal aortic aneurysm: A best-evidence systematic review for the u.s. preventive services task force, *Annals of Internal Medicine* 142(3): 203–211.

[26] Fung, Y. C., Fronek, K. & Patitucci, P. [1979]. Pseudoelasticity of arteries and the choice of its mathematical expression, *American Journal of Physiology* 237(5): AH620–31.

[27] Ganten, M. K., Krautter, U., von Tengg-Kobligk, H., H., D. B., Schumacher, Stiller, W., Delorme, S., Kauczor, H., Kauffmann, G. & Bock, M. [2008]. Quantification of aortic

distensibility in abdominal aortic aneurysm using ecg-gated multi-detector computed tomography, *Vascular-Interventional* 18(5): 966–73.

[28] Gasser, T. C. [2011]. An irreversible constitutive model for fibrouss of tbiological tissue: a 3d microfiber approach with demonstrative application to abdominal aorticaneurysms, *Acta Biomaterialia* 7(6): 2457–2466.

[29] Gasser, T. C., Auer, M., Labruto, F., Roy, J. & Swedenborg, J. [2009]. Using finite element analysis to assess rupture risk in abdominal aortic aneurysms including the effect of the intraluminal thrombus., *Journal of Vascular Surgery* 49(5): S29.

[30] Greenwald, S. E. [2007]. Ageing of the conduit arteries, *Journal of Pathology* 211: 157–172.

[31] Haskett, D., Johnson, G., Zhou, A., Utzinger, U. & Vande Geest, J. [2010]. Microstructural and biomechanical alterations of the human aorta as a function of age and location, *Biomechanics and Modeling in Mechanobiology* 9: 725–736. 10.1007/s10237-010-0209-7.

[32] He, C. M. & Roach, M. [1994]. The composition and mechanical properties of abdominal aortic aneurysms, *Journal of Vascular Surgery* 20(1): 6–13.

[33] Holzapfel, G. A. [2000]. *Holzapfel, G. A., 2000, Nonlinear Solid Mechanics: A Continuum Approach for Engineering, Wiley, England*, Wiley, England.

[34] Holzapfel, G. A., Gasser, T. C. & Ogden, R. W. [2000]. A new constitutive framework for arterial wall mechanics and a comparative study of material models, *Journal of Elasticity* 61: 1–48.

[35] Holzapfel, G. A., Gasser, T. C. & Stadler, M. [2002]. A structural model for the viscoelastic behavior of arterial walls: continuum formulation and finite element analysis, *European Journal of Mechanic–A/Solids* 21(3): 441–463.

[36] Humphrey, J. D. [1995]. Mechanics of the arterial wall: review and directions, *Critical reviewsinbiomedicalengineering* 23(1Ű2): 1–162.

[37] Humphrey, J. D. [2008]. Vascular adaptation and mechanical homeostasis at tissue, cellular, and sub-cellular levels, *Cell Biochem. Biophys.* 50: 53–78.

[38] Humphrey, J. D. & Rajagopal, K. R. [2002]. A constrained mixture model for growth and remodeling of soft tissues, *Mathematical Models and Methods in Applied Sciences* 12: 407–430.

[39] Humphrey, J. D. & Rajagopal, K. R. [2003]. A constrained mixture model for arterial adaptations to a sustained step change in blood flow, *Biomech Model Mechanobiol* 2(2): 109–26.

[40] Humphrey, J. D. & Yin, F. C. [1987]. A new constitutive formulation for characterizing the mechanical behavior of soft tissues, *Biophysical Journal* 52(4): 563–570.

[41] Kuhl, E. & Holzapfel, G. A. [2007]. A continuum model for remodeling in living structures, *Journal of Materials Science* 42: 8811–8823.

[42] Li, Z.-Y., Sadat, U., U-King-Im, J., Tang, T. Y., Bowden, D. J., Hayes, P. D. & Gillard, J. H. [2010]. Association between aneurysm shoulder stress and abdominal aortic aneurysm expansion. a longitudinal follow-up study, *Circulation* 122: 1815–1822.

[43] Länne, T., Sonesson, B., Bergqvist, D., Bengtsson, H. & Gustafsson, D. [1992]. Diameter and compliance in the male human abdominal aorta: influence of age and aortic aneurysm, *European Journal of Vascular Surgery* 6(2): 178–184.

[44] MacSweeney, S. T., Young, G., Greenhalgh, R. M. & Powell, J. T. [1992]. Mechanical properties of the aneurysmal aorta, *British Journal of Surgery* 79(12): 1281–4.

[45] Maier, A., Gee, M. W., Reeps, C., Eckstein, H. H. & Wall, W. A. [2010]. Impact of calcifications on patient-specific wall stress analysis of abdominal aortic aneurysms., *Biomech. Model. Mechanobiol.* 9(5): 511–21.

[46] McKay, M. D., Beckman, R. J. & Conover, W. J. [1979]. A comparison of three methods for selecting values of input variables in the analysis of output from a computer code, *Technometrics* 42: 55–61.
[47] Molacek, J., Baxa, J., Houdek, K., Treska, V. & Ferda, J. [2011]. Assessment of abdominal aortic aneurysm wall distensibility with electrocardiography-gated computed tomography, *Annals of Vascular Surgery* 25(8): 1036–1042.
[48] Murphy, S. L., Xu, J. & Kochanek, K. D. [2012]. Deaths: Preliminary data for 2010, *National Vital Statistics System* 60(4): 1–68.
[49] Nichols, W. W. & O'Rourke, M. [1997]. *Mcdonald's Blood Flow in Arteries: Theoretical, Experimental and Clinical Principles (4th ed.)*, Hodder Arnold Publication.
[50] Ogden, R. W. [2009]. Anisotropy and nonlinear elasticity in arterial wall mechanics, *in* G. A. Holzapfel, R. W. Ogden, F. Pfeiffer, F. G. Rammerstorfer, J. Salençon, B. Schrefler & P. Serafini (eds), *Biomechanical Modelling at the Molecular, Cellular and Tissue Levels*, Vol. 508 of *CISM Courses and Lectures*, Springer Vienna, pp. 179–258.
[51] O'Rourke, M. F. & Hashimoto, J. [2007]. Mechanical factors in arterial aging: A clinical perspective, *Journal of the American College of Cardiology* 50: 1–13.
[52] Polzer, S., Gasser, T., Swedenborg, J. & Bursa, J. [2011]. The impact of intraluminal thrombus failure on the mechanical stress in the wall of abdominal aortic aneurysms, *European Journal of Vascular and Endovascular Surgery* 41(4): 467–473.
[53] Raghavan, M. L. & da Silva, E. S. [2011]. *Studies in Mechanobiology, Tissue Engineering and Biomaterials*, Springer, chapter Mechanical Properties of AAA Tissue, pp. 139–162.
[54] Raghavan, M. L., Kratzberg, J., de Tolosa, E. M. C., Hanaoka, M. M., Walker, P. & da Silva, E. S. [2006]. Regional distribution of wall thickness and failure properties of human abdominal aortic aneurysm, *Journal of Biomechanics* 39: 3010–3016.
[55] Raghavan, M. L., Vorp, D. A., Federle, M. P., Makaroun, M. S. & Webster, M. W. [2000]. Wall stress distribution on three-dimensionally reconstructed models of human abdominal aortic aneurysm, *Journal of Vascular Surgery* 31: 760–769.
[56] Raghavan, M. & Vorp, D. [2000]. Toward a biomechanical tool to evaluate rupture potential of abdominal aortic aneurysm: identification of a finite strain constitutive model and evaluation of its applicability, *Journal of Biomechanics* 33(4): 475–82.
[57] Raghavan, M., Webster, M. & Vorp, D. [1996]. Ex vivo biomechanical behavior of abdominal aortic aneurysm: assessment using a new mathematical model, *Ann. Biomed. Eng* 24(5): 573–582.
[58] Reh, S., Beley, J.-D., Mukherjee, S. & Khor, E. H. [2006]. Probabilistic finite element analysis using ansys, *Structural Safety* 28: 17–43.
[59] Rissland, P., Alemu, Y., Einav, S., Ricotta, J. & Bluestein, D. . [2009]. Abdominal aortic aneurysm risk of rupture: patientspecific fsi simulations using anisotropic model, *Journal of Biomechanical Engineering* 131(3): 031001.
[60] Rizzo, R. J., McCarthy, W. J., Dixit, S. N., Lilly, M. P., Shively, V. P., Flinn, W. R. & Yao, J. S. T. [1989]. Collagen types and matrix protein content in human abdominal aortic aneurysms, *Journal of Vascular Surgery* 10: 365–373.
[61] Roach, M. R. & Burton, A. C. [1957]. The reason for the shape of the distensibility curves of arteries, *Canadian Journal of Biochemistry and Physiology* 35(8): 681–690.
[62] Rodríguez, J. F., Ruiz, C., Doblaré, M. & Holzapfel, G. A. [2008]. Mechanical stresses in abdominal aortic aneurysms: influence of diameter, asymmetry, and material anisotropy, *Journal of Biomechanical Engineering* 130(2): 021023.

[63] Rodríguez, J., Martufi, G., Doblaré, M. & Finol, E. [2009]. The effect of material model formulation in the stress analysis of abdominal aortic aneurysms, *Annals of Biomedical Engineering* 37: 2218–2221.
[64] Sacks, M. [2000]. Biaxial mechanical evaluation of planar biological materials, *Journal of Elasticity* 61($\aleph_0$): 199–246.
[65] Sakalihasan, N., Limet, R. & Defawe, O. [2005]. Abdominal aortic aneurysm, *Lancet* 365(9470): 1577–1589.
[66] Schriefl, A. J., Zeindlinger, G., Pierce, D. M., Regitnig, P. & Holzapfel, G. A. [2011]. Determination of the layer-specific distributed collagen fibre orientations in human thoracic and abdominal aortas and common iliac arteries, *Journal of The Royal Society Interface* doi:10.1098/rsif.2011.0727: on line.
[67] Scotti, C. M., Jimenez, J., Muluk, S. C. & Finol, E. A. [2008]. Wall stress and flow dynamics in abdominal aortic aneurysms: finite element analysis vs. fluid-structure interaction, *Computer Methods in Biomechanics and Biomedical Engineering* 11: 301–322.
[68] Speelman, L. A., Bohra, A., Bosboom, E. M. H., Schurink, G. W. H., van de Vosse, F. N., Makaroun, M. S. & Vorp, D. A. [2007]. Effects of wall calcifications in patient-specific wall stress analyses of abdominal aortic aneurysms., *Journal of Biomechanical Engineering* 129(1): 105–109.
[69] Spencer, A. J. M. [1984]. *Continuum Theory of the Mechanics of Fibre-Reinforced Composites*, Springer-Verlag, chapter Continuum Theory of the Mechanics of Fibre-Reinforced Composites, CISM Courses and Lectures No. 282, pp. 1–32.
[70] Thubrikar, M., Labrosse, M., Robicsek, F., Al-Soudi, J. & Fowler, B. [2001]. Mechanical properties of abdominal aortic aneurysm wall, *Journal of Medical Engineering & Technology* 25(4): 133–42.
[71] United Kingdom EVAR Trial Investigators, Greenhalgh, R., Brown, L., Powell, J., Thompson, S., Epstein, D. & Sculpher, M. [2010]. Endovascular versus open repair of abdominal aortic aneurysm, *New England Journal of Medicine* 362: 1863–1871.
[72] U.S. Preventive Services Task Force [2005]. Screening for abdominal aortic aneurysm: Recommendation statement, *Annals of Internal Medicine* 142(3): 198–202.
[73] Vaishnav, R. N., Young, J. T., Janicki, J. S. & Patel, J. S. [1972]. Non linear anisotropic elastic properties of the canine aorta, *Biophysical Journal* 12(8): 1008–1027.
[74] Valenta, J. [1993]. *Clinical Aspects of Biomedicine*, Elsevier.
[75] van Śt Veer, M., Buth, J., Merkx, M., Tonino, P., van den Bosch, H., Pijls, N. & van de Vosse, F. [2008]. Biomechanical properties of abdominal aortic aneurysms assessed by simultaneously measured pressure and volume changes in humans, *Journal of Vascular Surgery* 48(6): 1401–1407.
[76] Vande Geest, J. P., Sacks, M. S. & Vorp, D. A. [2004]. Age dependency of the biaxial biomechanical behavior of human abdominal aorta, *Journal of Biomechanical Engineering* 12: 815–822.
[77] Vande Geest, J. P., Sacks, M. S. & Vorp, D. A. [2006]. The effects of aneurysm on the biaxial mechanical behavior of human abdominal aorta, *Journal of Biomechanics* 39: 1324–1334.
[78] Vande Geest, J. P., Wang, D. H. J., Wisniewski, S. R., Makaroun, M. S. & Vorp, D. A. [2006]. Towards a noninvasive method for determination of patient-specific wall strength distribution in abdominal aortic aneurysms, *Ann. Biomed. Eng.* 34(7): 1098Ű106.
[79] Venkatasubramaniam, A., Fagan, M., Mehta, T., Mylankal, K., Ray, B., Kuhan, G., Chetter, I. & McCollum, P. [2004]. A comparative study of aortic wall stress using finite element

analysis for ruptured and non- ruptured abdominal aortic aneurysms, *European Journal of Vascular Surgery* 28: 168–176.

[80] Vito, R. P. & Dixon, S. A. [2003]. Blood vessel constitutive models: 1995Ű2002, *Annu. Rev. Biomed. Eng.* 5(No. 0): 413–439.

[81] Vorp, D. A. [2007]. Biomechanics of abdominal aortic aneurysm, *Journal of Biomechanics* 40: 1887–1902.

[82] Vorp, D. A., Raghavan, M. L., Muluk, S. C., Makaroun, M. S., Steed, D. L., Shapiro, R. & Webster, M. W. [1996]. Wall strength and stiffness of aneurysmal and nonaneurysmal abdominal aorta, *Annals of the New York Academy of Sciences* 800(1): 274–276.

[83] Vorp, D. A., Raghavan, M. L. & Webster, M. W. [1998]. Mechanical wall stress in abdominal aortic aneurysm: influence of diameter and asymmetry, *Journal of Vascular Surgery* 27: 632–639.

[84] Vorp, D., Lee, P., Wang, D., Makaroun, M., Nemoto, E., Ogawa, S. & MW., M. W. [2001]. Association of intraluminal thrombus in abdominal aortic aneurysm with local hypoxia and wall weakening, *Journal of Vascular Surgery* 34: 291–9.

[85] Wang, D. H. J., Makaroun, M. S., Webster, M. W. & Vorp, D. A. [2002]. Effect of intraluminal thrombus on wall stress in patient-specific models of abdominal aortic aneurysm, *Journal of Vascular Surgery* 36: 598–604.

[86] Wicker, B. K., Hutchens, H. P., Wu, Q., Yeh, A. T. & Humphrey, J. D. [2008]. Normal basilar artery structure and biaxial mechanical behaviour, *Computer Methods in Biomechanics and Biomedical Engineering* 11: 539–551.

[87] Zeinali-Davarani, S., Choi, J. & Baek, S. [2009]. On parameter estimation for biaxial mechanical behavior of arteries, *Journal of Biomechanics* 42: 524–530.

Chapter 2

Mineral Components in Aneurysms

Katarzyna Socha and Maria H. Borawska

Additional information is available at the end of the chapter

http://dx.doi.org/10.5772/47802

1. Introduction

Some studies reported imbalance of mineral components in patients with aneurysms [1-5]. The single available scientific reports from recent years describe the effect of certain dietary factors on the risk of aneurysm, such as eating high-cholesterol, fatty meat, alcohol consumption, inadequate intake of fruits and vegetables and also smoking. According to the authors of these papers it results in an increased incidence of aortic and cerebral aneurysms [6-9].

The objective of our research was investigation the relationships between content of selected mineral components: magnesium (Mg), copper (Cu), zinc (Zn), selenium (Se), lead (Pb) and cadmium (Cd) and dietary habits and smoking in patients with abdominal aortic aneurysm (AAA) and cerebral aneurysm (CA). We compared the status of examined elements in patients with aneurysm and healthy people in similar age (control group).

2. Material and methods

We examined 4 groups:

1. Patients with AAA (45 men and 5 women) aged 42-81 years, hospitalized at the Department of Vascular Surgery and Transplantology of Medical University of Bialystok, from which blood samples were taken. The samples of aortic wall and parietal thrombus were collected during surgery. The study included patients with an aneurysm diameter of 3.5 - 15 cm. In 33% of patients occurred aneurysm rupture, in 37% was inflammatory aneurysm, and in 45% of patients femoral artery aneurysm coexisted;
2. Patients with CA (27 men and 43 women) aged 16 - 73 years, hospitalized at the Department of Neurosurgery of Medical University of Bialystok, from which blood samples were taken in the early phase (up to 72 hrs.) after the aneurysmal rupture;

3. Healthy people (n = 22), appropriately matched to examined groups by age and gender, from which blood samples were taken – control group;
4. Aortic wall samples (n = 15) without aneurysm, taken from died people aged 39 – 79 years – control group.

Food-frequency questionnaires were implemented to collect the dietary data. The patients with aneurysms were asked to complete the questionnaire concerning the consumption frequency of food product and smoking by the National Food and Nutrition Institute and the National Cardiology Institute [10]. 28 patients with CA, due to poor health were disclosed from nutritional information collecting. The list of food commodities consisted of 36 food items (white bread, wholegrain bread, sweets, cereal products, grain products, pulses, milk, cottage cheese, other sorts of cheese, meat, poultry, offal, sausages, ham, meat products, bacon, tinned meat, tinned fish, fresh fish, eggs, butter, margarine, vegetable oils, potatoes, processed vegetables, fresh vegetables, fruit, sugar added to beverages, marmalade, honey, soft drinks, beer, wine, vodka, coffee, tea). The consumption frequency of different kind of food was estimated according to the following criteria: frequent consumption was defined as an intake of certain food products twelve to thirty days per month, except fish, that was eaten four to twelve a month. Food products eaten less frequently were classified into "sporadic consumption" group.

The concentration of mineral components in deproteinated blood and tissues, after microwave mineralization in concentrated nitric acid, was analyzed by flame (Mg, Zn) and electrothermal (Cu, Se, Pb, Cd) atomic absorption spectrometry method with Zeeman-effect background correction on Z-5000 and Z-2000 instrument (Hitachi). Certified reference materials: Seronorm – human serum and whole blood, BCR184 – bovine muscle were used to test the accuracy of this methods. The results of the quality control analyses were in agreement with reference values. The Department of Bromatology participates in a quality control program of the estimation of trace elements of the National Institute of Public Health and Institute of Nuclear Chemistry and Technology.

Statistical analyses were performed using Statistica v. 9.1 software. Differences between independent groups were tested by the Mann-Whitney U-test. The correlations were calculated and tested by the Spearman rank test. For estimation the influence of dietary habits on content of mineral components in the examined patients we have used multiple linear regression analysis. Values of $p<0.05$ were considered to be significantly different.

3. Results and discussion

3.1. Magnesium (Mg)

Mg as an activator of adenylate cyclase and ATPase cofactor is involved in most of the processes of the body. It participates in the synthesis and break-up of high-energy compounds, mainly ATP, activates enzymes involved in the metabolism of carbohydrates and fats, and is involved in protein synthesis [11]. Studies showed the efficacy of the compounds of Mg in the prevention and treatment of cardiovascular and nervous system, diabetes and some cancers, such as in the case of prostate cancer [12]. Mg decreases blood lipids, dilates blood vessels, reduces sensitivity to endogenous catecholamines, prevents hypercoagulability and reduces the sensitivity of the myocardium to hypoxia and also has anti-arrhythmic activity. In animal studies it was found that the deficiency of Mg causes hypercholesterolemia, hypertriglyceridemia and atherosclerosis [13]. Mg is one of the factors that modify the biosynthesis and degradation of elastin and collagen [14].

The average concentration of Mg in serum of patients with AAA was 21.88 ± 2.52 mg/L and did not differ significantly from the contents of this element in serum of healthy people: 21.09 ± 1.97 mg/L. The average content of Mg in the aortic wall with aneurysm: 191.40 ± 106.37 μg/g was significantly lower ($p < 0.03$) compared to the concentration of this element in normal aorta - average: 299.15 ± 234.98 μg/g (Table 1). The average content of Mg in the parietal thrombus was 47.63 ± 11.93 μg/g. There was no significant correlation between the content of Mg in examined tissues. We found that cigarette smoking decrease concentration of Mg in parietal thrombus of patients with AAA [15].

The average concentration of Mg in serum of patients with CA was 21.26 ± 3.10 mg/L and did not differ significantly ($p = 0.368$) on the content of this element in the serum of healthy people: 20.62 ± 2.06 mg/L - Table 1 [16].

Type of aneurysm	Concentration of Mg (average ± SD)		p
AAA	*Serum (mg/L)*		$p_{1/2} = 0.110$
	1. Control group (n = 22)	2. Examined group (n = 49)	
	21.09 ± 1.97	21.88 ± 2.52	
	Aortic wall (μg/g)		**$p_{3/4} < 0.03$**
	3. Without aneurysm (n = 14)	4. With aneurysm (n = 49)	
	299.15 ± 234.98	191.40 ± 106.37 ↓	
CA	*Serum (mg/L)*		$p_{5/6} = 0.368$
	5. Control group (n = 22)	6. Examined group (n = 65)	
	20.62 ± 2.06	21.26 ± 3.10	

SD – standard deviation, p – significance level, n – number of samples

Table 1. Concentration of Mg in patients with abdominal aortic aneurysm (AAA), cerebral aneurysm (CA) and in the control groups.

One of the factors that eliminate the development of the aneurysm may be proper diet [6-9], including adequate supply of mineral components, which are essential factors in numerous metabolic processes functioning as coenzymes or biologically active substances. Mg is absorbed from diet in about 50%, and there are many factors causing the negative balance of this element in the body. The source of Mg in the diet are: buckwheat, soya flour, cocoa, chocolate, seeds of legumes, spinach, wholegrain bread, nuts, figs, bananas, leafy vegetables, rice and fish [17].

Multiple regression analysis revealed a significant effect the dietary habits on Mg concentration in patients with the aneurysm. Dietary habits in about 50% ($R^2 = 0.50$) affected the concentration of Mg in the serum of the patients. Frequent consumption of fish and canned fish, grits, rice and legumes had the greatest influence on Mg status, but eating white bread, sweets and sugar was inversely correlated with concentration of Mg. A similar correlation in the case of frequent consumption of sweet bakery products and sweets we found in previous studies assessing the concentration of Mg in patients with larynx cancer [18]. It is known that one reason for the negative balance of Mg in the system are diabetes and eating foods rich in sugar [17]. Analysis of the Spearman rank correlation showed that people often consumed white bread (which significantly decreased serum Mg levels) did not consume wholegrain bread ($r = -.327$, $p < 0.05$), which is a good source of Mg.

3.2. Copper (Cu)

Imbalance in the concentrations of mineral elements in the human body is regarded as one of the risk factors for cardiovascular disease. The biological role of copper (Cu) is related to its participation in the structures and functions of many enzymes (tyrosinase, cytochrome c oxidase, Cu / Zn - superoxide dismutase, an antioxidant and anti-inflammatory). The role of Cu in the inflammation process has not been clearly defined. Significance for this process is its participation in the synthesis of prostaglandins in the arachidonic acid cascade. However, the greatest importance in influencing Cu in the inflammatory process has control of the synthesis of oxygen free radicals, resulting from the presence of this element in superoxide dismutase. In chronic inflammatory process associated with a severe phagocytosis generated free radical compounds that lead to tissue damage. Particularly susceptible to free radical attack are polyunsaturated fatty acids, which are then oxidized. This leads to damage of biological membranes and increase their permeability. Cu reducing the release of lysosomal enzymes by oxidation of membrane thiols to disulfides, to decrease the permeability of biological membranes. Cu also affects the inflammatory process by connecting to histamine, resulting in a decrease of its activity. This trace mineral plays an active role in the synthesis of collagen, elastin, myelin formation, affects bone formation and erythropoiesis [19]. The changes in the Cu content in the arterial wall are important because deficiency of this element may impair the formation of cross-links in collagen and elastin molecules, and thus cause a weakening of the elastic properties of elastin and collagen mechanical resistance and to increase the solubility of these proteins [20]. Cu promotion of angiogenesis is well documented. Cu stimulates endothelial cell proliferation and differentiation and promotes microtubule formation in cultured saphenous veins [21]. The enzyme lysyl oxidase (LOX) is a copper-dependent extracellular enzyme that catalyzes lysine-derived cross-links in collagen and elastin. LOX-mediated cross-linking of collagen types I and III fibrils leads to the formation of stiff collagen types I and III fibers and their subsequent tissue deposition. Evidence from experimental and clinical studies shows that the excess of LOX is associated with an increased collagen cross-linking and stiffness [22]. It has been suggested that ceruloplasmin, which binds more than 90% Cu contained in human plasma and delivers Cu ions play an important role in the oxidative modification of low density lipoprotein (LDL). LDL contributes to the arising and development of atherosclerotic lesions in the arterial wall [23]. It was found that Cu is essential for the initiation of endothelial cell proliferation by the activation of angiogenic factors. Carcinogenic properties of Cu may also be related to its ability to bind to some proteins, giving them angiogenic activity [24].

The average concentration of Cu in serum of patients with AAA: 1.16 ± 0.36 mg/L was significantly higher ($p < 0.03$) compared to the control group: 0.96 ± 0.16 mg/L (Table 2). The average content of Cu in the aneurysmal wall was 0.92 ± 0.36 μg/g, while in the parietal thrombus 1.50 ± 0.92 μg/g. We observed a significant correlation (correlation coefficient: $r = 0.453$, $p < 0.012$) between the content of Cu in the aortic wall and parietal thrombus in patients with AAA [25].

Our new research showed that average content of Cu in serum of patients with CA was significantly ($p < 0.00003$) lower (0.777 ± 0.32 mg/L) than in the control group (1.132 ± 0.41 mg/L) - Table 2. Imbalance in the concentration of Cu in the case of aneurysms have also been observed by other authors [1-2,4,5].

Type of aneurysm	Concentration of Cu (average ± SD)		p
	Serum (mg/L)		
TAB	1. Control group (n = 18)	2. Examined group (n = 34)	**$p_{1/2} < 0.03$**
	0.96 ± 0.16	1.16 ± 0.36 ↑	
CA	3. Control group (n = 22)	4. Examined group (n = 78)	**$p_{3/4} < 0.00003$**
	1.132 ± 0.41	0.777 ± 0.32 ↓	

SD – standard deviation, p – significance level, n – number of samples

Table 2. Concentration of Cu in patients with abdominal aortic aneurysm (AAA), cerebral aneurysm (CA) and in the control groups.

Dietary sources for Cu include whole grain cereals, legumes and green leafy vegetables, nuts, potatoes, oysters and other seafood, offal, poultry, cocoa, dried fruits such as prunes, raisins and yeast [26].

The increase of Cu concentration correlated positively with frequent consumption of ham, wholegrain products and negatively with frequent consumption of offal, probably due to higher concentrations of toxic elements in these products and their interactions [27].

3.3. Zinc (Zn)

The importance of zinc (Zn) in the human body is associated with its multidirectional biological activity by taking part in over 300 enzymatic reactions and metabolic disorders. Zn is a stabilizer or a catalyst for more than 200 enzymes that are involved in the processes of cellular respiration, protein and carbohydrate metabolism [28]. The most important biological role of Zn is to participate in the metabolism of nucleic acids and protein synthesis as an essential component of RNA and DNA polymerases [29]. Zn is involved in the metabolism of fatty acids n-3 prostaglandins, which, depending on the type and concentration may act anti-inflammatory, dilate blood vessels, lower blood pressure, prevent clotting, inhibit the synthesis of triglycerides and are essential in regulating the activity of T cells [30]. Zn is a protective factor in the structure and functioning of cell membranes, is involved in gene expression and cell differentiation. Due to the stabilizing properties of a protective effect on the integrity of the endothelial cell layer, which protects against harmful substances such as inflammatory cytokines and an excess of polyunsaturated fatty acids. It is suggest that an anti-arteriosclerosis role of Zn is related to prevention of this particular factors [31,32]. Zn also participates in the synthesis of collagen [33]. Due to antioxidant activity and anti-inflammatory properties Zn possesses anticancer activity. It was found that Zn supplementation has a beneficial effect on the reduction of angiogenesis and induction of inflammatory cytokines while increasing apoptosis in tumor cells [34,35]. Zn decreases absorption of Cu by competing for binding to metallothionein [36].

The average concentration of Zn in the serum of patients with AAA (0.653 ± 0.271 mg/L) was significantly lower ($p < 0.00007$) than the level of Zn in serum in the control group: 0.996 ± 0.260 mg/L. The average content of Zn in the aortic wall with aneurysm was 21.157 ± 12.582 μg/g, whereas in normal aorta: 23.318 ± 14.038 μg/g (Table 3). The average concentration of Zn in the parietal thrombus was 10.622 ± 6.799 μg/g There was no significant correlation between the content of Zn in examined tissues [37].

The average concentration of Zn in the serum of patients with CA was significantly ($p < 0.03$) lower (0.651 ± 0.20 mg/L) compared to the concentration of Zn in the serum of healthy subjects (0.761 ± 0.19 mg/L) - Table 3. We also showed that the level of Zn in the serum of patients who died during hospitalization was significantly ($p < 0.05$) lower (0.544 ± 0.19 mg/L) compared to the concentration of Zn in the serum of patients who survived (0.684 ± 0 20 mg/L). There was a significantly ($p < 0.003$) higher concentrations of Zn in serum of males (0.875 ± 0.17 mg/L) compared to the level of serum Zn in females (0.648 ± 0.13 mg/L) [38].

The absorption of Zn from food ranges from 10-40%. The diet and age have influence on the bioavailability of Zn. Excess of calcium, copper, iron and selenium in the diet decreases the bioavailability. Phytic acid and dietary fiber, found in plant food decrease its absorption, but amino acids increase the bioavailability of Zn. Food of animal origin (pork, poultry, fish, shellfish, oysters, offal, eggs, cheese) is one of the best sources of easily absorbed Zn. Plant products such as sunflower and pumpkin seeds, nuts, cereals with wholegrain bread, legume seeds, brown rice, onion, garlic and some mushrooms are also good sources of Zn [32,39,40].

Zn content significantly increased the frequent consumption of fish, canned fish and wholegrain breads, and decreased the frequent consumption of raw vegetables - probably due to the presence of these compounds impair the bioavailability [37,38,40].

Type of aneurysm	Concentration of Zn (average ± SD)		p
AAA	*Serum (mg/L)*		**$p_{1/2} < 0.00007$**
	1. Control group (n = 16)	2. Examined group (n = 42)	
	0.996 ± 0.260	0.653 ± 0.271↓	
	Aortic wall (µg/g)		$p_{3/4} = 0.650$
	3. Without aneurysm (n = 9)	4. With aneurysm (n = 42)	
	23.318 ± 14.038	21.157 ± 12.582	
CA	*Serum (mg/L)*		**$p_{5/6} < 0.003$**
	5. Control group (n = 22)	6. Examined group (n = 57)	
	0.761 ± 0.19	0.651 ± 0.20 ↓	

SD – standard deviation, p – significance level, n – number of samples

Table 3. Concentration of Zn in patients with abdominal aortic aneurysm (AAA), cerebral aneurysm (CA) and in the control groups.

3.4. Selenium (Se)

Se is a micronutrient essential to maintain normal physiological functions, but also has an excess of adverse effects on the body. Se content in food, and consequently in the body, is dependent on its presence in the environment. Poland is one of the regions with low content of Se in soil and its overdose of food practically does not happen. More common is deficiency of this micronutrient [41,42]. So far, about 20 selenoprotein, including glutathione peroxidase, selenoproteins P and W, iodothyronine deiodinase type 1,2 and 3, thioredoxin reductase, synthetase have been described [43]. Se is contained in the active center of glutathione peroxidase (GSH-Px) protecting the body against free radicals because of immunological and anti-inflammatory activities. Deficiency of Se can lead to cardiomyopathy and myocardial infarction, muscular dystrophy and fibrosis of pancreas [44]. Se is the element entered by selenocysteine into the genetic code and its low concentration may influence the increased risk of cancer (breast cancer, lung cancer) [45-48]. The metabolism of Se in the brain is different than in other organs - deficiency of this element causes accumulation of increasing quantities of Se in brain. Although the function of many selenoproteins are not yet exactly known, an important role of Se in the functioning of the brain in its normal development and disease states, such as schizophrenia, Parkinson's or Alzheimer's disease is suggested [49]. Se also shows a detoxifying effect in the case of exposure to toxic elements such as lead and cadmium; these metal ions readily form stable connection in a complex of poorly soluble selenides excluding those elements from the biochemical processes and improving their elimination from the body [44].

The average Se level in serum of patients with AAA (60.37 ± 21.2 μg/L) was significantly ($p < 0.008$) lower than in healthy volunteers (75.87 ± 22.4 μg/L). The average serum Se concentration in the examined group was below the reference range, which is 70-140 μg/L [50]. We have not found differences between the content of Se in the aortic wall of patients with AAA (52.31 ± 47.1 ng/g) and the control group: 55.44 ± 34.4 ng/g (died people) - Table 4. The average concentration of Se in parietal thrombus was 139.82 ± 44.6 ng/g. We have observed a significant correlation ($r = 0.69$, $p < 0.0001$) between the content of Se in serum and the parietal thrombus of examined patients. We observed a significantly lower ($p < 0.05$) concentration of Se in aortic wall of smoking than non-smoking patients [51].

The concentrations of Se in the serum of patients with CA (73.248 ± 13.30 μg/L) were similar to the average content of Se in the control group (75.789 ± 22.07 μg/L) - Table 4 [52].

Type of aneurysm	Concentration of Se (average ± SD)		p
AAA	*Serum (μg/L)*		**$p_{1/2} < 0.008$**
	1. Control group (n = 22)	2. Examined group (n = 49)	
	75.87 ± 22.4	60.37 ± 21.2 ↓	
	Aortic wall (ng/g)		$p_{3/4} = 0.839$
	3. Without aneurysm (n = 17)	4. With aneurysm (n = 40)	
	55.44 ± 34.4	52.31 ± 47.1	
CA	*Serum (μg/L)*		$p_{5/6} = 0.579$
	5. Control group (n = 22)	6. Examined group (n = 38)	
	75.79 ± 22.1	73.25 ± 13.3	

SD – standard deviation, p – significance level, n – number of samples

Table 4. Concentration of Se in patients with abdominal aortic aneurysm (AAA), cerebral aneurysm (CA) and in the control groups.

The content of Se in the diet depends on its content in foods. High-protein products such as meat, meat offal, fish, eggs and poultry are good sources of Se. Additionally plant foods like nuts (especially Brazil), tomatoes, cucumbers, onions, garlic, broccoli, cabbage, wheat germ, wholegrain cereals are also good sources of Se [44].

The frequent consumption of raw vegetables significantly increased the concentration of Se, which is consistent with the literature because it is known that the plant food, in which Se is present as a selenomethionine and selenocysteine, characterized by a higher bioavailability compared to animal products [44,53]. In addition frequent consumption of wholegrain bread, grits, rice, meat products, ham, poultry, eggs and honey increased levels of Se in the patients. Eggs, especially egg yolk and poultry in our country are a significant source of Se due to the addition of Se compounds to feed. We estimated the content of Se in different meats and the highest content of Se was in the poultry [54]. The consumption of offal, canned meat, vodka and wine was inversely correlated with Se concentration in examined patients. It is known that alcohol impairs the absorption of minerals; sulfur compounds added to wine as preservatives shows competitive effect to selenium [55].

3.5. Lead (Pb)

Pb is toxic elements, taken from food and drinking water. Pb may accumulate in selected organs, such as blood, liver, kidney, brain and bone [56]. Toxic effects of Pb reveal in disorders of the circulatory system in the form of inhibition of synthesis of hemoglobin [57]. In addition to inhibition of enzymes involved in heme synthesis, Pb compounds may impair the functions of central and peripheral nervous system. With chronic exposure, there is also damage kidneys and liver [58]. Pb is considered as a potential immunotoxic factor. It exerts a direct toxic effect on cells of the immune system or modulate the immune response to antigens and mitogens, and also causes contact allergy and induces autoimmune disease [59].

There were no significant differences in the concentration of Pb in blood and aortic wall of patients with AAA (27.96 ± 20.3 μg/L, 162.65 ± 157.2 ng/g, respectively) compared to controls (33.25 ± 11.1 μg/L and 137.16 ± 134.2 ng/g, respectively) - Table 5. The average concentration of Pb in the parietal thrombus was 7.97 9.6 ng/g. We found a significantly higher ($p < 0.05$) concentration of Pb in aortic wall samples of smoking than non-smoking patients [51].

In patients with CA the blood Pb concentration (48.98 ± 37.4 μg/L) was significantly higher ($p <0.028$) compared to healthy people (29.63 ± 22.8 μg/L) - Table 5 [60].

Approximately 80% of Pb absorbs to the body through food. The source of Pb in the diet is mostly plant food: leafy and root vegetables, potatoes, cereals, legumes, cucurbits and tomatoes. Offal, meat and fish also may be contaminated with Pb compounds and processes, and packaging add to the contents of Pb in food [56].

The concentration of Pb can increase the frequent consumption of wholegrain products, and cooked vegetables, but consumption of grits, rice and honey may have positively influence on Pb status [51,60].

3.6. Cadmium (Cd)

Cd, like Pb, is also a toxic element. Interaction of Cd with elements such as Zn, Cu, Fe, Mg, Ca, Se, which are essential for the body, causes morphological and functional changes in specific organs. Cd impairs carbohydrate metabolism, insulin secretion, inhibits the activity of oxidases and induces lipid peroxidation. Chronic exposure to Cd deteriorates kidney function, demineralization of bone, nervous system disorders, immune, and hyperglycemia [59,61,62]. Prolonged exposure to Cd can cause cardiovascular diseases. It is known that Cd can affect the formation of hypertension, which is probably caused by insufficient oxygen renin release from the kidney, which accumulate large amounts of metallothionein [63].

Type of aneurysm	Concentration of Pb (average ± SD)		p
AAA	*Blood (μg/L)*		$p_{1/2} = 0.327$
	1. Control group (n =22)	2. Examined group (n =49)	
	33.25 ± 11.1	27.96 ± 20.3	
	Aortic wall (ng/g)		$p_{3/4} = 0.562$
	3. Without aneurysm (n =17)	4. With aneurysm (n =40)	
	137.16 ± 134.2	162.65 ± 157.2	
CA	*Blood (μg/L)*		**$p_{5/6} < 0.03$**
	5. Control group (n =22)	6. Examined group (n =64)	
	29.63 ± 22.75	48.98 ± 37.36 ↑	

SD – standard deviation, p – significance level, n – number of samples

Table 5. Concentration of Pb in patients with abdominal aortic aneurysm (AAA), cerebral aneurysm (CA) and in the control groups.

The average blood Cd concentrations in AAA and CA patients were similar to the control groups. There was also no significant differences in content of Cd between aortic wall with aneurysm and normal aorta - Table 6 [60,64]. Cigarette smoking did not influence on content of Cd in examined patients.

Food is one of the sources of exposure to Cd, in addition to environmental and occupational exposure. High content of Cd may contain offal, fish and seafood and vegetable products from the areas contaminated with this element, such as leafy and root vegetables and mushrooms [56].

The frequent consumption of boiled and raw vegetables, and meat products contributed to the increase concentration of Cd, while frequent consumption of grits and rice decreased its level in the patients with aneurysms. Various species of grits and rice, especially brown rice, due to its high content of essential minerals can protect against the accumulation of toxic elements in the body [60,64].

Type of aneurysm	Concentration of Cd (average ± SD)		p
AAA	*Blood (μg/L)*		$p_{1/2}$ = 0.748
	1. Control group (n = 20)	2. Examined group (n = 42)	
	2.60 ± 2.42	3.22 ± 2.27	
	Aortic wall (ng/g)		$p_{3/4}$ = 0.824
	3. Without aneurysm (n = 6)	4. With aneurysm (n = 42)	
	75.47 ± 27.27	72.32 ± 32.69	
CA	*Blood (μg/L)*		$p_{5/6}$ = 0.342
	5. Control group (n = 22)	6. Examined group (n = 64)	
	1.652 ± 1.70	1.252 ± 1.14	

SD – standard deviation, p – significance level, n – number of samples

Table 6. Concentration of Cd in patients with abdominal aortic aneurysm (AAA), cerebral aneurysm (CA) and in the control groups.

4. Conclusions

Serum Zn concentration in patients with AAA and CA is significantly decreased. In turn, serum concentration of Cu in patients with AAA is increased, but decreased in the case of CA. On the other hand, serum concentration of Se in patients with AAA is lower when compared to healthy people, but does not change in the CA. The content of Mg is decreased only in the aortic wall with aneurysm, but its concentration in serum does not change in both types of aneurysms. The concentration of Pb is only increased in the blood of people with CA, while the concentration of Cd in the blood is comparable to healthy people in both types of aneurysms.

Dietary habits (frequency of consumption of each group of food products) may affect directly or indirectly on the content of the Mg, Cu, Zn, Se, Pb and Cd in people with AAA and CA.

Our results may help to explain the role of mineral components in case of aneurysms and be important in the prevention of this diseases.

Author details

Katarzyna Socha* and Maria H. Borawska
Department of Bromatology, Medical University of Bialystok, Poland

* Corresponding Author

Acknowledgement

We wish to thank our colleagues: Prof. Marek Gacko, Dr Andrzej Guzowski from Department of Vascular Surgery and Transplantology, Medical University of Bialystok and Prof. Zenon Mariak, Dr hab. Jan Kochanowicz from Department of Neurosurgery, Medical University of Bialystok; for cooperation and clinical consultations.

5. References

[1] de Figueiredo Borges L, Martelli H, Fabre M, Touat Z, Jondeau G, Michel JB (2010) Histopathology of an Iliac Aneurysm in a Case of Menkes Disease. Pediatr. dev. pathol. 13 (3): 247-251.

[2] Gacko M, Głowiński S, Worowska A (1999) Zawartość Cynku, Magnezu, Manganu, Miedzi i Żelaza w Ścianie Tętniaka Aorty (in Polish). Biul. magnezol. 4 (2): 322-324.

[3] Iskra M, Majewski W, Piorunska-Stolzmann M (2002) Modifications of Magnesium and Copper Concentrations in Serum and Arterial Wall of Patients with Vascular Diseases Related to Ageing, Atherosclerosis and Aortic Aneurysm. Magnes. res. 15 (3-4): 279-285.

[4] Iskra M, Patelski J, Majewski W (1997) Relationship of Calcium, Magnesium, Zinc and Copper Concentrations in the Arterial Wall and Serum in Atherosclerosis Obliterans and Aneurysm. J. trace elem. med. biol. 11 (4): 248-252.

[5] Koksal C, Ercan M, Bozkurt AK, Cortelekoglu T, Konukoglu D (2007) Abdominal Aortic Aneurysm or Aortic Occlusive Disease: Role of Trace Element Imbalance. Angiology 58 (2): 191-195.

[6] Gopal K, Kumar K, Nandini R, Jahan P, Kumar MJ (2010) High Fat Diet Containing Cholesterol Induce Aortic Aneurysm Through Recruitment and Proliferation of Circulating Agranulocytes in apoE Knock Out Mice Model. J. thromb. thrombolysis . 30 (2): 154-163.

[7] Kent KC, Zwolak RM, Egorova NN, Riles TS, Manganaro A, Moskowitz AJ, Gelijns AC, Greco G (2010) Analysis of Risk Factors for Abdominal Aortic Aneurysm in a Cohort of More Than 3 Million Individuals. J. vasc. surg. 52 (3): 539-548.

[8] Shiue I, Arima H, Hankey GJ, Anderson CS (2011) Dietary Intake of Key Nutrients and Subarachnoid Hemorrhage: a Population-based Case-control Study in Australasia. Cerebrovasc. dis. 31(5): 464-470.

[9] Wong DR, Willett WC, Rimm EB (2007) Smoking, Hypertension, Alcohol Consumption, and Risk of Abdominal Aortic Aneurysm in Men. Am. j. epidemiol. 165 (7): 838-845.

[10] Sygnowska E, Waśkiewicz A, Pardo B (1997) Zmiany Zwyczajowego Sposobu Żywienia Populacji Warszawy Objętej Programem Pol-MONICA w latach 1984-93 (in Polish). Żyw. człow. metab. 24: 234-248.

[11] Classen HG, Grimm P (1992) Pharmacokinetics of Magnesium Salts. Methods find. exp. clin. 14 (4): 261-268.

[12] Dai Q, Motley SS, Smith JA Jr, Concepcion R, Barocas D, Byerly S, Fowke JH (2011) Blood Magnesium, and the Interaction with Calcium, on the Risk of High-grade Prostate Cancer. PLoS One 6(4): e18237.

[13] Altura BT, Brust M, Bloom S, Barmour RL, Stempak JG, Altura BM (1990) Magnesium Dietary Intake Modulates Blood Lipid Levels and Artherogenesis. Proc. natl. acad sci. USA 87: 1840-1844.

[14] Gacko M (2000) Eksperymentalny Tętniak Aorty (in Polish). Post. hig. med. dośw. 54 (5): 699-722.

[15] Socha K, Borawska M, Gacko M, Guzowski A, Markiewicz R (2006) Dieta a Zawartość Magnezu w Surowicy, Ścianie i Skrzeplinie Przyściennej Tętniaka Aorty Brzusznej (in Polish). Bromat. chem. toksykol. 39: 655-658.

[16] Socha K, Borawska MH, Mariak Z, Kochanowicz J, Soroczyńska J (2009) Dieta a Zawartość Magnezu w Surowicy Pacjentów z Tętniakiem Mózgu (in Polish). Bromat. chem. toksykol. 42: 666-671.

[17] Ziemlański Ś (2001) Normy Żywienia Człowieka. Fizjologiczne Podstawy (in Polish). Warsaw: PZWL. pp. 349-362.

[18] Borawska MH, Czyżewska E, Łazarczyk B, Socha K (2005) Wpływ Nawyków Żywieniowych na Zawartość Magnezu u Ludzi z Nowotworami Krtani (in Polish). Bromat. chem. toksykol. 38: 639-642.

[19] Sobol G, Pyda E, Darmolińska B, Mizia A (2000) Biologiczna Rola Cynku i Miedzi i Ich Znaczenie dla Przebiegu Procesu Zapalnego (in Polish). Przeg. pediat. 30 (1): 7-9.

[20] Grant ME, Steven FS, Jakson DS (1971) Carbohydrate Content of Insoluble Elastins Prepared from Adult Bovine and Calf Ligamentum Nuchae and Tropoelastin Isolated from Copper-deficient Porcine Aorta. Biochem j. 121: 197-202.

[21] Kang YJ (2011) Copper and Homocysteine in Cardiovascular Diseases. Pharmacol. ther. 129(3): 321-31.

[22] López B, González A, Hermida N, Valencia F, de Teresa E, Díez J (2010) Role of Lysyl Oxidase in Myocardial Fibrosis: from Basic Science to Clinical Aspects. Am. j. physiol. heart circ. physiol. 299 (1): H1-9.

[23] Lamb DJ, Leake DS (1994) Acidic pH Enables Ceruloplasmin to Catalyse the Modification of Low Density Lipoprotein. FEBS lett. 338: 122-126.

[24] Nasulewicz A, Opolski A (2002) Rola Miedzi w Procesie Angiogenezy Nowotworowej – Implikacje Kliniczne (in Polish) Post. hig. med. dośw. 6: 691-705.

[25] Hukałowicz K, Borawska M, Gacko M, Guzowski A, Czyżewska E (2004) The Contents of Copper in Serum, Arterial Wall and Parietal Thrombus of Patients with Aortic Abdominal Aneurysm. Metal ions biol. med., 8: 456-459.

[26] Trumbo P, Yates AA, Schlicker S, Poos M (2001) Dietary Reference Intakes: Vitamin A, Vitamin K, Arsenic, Boron, Chromium, Copper, Iodine, Iron, Manganese, Molybdenum, Nickel, Silicon, Vanadium, and Zinc. J. am. diet. assoc. 101 (3): 294-301.

[27] Markiewicz R, Borawska MH, Socha K, Roszkowska M (2006) Content of Selenium and Lead in Some Tissues of Animals from Podlasie as an Indicator of Environmental Conditions. Pol. j. environ. stud. 15 (2a): 135-138.

[28] Nogowska M, Jelińska A, Muszalska I, Stanisz B (2000) Funkcje Biologiczne Makro- i Mikroelementów (in Polish). Farm. pol. 56 (21): 995-1004.

[29] Prasad AS (1983) Zinc Deficiency in Human Subjects. Prog. clin. biol. res. 129: 1-33.

[30] Bao B, Prasad AS, Beck FW. Fitzgerald JT, Snell D, Bao GW, Singh T, Cardozo LJ (2010) Zinc Decreases C-reactive Protein, Lipid Peroxidation, and Inflammatory Cytokines in Elderly Subjects: a Potential Implication of Zinc as an Atheroprotective Agent. Am. j. clin. nutr. 91 (6): 1634-1641.

[31] Kuliczkowski W, Jołda-Mydłowska B, Kobusiak-Prokopowicz M, Antonowicz-Juchniewicz J, Kosmala W (2004) Wpływ Jonów Wybranych Metali Ciężkich na Czynność Śródbłonka u Pacjentów z Chorobą Niedokrwienną Serca (in Polish). Pol. arch. med. wewn. 111 (6): 682-683.

[32] Puzanowska-Tarasiewicz H, Kuźmicka L, Tarasiewicz M (2009) Funkcje Biologiczne Wybranych Pierwiastków. III. Cynk – Składnik i Aktywator enzymów (in Polish). Pol. merk. lek. 161 (27): 419-421.

[33] Panek B, Gacko M, Pałka J (2004) Metalloproteinases, Insulin-like Growth Factor-I and its Binding Proteins in Aortic Aneurysm. Int. j. exp. pathol. 85 (3): 159-164.

[34] Prasad AS, Beck FW, Doerr TD, Shamsa FH, Penny HS, Marks SC, Kaplan J, Kucuk O, Mathog RH (1998) Nutritional and Zinc Status of Head and Neck Cancer Patients: an Interpretive Review. J. am. coll. nutr. 17 (5): 409-418.

[35] Prasad AS, Beck FW, Snell DC, Kucuk O (2009) Zinc in Cancer Prevention. Nutr. cancer.61 (6): 879-887.

[36] Milne D, Canfield W. Mahalko J (1984) Effect of Oral Folic Acid Supplements on Zinc, Copper and Iron Absorption and Excretion. Am. j. clin. nutr. 39: 535-539.

[37] Socha K, Borawska M, Gacko M, Guzowski A, Markiewicz R (2005) Dieta a Zawartość Cynku w Surowicy Krwi, Subkomórkowej Ścianie i Skrzeplinie Przyściennej Tętniaka Aorty (in Polish). Żyw. człow. metab. 32: 380-384.

[38] Socha K, Borawska MH, Mariak Z, Kochanowicz J, Markiewicz R (2009) Diet and Content of Zinc in Serum of Patients with Brain Aneurysm. Fresenius environ. bull. 18, 10a: 1932-1936.

[39] Koźlicka I, Przysławski J (2007) Wpływ Cynku na Występowanie i Przebieg Procesów Chorobowych u Osób Dorosłych (in Polish). Roczn. PZH 58 (3): 557-562.

[40] Schlegel-Zawadzka M (2001) Cynk: Źródła, Biodostępność, Metabolizm, Preparaty cynku. In: Nowak G, editor. Cynk w Fizjologii oraz w Patologii i Terapii Depresji (in Polish). Krakow: Instytut Farmakologii PAN. pp. 2007-2026.

[41] Wąsowicz W, Gromadzińska J, Rydzyński K, Tomczak J (2003) Selenium Status of Low - Selenium Area Residents: Polish Experience. Toxicol. lett. 137: 95-101.

[42] Zachara BA, Pawluk H, Bloch-Bogusławska E, Śliwka KM, Korenkiewicz-Skok Z, Ryć K (2001) Tissue Level, Distribution, and Total Body Selenium Content in Healthy and Diseased Humans in Poland. Arch. environ. health. 56 (5): 461-466.

[43] Holben DH, Smith AM (1999) The Diverse Role of Selenium within Selenoproteins. J. am. diet. assoc. 99 (7): 836-843.

[44] Wesołowski M, Ulewicz B (2000) Selen – Pierwiastek Śladowy Niezbędny dla Człowieka – Występowanie, Znaczenie Biologiczne i Toksyczność (in Polish). Farm. pol. 56 (21): 1004-1019.

[45] El-Bayoumy K (1994) Evaluation of Chemopreventive Agents Breast Cancer and Proposed Strategies for Future Clinical Intervention Trials. Carcinogenesis 15: 2395-2420.

[46] Gromadzińska J, Reszka E, Bruzelius K, Wąsowicz W, Akesson B (2008) Selenium and Cancer: Biomarkers of Selenium Status and Molecular Action of Selenium Supplements. Eur. j. nutr. 47 (2): 29-50.

[47] Jabłońska E, Gromadzińska J, Reszka E, Wąsowicz W, Sobala W, Szeszenia-Dąbrowska N, Boffetta P (2009) Association Between GPx1 Pro198Leu Polymorphism, GPx1 Activity and Plasma Selenium Concentration in Humans. Eur. j. nutr. 48: 383-386.

[48] Reid ME, Duffield-Lillico AJ, Garland L, Turnbull BW, Clark LC, Marshall JR (2002) Selenium Supplementation and Lung Cancer Incidence: an Update of the Nutritional Prevention of Cancer Trial. Cancer epidemiol. biomarkers prev. 11: 1285-1291.

[49] Benton D (2002) Selenium Intake, Mood and Other Aspects of Psychological Functioning. Nutr. neurosci. 5 (6): 363-374.

[50] Neumeister B, Besenthal I, Liebich H (2001) Diagnostyka laboratoryjna (in Polish). Wrocław: Urban & Partner. pp. 212-213.

[51] Socha K, Borawska MH, Gacko M, Guzowski A (2011) Diet and the Content of Selenium and Lead in Patients with Abdominal Aortic Aneurysm. VASA – European journal of vascular medicine 40 (5): 381-389.

[52] Borawska MH, Socha K, Konopka M, Mariak Z, Kochanowicz J (2010) Environmental Conditions and Selenium Status among Patients with Cerebral Aneurysms. Fresenius environ. bull. 19, 2a: 368-371.

[53] Ulewicz-Magulska B, Wesołowski M (2007) Selen jako Naturalny Składnik Mineralny Produktów Żywnościowych Pochodzenia Roślinnego (in Polish). Farm. pol. 63 (19): 869-876.

[54] Markiewicz R, Borawska MH (2005) Mięso jako Źródło Selenu w Diecie Mieszkańców Podlasia (in Polish). Bromat. chem. toksykol. 38: 249-252.

[55] Taylor D, Dalton C, Hall A, Woodroofe MN, Gardiner PH (2009) Recent Developments in Selenium Research. Br. j. biomed. sci. 66 (2): 107-116.

[56] Nabrzyski M (1998) Toksykologiczna ocena wybranych metali śladowych w żywności. In: Problemy jakości analizy śladowej w badaniach środowiska przyrodniczego (in Polish). Warsaw: Wydawnictwo Edukacyjne Zofii Dobkowskiej. pp. 13-40.

[57] Rogival D, Scheirs J, De Coen W, Verhagen R, Blust R (2006) Metal Blood Levels and Hematological Characteristics in Wood Mice (Apodemus Sylvaticus L.) Along a Metal Pollution Gradient. Environ. toxicol. chem. 25: 149-57.

[58] Seńczuk W (1999) Toksykologia (in Polish), Warsaw: PZWL. pp. 490-498.

[59] Zellikeff JT, Smiałowicz R, Bigazzi PE, Goyer RA (1994) Immunomodulation by Metals. Fundam. appl. toxicol. 22: 1-7.

[60] Socha K, Borawska MH, Mariak Z, Kochanowicz J, Markiewicz R, Bącławek E (2009) Dietary Habits and the Content of Lead and Cadmium in the Blood of Patients with Brain Aneurysms. Żyw. człow. metab. 36: 461-467.

[61] Brzóska MM, Jurczuk M, Moniuszko-Jakoniuk J (1997) Interakcje Kadmu z Wybranymi Biopierwiastkami (in Polish). Terapia 5: 28-30.

[62] Merali Z, Kacew S, Sibghal RL (1975) Response of Hepatic Carbohydrate and cAMP Metabolism to Cadmium Treatment in Rats. Can. j. physiol. pharmacol. 53: 174-184.

[63] Markiewicz J (1989) Wybrane Metale Ciężkie w Środowisku Człowieka (Rtęć, Ołów, Kadm). In: Gumińska M, editor. Ekologiczne Zagrożenia Zdrowia Człowieka (in Polish). Kraków: Nauka dla wszystkich, PAN. pp. 61-78.

[64] Socha K, Borawska MH, Gacko M, Guzowski A, Markiewicz R (2005) Dieta a Zawartość Kadmu w Krwi, Subkomórkowej Ścianie i Skrzeplinie Przyściennej Tętniaka Aorty Brzusznej (in Polish). Bromat. chem. toksykol. 38: 51-55.

Chapter 3

Main Models of Experimental Saccular Aneurysm in Animals

Ivanilson Alves de Oliveira

Additional information is available at the end of the chapter

http://dx.doi.org/10.5772/50310

1. Introduction

Intracranial saccular aneurysms are lesions of the arteries, the etiology of which remains controversial. Some evidence indicates that intracranial saccular aneurysms arise from a congenital deficiency of the smooth muscle of the arterial wall and local hemodynamic disorders particularly in areas of arterial bifurcation [1], [2]. These aneurysms are less commonly due to trauma, tumors, infections, use of drugs, and conditions associated with high arterial flow {e.g., arteriovenous malformations (AVM)} and connective tissue diseases [3-11]. Saccular aneurysms might be single or multiple and are mostly located in the Circle of Willis. These aneurysms are the most frequent cause of spontaneous subarachnoid hemorrhage (SAH) and primarily affect females. Patients become symptomatic after rupture, which usually occurs between ages 40 to 60 years old[12]. Because rupture is associated with high morbidity and mortality rates, appropriate treatment must be performed as soon as possible. The aim of the treatment is to exclude the aneurysm from the circulation to avoid further bleeding, while preserving the parent artery [13, 14]. Currently, two techniques are available for the treatment of saccular aneurysms: 1) microsurgery (developed by Yasargil), which is based on the placement of a metallic clip in the aneurysm neck [15], and 2) endovascular coiling (developed by Guglielmi), which is based on the introduction of platinum microcoils inside the aneurysms that induce thrombosis and thus isolate aneurysms from the circulation[16]. The continuous development of this latter technique has reduced the morbidity and mortality of the treatment of brain aneurysms [17]; however, improvement of models of experimental saccular aneurysms is needed to develop novel embolization techniques and to test new materials.

2. Selection of the animal species

2.1. Concept of experimental animal

The terms "laboratory animal" or "experimental animal" are somewhat inappropriate because in theory, any animal can be used in laboratory experiments. Nevertheless, both terms are frequently used in scientific literature to refer to animals exhibiting (natural or induced) diseases in which the mechanisms are similar to human diseases.

2.2. Types of experimental models with animals

Experimental models with animals are classified as: 1) induced, 2) spontaneous, 3) negative and 4) orphan[18]. In the induced animal models, the investigated condition is induced experimentally, which can be highly advantageous because these models allow for free selection of the animal species, for example, intake of beta-aminopropionitrile combined with arterial hypertension induces intracranial aneurysm formation in rats [19]. Induced animal models are very important in the development of novel surgical procedures, to assess the viability of procedures and their physiological consequences, and in therapeutic assays, for instance, the surgical creation of aneurysms on the lateral wall of the common carotid artery of dogs [20] and pigs [21]. In spontaneous models, the investigated disease occurs naturally, such as with prostatic hypertrophy in dogs and some diseases in animals with genetic mutations. The spontaneous occurrence of intracranial saccular aneurysms in animals is rare. Negative models involve a particular disease that does not develop in a particular species and, thus, these models are ideal to study mechanisms of resistance or a lack of reactivity to a given stimulus. For example, rabbits do not develop gonorrhea and vultures do no exhibit neoplasms. In orphan models, a disease (or condition) that occurs naturally in non-human species is "adopted" when a similar human disease is identified at a later time (e.g., bovine spongiform encephalopathy, which is also known as mad cow disease) [18].

2.3. Principles for animal selection

Experimental animals should only be used when there are limitations to the research with humans. In therapeutic assays, the use of animals is mandatory and constitutes an essential phase of the preclinical testing of embolization devices or materials. In general, small animals are the most frequently used for research purposes; mice, rats, rabbits, and guinea pigs correspond to 90% of scientific studies [22]. Larger animals such as dogs [20], pigs [21], or monkeys [23] are also used for research purposes, albeit less frequently. Such diversity of species that exhibit different characteristics makes it difficult to select a particular species for experimental aneurysm production. Although there are no specific guidelines on how to perform such a selection, three general principles must be considered: 1) the type of animal that will be used, 2) the type of aneurysm one seeks to simulate, and 3) the aims of the study.

Regarding the animal type, researchers should be thoroughly aware of its biological characteristics, behavior, vascular anatomy, and phylogenetic similarity with humans.

Among the biological characteristics, the size and metabolism of the animals exert a direct influence on the selection. Large animals are more difficult to handle and require more complex infrastructure (lodging, feeding, care, anesthesia, and specialized human resources), which increases the cost of research. In addition, size also influences the number of animals used in experiments. Thus, for ethical reasons, studies that use large animals such as dogs and monkeys restrict their number to the bare minimum needed to ensure the validity of the results. A reduced number of animals influences the statistical methods applied to the analysis, because small samples can reduce the statistical power of tests and lead researchers to infer inaccurate conclusions. In addition, the calculation of the minimum number of animals is difficult because unpredictable losses can also occur as a function of the initial training and pilot study.

With regard to metabolism, different animal species also exhibit different patterns of metabolic rate; for instance, the metabolism of rodents is often faster than that of humans. This metabolic power (also known as metabolic body weight) interferes with the effects of drugs on the organism, as well as with its processing, distribution across organic fluids and tissues, and modes of excretion. Thus, the calculation of experimental doses should be performed according to the metabolic weight rather than the absolute body weight of the animals. In surgical studies, different metabolic rates (influenced by factors such as age, gender, diet, and circadian rhythm) interfere with wound healing and regeneration of tissues and organs, thus encouraging researchers to learn the principles of veterinary anesthesia that correspond to the involved animals, the characteristics of the drugs that will be used, and more specifically, the potential interference of medications with the parameters analyzed in the study[18].

In addition to the biological characteristics, researchers must also be familiar with the intracranial and cervical arterial anatomy of each animal species, and the histology, diameters, flow patterns, and anastomoses of the vessels, because these are essential factors in the selection of the aneurysm construction technique.

The phylogenetic similarity between animals and humans is also important in species selection, but it does not suggest that the extrapolation of the results to humans will be reliable. For example, human immunodeficiency virus (HIV) does not induce immunodeficiency in monkeys, and thus, does not represent the ideal animal model to study acquired immunodeficiency syndrome (AIDS). Transgenic animals have been increasingly used in research studies; however, caution is needed because such animals might exhibit unknown disorders that may interfere with the extrapolation of the results to humans[18].

Once the animal model has been selected, the experiment performed, and the data selected, the stage of explaining the phenomena by means of induction begins. This process consists of verifying a particular fact and its adequation to a known general law. This mode of reasoning has inherent odds of error; thus, one must be cautious in the extrapolation of the results of experiments performed with non-human species to humans. In other words, compounds that might be noxious to a given non-human species might be innocuous or even beneficial to humans. For example, penicillin is lethal for guinea pigs, but is well tolerated and even beneficial for humans. In addition, aspirin is teratogenic in cats, dogs, rats, guinea pigs, mice, and monkeys, but it is innocuous in pregnant women. Thalidomide is teratogenic in human beings and monkeys, but innocuous in rats and other species. Therefore, phylogenetic proximity is not a fully reliable measure of similarity between the physiological phenomena of animals and humans [18].

To reduce the odds of selecting an inappropriate animal model for a given experiment, the ***multispecies approach*** is recommended. At least two different species including non-rodents must be used in studies employing drugs, whereas the use of more than one animal species is rare in studies of surgical techniques. Accordingly, some animal species have become traditional standard models for specific surgical procedures. However, surgical studies focusing on the physiological features of a disease require more than one animal species, which despite its usefulness, does not ensure the absolute reliability of the extrapolation of the results from animals to humans [18].

Regarding the aneurysm model, a comprehensive awareness of the available models is required, in addition to their construction techniques, advantages and disadvantages, and more specifically, which features of human aneurysms one seeks to simulate, that is, their histological, geometric, physiopathological, and hemodynamic characteristics (e.g., ruptured or not, small, medium-sized, large or giant, with or without thrombus, on the lateral wall or at a bifurcation, high or low hemodynamic tension, etc.).

Finally, the aims of the study are essential in the selection of the animal species and the techniques that will be used in aneurysm construction, e.g., verification of the physiopathological mechanisms, therapeutic assays, creation of novel surgical/endovascular techniques, or training of doctors in these therapeutic modalities. Regarding the latter issue, medical training using animals is justified as training on humans exposes patients to medical error. Thus, practical training using animal models is indispensable for medical education because it contributes to the development of psychomotor skills and enables physicians to safely perform invasive techniques.

2.4. Main animal species used in the construction of experimental saccular aneurysms

Despite all of the considerations above, the selection of the ideal animal species for studies on experimental saccular aneurysms is not yet well established. As spontaneous intracranial aneurysms rarely occur in animals, most studies employ induced models, which have the advantage of allowing for the free selection of species. Animals such as rats[19], rabbits[24], dogs[20], pigs[21], and monkeys[23] have been used in studies on physiopathology [25, 26], hemodynamics[27-31], and the training of surgical[32, 33] and endovascular techniques, in addition to the testing of embolization devices and new materials[21, 34-38]. In studies aimed at developing surgical/endovascular techniques, it is rare that more than one animal species is used in the same experimental model; therefore, there are no systematic comparative studies seeking to define which is the ideal animal species for the experimental production of intracranial saccular aneurysms. Nevertheless, in recent years, rabbits (*Oryctolagus cuniculus*) have been preferred for these studies because their coagulation system is very similar to that of humans. Rabbits are easy to handle, and the diameters of their extracranial carotid arteries are very similar to those of humans [39-44].

2.5. Cervicocerebral vascular anatomy of rabbits

Regarding the vascular anatomy of rabbits, knowledge of the cervicocerebral vessels and their connections is essential in the construction of experimental saccular aneurysms. Below, we present a summary of the cervical and intracranial vascular anatomy of rabbits together with their main anastomoses.

The innominate artery (3.5 mm in diameter) is the first branch of the aortic arch, and after running 6 mm, it divides into the right subclavian (2 mm in diameter) and right common carotid (2 mm of diameter) arteries. The left common carotid artery (2 mm in diameter) begins immediately next to or together with the innominate artery. The left subclavian artery (2 mm in diameter) is the last branch of the aortic arch, and it originates from the left vertebral (1 mm in diameter) and superficial cervical (1 mm in diameter) arteries[45]. In the second most frequent distribution type, the aortic arch can only be divided into three branches: the innominate, left common carotid, and left subclavian arteries. Lesser variations might also occur; for instance, the supreme intercostal and left vertebral arteries might originate directly from the aortic arch. The superior thyroid artery usually originates from the common carotid arteries; however, it emerges approximately between the 3rd and 6th tracheal rings and runs towards the thyroid gland, in some cases of only one common carotid artery[46]. Upon arriving at the isthmus, the superior thyroid artery divides into two branches: one ascending (cricothyroid branch) and the other descending (which runs inferiorly between the trachea and the esophagus). The bronchial branches stem from the right supreme intercostal and left common carotid arteries and lead to the tracheoesophageal branches, which run upwards between the trachea and the esophagus and anastomose with the descending branches of the superior thyroid artery[47] (figure 1). These branches rarely exhibit variations, and when they do occur, these variations are more common on the left side[48].

The common carotid artery (CCA) leads to only one branch, namely the thyroid artery, and immediately above it, the CCA divides into the internal and external carotid arteries. The main branches of the external carotid artery (ECA) are the occipital, lingual, external maxillary (facial), and anterior and posterior auricular arteries. Both the auricular and external maxillary arteries emerge separately or from a common trunk. At the level of the zygomatic arch, the ECA divides into the superficial temporal and transverse facial arteries and continues its course up to the pterygoid canal, where it divides into small branches to the posterior side of the orbit and originates the external ophthalmic artery, which in turn forms the lacrimal and frontal branches, and subsequently, the anastomose with the internal ophthalmic artery. The main branch of the internal maxillary artery is the middle meningeal artery. The intracranial internal carotid artery (ICA) divides into the ophthalmic arteries, cranial, and caudal branches. The cranial branch runs forward towards the uncus, where it divides into the anterior choroidal artery and middle cerebral artery (MCA) trunk, and then continues up to the chiasm, where it unites with the contralateral cranial branch to form a common anterior cerebral artery trunk that separates again at the level of the corpus callosum. The common anterior trunk originates from the lateral artery of the olfactory bulb, which leads to the ethmoidal branches of the cribiform plate. The MCA runs along the lateral cerebral sulcus and divides into the posterior ophthalmic artery, large posterior branch, and large anterior and middle branches, in addition to the small olfactory bulb branches. The caudal branch of the ICA supplies most of the blood flow of the basilar artery (BA) and leads to the following branches: posterior communicating artery, small medial geniculate body branches, large anterior quadrigeminal body, small branches of the posterior side of the uncus, and the posterior segment of the corpus callosum. The cerebellar artery might originate from the ending of the ICA or the BA and connects to several branches of the brainstem. The BA is formed by the fusion of the arteries of the first spinal nerves and divides (on the ventral surface of the trapezoid body) into two vessels that reunite at the upper margin of the pons. In addition, the BA gives small lateral branches, the cerebellar artery and the perforating branches. The arteries of the first spinal nerve then reunite at a lower level and form the ventral spinal artery[49].

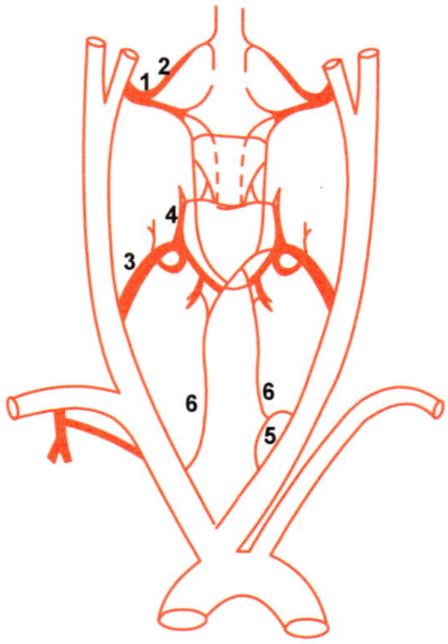

Figure 1. Graphic representation of the visceral vascularization of the neck of rabbits. 1- superior laryngeal artery, 2- superior branches, 3- superior thyroid artery, 4- cricothyroid branch, 5- bronchial branch and 6- tracheoesophageal branch. Modified from Bugge, 1967[2].

Regarding the system of intracranial anastomoses in rabbits, the collateral circulation is very different from that of dogs. The internal maxillary artery originates from the orbital branches, which end at the ophthalmic branch and represents an insufficient anastomotic pathway. The anastomotic branches between the orbital and internal carotid arteries are too small or are absent. A small branch links together the ICA and BA before they unite at the circle. Finally, when an occlusion of the common carotid artery occurs, the supply of blood is provided by the contralateral ICA (**figure 2**)[3].

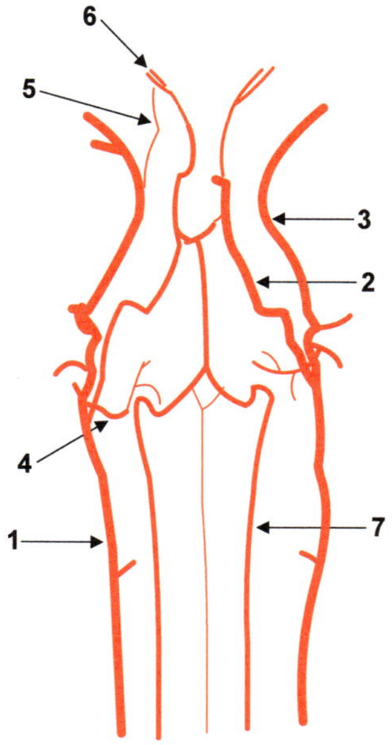

Figure 2. Graphic representation of the intracranial anastomosis system of rabbits. 1- common carotid artery, 2- internal carotid artery, 3- external carotid artery, 4- occipital artery, 5- orbital artery, 6 – internal ophthalmic artery and 7- vertebral artery. Modified from Chungcharoen, 1954[50].

3. Selection of an experimental saccular aneurysm model

3.1. Concept of experimental saccular aneurysm

Experimental saccular aneurysms are induced aneurysms intended to reproduce the histological, geometric, and hemodynamic characteristics of human intracranial aneurysms.

3.2. Characteristics of an ideal model of experimental saccular aneurysm

With the rise of endovascular treatment of human intracranial aneurysms – by means of embolization using platinum microcoils[16] – experimental models of saccular aneurysm are encouraged to adapt to this novel therapeutic modality by meeting the following criteria: 1) demonstration of long-term permeability in untreated control species, 2) development in animal species with a coagulation system similar to that of humans, 3) simulation of the morphology of arterial bifurcation, terminal artery, or other aneurysmal types that expose the aneurysm neck to high hemodynamic tension, 4) development in vessels with a similar size to human intracranial vessels, 5) development without the need of local surgery to minimize the repair/wound healing response, which might confound the results of the experiment with the natural increase of the biological activity characteristic of several embolization materials such as: coils, fluid agents, etc., and 6) simulation of the limitations met by embolization of human aneurysms using such materials[39].

3.3. Main models of experimental saccular aneurysm

German and Black (1954) were the first researchers to produce experimental aneurysms using a surgical construction of saccular aneurysms on the common carotid artery of dogs. Such aneurysms mimicked the ones occurring on the lateral wall and were frequently used in hemodynamic studies; however, they produced fibrosis at the suture site, which was a disadvantage[20]. Since then, surgical models have evolved with the culmination of the swine model (1994), consisting of a graft of the venous pouch onto the common carotid artery (CCA) of pigs. This method produces lateral wall aneurysms, but includes disadvantages such as venous histology, induction of intense fibrosis at the suture site, and low hemodynamic tension[16].

In addition to the surgical method, chemical induction might also be used in the construction of saccular aneurysms. The main proponent of this technique was Hashimoto (1970), who induced arterial wall weakening in rats by ingestion of 3-beta-aminopropionitrile, a toxic agent extracted from the seeds of the sweat pea (*Latyrus odoratus*), which destroys the elastic fibers and collagen of the arteries of rats[19]. In addition, Hashimoto ligated one of the common carotid arteries and induced arterial hypertension in rats (via nephrectomy, intake of saline solution, and high doses of corticosteroids) to cause greater hemodynamic tension on the weakened arterial wall[30]. This technique was the first to produce successful intracranial saccular aneurysms at the bifurcations of the cerebral arterial circle. Nonetheless, the aneurysms were too small and were not useful for the development of surgical techniques nor for the study of intra-aneurysmal hemodynamic alterations[26, 29].

3.3.1. Surgical models

The technique used in the surgical construction of experimental aneurysm is based on grafting a venous pouch (usually taken from the external jugular vein) onto the common carotid artery. The main advantage of this approach is that the constructed aneurysms exhibit hemodynamic features that are very similar to those of humans. the disadvantages of constructed aneurysms include their venous histology and resistance to rupture.

With regard to the construction site, the graft might be placed on the lateral wall or at bifurcations. There are five main techniques to construct lateral wall aneurysms:

1. Non-ligated venous pouch with end-to-side anastomosis to the artery.
2. Non-ligated venous pouch with side-to-side anastomosis to the artery (variation of the former).
3. End-to-side anastomosis of the vein onto the artery with ligated venous pouch.
4. Side-to-side anastomosis of the vein onto the artery with ligated venous pouch.
5. End-to-side anastomosis of the venous pouch. The main advantage of this technique is the short-lasting clamping of the common carotid artery that thus avoids endothelial damage and vasospasm[21].

The main model for the construction of bifurcation aneurysms was performed using Forrest and O'Rielly's technique, in which the left common carotid artery of rabbits was partially anastomosed with the right common carotid artery. Next, a venous pouch (taken from the external jugular, anterior facial, or posterior facial vein) was grafted onto the knot formed by the union of the arterial anastomoses. The advantage of this technique was that unlike the lateral wall aneurysms, it did not induce aneurysmal thrombosis (**figure 3**)[24].

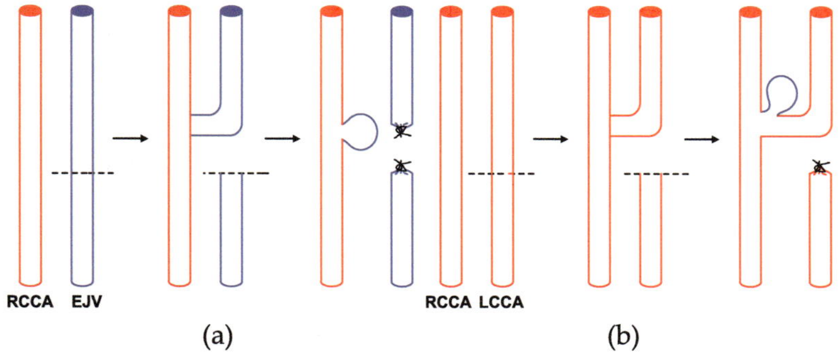

Figure 3. Graphic representation of the main surgical models of experimental saccular aneurysm. (a) Lateral wall, (b) bifurcation (RCCA – right common carotid artery, EJV – external jugular vein, LCCA – left common carotid artery).

3.3.2. Other experimental models of aneurysms

In addition to the abovementioned techniques, other methods have been attempted to construct saccular aneurysms, such as hyper-flow (through the creation of arteriovenous fistulas), trauma (traumatic puncture of the arterial wall or using CO_2 laser), and chemical wall injury (by injecting nitrogen mustard or other substances directly inside the arterial wall) [51]. All of these techniques are less efficient than chemical induction and surgical construction. Despite these attempts at the construction of an experimental model of saccular aneurysm, none of these methods was able to reproduce all of the histopathological, geometric, and hemodynamic features of human intracranial saccular aneurysms [51-54]. Nevertheless, the enzymatic method has stood out in recent years.

3.3.3. Enzymatic models

3.3.3.1. Elastase-induced model

3.3.3.1.1. Mechanisms of action of elastase in aneurysm formation

The formation of saccular aneurysms depends on several mechanisms, including inflammatory reaction, weakening of the arterial wall, and hemodynamic tension. Enzymatic imbalance and inflammatory activity are some of the potential causes involved in aneurysm formation in humans. Anidjar (1992) perfused the abdominal aorta of a group of Wistar rats with pancreatic elastase from swine and used thioglycollate plus plasmin (activators of the inflammatory response) in another group of animals. Both groups exhibited an inflammatory reaction, elastic lamina fragmentation, and formation of fusiform aneurysms similar to those that occur in humans. The inflammatory activity was stronger in the elastase group (achieving its peak on the sixth day) and produced macrophages, polymorphonuclear cells, helper and suppressor T lymphocytes in the arterial wall. Combined with the progression of the inflammatory activity, the diameter of the abdominal aorta increased[55]. Halpern (1994) established the sequence and synchrony of induction of the inflammatory response. Elastase induces injury of the arterial wall, which triggers an initial inflammatory response. The inflammatory cells then activate endogenous proteinases (molecular weight between 50 and 90 kD) and the destruction of elastin and collagen, in addition to aortic dilation. Halpern's study showed that the rupture of elastin and its contact with macrophages are the main events in the activation of endogenous proteinases, which results in increased tissue destruction [56].

Although inflammatory activity might lead to destruction of the elastic fibers and a weakening of the arterial wall, its role in the development of saccular aneurysms has not been fully established. Other mechanisms may also participate in aneurysm formation such as alterations of the mechanical properties of arteries together with the hemodynamic tension on the vascular wall, which can produce aneurysms by themselves. Miskolczi (1997) demonstrated this phenomenon in an in vitro study, in which the common carotid arteries of swine and sheep were isolated and their walls were digested using pancreatic elastase from swine. Next, the arterial segments were placed between a pulsatile flow artificial pump and a series of test tubes, which allowed the control of variables such as flow, pulsation, and pressure without inducing the inflammatory response that occurs in in vivo studies. Consequently, small saccular aneurysms appeared at the sites where the elastin was damaged and hemodynamic tension was exerted on the weakened arterial wall[57].

3.3.3.1.2. Creation and improvement of the elastase-induced model

Based on studies of experimental aneurysm creation using elastase [55, 56], Cawley et al. (1996) developed a new experimental model of lateral wall aneurysms in rabbits. This model consisted of dissecting the neck of rabbits, ligating the proximal segment of the external carotid artery, and performing intra-arterial perfusion of pancreatic elastase from swine. Three weeks later, saccular aneurysms were formed, which, from angiographic and histological perspectives, were very similar to those in humans. However, the lumen remained patent in only 40% of the aneurysms, because lateral aneurysms do not originate from the type of hemodynamic stress and intra-aneurysmal blood flow that occur at the bifurcations of the human cerebral arteries[58].

Cloft et al. (1999) improved this model by producing greater hemodynamic stress on the left common carotid artery (LCCA), which was directly hit by the blood flow from the ascending aorta in two-thirds of the rabbits. This technique is fully endovascular and consists of insufflating a balloon at the origin of the LCCA and isolating a small arterial segment for intraluminal infusion of bovine pancreatic elastase for 30 minutes. Angiographic control was performed by the dissection and retrograde puncture of the femoral arteries. This method succeeded in producing aneurysms with an average size of 3.0 mm x 5.0 mm whose lumen remained patent up to three months after creation. From a microscopic point of view, all of the aneurysms exhibited intact endothelium, the absence of an inflammatory response, moderately damaged elastic lamina inside of the aneurysm (but undamaged at the neck), and apical thrombus. No animal exhibited neurological sequelae (due to the intracranial collateral vessels network) or showed systemic signs of elastase intoxication[59].

Kallmes et al. (1999) modified this method by creating additional hemodynamic tension on the proximal segment of the right common carotid artery (RCCA), which is located between the brachiocephalic artery and ascending aorta, and mimics a "bifurcation aneurysm." In addition, the long curvature of the brachiocephalic artery increased the hemodynamic tension at the origin of the RCCA compared to the LCCA. Further modification of this model consisted of reducing the time of enzymatic digestion to 20 minutes (**figure 4**).

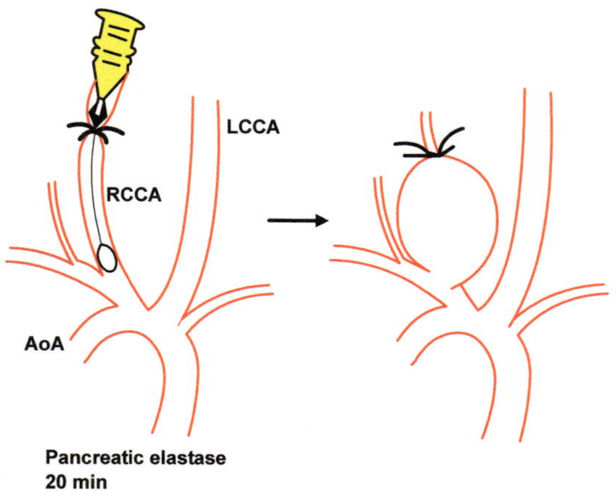

Figure 4. Graphic representation of the endovascular elastase-induced aneurysm construction technique. AoA – aortic arch, RCCA – right common carotid artery and LCCA – left common carotid artery. Modified from Hoh, 2004[60].

These technical modifications resulted in experimental aneurysms similar to those observed in humans with regard to the arterial origin, shape, hemodynamics, and patency. The high hemodynamic tension caused by the long curvature of the brachiocephalic artery makes these experimental aneurysms similar to those occurring in the ophthalmic segment of the human internal carotid artery[40]. Altes et al. (2000) used the RCCA for the intraluminal infusion of pancreatic elastase from swine in rabbits and obtained aneurysms in 89% of the animals. Two weeks later, the elastic lamina ruptured and aneurysms were formed (average dimensions of 4.5 mm x 7.5 mm), with organized thrombus in the aneurysm dome, whereas the elastic lamina was undamaged in the walls of the parent arteries. The cells present in the organized thrombus exhibited features of smooth muscle cells and fibroblasts. Ten weeks later, no significant alterations were observed. The execution of this technique required less than one hour, and although it included surgical procedures (e.g., section of the RCCA), this technique exhibited lower morbidity and mortality compared to the use of the LCCA[43].

From a technical perspective, it is noteworthy that the concentration of elastase and the time of incubation exert a partial effect on the size of the aneurysms. One study compared animals that were not subjected to elastase to animals that were subjected to low, medium, and high concentrations of this drug, under variable durations. The rabbits that were not subjected to elastase exhibited complete thrombosis of the arterial stump and did not form aneurysms, whereas the rabbits that were given elastase in progressive concentrations formed aneurysms. The increase of the elastase dose above a given value did not influence the size of the aneurysms; however, high concentrations of elastase induced the dilation of the parent artery and resulted in a more complex geometry of the aneurysm neck, which is closer to that observed in human aneurysms. Low concentration (25%) of elastase induced aneurysms without dilation of the adjacent artery[61].

Hoh et al. (2004) developed a simpler technique of construction and obtained aneurysms similar to those previously mentioned. The first simplification consisted of the use of a 24-gauge angiocatheter (instead of an introducer) and transitory occlusion of the origin of the RCCA using a neurosurgical clamp (instead of a balloon)[60]. The second simplification was achieved using an accurate neurological assessment of the rabbits using a four-point scale to rate the observed movements of the rabbits on a flat surface to verify whether paresis of the legs or abnormal gait occurred (movements in a circle or difficulty to walk). Accordingly, the animals were rated as grade I – no neurological deficit; grade II: minimal of suspected neurological deficit; grade III: mild neurological deficit without abnormal motion; and grade IV: remarkable neurological deficit and abnormal motion[62].

Although the studies performed to date have not reported any loss of animals, Möller-Hartmann et al. (2003) found a mortality of 25% due to the accidental passage of elastase into the superior thyroid artery with an aberrant origin or into the tracheoesophageal branch, which originated in the common carotid artery, resulting in hemorrhagic necrosis of the trachea[63]. Another source of undesirable distribution of elastase and tracheal necrosis is the anomalous origin of the tracheobronchial artery, which can be identified in angiographies as a small branch perpendicular to the proximal part of the RCCA, and runs medially towards the trachea[64]. Therefore, the elimination of those anomalous vessels (by ligation, coagulation or placing of the introducer lower inside the RCCA) is crucial for success in aneurysm creation by intraluminal infusion of elastase[63].

In addition to the problem posed by aberrant vessels, Krings et al. (2003) identified two additional potential causes of failure of the elastase model. The first potential cause depends on how elastase is injected through the introducer. Thus, instead of elastase, the blood column of the introducer dead space is pushed into the arterial lumen. Furthermore, the authors observed that doses of 100U of elastase were usually lethal. To address these problems, the authors reduced the dose of elastase to 20 U and performed a contrast injection test to detect aberrant arteries as follows: after occluding with a balloon in the proximal area of the RCCA, a non-ionic contrast material was injected (by means of an introducer) inside the RCCA, and the contrast column was verified for two minutes. If the contrast material remained, without washing out or dilution for two minutes, the test was deemed to be negative, i.e., there were no anomalous vessels. Otherwise, the test was deemed to be positive, and the introducer was advanced to a more proximal site of the RCCA where the contrast washing out or dilution no longer occurred. When these procedures were applied, none of the animals died, and all developed aneurysms. The full duration of this procedure was 40 minutes. The problem posed by the blood column and contrast material inside of the introducer was resolved by performing continuous suction using a syringe[65].

Prospective studies on the morphology and viability of elastase-induced aneurysms in rabbits require serial high-quality angiographic control. Three routes are currently used: the femoral arteries, left external auricular vein, and left central auricular artery. Miskolczi et al. (2005) suggested performing a retrograde puncture of the left central auricular artery as the best route, because the femoral artery is narrow and fragile and thus exhibits a high risk of injury and definitive loss. In addition, retrograde femoral catheterization requires the dissection of the groin, arteriotomy, and subsequent ligation with permanent vascular occlusion, thus making subsequent angiography at this site impossible. Puncture of the left external auricular vein allows for repeated injections of contrast material, but the resulting images exhibit low spatial resolution and frequent motion-related artifacts. In contrast, the left central auricular artery allows for repeated injections, high-quality images, and excellent visualization of the brachiocephalic trunk vessels because rabbits usually exhibit LCCA of bovine origin; thus, when the contrast material is injected into the left central auricular artery, the brachiocephalic trunk and its branches immediately become filled. When the LCCA originates directly from the aortic arch or from a common origin with the brachiocephalic trunk, but the angle is unfavorable, the contrast material only fills the distal aortic arch. The anatomy of approximately 70% - 80% of white New Zealand rabbits is favorable for retrograde injection in the left central auricular artery; therefore, pre-selection is important to exclude animals with unfavorable anatomy from studies[66].

3.3.3.1.3. Morphological and geometric features

The elastase model efficiently reproduces aneurysms similar to ones that occur in the ophthalmic segment of the human internal carotid artery with regard to width, height, neck size, and diameter of the parent artery. These characteristics were very well established by Short et al. (2001), who prospectively studied 40 rabbits and observed that the size of the aneurysmal cavities afforded by the elastase model was appropriate for preclinical tests of endovascular occlusion techniques and devices. The authors measured the width (points in the cavity exhibiting the maximal width), height (measurement of the aneurysmal dome to the mid-portion of a line connecting the proximal and distal portions of the aneurysm neck), neck (maximal diameter between the proximal and distal portions of the aneurysm orifice), the diameter of the parent artery (diameter of the artery just proximal to the aneurysm neck), and the dome/neck ratio (maximal dome width/neck width). In addition, they classified the aneurysms as small (2.0 mm – 4.9 mm), medium-sized (5.0 mm – 9.9 mm), or large (10.0 – 16.0 mm). Moreover, the neck was classified as small (< 4 mm) or wide (> 4 mm). Two weeks later, all of the animals had survived, none showed clinical evidences of neurological insult, and exhibited aneurysms at the apex of the long curve of the brachiocephalic artery, with an elongated shape, and a height greater than the width. Medium-sized (50%) and large (42.5%) aneurysms with small necks (55%) prevailed. The average width of the cavity was 4.1 ± 1.2 mm, which varied between 2.5 and 7.1 mm, and the average height was 8.8 ± 2.6 mm, which varied between 3.0 and 15.6 mm. A dome/neck ratio > 1 was observed in 50% of the aneurysms with an average value of 1.13 ± 0.5, and the average diameter of the parent artery was 4.3 ± 1.4 mm. Although these measures were similar to those of human aneurysms, they did not reproduce all of the corresponding morphological characteristics, which are difficult to quantify for many reasons[44].

Short-term follow-up of elastase-induced aneurysms showed that their dimensions increased gradually up to the end of the first month after creation and then become stable. The average measurements of the dome width and length at days 3 and 28 after induction were (3.2 ± 0.6 mm; 5.0 ± 0.9 mm) and (6.0 ± 1.3 mm; 10.0 ± 2.2 mm), respectively. Conversely, the aneurysms that were not incubated with elastase progressively retracted and formed thrombi inside. Because a millimeter-scale was used and the differences found were small, the authors considered the low resolution of intravascular angiography, radiographic projections used, and variations of the cardiac cycle that promoted different intra-aneurysmal pressures to be potential sources of variation and the lack of histological correlation to be a limitation of the study[67]. Ding et al. (2006) studied the long-term permeability of elastase-induced aneurysms and observed that the aneurysmal cavity remained patent and without thrombi for up to two years after creation and that after the first month, their dimensions (width, height, and neck width) did not exhibit significant variation [68].

The size of the neck has paramount importance when testing endovascular devices, as well as in the study of the physiopathology of aneurysms, and might be modified during the construction of experimental aneurysms. This finding was revealed by Ding et al. (2005), who observed that the size of the neck might be controlled by adjusting the position of the balloon during incubation with elastase. When the balloon is placed high, that is, half inside the proximal RCCA and half inside the subclavian and brachiocephalic arteries, the neck of the resulting aneurysms is narrow (< 4 mm). When the balloon is placed low, that is, exclusively inside of the subclavian and brachiocephalic arteries, the neck of the resulting aneurysms is wide (> 4 mm). The authors further observed that the position of the balloon did not influence the length of the aneurysms and that the balloons that were placed low did not always result in wide necks[69].

In addition to the low position of the balloon, the geometric relationship between the longest axis of the aneurysms and the axis of the parent artery played an important role in the determination of local hemodynamics and the final architecture of aneurysms. Onizuka et al. (2006) compared the angle formed by the longest axis of aneurysms and the axis of the parent artery immediately and three months after aneurysm construction. The authors found a positive correlation between the neck size and the dome height. In addition, the dome height was proportional to the angle formed by the brachiocephalic artery and the aneurysm neck. Therefore, the authors concluded that the larger the angle, the greater the hemodynamic stress caused by the blood flow on the distal neck and the aneurysm bottom[70].

The volume of elastase-induced aneurysms might also be adjusted by the position of the RCCA ligation so that high ligations might create relatively larger aneurysms compared to the ones produced by low ligations. Ding et al. (2007) prospectively studied the influence of the height of the RCCA ligation on the volume of aneurysms. Ligations were rated lower when the height of the ligation point was 10-mm away from the origin of the RCCA and high when the ligation point was 15-mm away from the origin of the RCCA. The same authors applied the formula for the volume of cylinders to calculate the volume of aneurysms because the shape of the created aneurysms was cylindrical. The aneurysms with higher ligations exhibited larger volumes (102.4 ± 54.8 mm^3) compared to the ones with lower ligations (36.6 ± 26.8 mm^3). In addition, the aneurysms with higher ligations exhibited larger dimensions such as the neck (3.3 ± 0.8 mm), width (3.7 ± 0.7 mm), and height (9.0 ± 1.7 mm). The authors attributed these results to a larger cavity space of aneurysms with higher ligation, in addition to probable greater hemodynamic stress on the aneurysms. Finally, according to those authors, no animals died due to the accidental passage of elastase (through aberrant vessels) in the case of aneurysms with higher ligation[69].

3.3.3.1.4. Histology

Abruzzo et al. (1998) compared the histological characteristics between lateral wall aneurysms (produced by means of elastase incubation in the external carotid artery of rabbits) and lateral wall aneurysms constructed by grafting a venous pouch onto the common carotid artery of pigs. Both experimental aneurysms were compared to human aneurysms with 5 – 10 mm of diameter (recently ruptured and obtained at autopsy), whose main characteristics included: 1) a complete absence of the internal elastic lamina in the aneurysms, and abrupt termination of the internal elastic lamina of the parent artery at the margins of the saccular orifice; 2) complete absence of the tunica media in the aneurysms and abrupt termination of the tunica media of the parent artery at the margins of the aneurysmal orifice; 3) absence of intramural inflammatory reaction in the aneurysms; 4) absence of neointimal fibromuscular proliferation; 5) a sac wall thickness of 51 μm and a neck thickness of 52 μm. In three out of the five studied aneurysms, one-third of the aneurysmal cavity was filled by a thrombus at different stages of organization and firmly adhered to the point of rupture. The elastase-induced aneurysms exhibited an abrupt termination of the internal elastic lamina at the margins of the saccular orifice, but the tunica medica was undamaged and continued into the interior of the saccular part of the aneurysms. The sac walls exhibited a mild to moderately inflammatory cellular (monocytes and neutrophils) response and a mild fibromuscular response. The thickness of the neck was 49 μm, and the thickness at the sac wall was 44 μm. An unorganized thrombus filled one-third of the aneurysmal cavity in two out of the four investigated rabbits. The aneurysms constructed using a venous pouch exhibited a well-developed elastic lamina, and the tunica media extended into the sac wall. The wall of the venous pouch contained remarkable inflammatory infiltrate (monocytes and neutrophils) and extreme degrees of fibromuscular proliferation completely across the aneurysm wall, resulting in a remarkable neointimal thickening and luminal narrowing. The thickness of the dome wall was 228 μm, and the thickness at the neck was 350 μm. Thus, the authors concluded that from a histological perspective, the elastase-induced aneurysms were the ones most similar to human aneurysms, in addition to exhibiting little spontaneous fibromuscular response compared to the surgical model with venous pouch grafting[71]. Accordingly, the elastase-induced model is currently used in tests for endovascular devices[39-42].

3.3.3.2. Papain-induced model

Although the damage of elastic fibers induced by swine pancreatic elastase resulted in experimental aneurysms similar to those appearing in the ophthalmic segment of the human internal carotid artery, they are small (<5 mm), which is not completely consistent with the actual clinical characteristics of human aneurysms, where the aneurysms are larger than 5 mm. To overcome this limitation, Chinese researchers tested an association between elastase and collagenase in the *in vitro* pre-digestion of an arterial pouch grafted onto the aortic arch of rabbits; however, that model exhibited a higher tendency to spontaneously rupture[72]. To produce saccular aneurysms larger than 5 mm, De Oliveira et al. (2011) infused the papain enzyme successfully inside the right common carotid artery of rabbits[73].

3.3.3.3. Mechanisms of action of papain

Papain is a cysteine-proteinase type of endolytic enzyme extracted from the latex of green papaya (*Carica papaya*). It weighs 23,000 Da , and its molecules form a single peptide chain with 211 amino acid residues that fold into two distinct parts, which are divided by a cleft that represents its active site[74]. In addition to papain, the latex contains three additional enzymes (chymopapain, caricain, and glycil endopeptidase), which together with papain represent 80% of the enzymatic fraction, where papain corresponds to the smallest enzymatic fraction (5-8%). Although purification of papain is usually performed using precipitation techniques, it remains contaminated by other proteases[75]. With regard to its enzymatic activity, papain is activated by the addition of substances such as cyanide, reduced glutathione, and sulfate and is inactivated by oxidants. The maximal enzymatic activity occurs with a pH between 5 and 7.5. With regard to its specificity, in addition to hydrolyzing several substances, papain exhibits strong esterase activity, which makes its scope of action even wider to the point of acting on the very same substrates as pancreatic proteolytic enzymes with esterase activity[76].

Regarding its biological effects, papain exhibits remarkable elastolytic properties and has been successfully used in the production of experimental lung emphysema in animals[77, 78]. In addition to digesting elastic fibers, papain is also able to destroy collagen. Junqueira (1980) studied the ability of papain to destroy the collagen fibers of several tissues (cartilage, bone, skin, and blood vessel) from several animal species, such as *Gallus gallus* (chicken), *Canis familiaris* (dog), *Oryctolagus cuniculus* (rabbit) and *Sus scrofa* (pig), and observed that the degree of collagen destruction varies according to the type of tissue[79]. Ionescu (1977) used papain to de-antigenize a venous heterograft to subsequently graft it onto the common carotid artery of dogs and observed that papain caused an excessive weakening of the graft with a tendency to form venous aneurysms. To overcome this problem, the author subjected the grafts to a previous treatment with formol to maintain their rigidity and flexibility and not form aneurysms[80].

With regard to commercial presentation, papain is found as raw latex (~ 12 U/mg), lyophilized powder (10 U/mg) and aqueous suspension (16-40 U/mg)[81].

3.3.3.4. Creation of papain-induced aneurysms

The technique applied in the construction of papain-induced aneurysms uses the right common carotid artery of rabbits and is fully surgical, based on the study by Hoh et al. However, this technique does not use angiography during the puncture of the right common carotid artery and injection of the enzyme. This simplification proved to be safe and efficacious, and no animal exhibited complications due to the unduly passage of papain to an aberrant vascular branch that was accidentally present in the neck of the animals. Other innovations were the removal of the aortic arch and the supra-aortic trunks, direct measurement of the macroscopic dimensions of aneurysms and vessels using a caliper, and quantitative histological studies by means of histomorphometry in addition to a qualitative histological analysis[60,73].

3.3.3.5. Morphologic and geometric features

Papain-induced aneurysms exhibited a size similar to the elastase-induced aneurysms described in previous studies. Nevertheless, it is noteworthy to stress that the papain-induced aneurysms were measured directly on the right common carotid artery. This is an important point because most of the studies performed using elastase employed digital subtraction angiography to measure the aneurysms, which led to an overestimate of the aneurysm size. Thus, if papain-induced aneurysms were also measured by means of digital subtraction angiography, then their size would have most likely been overestimated. Independent from the method used, papain was efficacious in producing saccular aneurysms with an average diameter of 3.8 +/- 1.4 mm (2.5-7.0 mm), similar to those appearing in the ophthalmic segment of the human internal carotid artery.

3.3.3.6. Histology

From a histological perspective, papain caused the destruction of elastic fibers, endothelial damage, thrombosis, and intimal fibrosis. These alterations are similar to those found in elastase-induced aneurysms, in which the only difference is the degree of thrombosis, which was more remarkable in the papain-induced aneurysms[73].

3.3.3.7. Future of the enzymatic model

Currently, there are no ideal animal models of experimental saccular aneurysms available. From a practical perspective, it is impossible for one single model to reproduce the full histological, geometric, and hemodynamic characteristics of the wide variety of aneurysms and human-related conditions. Nevertheless, the enzymatic model has been increasingly used in the production of saccular aneurysms due to its simplicity, easy execution, and lower cost, resulting from the use of small animals such as rabbits, in addition to allowing the control of height, width, and size of the aneurysm neck. Furthermore, the enzymatic model can be improved, as a wide variety of enzymes have not yet been tested. Despite the advantages of the enzymatic model, the use of both elastase and papain exhibits some limitations, such as an intramural inflammatory response, endothelial damage, and thrombosis. Indeed, thrombosis is the most important effect because it hinders the interpretation of the results of the embolization materials tested. However, even when they are present, the intra-aneurysmal thrombi do not invalidate this experimental model because under actual clinical conditions, most human aneurysms have thrombi present. Therefore, although they are not ideal for preclinical tests of embolization materials, enzymatic models most closely mimic the actual clinical conditions and thus exhibit a high potential to contribute to the study of the physiopathology of human intracranial aneurysms and testing of embolization materials and endovascular devices.

Author details

Ivanilson Alves de Oliveira
Neuroradiology, Experimental Medicine Laboratory, Universidade Federal de Sergipe-UFS, Brazil

4. References

[1] Nyström H.S.M. Development of intracranial aneurysms as revealed by electron microscopy. J Neurosurg, 1963. 20: p. 329-337.

[2] Rhoton A.L., Jr. Anatomy of saccular aneurysms. Surg Neurol, 1980. 14(1): p. 59-66.

[3] Senegor M. Traumatic pericallosal aneurysm in a patient with no major trauma. Case report. J Neurosurg, 1991. 75(3): p. 475-7.

[4] Barker C.S. Peripheral cerebral aneurysm associated with a glioma. Neuroradiology, 1992. 34(1): p. 30-2.

[5] Frazee J.G., Cahan L.D. and Winter J. Bacterial intracranial aneurysms. J Neurosurg, 1980. 53(5): p. 633-41.

[6] Lee K.S., Liu S.S., Spetzler R.F., Rekate H.L. Intracranial mycotic aneurysm in an infant: report of a case. Neurosurgery, 1990. 26(1): p. 129-33.

[7] Bohmfalk G.L., Story J.L., Wissinger J.P., Brown, W.E. Bacterial intracranial aneurysm. J Neurosurg, 1978. 48(3): p. 369-82.

[8] Brown R.D., Jr., Wiebers D.O. and Forbes G.S. Unruptured intracranial aneurysms and arteriovenous malformations: frequency of intracranial hemorrhage and relationship of lesions. J Neurosurg, 1990. 73(6): p. 859-63.

[9] Brown B.M. and Soldevilla F. MR angiography and surgery for unruptured familial intracranial aneurysms in persons with a family history of cerebral aneurysms. AJR Am J Roentgenol, 1999. 173(1): p. 133-8.

[10] Schievink W.I., Parisi J.E, Piepgras D.G., Michels V.V. Intracranial aneurysms in Marfan's syndrome: an autopsy study. Neurosurgery, 1997. 41(4): p. 866-70; discussion 871.

[11] Heiserman J.E., Drayer B.P., Fram E.K., Keller P.J. MR angiography of cervical fibromuscular dysplasia. AJNR Am J Neuroradiol, 1992. 13(5): p. 1454-7.

[12] Kopitnik T.A. and Samson D.S. Management of subarachnoid haemorrhage. J Neurol Neurosurg Psychiatry, 1993. 56(9): p. 947-59.

[13] Dix G.A., Gordon W., Kaufmann A.M., Sutherland I.A., Sutherland G.R. Ruptured and unruptured intracranial aneurysms--surgical outcome. Can J Neurol Sci, 1995. 22(3): p. 187-91.

[14] Winn H.R., Almaani W.S., Berga S.L., Jane J.A., Richardson A.E. The long-term outcome in patients with multiple aneurysms. Incidence of late hemorrhage and implications for treatment of incidental aneurysms. J Neurosurg, 1983. 59(4): p. 642-51.

[15] Yasargil M.G. and Fox J.L. The microsurgical approach to intracranial aneurysms. Surg Neurol, 1975. 3(1): p. 7-14.

[16] Guglielmi G., Vinuela F., Dion J., Duckwiler G. Electrothrombosis of saccular aneurysms via endovascular approach. Part 2: Preliminary clinical experience. J Neurosurg, 1991. 75(1): p. 8-14.

[17] Derdeyn C.P., Barr J.D., Berenstein A., Connors J.J., Dion J.E., Duckwiler G.R., Higashida R.T., Strother C.M., Tomsick T.A., Turski P. The International Subarachnoid Aneurysm Trial (ISAT): a position statement from the Executive Committee of the American Society of Interventional and Therapeutic Neuroradiology and the American Society of Neuroradiology. AJNR Am J Neuroradiol, 2003. 24(7): p. 1404-8.

[18] Fagundes D.J., Taha M.O. Modelo animal de doença:critérios de escolha e espécies de animais de uso corrente. Acta Cirúrgica Brasileira, 2004. 19(1): p. 59-65.
[19] Hashimoto N., Handa H. and Hazama F. Experimentally induced cerebral aneurysms in rats. Surg Neurol, 1978. 10(1): p. 3-8.
[20] German W.J. and Black S.P.W. Experimental production of carotid aneurysms. N Engl J Med, 1954. 250(3): p. 104-6.
[21] Massoud T.F., Guglielmi G., Ji C., Vinuela F., Duckwiler G.R. Experimental saccular aneurysms. I. Review of surgically-constructed models and their laboratory applications. Neuroradiology, 1994. 36(7): p. 537-46.
[22] Schanaider A., Silva P.C., The use of animals in experimental surgery. Acta Cirúrgica Brasileira, 2004. 19(4): p. 1-9.
[23] Hashimoto N., Kim C., Kikuchi H., Kojima M., Kang Y., Hazama F. Experimental induction of cerebral aneurysms in monkeys. J Neurosurg, 1987. 67(6): p. 903-5.
[24] Forrest M.D. and O'Reilly G.V. Production of experimental aneurysms at a surgically created arterial bifurcation. AJNR Am J Neuroradiol, 1989. 10(2): p. 400-2.
[25] Hashimoto N., Handa H. and Hazama F. Experimentally induced cerebral aneurysms in rats: part II. Surg Neurol, 1979. 11(3): p. 243-6.
[26] Hashimoto N., Handa H. and Hazama F. Experimentally induced cerebral aneurysms in rats: Part III. Pathology. Surg Neurol, 1979. 11(4): p. 299-304.
[27] Kerber C.W. and Buschman R.W. Experimental carotid aneurysms: I. Simple surgical production and radiographic evaluation. Invest Radiol, 1977. 12(2): p. 154-7.
[28] Nagata I., Handa H. and Hashimoto N. Experimentally induced cerebral aneurysms in rats: part IV--cerebral angiography. Surg Neurol, 1979. 12(5): p. 419-24.
[29] Hashimoto N., Handa H. Nagata I., Hazama, F. Experimentally induced cerebral aneurysms in rats: Part V. Relation of hemodynamics in the circle of Willis to formation of aneurysms. Surg Neurol, 1980. 13(1): p. 41-5.
[30] Nagata I., Handa H., Hashimoto N., Hazama F. Experimentally induced cerebral aneurysms in rats: Part VI. Hypertension. Surg Neurol, 1980. 14(6): p. 477-9.
[31] Nakatani H., Hashimoto N., Kikuchi H., Yamaguchi S., Niimi H. In vivo flow visualization of induced saccular cerebral aneurysms in rats. Acta Neurochir (Wien), 1993. 122(3-4): p. 244-9.
[32] Stehbens W.E. Experimental production of aneurysms by microvascular surgery in rabbits. Vasc Surg, 1973. 7(3): p. 165-75.
[33] de los Reyes R.A., Boehm F.H., Boehm F.H., Ehler W., Kennedy D., Shagets F., Woodruff W., Smith T. Direct angioplasty of the basilar artery in baboons. Surg Neurol, 1990. 33(3): p. 185-91.
[34] Yoshino Y., Niimi Y., Song J.K., Khoyama S., Shin Y.S., Berenstein A. Endovascular treatment of intracranial aneurysms: comparative evaluation in a terminal bifurcation aneurysm model in dogs. J Neurosurg, 2004. 101(6): p. 996-1003.
[35] Graves V.B., Strother C.M., Partington C.R., Rappe A. Flow dynamics of lateral carotid artery aneurysms and their effects on coils and balloons: an experimental study in dogs. AJNR Am J Neuroradiol, 1992. 13(1): p. 189-96.

[36] Spetzger U., Reul J., Weis J., Bertalanffy H., Thron A., Gilsbach J.M. Microsurgically produced bifurcation aneurysms in a rabbit model for endovascular coil embolization. J Neurosurg, 1996. 85(3): p. 488-95.

[37] Spetzger U., Reul J., Weis J., Bertalanffy H., Gilsbach J.M. Endovascular coil embolization of microsurgically produced experimental bifurcation aneurysms in rabbits. Surg Neurol, 1998. 49(5): p. 491-4.

[38] Raymond J., Salazkin I., Metcalfe A., Robledo O., Gevry G., Roy D., Weill A., Guilbert F. Lingual artery bifurcation aneurysms for training and evaluation of neurovascular devices. AJNR Am J Neuroradiol, 2004. 25(8): p. 1387-90.

[39] Kallmes D.F., Helms G.A., Hudson S.B., Altes T.A., Do H.M., Mandell J.W., Cloft H.J. Histologic evaluation of platinum coil embolization in an aneurysm model in rabbits. Radiology, 1999. 213(1): p. 217-22.

[40] Kallmes D.F., Williams A.D., Cloft H.J., Lopes M.B., Hankins G.R., Helm G.A. Platinum coil-mediated implantation of growth factor-secreting endovascular tissue grafts: an in vivo study. Radiology, 1998. 207(2): p. 519-23.

[41] Hans F.J., Krings T., Möller-Hartmann W., Thiex R., Pfeffer J., Cherer K., Brunn A., Dreeskamp H., Stein K.P., Meetz A., Gilsbach J.M., Thron A. Endovascular treatment of experimentally induced aneurysms in rabbits using stents: a feasibility study. Neuroradiology, 2003. 45(7): p. 430-4.

[42] Struffert T., Roth C., Romeike B., Grunwald I.O., Reith W. Onyx in an experimental aneurysm model: histological and angiographic results. J Neurosurg, 2008. 109(1): p. 77-82.

[43] Altes T.A., Cloft H.J., Short J.G., DeGast A., Do H.M., Helm G.A., Kallmes D.F. 1999 ARRS Executive Council Award. Creation of saccular aneurysms in the rabbit: a model suitable for testing endovascular devices. American Roentgen Ray Society. AJR Am J Roentgenol, 2000. 174(2): p. 349-54.

[44] Short J.G., Fujiwara N.H., Marx W.F., Helm G.A., Cloft H.J., Kallmes D.F. Elastase-induced saccular aneurysms in rabbits: comparison of geometric features with those of human aneurysms. JNR Am J Neuroradiol, 2001. 22(10): p. 1833-7.

[45] Adams D.F., Olin T.B. and Redman H.C. Catheterization of Arteries in the Rabbit. Radiology, 1965. 84: p. 531-5.

[46] Angel-James J. Variations in the vasculature of the aortic arch and its major branches in the rabbit. Acta Anat, 1974. 87: p. 283-300.

[47] Bugge J. Arterial supply of the cervical viscera in the rabbit. Acta Anat (Basel), 1967. 68(2): p. 216-27.

[48] Blanding J.D., Jr., Ogilvie R.W., Hoffman C.L., Knisely W.H. The Gross Morphology of the Arterial Supply to the Trachea, Primary Bronchi, and Esophagus of the Rabbit. Anat Rec, 1964. 148: p. 611-4.

[49] Du Boulay G.H. Comparative neuroradiologic vascular anatomy of experimental animals. In: Newton D.G. and Potts T.H. (ed.) Radiology of the skull and brain. Saint Louis: Mosby; 1974. p. 2763-86.

[50] Chungcharoen D., Daly M.B.; Neil E. The efect of occlusion upon the intrasinusal presure with special reference to vascular communications between the carotid and vertebral circulations in the dog, cat, and rabbit. J Physiol, 1952. 117: p. 56-76.

[51] Stehbens W.E. Evaluation of aneurysm models, particularly of the aorta and cerebral arteries. Exp Mol Pathol, 1999. 67(1): p. 1-14.

[52] Nishikawa M., Smith R.D. and Yonekawa Y. Experimental intracranial aneurysms. Surg Neurol, 1977. 7(4): p. 241-4.

[53] TerBrugge K.G., Lasjaunias P. and Hallacq P. Experimental models in interventional neuroradiology. AJNR Am J Neuroradiol, 1991. 12(6): p. 1029-33.

[54] Powell J. Models of arterial aneurysm: for the investigation of pathogenesis and pharmacotherapy--a review. Atherosclerosis, 1991. 87(2-3): p. 93-102.

[55] Anidjar S., Dobrin P.B., Eichorst M., Graham G.P., Chejfec G. Correlation of inflammatory infiltrate with the enlargement of experimental aortic aneurysms. J Vasc Surg, 1992. 16(2): p. 139-47.

[56] Halpern V.J., Nackman G.B., Gandhi R.H., Irizzary E., Scholes J.V., Ramey, W.G. The elastase infusion model of experimental aortic aneurysms: synchrony of induction of endogenous proteinases with matrix destruction and inflammatory cell response. J Vasc Surg, 1994. 20(1): p. 51-60.

[57] Miskolczi L., Guterman L.R., Flaherty J.D., Hpkins L.N. Saccular aneurysm induction by elastase digestion of the arterial wall: a new animal model. Neurosurgery, 1998. 43(3): p. 595-600; discussion 600-1.

[58] Cawley C.M., Dawson R.C., Shengelaia G., Bonner G., Barrow D.L., Colohan A.R. Arterial saccular aneurysm model in the rabbit. AJNR Am J Neuroradiol, 1996. 17(9): p. 1761-6.

[59] Cloft H.J., Altes T.A., MArx W.F., Raible R.J., Hudson S.B., Helm G.A., Mandell J.W. Jensen M.E., Dion J.E., Kallmes D.F., Endovascular creation of an in vivo bifurcation aneurysm model in rabbits. Radiology, 1999. 213(1): p. 223-8.

[60] Hoh B.L., Rabinov J.D., Pryor J.C., Ogilvy C.S. A modified technique for using elastase to create saccular aneurysms in animals that histologically and hemodynamically resemble aneurysms in human. Acta Neurochir (Wien), 2004. 146(7): p. 705-11.

[61] Kallmes D.F., Fujiwara N.H., Berr S.S., Helm G.A., Cloft H.J. Elastase-induced saccular aneurysms in rabbits: a dose-escalation study. AJNR Am J Neuroradiol, 2002. 23(2): p. 295-8.

[62] Endo S., Branson P.J. and Alksne J.F. Experimental model of symptomatic vasospasm in rabbits. Stroke, 1988. 19(11): p. 1420-5.

[63] Möller-Hartmann W., Krings T., Stein K.P., Dreeskamp A., Meetz A., Thiex R., Hans F.J., Gilsbach J.M., Thron A. Aberrant origin of the superior thyroid artery and the tracheoesophageal branch from the common carotid artery: a source of failure in elastase-induced aneurysms in rabbits. AJR Am J Roentgenol, 2003. 181(3): p. 739-41.

[64] Thiex R., Hans F.J., Krings T., Möller-Hartmann W., Brunn A., Scherer K., Gilsbach J.M., Thron A. Haemorrhagic tracheal necrosis as a lethal complication of an aneurysm model in rabbits via endoluminal incubation with elastase. Acta Neurochir (Wien), 2004. 146(3): p. 285-9; discussion 289.

[65] Krings T., Möller-Hartmann W., Hans F.J., Thiex R., Brunn A., Scherer K., Meetz A., Dreeskamp H., Stein K.P., Gilsbach J.M., Thron A. A refined method for creating saccular aneurysms in the rabbit. Neuroradiology, 2003. 45(7): p. 423-9.

[66] Miskolczi L., Nemes B., Cesar L., Masanari O. Gounis M. Contrast injection via the central artery of the left ear in rabbits: a new technique to simplify follow-up studies. AJNR Am J Neuroradiol, 2005. 26(8): p. 1964-6.
[67] Fujiwara N.H., Cloft H.J., Marx W.F., Short J.G., Jensen M.E., Kallmes D.F. Serial angiography in an elastase-induced aneurysm model in rabbits: evidence for progressive aneurysm enlargement after creation. AJNR Am J Neuroradiol, 2001. 22(4): p. 698-703.
[68] Ding Y.H., Dai D., Lewis D.A., Danielson M.A., Kadirvel R., Cloft H.J., Kallmes D.F. Long-term patency of elastase-induced aneurysm model in rabbits. AJNR Am J Neuroradiol, 2006. 27(1): p. 139-41.
[69] Ding Y.H., Dai D., Danielson M.A., Kadirvel R., Lewis D.A., Cloft H.J., Kallmes D.F. Control of aneurysm volume by adjusting the position of ligation during creation of elastase-induced aneurysms: a prospective study. AJNR Am J Neuroradiol, 2007. 28(5): p. 857-9.
[70] Onizuka M., Miskolczi L., Gounis M.J., Seong J., Lieber B.B., Wakhloo A.K. Elastase-induced aneurysms in rabbits: effect of postconstruction geometry on final size. AJNR Am J Neuroradiol, 2006. 27(5): p. 1129-31.
[71] Abruzzo T., Shengelaia G.G., Dawson R.C., Owens D.S., Cawley C.M., Gravanis M.B. Histologic and morphologic comparison of experimental aneurysms with human intracranial aneurysms. AJNR Am J Neuroradiol, 1998. 19(7): p. 1309-14.
[72] Yang X.J., Li L. and Wu Z.X. A novel arterial pouch model of saccular aneurysm by concomitant elastase and collagenase digestion. J Zhejiang Univ Sci B, 2007. 8(10): p. 697-703.
[73] de Oliveira I.A., Mendes Pereira Caldas J.G., Oliveira H.A., Brito E.A.C. Development of a new experimental model of saccular aneurysm by intra-arterial incubation of papain in rabbits. Neuroradiology, 2011. 53(11): p. 875-81.
[74] Drenth J., Jansonius J.N., Koekoek R., Swen H.M., Wolthers B.G. Structure of papain. Nature, 1968. 218(5145): p. 929-32.
[75] Nitsawang S., Hatti-Kaul R., Kanarawud P., Purification of papain from Carica papaya latex: aquous two-phase extraction versus two-step salt precipitation. Enzime and Microbiolol technology., 2006: p. 1-5.
[76] Kimmel J.R., Smith E.L. Crystaline papain. I. Preparation,specificity and activation. J Biol Chem, 1954. 207(2): p. 515-531.
[77] Johanson W.G., Jr. and Pierce A.K. Effects of elastase, collagenase, and papain on structure and function of rat lungs in vitro. J Clin Invest, 1972. 51(2): p. 288-93.
[78] Gross P., Babyak M.A., Tolker E., Kaschak M. Enzymatically Produced Pulmonary Emphysema; a Preliminary Report. J Occup Med, 1964. 6: p. 481-4.
[79] Junqueira L.C., Bignolas G., Mourão P.A.S., Bonetti S.S., Quantitation of collagen - proteoglycan interaction in tissue sections. Connect Tissue Res, 1980. 7(2): p. 91-6.
[80] Ionescu G., Neumann E., Domokos M., Andercou A., Cardan E., Cucu A. Experimental preparation of deantigenized vascular heterografts and study of tolerance after transplantation. Acta Chir Belg, 1977. 76(4): p. 393-9.
[81] Sigma-Aldrich. Reagentes bioquímicos e kits para pesquisa em ciências da vida. Sigma-Aldrich (ed.); Brasil. 2006:p. 1812-1813.

Chapter 4

The Role of Metalloproteinases in the Development of Aneurysm

Krzysztof Siemianowicz

Additional information is available at the end of the chapter

http://dx.doi.org/10.5772/47792

1. Introduction

Matrix metalloproteinases (MMPs) were first described by Gross fifty years ago. They are a family of zinc-dependent endopeptidases. They comprise a group of 25 enzymes. Metalloproteinases were first described as proteases degrading extracellular matrix (ECM) proteins such as collagens, elastin, proteoglycans and laminins, hence they were named matrix meatalloproteinases. MMPs were divided according to their substrate specificity into collagenases, gelatinases, stromolysins and matrilysins. This classification was later replaced by numbering the enzymes according to the chronology of their identification. Metalloproteinases are also called metalloproteases.

Four metalloproteases (MMP-14, MMP-15, MMP-16 and MMP-24) have a transmembrane and cytosolic domains. They constitute a subgroup of membrane-type metalloproteases (MT-MMPs) [1, 2].

2. Physiological role of metalloproteinases

MMP-1 (collagenase 1) hydrolyzes collagen types I, II, III, VII, VIII, X and XI, as well as gelatin, fibronectin, vitronectin, laminin, tenascin, aggrecan, links protein, myelin basic protein and versican. MMP-2 (gellatinase) degrades collagen types I, II, III, IV, V, VII, X and XI, gelatin, elastin, fibronectin, vitronectin, laminin, entactin, tenascin, SPARC and aggrecan, links protein, galectin-3, versican, decanin and myelin basic protein. One of the most important differences between theses two metalloproteinases is the possibility of the hydrolysis of elastin and collagen type IV by MMP-2, but not by MMP-1. Researches have also focused their interest on MMP-9 which can degrade collagen types IV, V, VII, X and XIV, fibronectin, laminin, nidogen, proteoglycan link protein and versican.

For a long time metalloproteinases have been vied solely as enzymes of matrix proteins breakdown. Results of researches performed in recent years indicate that there is a group of non-matrix proteins which can be substrates for various MMPs. Metalloproteinases are involved in the activation of latent forms of effective proteins. For example, MMP-2, MMP-3 and MMP-9 can activate interleukin 1β (IL-1β). They can also act on active cytokines, IL-1β undergoes subsequent degradation catalyzed by MMP-3. Metalloproteinases can alter cell surface proteins such as receptors and act on microbial peptides.

Metalloproteinases are not indiscriminately released by cells. They are secreted to or anchored to cell membrane. MT-MMPs have a specific transmembrane domain placing them in a certain position. Other metalloproteinases can be bound by specific cell-MMP interactions. This phenomenon allows an exact localization of their proteolytic activity [1,2].

3. Activation of metalloproteinases

Metalloproteinases are encoded as inactive proenzymes, zymogens. They undergo proteolytic activation. This process can take place either intracellulary or extracellulary. One third of MMPs are activated by intracellular serin protease, furin. This process takes place in trans-Golgi network. A number of MMPs has a cleavage site for other metalloproteinases. MMP-3 activates proMMP-1 and pro-MMP-7. Some metalloproteinases have been described to be activated by kallikrein or plasmin.

In vivo studies indicate that reactive oxygen species (ROS) generated by neutrophils can both activate and subsequently inactivate MMPs. Hypochlorus acid (HClO) generated by neutrophil myeloperoxidase and hydroxyl radicals can activate proMMP-1, proMMP-7 and proMMP-9, whereas peroxynitrate can activate proenzymes of MMP-1, MMP-2 and MMP-9. This process enables a control of burst of proteolytic activity within an inflammatory setting.

Like some other proteases, activity of MMPs is controlled also by two other mechanisms, regulation of gene expression and specific inhibitors. MMP-2 is constitutively expressed and regulation of its activity occurs by either activation or inhibition. Expression of a number of metalloproteinases is up-regulated during various pathological conditions. Among them inflammation is the most studied setting. MMPs are inhibited by α-2 macroglobulin and tissue inhibitors of metalloproteinases (TIMPs). There are four TIMPs. Their secretion is also regulated and represents another point in a network of control of the activity of metalloproteinases. TIMP-3 is primarily bond to ECM and allows a regulation of MMPs' activity in the very site of their action. The network of the control of the activity of metalloproteinases is complex and very precise. Sometimes TIMP interacts with proMMP and inactivate other MMP, e.g. a complex of TIMP-1 and proMMP-9 inactivates MMP-3.

Protection from MMP degradation represents the next step in this sophisticated network of diverse interactions. Neutrophil gelatinase-associated lipocalin (NGAL) bounds to MMP-9 protecting this metalloproteinase from its degradation [1,2].

4. Localisation of metalloproteinases in a vascular wall

Metalloproteinases can be detected in all three layers of a vascular wall. Endothelium can produce MMP-1 and MMP-2. Smooth muscle cells (SMC) of both intima and media are the next source of MMPs. They can secrete MMP-2 and MMP-9. SMC can also produce TIMP-1 and TIMP-2. Adventitia is the layer where MMP-9 can be synthesized. Apart from these most studied metalloproteinases some other MMPs can be detected in a vascular wall: MT1-MMP, MMP-3, MMP-8, MMP-10, MMP-12 and MMP-13. Metalloproteinases are found not only in a wall of arterial wall, but in veins as well.

The balance between the expression of MMPs and TIMPs plays a vital role in preserving the proper and health state of the vascular wall. This equilibrium between activation and inactivation of MMPs is a part of a balance between synthesis and degradation of collagen and elastin, two proteins which have various properties and functions in the arterial wall. Both proteins are crucial for a proper function of the arterial wall. An interruption of these two balances may lead to a development of various vascular pathologies including atherosclerosis, formation of aneurysm and inflammation [3-5].

5. Metalloproteinases and aneurysms

The most studied aneurysm is abdominal aortic aneurysm (AAA), far less research has been focused on aneurysms of cerebral arteries and thoracic aortic aneurysm. All aneurysms are characterized by the destruction of the structural integrity of the extracellular matrix proteins, mainly collagens and elastin. MMPs involved in this pathology can origin both from the cells that physiologically constitute the arterial wall and are stimulated to secrete MMPs, i.e. endothelium, SMC and cells that infiltrate the arterial wall in a response to various stimuli [1, 3, 6-9].

Many scientists points out that cells constituting an inflammatory infiltrate are the major source of metalloproteinases involved in the development of aneurysms. Studies of samples derived from patients undergoing surgery for AAA demonstrated that macropgages from the inflammatory infiltrate can express MMP-1, MMP-2, MMP-3, MMP-9 and MT-1MMP. Metalloproteinase-2 was often detected in cells physiologically constituting the arterial wall, but was absent in macrophages within aneurysms. The pathogenesis of AAA and aneurysms of cerebral arteries differs as these vessels present different types of arteries and there are some differences in the physical characteristic of blood flow in them. Recent experimental studies carried on animals confirmed the role of macrophage infiltration in the formation of intracranial aneurysms. A degranulation of mast cells induces the expression and activation of MMP-2 and MMP-9. Inhibitors of mast cell degranulation inhibited the development of cerebral aneurysms in experimental rats [10, 11].

Human studies confirmed that the expression of metalloproteinases within the AAA is greater than in other sites, remote from the dissection. Nishimura *et al.* observed a different profile of MMP activation in small size abdominal aortic aneurysms, less than 45 mm and large size AAA with diameter exceeding 45 mm. In small size AAA MMP-2 and MMP-9 presented greater gene expression whereas in large size AAA membrane type-1 metalloproteinase and MMP-9 had greater expression. The same study demonstrated also differences in the distribution of the metalloproteinases in the arterial wall. MMP-2 was detected mainly in the intima, whereas MMP-9 was present both in intima and adventitia.

Nishimura *et al.* also observed a significant correlation of the expression of MMP-2 and MMP-9 and between each of these metalloproteinases and TIMP-1 [6].

The degeneration of collagen and elastin leading to the development of aneurysms is a multifactorial process. Various factors may take part in the stimulation of both cells constituting the arterial wall and cells infiltrating it to produce MMPs. Aortic wall is subjected to cyclic stretching because of pulsative blood flow which is a normal physiological condition. AAA is often accompanied by an intraluminal thrombus. It causes that some cells within the aneurysm may be subjected to hypoxia. Experimental study of Oya *et al.* revealed that macrophages cultured in conditions subjected to cyclic stretching under normoxia and hypoxia which simulated the pulsative blood flow and hypoxia due to thrombus presented an increased MMP-9 production. These macrophages produced interleukin-8 (IL-8) and tumor necrosis factor-α (TNF-α) leading to increased apoptosis of vascular smooth muscle cells. Hypoxia was also demonstrated to augment the expression of MMP-1, MT-1 MMP, MMP-2, MMP-7 and MMP-9 in SMC derived from human aorta [12, 13].

Nowadays many scientists focus their research on finding new factors which may augment the secretion of metalloproteinases by the cells present in aneurysms. Experimental studies confirmed that stenosis resulting in a turbulent blood flow can be the next factor increasing expression of MMP-2 and MMP-9 within abdominal aortic aneurysm. Interesting results were obtained by Stolle *et al.* Mice exposed to cigarette smoke and angiotensin II treatment had increased the incidence of AAA and higher gene expression of MMP-2, MMP-3, MMP-8, MMP-9 and MMP-12 in aorta and increased proteolytic activity of two most investigated metalloproteinaes, MMP-2 and MMP-9. Although each of this two factors alone induced minor changes, their combination accelerated the pathologic process. Exposure of the arterial wall to an increased concentration of angiotensin II represents conditions that may be observed in patients with arterial hypertension. This experiment demonstrates that coexistance of arterial hypertension and smoking augments the risk of a development of aneurysm [14, 15].

Studies of Zhang *et al.* demonstrated that human AAA tissues had elevated levels of advanced glycation end products (AGEs) and their receptor (RAGE). In experimental model this group of researchers observed that AGEs induce the production of MMP-9 by macrophages. An increased serum concentration of AGEs accompanies poorly controlled diabetes mellitus. These results indicate that such patients may be at a greater risk of a development of AAA [16].

Abdominal aortic aneurysm is characterized not only by the destruction of its structural integrity of the extracellular matrix protein and inflammatory infiltrate but also by intensive neovascularisation. These new blood vessels developing inside the arterial wall in a place of growing aneurysm are the next source of metalloproteinases degrading ECM. Immature neovessels express MMP-1, MMP-2, MMP-3, MMP-7, MMP-8, MMP-9 and MMP-12 [8].

Polish scientists have observed that the intraluminal thrombus occurring within AAA may modulate the activity of MMP-8, MMP-9, neutrophil elastase and TIMP-1. Specimens from patients with thin, less than 10 mm, thrombus-covered wall of AAA presented significantly higher activity of 3 evaluated metalloproteinases and lower TIMP-1 concentration than thick, exceeding 25 mm, thrombus-covered wall. The intraluminal thrombus may exert its pathological effect through trapping erythrocyte and neutrophils and monocytes. The exact mechanism of activation of MMP in these conditions has not been fully elucidated. Scientists consider various factors activating metalloproteinases, such as hypoxia caused by reduced blood flow or oxidative stress in trapped blood cells. This aspect needs further evaluation [17].

Japanese researchers compared the activity of MMP-2 and MMP-9 in ruptured and unruptured middle cerebral artery dissections obtained during neurosurgery in the same patient. Both metalloproteinases presented greater expression in the ruptured dissection [9].

6. Possible diagnostic markers

The results of scientific researches discussed so far concern the evaluation of either expression or activity of MMPs in the tissue obtained from aneurysms in humans or experimental animals. These measurements have the scientific importance but cannot serve as a diagnostic marker. A growing interest is focused on finding circulating predictors of risk of the development of aneurysm or plasma markers of existing, yet undiagnosed aneurysm. Plasma levels of MMPs are of great interest. MMP-2 and MMP-9 are the candidates for such markers. Polish researchers observed significantly higher plasma concentration of MMP-9 in patients with AAA and thin intraluminal thrombus than in patients with abdominal aortic aneurysm and thick thrombus. Hellenthal *et al.* points out that plasma level of MMP-9 may serve as a marker discriminating patients with and without endoleak within AAA [18-20].

Several polymorphisms of metalloproteinases have been discovered. Their role in the development of AAA is being studied. The polymorphisms of MMP-2 (1306C/T), MMP-3 (5A/6A) and MMP-13 (77A/G) may contribute to the pathogenesis of AAA. The studies of circulating markers of aneurysms give promising results but further research is still required [21].

7. Visualisation of metalloproteinases in aneurysm

Several studies have been aimed at imaging of matrix metalloproteinases and quantifying the inflammatory process that drives abdominal aortic aneurysm development. American scientists developed the MMP-activated probe, MMP Sense 18[20] (VisEn Medical, Woburn, USA) that was used for the *in vivo* and *ex vivo* macroscopic scale imaging. This method based on fluorochromes may be used intravascularly. A new magnetic resonance imaging contrast agent, P947, has been tested for its capabilities of targeting MMPs *in vivo* in expanding experimental AAA. This method allows the detection of MMP activity within the inflammatory infiltrate within AAA and may become a potential non-invasive method to detect AAA at a high risk of rupture [22, 23].

8. Possibilities of pharmacological modulation of metalloproteinases activity

Patients with a high activity of MMPs within the aneurysm are at increased risk of its rupture leading to serious clinical consequences including death. It is of a great importance to find agents which can inhibit MMPs activity and reduce this risk.

Doxycycline, a tetracycline antibiotic, is a known inhibitor of metalloproteinases activity with a growing body of evidence of its beneficial effects observed in animal studies. However data from human studies comprising 6 controlled trials and 2 cohort studies gave conflicting results. The safety of long term use of doxycycline needs evaluation [24].

Statins are a well known group of drugs lowering plasma cholesterol level used to reduce the risk of a coronary heart disease. They have a pleiotropic mode of action reducing the progress of atherosclerosis. Experimental studies indicate that simvastatin can reduce the activity of MMP-2 and MMP-9 in AAA and suppress the development and expansion of abdominal aortic aneurysm. A study performed on samples derived from patients receiving atorvastatin and undergoing surgical treatment for AAA gave promising results demonstrating a significantly reduced activity of MMP-13. Another study with short term, 4 weeks, administration of atorvastatin preceding the operation did not show any differences in the activity of MMP-2, MMP-8, MMP-9, TIMP-1 or TIMP-2. These data indicate that statins may require a long term use to develop their beneficial influence on MMPs' activity [25-27].

Drugs which are administered for a long time focus the scientists' interest. Anti-hypertensive drugs have been studied in this aspect. Calcium channel blocker, azelnidipine, decreased the activity of MMP-2 and MMP-9. The similar influence of angiotensin II receptor blockers, olmesartan and losartan, was observed. The latter was also shown to act synergistically with doxycycline. Perindopril, an angiotensin converting enzyme inhibitor, is known as an anti-hypertensive agent with an ability to affect vascular wall remodeling. In an experimental study perindopril significantly reduced the activity of MMP-2 and MMP-9. In animal studies the activity of MMP-2 and MMP-9 were also decreased by edaravone, a scavenger of reactive oxygen species, resveratrol, a plant derived polyphenolic compound. Two inhibitors of cyclic adenosine monophosphate phosphodiesterase (PDE) were also shown to inhibit the activity of metalloproteinases. Cilostazol, the inhibitor of PDE-3 decreased the activity of MMP-2 and MMP-9, whereas ibudilast, which predominantly blocked PDE-4, decreased the expression of MMP-9 [28-37].

Although the experimental studies indicate that various drugs can reduce the expression and activity of metalloproteinases, their potential use in humans to protect from AAA or inhibit its development requires further studies. Their efficacy and safety of a long term administration must be proven.

Author details

Krzysztof Siemianowicz
Medical University of Silesia, Department of Biochemistry, Poland

9. References

[1] Pearce W.H. & Shively V.P. (2006). Abdominal aortic aneurysm as a complex multifactorial disease. *Annals of New York Academy of Sciences* (1085): 117-132

[2] Ra H-J. & Parks W.C. (2007). Control of matrix metalloproteinase catalytic activity. *Matrix Biology* (26): 587-596

[3] Goodall S. & Crowther M. & Hemingway D.M. &Bell P.R. & Thompson M.M. (2001). Ubiquitous elevation of matrix metalloproteinase-2 expression in the vasculature of patients with abdominal aneurysms. *Circulation* (104): 304-309

[4] Ishii T. & Asuwa N. (2000). Collagen and elastin degradation by matrix metalloproteinases and tissue inhibitors of matrix metalloproteinases in aortic dissection. *Human Pathology* (31): 640-646

[5] Siemianowicz K. & Gminski J. & Goss M. & Francuz T. & Likus W. & Jurczak T. & Garczorz W. (2010). Influence of elastin-derived peptides on metaloprotease production in endothelial cells. *Experimental and Therapeutical Medicine* (1): 1057-1060

[6] Nishimura K. & Ikebuchi M. & Kanaoka Y. & Ohgi S. & Ueta E. & Nanba E. & Ito H. (2003). Relationship between matrix metalloproteinases and tissue inhibitors of metalloproteinases in the wall of abdominal aortic aneurysms. (2003). *International Journal of Angiology* (22): 229-238

[7] Michel J.B. & Martin-Ventura J.L. & Egido J. & Sakalihasan N. & Treska V. & Lindholt J. & Allaire E. & Thorsteinsdottir U. & Cockerill G. & FAD UE consortium. (2011). Novel aspects of the pathogenesis of aneurysms of the abdominal aorta in humans. *Cardiovascular Research* (90): 18-27

[8] Reeps C. & Pelisek J. & Seidl S. & Schuster T. & Zimmerman A. & Kuehnl A. & Eckstein H.H. (2009). Inflammatory infiltrates and neovessels are relevant sources of MMPs in abdominal aortic aneurysm wall. *Pathobiology* (76): 243-252

[9] Saito A. & Fujimura M. & Inoue T. & Shimizu H. & Tominada T. (2010). Lectin-like oxidized low-density lipoprotein receptor 1 and matrix metalloproteinase expression in ruptured and unruptured multiple dissections of distal middle cerebral artery: case report. *Acta Neurochirurgica* (Wien) (152): 1235-1240

[10] Kanematsu Y. & Kanematsu M. & Kurihara C. & Tada Y. & Tsou T.L. & van Rooijen N. & Lawton M.T. & Young W.L. & Liang E.L. & Nuki Y. & Hashimoto T. (2011). Critical roles of macrophages in the formation of intracranial aneurysm. *Stroke* (42): 173-178

[11] Ishibashi R. & Aoki T. & Nishimura M. & Hashimoto N. & Miyamoto S. (2010). Contribution of mast cells to cerebral aneurysm formation. *Current Neurovascular Research* (7): 113-124

[12] Oya K. & Sakamoto N. & Ohashi T. & Sato M. (2011). Combined stimulation with cyclic stretching and hypoxia increases production of matrix metalloproteinase-9 and cytokines by macrophages. *Biochemical and Biophysical Research Communications* (412): 676-682

[13] Erdozain O.J. & Pegrum S. & Winrow V.R. & Horrocks M. & Stevens C.R. (2010). Hypoxia in abdominal aortic aneurysm supports a role for HIF-1α and Ets-1 as drivers of matrix metalloproteinase upregulation in human aortic smooth muscle cells. *Journal of Vascular Research* (48): 163-170

[14] Mata K.M. & Prudente P.S. & Rocha F.S. & Prado C.M. & Floriano E.M. & Elias J. Jr & Rizzi E. & Gerlach R.F. & Rossi M.A. & Ramos S.G. (2011). Combining two potential causes of metalloproteinase secretion causes abdominal aortic aneurysms in rats: a new experimental model. *International Journal of Experimental Pathology* (92): 26-39

[15] Stolle K. & Berges A. & Lietz M. & Lebrum S. & Wallerath T. (2010). Cigarette smoke enhances abdominal aortic aneurysm formation in angiotensin II-treated apolipoprotein E-defficient mice. (2010). *Toxicology Letters* (199): 403-409

[16] Zhang F. & Banker G. & Liu X. & Suwanabol P.A. & Lengfeld J. & Yamanouchi D. & Kent K.C. & Liu B. (2011). The novel function of advanced glycation end products in regulation of MMP-9 production. *Journal of Surgical Research* (171): 871-876

[17] Wiernicki I. & Stachowska E. & Safranow K. & Cnotliwy M. & Rybicka M. & Kaczmarczyk M. & Gutowski P. (2010). Enhanced matrix-degradating proteolytic activity within the thin thrombus-covered wall of human abdominal aortic aneurysms. *Atherosclerosis* (212): 161-165

[18] Hellenthal F.A. & Ten Bosch J.A. & Pulinx B. & Wodzig W.K. & de Haan M.W. & Prins M.H. & Welten R.J. & Teijink J.A. & Schurink G.W. (2012). Plasma levels of matrix metalloproteinase-9: a possible diagnostic marker of successful endovascular aneurysm repair. *European Journal of Vascular and Endovascular Surgery* (43): 171-172

[19] Wiernicki I. & Millo B. & Safranow K. & Gorecka-Szyld B. & Gutowski P. (2011). MMP-9, homocysteine and CRP circulating levels are associated with intraluminal thrombus thickness of abdominal aortic aneurysms: a new implication of the old biomarkers. *Disease Markers* (31): 67-74

[20] Wen D. & Zhou X.L. & Li J.J. & Hui R.T. (2011). Biomarkers in aortic dissection. *Clinica Chimica Acta* (412): 688-695

[21] Saracini C. & Bolli P. & Sticchi E. & Pratesi G. & Pulli R. & Sofi F. & Pratesi C. & Gensini G.F. Abbate R. & Giusti B. (2012). Polymorphisms of genes involved in extracellular matrix remodeling and abdominal aortic aneurysm. *Vascular Surgery* (55): 171-179

[22] Sheth R.A. & Maricevich M. & Mahmood U. (2010). In vivo optical molecular imaging of matrix metalloproinase activity in abdominal aortic aneurysms correlates with treatment effects on growth rate. *Atherosclerosis* (212): 181-187

[23] Bazeli R. & Coutard M. & Duport B.D. & Lancelot E. & Corot C. & Laissy J.P. & Letourneur D. & Michel J.B. & Serfaty J.M. (2010): In vivo evaluation of a new magnetic

resonance imaging contrast agent (P947) to target matrix metalloproteinases in expanding experimental abdominal aortic aneurysms. *Investigative Radiology* (45): 662-668

[24] Dodd B.R. & Spence R.A. (2011). Doxycycline inhibition of abdominal aortic aneurysm growth: a systemic review of literature. *Current Vascular Pharmacology* (9): 471-478

[25] Mastoraki S.T. & Toumpoulis I.K. & Anagnostopoulos C.E. & Tiniakos D. & Papalois A. & Chamogeorgakis T.P. & Angouras D.C. & Rokkas C.K. (2012). Treatment with simvastatin inhibits the formation of abdominal aortic aneurysms in rabbits. *Annals of Vascular Surgery* (26): 250-258

[26] Schweitzer M. & Mitmaker B. & Obrand D. & Sheiner N. & Abraham C. & Dostanic S. & Meilleur M. & Sugahara T. & Chalifour L.E. (2010). Atorvastatin modulates matrix metalloproteinase expression, activity, and signaling in abdominal aortic aneurysms. *Vascular and Endovascular Surgery* (2010): 116-122

[27] Rahman M.N. & Khan J.A. & Mazari F.A. & Mockford K. & McCollum P.T. & Chetter I.C. (2011). A randomized placebo controlled trial of the effect of preoperative statin use on matrix metalloproteinases and tissue inhibitors of matrix metalloproteinases in areas of low and peak wall stress in patients undergoing elective open repair of abdominal aortic aneurysm. (2011). *Annals of Vascular Surgery* (25): 32-38

[28] Nakamura E. & Akashi H. & Hiromatsu S. & Tanaka A. & Onitsuka S. & Aoyagi S. (2009). Azelnidipine decreases plasma matrix metalloproteinase-9 levels after endovascular abdominal aortic aneurysm repair. *Kurume Medical Journal* (56): 25-32

[29] Yokokura H. & Hiromatsu S. & Akashi H. & Kato S. & Aoyagi S. (2007). Effects of calcium channel blocker azelnidipine on experimental abdominal aortic aneurysms. *Surgery Today* (37): 468-473

[30] Yang H.H. & Kim. J.M. & Chum E. & van Breemen C. & Chung A.W. (2009). Long-term effects of losartan on structure and function of the thoracic aorta in a mouse model of Marfan syndrome. *British Journal of Pharmacology* (158): 1503-1512

[31] Yang H.H. & Kim J.M. & Chum E. & van Breemen C. & Chung A.W. (2010). Effectiveness of combination of losartan potassium and doxycycline versus single-drug treatments in the secondary prevention of thoracic aortic aneurysm in Marfan syndrome. *Journal of Thoracic and Cardiovascular Surgery* (140): 305-312

[32] Alsac J.M. & Journe C. & Louedec L. & Dai J. & Fabiani J.N. & Mitchel J.B. (2011). Downregulation of remodelling enzymatic activity induced by angiotensin-converting enzyme inhibitor (perindopril) reduces the degeneration of experimental abdominal aortic aneurysms in a rat model. *European Journal of Vascular and Endovascular Surgery* (41): 474-480

[33] Hosokawa Y. (2010). Effects of angiotensin receptor blocker and calcium channel blocker on experimental abdominal aortic aneurysms in a hamster model. *Kurume Medical Journal* (57): 1-8

[34] Morimoto K. & Hasegawa T. & Tanaka A. & Wulan B. & Yu J. & Morimoto N. & Okita Y. & Okada K. (2012). Free radical scavenger receptor edaravone inhibits both formation and development of abdominal aortic aneurysm in rats. *Journal of Vascular Surgery* (Epub ahead of print)

[35] Kaneko H. & Anzai T. & Morisawa M. & Nagai T. & Anzai A. & Takahashi T. & Shimoda M. & Sasaki A. & Maekawa Y. & Yoshimura K. & Aoki H. & Tsubota K. & Yoshikawa T. & Okada Y. Ogawa S. & Fukuda K. (2011). Resveratrol prevents the development of abdominal aortic aneurysm through attenuation of inflammation, oxidative stress, and neovascularisation. *Atherosclerosis* (217): 360-367

[36] Zhang Q. & Huang J.H. & Xia R.P. & Duan X.H. & Jiang Y.B. & Jiang Q. & Sun W.J. (2011). Suppresion of experimental abdominal aortic aneurysm in a rat model by phosphodiesterase 3 inhibitor cilostazol. *Journal of Surgical Research* (167): 385-393

[37] Yagi K. & Tada Y. & Kitazato K.T. & Tamura T. & Satomi J. & Nagahiro S. (2010). Ibudilast inhibits cerebral aneurysms by down-regulating inflammation-related molecules in the vascular wall of rats. *Neurosurgery* (66): 551-559

Section 2

Abdominal Aneurysm

Chapter 5

Biomechanical Approach to Improve the Abdominal Aortic Aneurysm (AAA) Rupture Risk Prediction

Guillermo Vilalta, Félix Nieto, Enrique San Norberto,
María Ángeles Pérez, José A. Vilalta and Carlos Vaquero

Additional information is available at the end of the chapter

http://dx.doi.org/10.5772/46030

1. Introduction

It is well known that the human body operates under a continuous interaction of complex processes taking place at multiple dimensional and temporal scales. While biomedical research is slowly elucidating many of these processes, it remains mostly unclear how they interact in the production of the global physiological or pathological conditions we observe [1]. The cardiovascular system in general and the Abdominal Aortic Aneurysms (AAA) in particular is a good example.

Aneurysm is a pathology that can affect most blood vessels, arteries or veins, and it commonly occurs in the cerebral vasculature and the thoracic aorta even if the vast majority of cases occur in the abdominal aorta and are termed AAA.

In its most accepted definition, AAA is a localized, progressive and permanent dilation (usually larger than 3 cm in diameter) of the aortic wall. Under specific conditions mainly associated with an irreversible pathological remodelling of arterial connective tissue, the aneurysm tends to increase in size, with an increased risk of rupture which can cause death. Atherosclerosis is the most common cause of aortic aneurysm. However the causes are usually multifactorial: environmental, genetic, autoimmune or infectious.

AAA has increasingly been recognized as an important health problem in the last decades. The statistics associated with this pathology are the major concern: AAA has been estimated to occur in 3-9% of the population [2], with a mortality rate on rupture between 78-94% [3] producing more than 15,000 deaths annually in the US and 8,000 in England. The mean age of patients with AAA is 67 years and men are affected more than women by a ratio 4:1 with prevalence up to 5% [4].

The majority of studies found in medical literature report this increase in the incidence of aortic aneurismal disease, which is expected in a continuously aging population in developed countries. In spite of significant improvement in surgical procedures and technological advancements in imaging devices in recent years, the associated aneurysm mortality and morbidity rate have also risen concomitantly.

Currently, the lack of an accurate AAA rupture risk index remains an important problem in the clinical management of the disease. The main clinical criteria in deciding on the treatment of AAA patients are: a) the peak transverse diameter and b) the growth rate. If the peak diameter reaches the upper threshold (5-5.5 cm) or the maximum diameter expansion rate is > 0.5 cm/yr for smaller AAAs the patient may be submitted for surgical intervention, also depending on the state of health and willingness of the patients. The main limitation of this practice is that these criteria, although have a significant empirical basis, can be considered insufficient because they have not a physically sound theoretical basis. This statement should not be surprising; approximately 33% of ruptured AAAs have diameters smaller than 50 mm [5] which is indicative of the complex pathogenesis of the disease progression that cannot be capture by traditional indicators.

Due to these observations, recently researches have been focused at improving the knowledge and the understanding of the phenomena associated with the formation and evolution of aneurysm pathology in order to define whether other variables could be predictive of rupture. The literature begins to reflect the existence of a consensus that, rather than empirical criteria, the develop of a biomechanical approach based on a multiscale model can be a significant step for the accurate assessment of the rupture risk.

This chapter examines the basis of the biomechanical approach. The main aim is to support the hypothesis that biomechanical considerations may become into powerful tool for a reliable patient-specific prediction of AAA rupture risk.

2. Biomechanical approach. Method grounds

This new approach has its foundation in the integration, through appropriate relations, of factors from different natures (biological, structural and geometric) and scales (temporal and dimensional) at the molecular, cellular, tissue and organ levels (from bottom level to top level), which allow to describe, from quantitatively point of view, the aneurysm progression and its rupture potential.

These defined relations are known as biomechanical factors or biomechanical determinants (BDs).

The basic premise of the biomechanical approach to estimate the AAA rupture risk, is that this phenomenon follows the principle of material failure, that is, an aneurysm ruptures when the stresses acting on the arterial wall exceeding its failure strength, reflecting the interaction between the arterial wall structural remodelling and the forces generated by blood flow within the AAA.

3. Remodeling history model. Biological Biodeterminants, BBDs

Most investigators would agree that the pathogenesis of the abdominal aortic aneurysm (AAA) is multifactorial. There appear to be environmental, genetic, autoimmune, inflammatory, and structural factors.

The term "atherosclerotic AAA" is misleading because it suggests that atherosclerosis is a necessary cause of AAA disease. While some patients with have atherosclerotic occlusive peripheral vascular disease, others have minimal atherosclerotic disease. For this reason, the Joint Committee of the Society for Vascular Surgery recommending that the term "non-specific AAA" be used since 1991.

The definition of AAA has varied in the literature over the years, but all definitions have in common a specification of the degree of aortic dilatation. So, the definition is a permanent localized dilatation of an artery having at least a 50% increase in diameter compared with the expected normal diameter of the artery or of the diameter of the segment proximal to the dilatation. According to this definition, an infrarenal AAA could then be defined as 3.0 cm if 2.0 cm is the expected maximal diameter of the infrarenalaort in an individual of a specific body scale.

Risk factors

The four principal positive risk factors for AAA are smoking, age, male sex, and family history. While smoking clearly seems to be an environmental factor, issues related to addiction and dose-effect responses are doubtless modified by genetic influences. The three principal negative risk factors for AAA are diabetes, female sex, and African-American descent, all of which are genetically determined.

There is a more complicated relationship between plasma lipid levels and the risk of AAA. Blanchard et al [6], failed to show any correlation between cholesterol levels, low-density lipoprotein (LDL) or high-density lipoprotein (HDL) and aneurysm risk (Blanchard). However, it have been showed an increased risk in patients whose plasma cholesterol was high and a protective effect was seen in patients whose serum HDL was high [7]. Low serum HDL gave an increased risk of AAA [8].

There is some disagreement in the literature regarding the effect of hypertension on aneurysm risk. The American Veterans study represented the largest of its type and showed hypertension to be an independent risk factor. Taking medication for high blood pressure was a risk factor, whereas hypertension itself was significant in women. Tornwall and Blanchard both showed both systolic and diastolic hypertension to be risks [6]. A study of all men born in Malmo in the year 1914 failed to demonstrate hypertension as a risk factor at all [9]. Experimentally, AAAs artificially induced into hypertensive rats were found to grow larger than those in normotensives [10] and the dilatation correlated well with systolic pressure.

Molecular genetics

Epidemiologic review indicates an aneurysm gene expression that is typically delayed until at least the sixth decade. There is strong evidence for inherited predisposition, and possibly an association with generalized arteriomegaly. It have been demonstrated an incidence of 20% aortic aneurysms among first order relatives of aneurysm patients [11]. In [12] was showed genetic linkages, accounting for abdominal aneurysm formation in 50 families, who had clustering of the lesion in two or more first order relatives. Possibly, they possessed a common metabolic disorder affecting the arterial wall.

A retrospective study of hospital patients in Zimbabwe demonstrated a higher incidence of aneurysms among whites than Africans [13]. By using ultrasound screening of first degree relatives demonstrated aortic aneurysms in 20–30% of male siblings over 55 years of age [14]. Case reports of familial aneurysm disease in patients without connective tissue or vascular diseases add validity to the theory of genetic linkage. The occurrence of multiple aneurysms in individuals is consistent with a genetic foundation. Many authors suggest aneurysm disease is a systemic process. Frequently, patients suffer from generalized arteriomegaly; often this is accompanied by multiple aneurysms.

Several cross-linking defects have been associated with aneurysm formation. Tilsonstudied the biochemistry of a collagen component deficiency that predisposes to aneurysms [12]. They evaluated pyridine cross-linkages and found fewer cross-linkages per collagen molecule in human skin samples. This suggests a genetic basis for aneurysm disease. Experiments with sex-linked defects of collagen and elastin demonstrate the blotchy BLO allele. These models exhibit aortic aneurysms and diminished skin tensile strength. The pattern of expression indicates the trait is related to the X chromosome. In [15] it was reviewed the literature and found clear evidence for an independent genetic defect in most AAAs. Their work centered on a genetic analysis of collagen genes. Genetic collagen defects causing architectural defects are established in osteogenesisimperfecta (type I collagen of bone) and chondrodysplasias (type II collagen of cartilage). New evidence implicates mutations in the type III procollagen gene in the pathogenesis of aneurysmal disease. Various mutations have been confirmed in studies of patients with type IV Ehlers–Danlos syndrome (EDS) [16].

Studies of patients with aneurysms clearly demonstrate family linkage, and the data strongly suggest a genetic defect. Statistical analysis supports a recessive inheritance pattern in approximately 10% of men who have aneurysms. Research in this area is active and implicates an autosomal diallelic major locus.

The two genes with the strongest supporting evidence of contribution to the genetic risk for AAA are the CDKN2BAS gene, also known as ANRIL, which encodes an antisense ribonucleic acid that regulates expression of the cyclin-dependent kinase inhibitors CDKN2A and CDKN2B, and DAB2IP, which encodes an inhibitor of cell growth and survival. Functional studies are now needed to establish the mechanisms by which theses genes contribute toward AAA pathogenesis [17].

Structural pathophysiology

Atherosclerosis

The traditional view of aneurysm formation is that arterial dilation is a consequence of degenerative atherosclerotic disease, which results in acquired wall weakness. The experienced vascular surgeon is well aware that peripheral arteriosclerosis and aneurysmal disease often coexist. Severe atherosclerotic calcification in the aortoiliac vessels presents a technical challenge in aneurysm surgery. Epidemiologic, radiographic, and histologic data support the association between aneurysm disease and atherosclerosis [18].

AAAs and atherosclerosis share many risk factors and frequently occur simultaneously. The frequency of aortic aneurysms closely parallels the prevalence of atherosclerosis; for example, the low abdominal aneurysm rate in Asia correlates with the decreased incidence of atherosclerosis. Radiographic and histopathologic studies support the link between atherosclerosis and aneurysms. Ultrasound screening of patients with peripheral vascular disease detects a 5.9% rate of AAA, double that of the general population [19]. Studies of patients suffering from coronary and carotid artery occlusive disease detect an aortic aneurysmal rate of 11–13.5% [9]. Histologic evaluations of sections from aortic aneurysms show atherosclerotic changes and thinning of the media.

Pathophysiologic principles also support the concept that atherosclerosis contributes to aneurysm formation. Atherosclerotic plaques may obstruct nutrient diffusion from the lumen to the media. The needs of the media must then be supplied exclusively by vasa vasorum from the adventitia. However, this may be inadequate due to incomplete distribution of vasa vasorum throughout the human arterial system [20]. Aortic vasa vasorum usually arise from the renal arteries, accounting for the relative sparing of the perirenal aorta from aneurysm formation.

Structural changes induced by atherosclerosis may contribute to aneurysm formation. As atherosclerosis progresses in humans, friable type I collagen replaces native type III collagen [21].Thus, the architectural integrity of the vessel is impaired, leading to a predilection to aneurysm formation. An association between aortic aneurysms and atherosclerosis is not surprising since the geometry and hemodynamics of arterial dilation predispose to atherosclerosis formation. Aneurysms have increased in incidence, prevalence, and mortality over the last 30 years, while coronary artery and cerebrovascular diseases have not. The divergence of these diseases in prevalence and mortality indicates that while risk factors are shared, the development of aneurysm disease is not entirely explained by atherosclerosis.

Although the epidemiologic link between the two is strong, it is propose that occlusive atherosclerotic aortic disease and aortic aneurysmal disease are distinct entities [12]. This is based on the different characteristics of these groups including age of onset, male–female ratio, clinical course, and prognosis. Evidence found to correlate with the size and state of aneurysm indicates that aneurysms reflect a heterogeneous disease with multiple forms and etiologic factors.

Autoimmunity

Autoimmunity may precipitate the inflammatory cascade. Aneurysm aortic extract was studied and noted to contain large quantities of IgG. Further studies revealed that the IgG from AAA patients was present and reactive against various proteins present in the aneurysmal aorta [22]. One of the initial putative autoantigen extracts was an 80-kDa dimer, designated aortic aneurysm associated protein-40 (AAAP-40). AAAP-40 was reactive with 79% (11 of 14) of AAA IgG preparations, and 11% (1 of 9) of controls ($p = 0.002$) (Gregory). Other autoantigens have subsequently been found, and are currently under investigation in our laboratory. Evidence continues to accumulate to support the notion that autoimmunity may play an important role in aneurysmal degeneration of the aorta. Some of these autoantigens are absent in the external iliac artery, perhaps explaining why this artery rarely becomes aneurismal.

Triggering of autoimmunity can be brought about by autoantigens or molecular mimics. For example, molecular mimicry may occur with cytomegalovirus and clone 1. Also, rabbit antibody against *Treponemapallidum*and herpes simplex have been shown to bind to the adventitial elastin-associated microfibrils. The putative autoantigen AAAP-40 has homologies with *Treponemapallidum*and herpes. The hypothesis is that there are epitopes in the microbial proteins that are similar to the AAAP-40, thereby triggering an autoimmune response. Tanaka et al [23] detected herpes simplex viral DNA in 12 of 44 AAA specimens, compared with 1 of 10 normal subjects.

Inflammation

The normal aorta has few inflammatory cells within in its wall. An influx of CD3+ cells and lymphocytes is seen in AAA tissues Although 66% of all lymphocytes in AAAs are in the adventitia, polyclonal B-lymphocytes are abundant in the media. IgG is elevated in AAA specimens. In [24] it was showed an inflammatory infiltrate in the adventitia in 68% of 156 AAA resection specimens examined retrospectively. Macrophages are found throughout the wall of AAA specimens. The macrophage Fc receptors regulate the secretion of proteinases by receptor specific mechanisms. Phagocytes produce proteinases such as elastase and collagenase. On the other hand, it have been implicated the collagenase, stromelysin, and gelatinase-B (MMP-1,3,9) in the destruction of the aorta matrix [25]. Cytokines are released by inflammatory cells and smooth muscle cells in the aorta. They are predominantly: interleukin 1 (IL-1), IL-6, IL-8, monocyte chemoattractant protein (MCP-1), tumor necrosis factor (TNF), and interferon (IFN). These cytokines, to varying degrees, cause MMP expression, TIMP reduction, induction of prostaglandin synthesis, lymphocyte proliferation, and chemotaxis. An autoimmune or inflammatory cascade, as proposed in some etiologies of AAAs, is perpetuated via the use of cytokines [26].

Enzymatic degradation

The elastin: collagen ratio has consistently been shown to be reduced in AAAs when ompared with normal aortas, leading to loss of elasticity and weakening of the aneurysmal wall. This may not be simply due to increased elastin degradation, as Minion et al. have shown that the total elastin content of the aneurismal wall may actually increase, but that the corresponding increase in collagen is much greater (Minion). Despite this evidence, there is little doubt that proteolysis plays an important role in aneurysm development. Aneurysmal disease differs from stenotic disease by the intensity of proteolytic activity within the extracellular matrix. The established association with chronic lung disease supports the argument that elastolysis is a major contributory factor, and indeed this is an area in which there has been much research. For some time, the cause of elastin degradation remained unknown, but even as early as 1980 when it was described increased collagenase activity [27]. In 1991, it was found a spectrum of collagenase activity in the aortic wall of both atherosclerotic and aneurysmal vessels ranging from 55–92 kDa [29].

Importantly, although the collagenase activity was limited, it increased dramatically when tissue inhibitors of metalloproteinases (TIMPs) were destroyed. In [30], it wasalso described the increased expression of a 92 kDagelatinase in AAAs when compared with both normal aortas and aorto-occlusive disease, and localized this to the area around infiltrating macrophages. This gelatinase is part of a family of zinc-dependent proteolytic enzymes, the matrix metalloproteinases (MMPs), now known as MMP9. In the same year, Freestone et al [31],further elucidated the relative amounts of both MMP9 and MMP2 by a combination of gelatinzymography and immunoblotting. This study demonstrated that the principal gelatinase in smaller aneurysms was MMP2, but that in larger aneurysms MMP9 predominated. McMillan et al [21],investigated mRNA levels for MMPs in AAAs and found that MMP9 was maximally expressed in moderate diameter (5–6.9 cm) rather than large (>7 cm) or small (<4 cm) aneurysms. These findings suggested that whilst MMP9 was responsible for the rapid growth that was seen in this size of aneurysm, other enzymes were responsible for initiation and rupture. Pyoet al.'s paper elegantly proves a link between MMP9 and aneurysm pathogenesis by looking at the effect of inhibiting it both pharmacologically and by targeted gene disruption [32]. Mice that were deficient in the MMP9 gene failed to develop aneurysms as their wild-type counterparts did when subjected to elastase perfusion of the aorta. Bone marrow transplants from each group to the other reversed the response to elastase infusion, demonstrating that the expression of MMP9 by inflammatory cells is crucial to aneurysm development. Other MMPs have also been implicated in the development of AAAs, particularly MMP1 and MMP3. Vine and Powell also found immunoreactive MMP1 in extracts from AAAs (Vine). And more recently the expression of MMP3, as measured by reverse transcriptase polymerase chain reaction (rt-PCR), was found to be elevated in AAAs when compared to aorto-occlusive disease.

Matrix metalloproteinase 13 is a recently described enzyme also known as collagenase-3 and its expression is tightly regulated. Whilst MMP13 was not expressed at all in normal tissue, it was found in atherosclerotic disease and in significantly higher concentrations in AAAs. Expression was localized to medial smooth muscle cells in the aortic tissue, and could also be detected in human vascular smooth muscle cells in culture. Membrane type MMP1 (MT MMP1) is an activator of MMP2 and was found to be increased in aneurismal aorta when compared to normal or atherosclerotic aorta. Membrane type MMP1 was localized to aortic smooth muscle cells and macrophages in aneurysmal tissue by immunohistochemical analysis. The ability to activate MMP2 was confirmed by the addition of radiolabelled pro-MMP2, and determination of the subsequent amount of radiolabelled active MMP2. In vivo, the activity of MMPs is tightly controlled by their natural inhibitors, the TIMPs. In 2000, it was demonstrated that TIMP-1 bound to both the monomeric and dimeric forms of MMP9, whereas TIMP-2 bound only to the active form. Whilst it has been shown that the TIMPs are present in large quantities in AAAs, it has been suggested that itis an imbalance between MMPs and TIMPs that leads to the net increase in proteolysis seen. Tamarinaet al also showed that the TIMP: MMP ratio was actually decreased in AAAs, despite an absolute increase in TIMP levels [33].

Whilst there has been considerable work published in the area of collagenases and other metalloproteinases in AAAs, less is known about the role of serine proteases. Elastases of approximately 20–30 kDa have been demonstrated in the inner aspect of the media in AAAs. This elastase works best in the alkaline range, and is inhibited by α-1 anti-trypsin. The fact that it is also inhibited by phenylmethylsulphonyl fluoride (PMSF) confirms that it is indeed a serine protease. Five distinct serine proteases have been separated by gel electrophoresis from aortic aneurysm tissue, suggesting there is a spectrum of enzymes at work. In addition to MMPs and serine proteases, there is also the cysteine protease group. These differ from serine proteases by the substitution of an Asn residue for an Asp in the catalytic triad. Cathepsins S and K are examples of this type of elastase and have been shown to be produced in abundance by smooth muscle cells in atheroma. They are inhibited by cystatin C, the expression of which is governed by a polymorphism of its signal peptide. As discussed previously, patients in whom the cathepsins were not inhibited displayed faster growing aneurysms.

AAA is a multifactorial disease with genetic risk factors and an immunologic component. Immune cells, including macrophages, neutrophils, mast cells, B- and T- lymphocytes, along with vascular smooth muscle cells and adventitial fibroblasts, produce cytokines and enzymes, promoting an inflammatory reaction, extracellular matrix degradation, and neovascularization. Among the different enzymes secreted by immune and stromal cells, matrix metalloproteinase (MMP)-2, MMP-9, MMP-12, cathepsins, and neutrophil elastase cause medial degeneration. Chymase causes smooth muscle cell apoptosis, and MMP-3, MMP-8, and MMP-13 cause adventitial collagen degradation, promoting abdominal aortic aneurysm rupture [34].

Oxidative stress

The action of reactive oxygen species has been implicated in the etiology of many disease processes. In particular, the effect of oxidative stress on many aspects of vascular biology has come under intense scrutiny over the past few years. The addition of antioxidants significantly reduced the activity of MMP9, whereas the addition of inhibitors of protein kinase C had no effect. These results suggest that the increased proteolytic activity seen in the extracellular matrix in patients with diabetes mellitus is due, at least in part, to the effects of oxidation, and may help to explain a link between aneurysm formation and oxidative stress. A further series of aortic banding experiments have demonstrated that in areas of high pressure there is an up-regulation of endothelial nitric oxide synthase (eNOS) when compared with tissues downstream of the artificial coarctation [35].

Measuring nitrotyrosine in the same tissues gave some indication of the degree of nitric oxide breakdown and sequestration by reactive oxygen species. In the areas above the banding (heart, brain and thoracic aorta) the levels of nitrotyrosine were much higher than in areas not exposed to high pressures (distal aorta). The inactivation of nitric oxide due to oxidative damage in areas of high pressure is another indication of vascular endothelial dysfunction, which may contribute to the pathogenesis of aneurysms. Combining the in vitro elastase perfusion rat model of Anidjaret al [10],with modern cDNAmicroassay analysis,looked at the expression of 8799 genes in rats with induced aortic aneurysms, and compared them with genes expressed in rats that had undergone sham operations [36]. Using this technique they were able to identify over 200 genes whose expression had more than doubled in the aneurysm group. Significantly, this included many genes reflecting an increase in oxidative stress, notably hemeoxygenase, inducible nitric oxide synthase (iNOS), 12-lipoxygenase and heart cytochrome C oxidase, subunit VIa. Conversely, antioxidant genes such as superoxide dismutase, reduced NAD-cytochrome b-5 reductase and glutathione S reductase werefound to be down-regulated. These two complementary findings both point to oxidative stress playing a major role in AAA development.

Infection

Infected aortic aneurysms are uncommon, and infrequently have their pathological features been described. Panneton and Edwards evaluated clinical and histopathologic features in patients undergoing surgical repair of infected aneurysms of the descending thoracic or abdominal aorta over a 24-year period [37]. The results showed that among cases with an identifiable causative organism, staphylococcus accounted for 30%, streptococcus for 20%, salmonella for 20%, Escherichia coli for 15%, and other organisms for 15%.

During recent years, attention has been paid to the role of atypical bacterial infections, including Chlamydia and Helicobacter pylori, in the process of atherogenesis and arterial disease development. The reported rates of detection within atherosclerotic lesions by PCR vary widely. Regarding Chlamydia, several studies hypothesized this organism as a possible source of vascular disease, including carotid, coronary, and aortic pathology. Its role in the pathogenesis of aortic aneurysms, however, has been controversial. Sodecket al [38],investigated the presence of C. pneumoniae in 148 tissue samples excised from control and diseased aortas. DNA of C. pneumoniae, C. trachomatis and C. psittaci were assessed by highly sensitive and specific real time polymerase chain reaction (PCR). C. trachomatis-DNA was detected in 1/65 diseased patients and in none of 83 controls (P=0.43). In a similar study, surgical specimens derived from aneurysm or aorta fragments were investigated for C. pneumoniae utilizing PCR. In asymptomatic aneurysms, DNA was found in 9 cases (29%), and in ruptured aneurysms in 14 cases (49%). In the control group, C. pneumoniae DNA was not detected in the aortic wall. Conflicting data has failed to show a clear relationship between chlamydia infection and aortic pathology.

Cytomegalovirus (CMV)-induced arterial disease has also been linked to aortic pathology. To further elucidate the mechanism by which CMV may promote atherosclerosis, Westphalet al.(Westhpal), studied the expression pattern of cellular inflammatory and proliferative signals in the aortic wall of CMV (+) and CMV (−) patients undergoing coronary artery bypass grafting (CABG). CMV-DNA in smooth muscle cells was thought to induce local growth factor expression as well as endothelial activation, both of which can promote the progression of atherosclerosis. Since traditional atherogenic risk factors increase the likelihood of aortic CMV manifestation, CMV may play a crucial role in mediating the progression of atherosclerosis. The persistent expression of CMV-gene in the vessel wall plays a role in the vascular cellular response, including progression of atherosclerosis or vasculitis in vivo. Kilicet al [39], performed PCR analysis to demonstrate the relationship between CMV and atheromathosis at the aortic wall. CMV DNA was found in 37.9% atherosclerotic and 32.7% non-atherosclerotic vascular wall specimens.

Vitamin E deficiency

Studies have pointed to an inverse relationship between vitamin E (a-tocopherol) levels and the incidence of arterial disease. Vitamin E is an important lipid-soluble antioxidant that localizes to the hydrophobic area of biologic membranes [40]. In terms of AAA, it is hypothesized that activated polymorphonuclear cells (PMNs) release proteinases which degrade the aortic wall matrix. These same PMNs would also release oxidative enzymes, generating toxic oxygen species such as hydrogen peroxide which would lead to lipid peroxidation. Vitamin E is considered a specific, though indirect, index of in vivo peroxidation. They also showed that a small group of AAA patients had decreased vitamin E levels but not decreased vitamin E/total lipid ratios compared with controls (coronary artery disease and normal patients). Accordingly, the AAA patients may be under increased oxidative stress (e.g., increased inflammation or PMN activation) but do not have decreased concentrations of plasma vitamin E carriers.

This analysis reveals how the biological information associated with AAA pathogenesis constitute the foundation on which can be defined the destructive remodeling of the aortic wall and its influence in AAA rupture.

4. Morphological Biodeterminants, MBDs

After its formation, the aneurysm trends to increase in size and change its shape as consequence of the arterial wall destructive remodeling. This phenomenon, which occurs along many years in asymptomatic way, characterizes the AAA morphology and morphometry. Aneurysm geometric characteristics have been reported to be a significant predictors of the tendency for expansion or subsequent risk of rupture [41, 42] and can be the deciding factors in the clinical management of the disease. The correlation of the rupture risk with the aneurysm geometry has been clearly depicted in cases of intracranial aneurysms, where various shape indices were proven to discriminate sufficiently between rupture and unrupture aneurysms.

For AAAs, a pioneer work to assess the rupture risk based using the biomechanical concept was recently presented [43]. The authors combined geometrical and structural factors to obtain a dimensionless severity parameter, from which, they could estimate the potential risk of a specific aneurysm in any stage of development. Later, this concept it was modified for only considering the main geometric parameters of the aneurysm which can be easily determined by computed axial tomography (CT) or magnetic resonance imaging (MRI) obtained during periodic check-up [44]. The basic idea of the method was to correlate the main simple geometric parameters of the aneurysm in order to obtain the morphologic biomechanical determinants, MBDs. This idea is supported by the hypothesis that the aneurysm shape is strongly related with its rupture potential. Here, it is important to take into consideration that this method is a baseline for the determination of a rupture risk predictor and that such a treatment decision must be made within a reasonable turnaround time. Therefore, the precision of the method should be smaller than the clinical scale of evolution of the pathology and justifies the utilization of the aneurysm morphology based on simple geometric parameters as a rupture risk predictor.

Figure 1 shows an AAA schematic representation where the simple geometric parameters involved in this method are defined. D is the diameter at the plane of maximum diameter, D_L is the lumen diameter, L is the aneurysm length which is measured from proximal neck to distal neck, L_A is the anterior length measured from point of intersection O to anterior wall and L_P is the posterior length measured from point of intersection O to posterior wall. During the follow up treatment the current clinical practice establishes that only three parameters are controlled: sagittal and coronal maximum diameter and length.

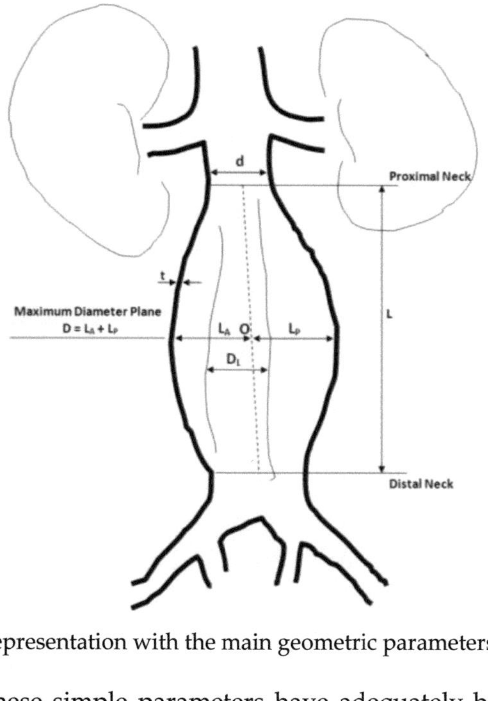

Figure 1. AAA schematic representation with the main geometric parameters.

After careful analysis, these simple parameters have adequately been combined to define the proposed geometric biomechanical factors. Some considerations about them are listed below:

1. Deformation Rate, χ.Characterizes the actual deformation of the aorta. It is defined as a ratio between the maximum transverse diameter D and infra-renal aorta diameter, d.

This concept considers that the aorta diameters range between 1.5 and 2.5 cm for any patient. The value that defines a low rupture risk is taken as the lower deformation condition of the artery (lower values D and higher d), and for the most critical condition, as the higher deformation (higher values *D* and lower *d*).

2. Asymmetry, β.A characteristic feature of an aneurysm is its asymmetry, which can be attributed to the non-symmetry expansion of the aneurysm sac as a result of the expansionconstraints introduced by the proximity to the spinal column. Due to this, AAA geometry exhibits a high surface complexity and a significant tortuosity of the inflow conduit and the segments of the iliac arteries. An aneurysm has lower rupture risk if it is more symmetric (β=1) and the risk increases as L_P tends to be lower than L_A, which means that β trend to 0.
3. Saccular Index, γ. This factor assesses the portion of the aorta, with length (*L*), which is affected by the formation and further development of the aneurysm. This means that long aneurysms have more rupture possibilities than a short one. Typical values of *L* are ranged from 90 to 140 mm (some works have reported values of *L*, higher). The calculation condition of the upper threshold value is the higher value of *L* and the peak value of *D* (typical for elective repair).
4. Relative Thickness, ι. The aneurysm geometric characterization determines the existence of a variable wall thickness; both between the anterior and posterior walls and between the aneurysmatic sac and the regions close to the distal and proximal ends.◎ Initial studies have used uniform wall thickness in their attempt to characterize aneurysm shape. Although wall thickness was not one of the highest ranked features chosen with the feature selection algorithm based on the χ^2–test, its effect on aneurysm rupture cannot be ignore [45]. Typical values of wall thickness (*t*) in aneurysmatic arteries are ranged from 0.5 to 1.5 mm [46]. This general range may vary from 0.23 mm to 4.26 mm at a calcified site [47]. The danger of aneurysm rupture will be greater when the thickness is low in the peak diameter region. This trend falls with the increase of the wall thickness.
5. ILT/AAA area ratio,λ. Although 70% of AAA includes thrombus [48], there isnot consensus about its real influence in the AAA rupture phenomenon. Some investigators state that ILT may reduce the stress in the AAA wall, improving its compliance and significantly preventing AAA rupture. Other declared that ILT could accelerate AAA rupture. Hence, it is very important to consider the effects of ILT in the rupture potential, by means of the parameter ILT/AAA area ratio.
6. Growth rate,ε.It is considered as an important indicator for AAA rupture. A high expansion rate of 0.5-1.0 cm/year is often associated with a high risk of rupture, and an elective repair should be considered even if the maximum diameter is lower than 5 cm. The value indicating that an aneurysm is in rupture risk has been determined regarding to the worst situation (the lowest value inside the range of high growth rate (0.5cm/year), the peak diameter D and the time *T* between periodic check-up (0.5 year). The low rupture risk limits were determined for aneurysm formation conditions.

Once these factors were defined, it was necessary to evaluate their weight in the rupture phenomenon by means of the definition of the weighted coefficient ωi and of the weighted level risk *WLRi*.

The weighted coefficient takes into consideration the weight of a specific factor on the frequency of occurrence of the AAA rupture. The initial values of the coefficients ωi have been obtained from the opinion of a group of surgeons about the importance of each factor. Furthermore, the weighted level risk considers the impact of a factor in the probability of AAA rupture and was sorted in four intervals: low impact, middle, high and dangerous. The *WLRi* have been obtained from considerations made in open literature when the importance of a factor's value is given according to the level of risk.

Table 1 shows the threshold values assigned to each geometric biomechanical factor and their related weighted coefficient and level risk.

MDDs	Definition	Threshold values Low Risk	Middle Risk	High Risk	Dangerous	Weighted Coefficient, ωi
Deformation Rate, χ	$\frac{D}{d}$	1.20-1.70	1.71-2.30	2.31-3.29	≥ 3.3	0.35
Asymmetry, β	$\frac{(D-L_A)}{L_A}$	1-0.9	0.8-0.7	0.6-0.5	≤ 0.4	0.10
Saccular Index, γ	$\frac{D}{L}$	≥ 0.75	0.74-0.69	0.68-0.61	≤ 0.6	0.10
ILT/AAA ratio, λ	$\frac{(D^2-D_L^2)}{D^2}$	0.1-0.24	0.25-0.44	0.45-0.61	≥ 0.62	0.10
Relative Thickness, ι	$\frac{t}{D}$	0.05-0.04	0.04-0.02	0.02-0.11	≤ 0.01	0.10
Growth rate, ε	$\frac{(D_A-D_P)}{T}$	0.1-0.17	0.18-0.3	0.31-0.49	≥ 0.5	0.25
Weighted Level Risk, *WLRi*		0.1	0.3	0.7	1	

Table 1. Geometric biomechanical factors characterization.

Hence, rupture risk quantitative indicator defined in term of AAA morphology, can be expressed as the sum of each weighted coefficient ωi multiplied by the corresponding *WLRi*:

$$RI(t) = \sum_1^6 \omega_i WLR_1 \tag{1}$$

Regarding the results of *RI*(*t*), it is possible to advise several actions and suggestions to physicians. This is shown in Table 2.

As above indicated, the proposed method is based on six geometric biomechanical factors. But, it is possible that, for any reason, the information about some parameters is not available. In this case, the method fits its algorithm to calculate only the factors associated with the existing geometric parameters and it is able to weights the final result according to the amount of parameters taken into account.

An initial limitation of the method is associated with indirect errors in obtaining the MBDs, due to the difficulty in extracting exact values from the geometric parameters needed in determining these MBDs. The measurements of the simple geometric parameters is, usually, carried out by a radiologist, a human being with its professional customs and resources,

RI(t)	Actions/Suggestions
< 0.2	Rupture risk is very low. No action is suggested.
0.2 ÷ 0.45	Rupture risk is low. A close observation is required.
÷ 0.7	Elective repair should be considered. Other symptoms such a back and abdominal pain, syncope or vomiting, should be observed.
> 0.7	Rupture risk is very high. Surgical intervention must be necessary.

Table 2. *RI*(*t*) intervals and actions and suggestions offered by method to physicians.

with best and/or worst days, with/without personal and labor problems. Therefore, it is important to assess the influence of all these (and others) conditions on the precision of the results.

The ANSI-ASME PTC 85, ISSO 5167 standard was used to determine the indirect errors in the calculation of GBDs due to the direct measurements of the simple geometric parameters. The methodology was applied to data-base which was used for validation tests. The results that are shown in Table 3 correspond to higher values for the errors obtained. The bias limit in measuring of the geometric parameters for all parameters was considered 0.001m. The main conclusion that can be drawn from Table 3 is that the errors in determining the MBDs, are not significant.

MDBs	Uncertainty, *Uz*	Relative uncertainty, *U* (%)
Deformation Rate, χ	1.81E-01	0.0464
Asymmetry, β	2.55E-02	0.075
Saccular Index, γ	1.23E-02	0.022
ILT/AAA ratio, λ	1.81E-03	3.13E-03
Relative Thickness, ι	1.18E-02	1.8
Growth rate, ε	1.67E-02	0.027

Table 3. Indirect errors obtained in determining the GBDs.This standard allows defining the experimental uncertainty, *U* in determining a variable *Z*, as:

This initial set of values was validated by using one clinical case and three cases from literature.

In shortly. In the clinical case, the state of a 74 year-old male patient with an aneurysm was assessed. The geometrical characterization shows that the peak diameter is lower than the threshold value (50 mm), therefore under current medical practice; the patient should be kept under observation. But, on the other hand, the values of the deformation rate and the asymmetry index fall into the high risk level interval. It must be noticed that by means of statistical analysis these geometric biomechanical factors are considered as the most influential factors on the aneurysm potential rupture.Other two MBDs are also sorted as high risk level, although their weight on the rupture phenomenon is lower. Therefore, the value of the patient-specific quantitative predictor calculated by equation (1) is *RI*(t)=0.64, which indicates that the elective repair should be considered. This result was confirmed because, during the period of check-up examination, the patient underwent an emergency surgical procedure for aneurysm rupture in the posterior wall.

In another test, a triple validation was performed comparing the results documented in the original papers [49], [50] and [51], the results presented by [43] and the results obtained with the proposed set of values [52]. The geometries of the different analyzed AAAs are very different, however the value of RI(t) is able to sort patients correctly. In the model presented in [49], it is noticed that the aneurysm affects a significant region of the aorta and has a high rate of growth, which has a high relative importance in the value of *RI*(*t*). In the model [50], the two biomechanical factors that have more influence in the deterioration of the aneurysm increase in comparison with the previous one, but they stay in the range of elective repair, although it was expected that the indicator value would be higher.

Analyzing the model [51], it is noticed that there is a worsening of most of the geometric parameters; the most important are a high growth rate, a maximum diameter 20% greater than the threshold value and an aneurysm affecting a significant region of the artery. This behavior justifies that the value of the rupture risk indicator falls into the category of possible rupture.

These results encouraged the implementation of another validation test: a broader control study with a population of two hundred and one patients at the Clinic Hospital of Valladolid-Spain, who were submitted to Endovascular Aneurysm Repair (EVAR) treatment.Previously, a new the set of values for the weighted coefficient was defined by using a statistical tool to contrast the hypothesis that certain events have a probability of occurring. In this case, the event is associated to the AAA rupture due to a specific MBD.

According to this statistical tool, the new set of values resulting for ωi is: Deformation Rate= 0.35, Asymmetry=0.07, Saccular Index=0.1, Relative Thickness=0.07, ILT/AAA area ratio=0.07 and Growth rate=0.34.

For this new test, the population of the sample was divided in three groups: Group I (n=174) - patients without later consequences after EVAR treatment; Group II (n=5) - patients who died from causes associated with the AAA pathology; Group III (n=22) - patients whose AAA ruptures. As all these patients were submitted to EVAR treatment, the main objective of this test is to verify if some of the surgical procedures in patients whose aneurysm has a maximum diameter higher than threshold value could have been avoided, and/or if the method can predict the rupture of aneurysm with a diameter less than the threshold value.

The results showed that in 88% of the patients who belongs to group I is justified the surgical procedure, because the *RI(t)* values fall into dangerous and high level rupture risk. In the group II, the results suggest that the five patients should be submitted to surgical procedure because their rupture risk index is dangerous + high risk condition. All these patients died either during repair treatment or during recovering of it. The state of health of all these patients was not good, because they presented other diseases like renal chronic insufficiency, atheromatic plaque, previous complications related with cardiovascular diseases, digestive hemorrhages.

Very interesting results are obtained in the analysis of the group III. The values of *RI(t)* indicate that95.4% of the patients, present levels of rupture risk sorted as dangerous and high and the surgical procedure could have been considered before rupture. All these patients had aneurysms whose maximum diameter was less than the threshold value for surgical treatment and a systematic (time between two consecutive revisions lower than 1 year) follow-up check are suggested to diminishing the risks associated to emergency surgery by ruptures.

The fact that one patient presented a middle rupture index was somewhat unexpected and it is probably attributable to a combination of other factors not considered here, associated to factors of biological and/or structural nature. It was verified that the geometric parameters are lower than the threshold values.

The obtained outcomes are promising and have motivated further actions. Recent studies [53] have identified other MBDs based on the lumen centerline geometry. According to [54], the resulting centerline is a piecewise linear line defined on the Voronoi diagram, whose vertices lie on Voronoi polygon boundaries [55]. Values of Voronoi sphere radius $R(\mathbf{x})$ are therefore defined on centerlines, so that centerline points are associated with maximal inscribed spheres. Since centerlines were constructed to lie on local maxima of distance from the boundary, there is a tight connection between maximal sphere radius and minimum projection diameter used in clinical evaluation. In fact, classic angiographic vessel diameter evaluation is performed considering the minimum diameter obtained by measurements on different projections. The availability of a robust method for centerline computation and diameter measurement allows to characterize blood vessel geometry in a synthetic way, therefore giving the opportunity of performing a study on a population of models. Since it has been shown that planarity, tortuosity and branching angles have a major influence on complex blood flow patterns, such a study may reveal if particular vessel configurations are involved in vascular pathology.

Three MBDs have been defined using this approach: tortuosity, curvature and torsion centerline. Today, VMTK software havebeen developed to 3D reconstruction of the lumen centerline geometry. Figure 2 shows the visual representation of these determinants. Tortuosity, an absolute number, expresses the fractional increase in length of a tortuous vessel in relation to the imaginary straight line and has been described in [55]. Torsion is measured in $1/cm^2$ and curvature is measured in 1/cm.

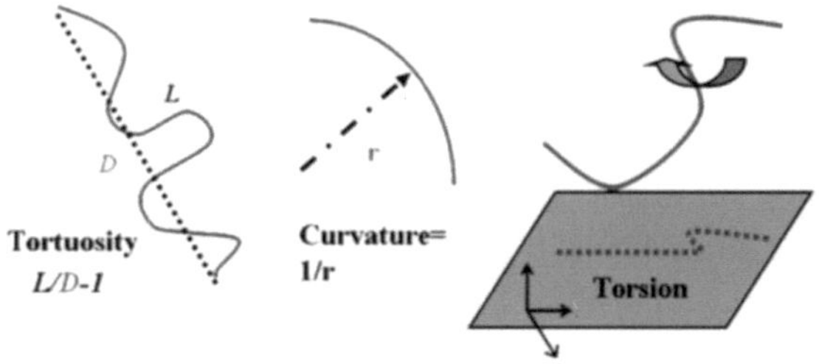

Figure 2. Schematic visualization of tortuosity, curvature and torsion [53].

Recently, it has been postulated that aneurysm peak wall stress (PWS) may be superior to diameter as predictor of the rupture risk. This statement has its theoretical foundation in the physical principle of the aneurysm rupture. Complex AAA geometry contributes to equivalent complex wall stress distribution over the entire AAA, with the higher stresses associated with regions of high curvature [56].

The role of these geometric biodeterminants in the prediction of AAA it has been assessed taking into consideration the presence of intra-luminal thrombus (ILT) [53]. In the study were included nineteen patients whose-which AAA maximum diameters ranged from 5 to 12 cm. Statistical analysis confirmed that the maximum diameter significantly influenced PWS and the tortuosity may also affect PWS values in models with ILT in the same direction.

On the other hand, it has been demonstrated [57] that PWS is strongly correlated with the maximum diameter as well as the centreline asymmetry. It is notable, however, that in 73% of the analyzed models in this work a significant correlation was found between asymmetry and maximum diameter. Therefore, if diameter strongly correlated with peak stress then asymmetry would also score high.

Perhaps one of the most ambiguous issues in the assessment of rupture risk is the existence as well as the develop of the ILT. Despite ILT´s impact on aneurysm disease, little is known about its development, and it is unclear whether it increases or decreases the risk of aneurysm rupture. That is, the ILT reinforces proteolytic activity [58], which weakens the wall [59], or buffers against wall stress [50]. It has been hypothesized that ILT develops either from rupture of vulnerable plaques or as a more continuous process characterized by blood-flow induced activation of platelets and their deposition at non-endothelialized sites of the wall exposed to low (sub-physiological) wall shear stress [60].

Recently, the investigationsare addressed to the integration of ILT in the computational models and, consequently, its effects in patient-specific on PWS values and distribution. A significant difference in PWS when including the ILT in 3D AAA computational model it has been reported [61]. Wang et al [50] showed that computational integration of ILT in 3D models could actually modify not only the value but also the distribution of PWS, thus playing a protective role against rupture but this conclusion was not supported in [62]. On the other hand, there is still some concern regarding the protective role of ILT, since many authors who evaluate the influence of ILT on hemodynamic stress transmission, reported that he presence of ILT fails to reduce the transmission of this stress on the AAA wall, consequently, leaving the AAA rupture risk equalled [63]. AAAs can experience higher stresses at regions of inflection, regardless of wall thickness variation. In such cases, the concentric or eccentric location of ILT in the AAA sac cannot be effectively reduce PWS values or changes its distribution [64]. A question of interest arises here, regarding whether such PWS values derived from computational estimation should be taken into consideration, since AAA rupture rarely takes places at these sites, reserving this possibility only for thrombosed AAAs [65]. Therefore, all these ideas reinforce the need to quantify and take into consideration the effect of the ILT.

Finally, it is important to address the topic related to the use either simple geometric parameters or biodeterminants in the AAA rupture risk assessment. To answer this question some aspects should be analyzed. The first one is related to the temporal scales of the disease progression which is higher than the results′ precision in the determination of the geometric parameters. This conclusion justify the use of morphological determinants. On the other hand, is the fact that aneurysm shape has a significant influence on flow patterns and consequently in its rupture potential. Recent findings have shown that the aneurysm geometrical shape may be related to the rupture risk. The morphological nature determinants (MBDs) are defined by appropriate relations among simple geometric parameters to characterize the influence of the aneurysm morphology on its rupture potential.

Utilizing idealized aneurysm models of the true vessel lumen surface geometry, the role of the geometric characteristics in the hemodynamic stresses prediction by using of Pearson′s rank correlation coefficients was assessed [66]. In this work, the model was modified to allow the parametrization of the main parameters assessed: maximum diameter D, length L and asymmetry, β. Figure 3, shows a schematic view of the models used in this study.

The results show that hemodynamics stresses correlate better with MBDs. For hemodynamic pressure, the relation with saccular index and deformation rate are strong and negative ($r=-0.75$, $p=0.000$ and $r=-0.7$, $p=0.000$ respectively). The asymmetry coefficient has no-significant correlation ($r=-0.25$, $p=0.00$).

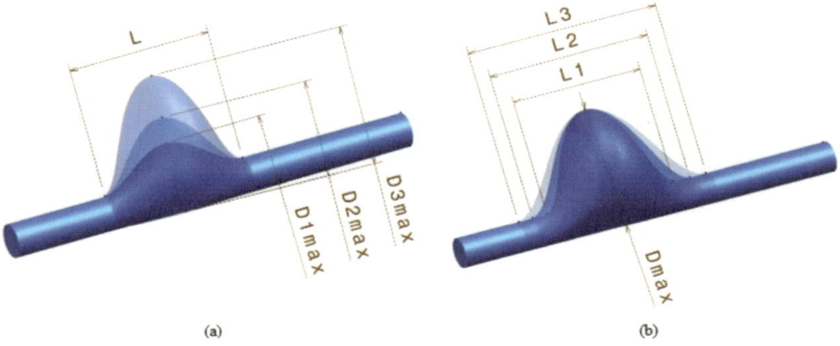

Figure 3. Schematic view of the parametrized aneurysm models. a) *L* and β are constant and *D* varies; b) *D* and β are constant and L varies.

The relation of asymmetry and deformation rate with WSS is weak with significance less than 15% and saccular index is no significant.

The main conclusions of this study are: luminal pressure is the primary mechanical load on the aneurismal wall and that MBDs are better predictors than simple parameters of the hemodynamic stresses.

On the other hand, Raghavanet al [67], showed that the deviation of the aneurysm shape from spherical configuration, the level of its surface ondulation or ellipticity and the norm of the surface mean curvature are a good predictors of rupture.

This analysis confirms that MBDs may become a useful addition to current clinical criteria, mainly maximum diameter, in the decision-making process of the aneurysm treatment. Certainly, as in the same way that other biomechanical consideration, the suggested models require further studies.

5. Structural Biodeterminants, SBDs

In addition to morphological factors, numerically predicted wall stress, finite element analysis rupture index, rupture potential index and severity parameters have been proposed as alternative approaches to assessing rupture risk [68].

The criterion currently used by the medical community is that you can relate directly the risk of rupture with the maximum diameter of the aneurysm. However, as noted above, the biomechanics states that rupture occurs when wall stress exceeds its strength. This assumes a linear relationship between the maximum stress and the maximum diameter of the aneurysm. Thus, we propose an equation to describe this approach.

$$\sigma_{max} = kR_{max} \tag{2}$$

where σ_{max} is the maximum stress in the aneurysm, k is a constant determined by experience, and R_{max} the maximum radius of the aneurysm. The maximum diameter criterion has many limitations.

Since there is currently no method to determine the stresses in the wall in vivo, it is necessary to develop models of the mechanical behavior of the arterial wall. These models can be generated from ideal parameterized geometries created by three-dimensional design software (CATIA, SolidWorks, etc.), or can be obtained through the processing of medical images.

Once the geometry is generated, we calculate using finite element method software (ANSYS, ABAQUS, etc.) in order to determine the stress distribution in the wall of AAA.

Structural biomechanical determinant of VandeGeest

After evaluating the stresses, and using the ultimate strength of arterial tissue or an assessment of the strength of the wall, you can define a structural biomechanical factor. This factor or biodeterminant, can allow us to estimate how close an aneurysm can be of the rupture and, consequently, the appropriateness of the surgical procedure in the patient.

Thus, it is proposed [69] the following factor:

$$RI(t) = \frac{Stress_i}{Strength_i} \tag{3}$$

where$i$is the chosen point on aneurysm geometry.

It is noted that when the rupture index approaches the value of 1, the state of risk of aneurysm rupture increases, ie when the stress observed in the wall reaches the value of strength.

If the strength is only an estimated value for the entire aneurysm, use the maximum stress given by the simulation. But, when using the strength distribution in the whole geometry, the rupture index is evaluated at each point of the geometry of the aneurysm.

Rupture criterion of Li and Kleinstreuer

This approach [70] is based not only on statistical analysis of some cases of abdominal aortic aneurysms, but also on results of numerical simulations. To do so, tests were conducted with 10 patients whose data were known, in order to verify the accuracy criterion used to calculate σ_{max}:

$$\sigma_{max} = 0.006\frac{(1-0.68\lambda)e^{\left(0.0123(0.85P_{sist}+19.5D)\right)}}{t^{0.63}\beta^{0.125}} \quad (4)$$

where σ_{max} is the maximum stress that appears frequently in an area whose diameter is equal to two thirds of the maximum diameter of AAA, λ is the ratio of the areas in the plane of maximum diameter ($\lambda = A_{ILT,\max} / A_{AAA,max}$), β is the coefficient of asymmetry, *Psis* is the systolic blood pressure (mmHg), D is the maximum diameter of AAA (cm) and t is the thickness of the wall in the plane of maximum diameter.

If the thickness of the arterial wall cannot be determined from images taken by the TAC, can be approximated by the following equation:

$$t = 3.9\left(\frac{D}{2}\right)^{-0.2892} \quad (5)$$

According to the authors, this approach presents a very low error in the determination of the maximum stress compared to other models. Whatever the feature is used to calculate stress, the results are very similar to the stress determined by finite element method software.

Clearly, the geometry should not be too complex, which is a limitation. Furthermore, the location of the maximum stress cannot determine, although the value is known.

This approach appears to be quite accurate results, and its application is very simple. So it could be used to determine the maximum stress of the aneurysm with a very simple approach. However, we emphasize that in no other study has been applied.

Rupture criterion based on remodeling history model

These models allow determining a stress value, which is compared with the strength of the arterial wall to evaluate if the break is close or not.

The value of strength can be obtained:

- Form literature, which are based on uni-axial tests aneurysmal tissue of patients.
- By an empirical approach based on an expression that takes into account the patient's personal information.

Criteria based on two-dimensional modeling

- It is a very simple model in two dimensions of the arterial wall;

- The maximum stress is located at the maximum diameter;
- The aneurysm is cylindrical (or spherical);
- Wall thickness constant E;
- Linear elastic behavior.

From these criteria leads to a simple equation that relates the pressure P, the wall thickness t and the maximum radius R_{max} of the aneurysm:

$$\sigma_{max} = P\frac{R_{max}}{t} \tag{6}$$

This modeling, which leads to the stress calculation, presents the following limitations:

- The geometry is very simple, which influences the results.
- Although you can adjust the value of the pressure acting on the wall, assigning the value at the studied patient's blood pressure, stress is always proportional to the radius of the aneurysm.

This approach is similar to the criterion of maximum diameter used today.

Criteria based on three-dimensional modeling

a. Modeling of material behavior: linear elasticity.

Many authors have used an elastic model of the arterial wall in their research [71, 72]

Commenting on the approach proposed in [73], the authors have attempted to determine the influence of the diameter and symmetry in the mechanical stress of the arterial wall of abdominal aortic aneurysm using an elastic behavior of the wall.

This approach has the merit of taking into account the behavior of the material used, and the authors are aware of the limits of their model, since the aim of their study was to show the influence of symmetry. However, other studies [74, 75] showed that the hyperelastic behavioral model is more suitable for simulating an aneurysm under pressure due to the large strains that can undergo aneurysmal arterial wall (20-40%).

b. Modeling of material behavior: hyperelasticity.

Given the fact that the tissue of the aneurysmal arterial wall can be deformed the order of 20-40%, the behavior can no longer be considered as elastic.

Hyperelastic materials are characterized by the existence of an energy function W, which depends on the state of deformation.

Tensions can be calculated with this energy function *W*, which depends on the material, which can be isotropic or anisotropic, which will influence in *W*.

b.1) Isotropic hyperelasticity

In 1940, Mooney and Rivlin established a behavioral model for the material like rubber, whose behavior is similar to the tissue of the arterial wall due to the incompressibility of both materials.

Heng et al. [76], used the Mooney-Rivlin equation to establish one of the simplest hyperelastic models. The problem with this model with only two parameters is that is more suited to the study of polymers. This law was made by Mooney to model the behavior of rubbers, and it seems too simple for the study of tissues, whose behavior seems much more complex because its composition is not homogeneous.

You can also use a more complex form of Mooney-Rivlin model. In [77] it is performed a study which uses this model and the results seem that calculate appropriately the real tensions of the arterial wall. This form uses 9 parameters addition to the incompressibility parameter.

In 2000, it is defined a mathematical model using a regression from experimental results [75]. This is part of the theory of finite deformations and is based on the first principle of mechanics of continuous media. The assumptions underlying this model were that the wall is non-linear, homogeneous, incompressible and isotropic.

In 2006, this model is modified using another form of the density function [78]. It is observed that for incompressible materials considered, this equation is the same as proposed in [75].

In 2008, it is proposed a model based on the concept of material failure energy Φ [79]. This energy is the maximum amount of energy that the wall can withstand before breaking, because of the deformations. This value depends on the atomic or microscopic structure of the wall of an AAA.

b.2) Anisotropic hyperelasticity

- single transverse anisotropy.

In 1976, Tong and Fung [80], developed a cross-anisotropic hyperelastic model, which allows a behavioral model of the arterial wall aneurysm.

- Anisotropy with two families of fibers
  - Rodríguez anisotropichyperelasticmodel [81];
  - Holzapfel anisotropic hyperelastic model [82]. Proposed model for biological materials with two families of collagen fibers, as they really are the arterial walls.

The anisotropic hyperelastic behavior models better approximate the actual behavior of the aneurysmal arterial wall, but according to the model used, the results can be very different. One can see that the Rodríguez hyperelastic anisotropic model is closer (at the level of stress distribution) to an isotropic hyperelastic that the Holzapfelhyperelastic anisotropic model, as shown in Figure 4.

c. Fluid-Structure Interaction

All approaches that have been presented are based on the physical principle of fault material of aortic wall. However, all these approaches use a constant pressure value (often the peak systolic pressure), whereas, in reality, not only the pressure varies, but also the blood moves. In an attempt to make models as realistic as possible, we have developed the modeling fluid-structure interaction (FSI), in which the model considers simultaneously the effect of blood flow on the arterial wall and vice versa.

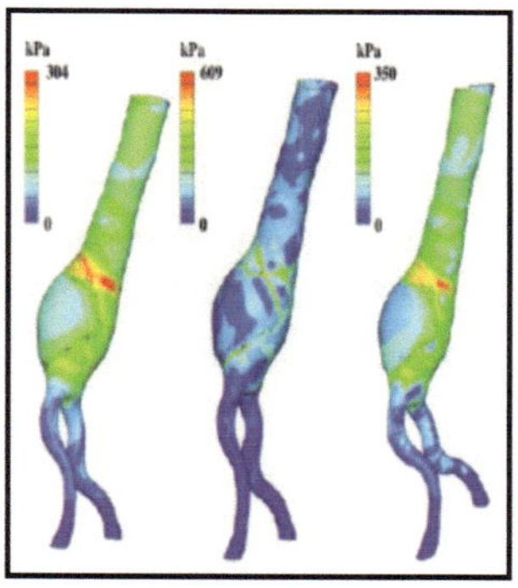

Isotropic Holzapfel Rodríguez

Figure 4. Stress in different models.

Some authors try to use a method of modeling of blood flow, to study its influence on the stresses of the aneurysm wall. These approaches are also used mechanical simulations to assess the stress in the wall of the aneurysm.

From the results obtained with FSI simulations [46], has been determined that in the simulations using the computational analysis of the static stress incurred in an underestimation of wall tension, which is shown in Figure 5. This value can reach 12.5%, as reported [83].

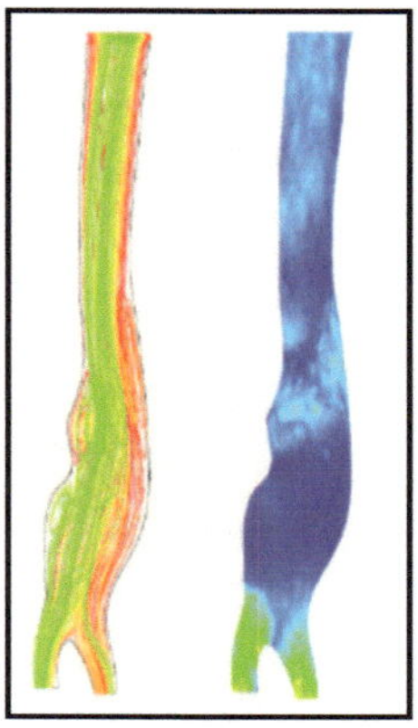

Figure 5. Stream lines which characterize the blood flow inside the aneurysm and surface distribution of stresses, obtained using a modeling FSI.

In 2006, a simulation of aneurysm under pressure [41] and blood flow was carried out in addition to demonstrating that when taking into consideration the bloodstream, the stresses change little while the time required for the simulation is three to four times greater.

The authors concluded that the fluid-structure interaction approach is interesting, but a modeling of the wall with the systolic pressure is sufficient to calculate the stresses in it.

After the revision presented we can conclude that an anisotropic hyperelastic model, using systolic pressure load, and geometry with the important details of the AAA, is the best choice for calculating the stresses in aneurysmal wall.

Evaluation of the arterial wall strength.

At this point, is already known that the evaluation of the wall stress cannot be considered as an isolated indicator to assess the risk of rupture of AAAs, as an aneurysmal wall region which is subjected to high stresses, may also have a high strength, thus equalizing potential rupture. According to the remodeling history model, the strength of the wall is different from patient to patient and in the same patient at different regions and time scales. To resolve this situation, has been developed a technique for noninvasive estimation of the distribution of strength, defining a potential rupture index (RPI)[84], with equation:

$$Strength = 141.26 - 17.16ILT + 3.39AGE - 257.3NORD - 69.5HIST \quad (7)$$

where *ILT* is the thickness of the *ILT* (in cm), *AGE* is the patient age in years, *NORD* is the diameter normalized to the maximum diameter of AAA, *HIST* is ± ½ according to family history (½ if the history is positive, - ½ if no background) and *SEX* is ± ½ by sex of the patient (½ if the patient is a man, - ½ for women).

These authors have increasingly improved this criterion, being the last, expressed by equation 8, thatbest approximates the strength of the wall.

$$Strength = 72.9 - 33.5\left((ILT^{0.5}) - 0.79\right) - 12.3(NORD - 2.31) - 24HIST + 15SEX \quad (8)$$

Rupture of aneurysm prediction

The logical process for estimating the risk of aneurysm rupture using structural biomechanical factors would be the one described below:

1. Obtain the blood pressure of the patient.
2. CT of the patient's aneurysm.
3. Geometric model of the aneurysm from medical imaging.
4. Simulation of the aneurysm using data specific to the patient.
5. Estimating the strength of the arterial wall aneurysmal of the patient.
6. State estimation of risk of rupture of the aneurysm.

Subsequently, using the Rupture Index (*RI*) proposed in Equation 1 can be estimated if a ruptured aneurysm is close. Obviously, it will require a medical evaluation of patient state of health (PSH).

Simulation using the Finite Element Method (FEM)

Unable to provide a method for determining the in vivo distribution of wall stress, nowadays it is used the finite element method (FEM), which is recognized as a very precise technique, which aims to find approximate solutions of partial differential equations and integral equations. Equations are solved at the nodes of the meshes that are generated and interpolated within the element, generating a continuous solution throughout the domain.

Overall analysis by using Finite Element Method is an orderly process that will include the following steps:

1. Generation of geometry. The geometry can be generated or imported. In the case of aneurysm geometry is imported directly from the patient CT using some of the commercial software or open source currently available, so it has the actual geometry of the aneurysm affecting the patient under study. Figure 6, shows the geometric model of AAA obtained by the processing of medical images using the public software MeVisLab.

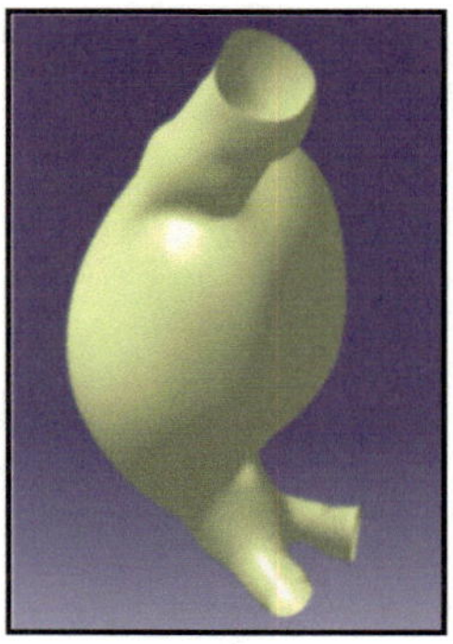

Figure 6. Geometric model of AAA obtained from the processing of medical images.

2. Discretization of meshing domain: The structure or part is divided into elements and modeled as a finite element mesh. In this step the analyst must decide the type, number, size and order of items to be used. This decision will characterize the degree of confidence results thereafter. An example that represents the arterial wall mesh is presented in Figure 7.

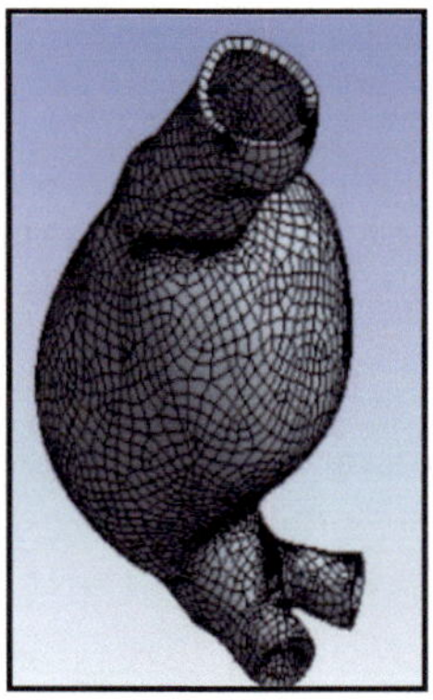

Figure 7. Mesh representation of a geometry that represents the arterial wall of an AAA.

3. Application of the boundary conditions: apply the loads which will be under the model (in this case the blood pressure) and the restrictions of the same (in this case is assumed to be attached to the remainder of the artery limiting their movement and must be taken into account if organs or body parts that limit their movement).

4. Solution of unknown nodal displacements: The global balance equation is modified to take into account the boundary conditions of the problem and to obtain algebraic equations where the unknowns are nodal displacements.
5. Calculation of stresses and strains of the elements: Knowing the nodal displacements resulting from the previous stage, it could be calculated the stresses and strains using the corresponding mechanical equations.
6. Evaluation of results: the stresses solutions are obtained (and displacements in some models) along theaneurysm. It is possible to locate the exact point of the aneurysm where it produces the maximum stress and the value thereof. Figure 8, shows the surface distribution of stresses. The red color indicates the region with higher values of stress and therefore, with greater risk of rupture.

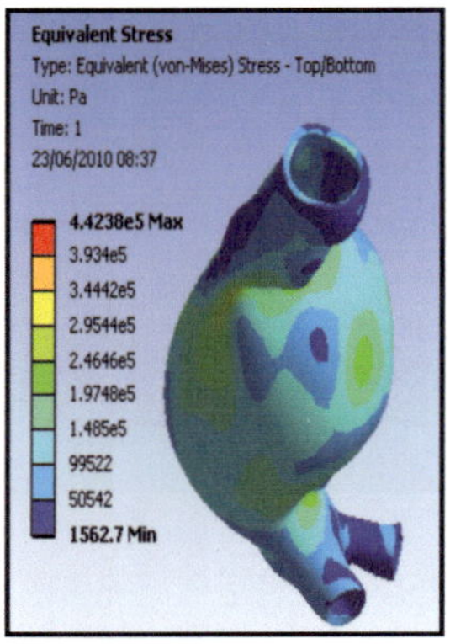

Figure 8. Stress distribution in the arterial wall obtained by finite element simulation.

6. General

At this point, it is important to highlight two aspects. The first one is that the accumulation of knowledge around the topic of accurate prediction of AAA rupture is large enough and significant advances have been achieved in last years although the physicians continue using the same criteria. The second one is related to the growing consensus that it is possible to improve the reliability of the AAA rupture assessment by means of the biomechanical approach.

Despite the growing interest for the behaviour of all these factors, many physicians question its clinical utility advocating the difficulties in its assessing during the everyday clinical practice. Often, these procedures require sophisticated software, very specific and accurate correlations and highly qualified personnel. This feeling appears clearly reflected in a survey carried out among vascular surgeons [85], whose outcomes are summarized in:

90% of the institutions rely their rupture risk estimation on the maximum diameter and the expansion rate, whereas only 15% use the high mechanical stress criteria;

40% of the institutions think that using their criteria, the rupture risk of AAAs is reliable in up to 75% of all cases;

18% of surveyed know and are familiar with the biomechanical criteria to estimate the aneurysm rupture risk, 63% know it but are not familiar with these criteria, where the other percentage has never heard about it.

Seems to be unlikely this knowledge replace the use of current criteria. Clinicians will always feel that large AAAs represent a rupture-threat and should be repaired. It is the small and medium size AAAs that could be examined by using these alternative diagnostic tools which, in the future, may prove to be useful adjunct to maximum diameter.

7. Conclusions

Aneurysmal disease and its progression is a very complex multifactorial process and its statistics are of great concern. The biomechanical approach here developed and substantiated can predict the rupture potential of a patient-specific AAA in any stage of evolution with sufficient accuracy to be clinically relevant. This predictive model is conceived by the integration of biological, morphological and structural information and can constitute a significant step in the clinical management of patients with aneurysm. Nowadays, we are developing a broader validation test of the proposed model by establishing its statistical significance with a large enough number of AAA cases.

Author details

Guillermo Vilalta* and Félix Nieto
Mechanical Engineering Division, CARTIF Centro Tecnológico, Boecillo (Valladolid), Spain

Enrique San Norberto and Carlos Vaquero
Angiology and Vascular Surgery Service,
University and Clinic Hospital of Valladolid, Valladolid, Spain

María Ángeles Pérez
ITAP Institute, University of Valladolid, Valladolid, Spain

José A. Vilalta
Industrial Engineering Department, Polytechnical University of Havana, Havana, 19340, Cuba

8. References

[1] Viceconti M, Taddei F, Van Sint Jan S, Leardini A, Critofolini L, Stea S, Baleani M (2008) MultiscaleModelling of the Skeleton for the Prediction of the Risk of Fracture. Clinical Biomechanics. 23: 845-852.

[2] Newman AB, Arnold AM, Burke GL, O'Leary DH, Manolio TA (2001) Cardiovascular Disease and Mortality in Older Adults with Small Abdominal Aortic Aneurysms Detected by Ultrasonography: the Cardiovascular Health Study. Annals of Internal Medicine. 134: 182–190.

* Corresponding Author

[3] Johansson G, Swedenborg J (1986) Rupture Abdominal Aortic Aneurysms: A Study of Incidence and Mortality. Br. J. Surg. 73: 101-103.

[4] Karkos C, Mukhopadhyay I, Papakostas I, Ghost J, Thomson G, Hughes R (2000) Abdominal Aortic Aneurysm: the Role of Clinical Examination and Opportunistic Detection. Eur. J. Vasc. Endovasc Surg. 19: 299-303.

[5] Vorp DA (2007) Biomechanics of abdominal aortic aneurysm. J. Biomech. 40(9): 1887–1902.

[6] Blanchard JF, Armenian HK, Friesen PP (2000) Risk factors for abdominal aortic aneurysm: results of a case-control study. Am J Epidemiol. 151: 575–83.

[7] Tornwall ME, Virtamo J, Haukka JK, Albanes D, Huttunen JK (2001) Life-style factors and risk for abdominal aortic aneurysm in a cohort of Finnish male smokers. Epidemiology. 12: 94–100.

[8] Singh K, Bonaa KH, Jacobsen BK, Bjork L, Solberg S (2001) Prevalence of and risk factors for abdominal aortic aneurysms in a population-based study: the Tromso study. Am J Epidemiol. 154: 236–244.

[9] Bengtson H, Ekberg O, Aspdlin P, TakoLander R, Bergqvist D (1988) Aneurysmal disease: abdominal aortic dilatation in patients operated on for carotid artery stenosis. Acta Chit Scand. 143: 441-444.

[10] Anidjar S, Osborne-Pellegrin M, Coutard M, Michel JB (1992) Arterial hypertension and aneurismal dilatation. Kidney Int. 37 S61–66.

[11] Johansen K, Koepsell T (1986) Familial tendency for abdominal aortic aneurysms. JAMA. 256: 1934-1936.

[12] Tilson M (1985) Further studies of a putative crosslinking amino acid (3-deoxy-pyridinoline) in skin from patients with AAAs. Surgery. 98: 888-893.

[13] Kitchen ND (1989) Racial distribution of aneurysms in Zimbabwe. JR Soc Med. 82: 136-145.

[14] Webster MW, Ferrel RE, St Jean FL, Majuroder et al (1991) Ultrasound screening of first-degree relatives of patients with abdominal aortic aneurysm. J Vasc Surg. 12: 9-13.

[15] Kuivarilemi H, Tromp G, Prockop DJ (1991) Genetic causes of aortic aneurysms: unlearning at least part of what the textbooks say. J Clin Invest. 88: 1441-1445.

[16] Tromp G, Kuivaniemi H, Shikata H, Prockop DJ (1989) A single basemutation that substitutes serine for glycine 790 of the a 1 (III) chain of type III procollagen exposes an arginine and causes Ehlers–Danlos syndrome IV. J Biol Chem. 264: 1349-1356.

[17] Hinterseher I, Tromp G, Kuivaniemi H (2011) Genes and abdominal aortic aneurysm. Ann Vasc Surg. 25: 388-412.

[18] Nordon IM, Hinghliffe RJ, Holt PJ, et al (2009) Review of current theories for abdominal aortic aneurysm pathogenesis.Vascular. 17: 253-263.

[19] Shapira OM, Pakis S, Wassermann JP, Barzlllai N, Mashlah A (1990) Ultrasound screening for abdominal aortic aneurysms in patients with atherosclerotic peripheral vascular disease. J Cardiovasc Surg. 31: 170-175.

[20] Heistad DD, Marcus ML, Carsen GE et al (1981) Role of vasa vasorum in nourishment of the aortic wall. Am J Physiol. 240: 11781-11783.

[21] McMillan WD, Tamarina NA, Cipollone M (1997) Size matters: the relationship between MMP-9 expression and aortic diameter. Circulation. 96: 2228–2232.

[22] Jagadesham VP, Scott DJ, Carding SR (2008) Abdominal aortic aneurysms: an autoimmune disease? TrensMol Med. 14: 522-529.

[23] Tanaka S, Komori K, et al (1994) Detection of active cytomegalovirus infection n inflammatory aortic aneurysms with RNA polymerase chain reaction. J Vasc Surg. 20: 235-243.

[24] Beckman EN (1986) Plasma cell infiltrates in atherosclerotic in abdominal aortic aneurysms. Am J ClinPathol. 85: 21-24.

[25] Newman KM, Jean-Claude J, et al (1994) Cellular localization of matrix metalloproteinases in the abdominal aortic aneurysm wall. J Vasc Surg. 20: 814-820.

[26] Nanda S, Sharma SG, Longo S (2009) Molecular targets and abdominal aortic aneurysms. Recent Pat Cardiovasc Drug Discov. 4: 150-159.

[27] Busuttil RW, Abou-Zamzam AM, Machleder HI (1980) Collagenase activity of the human aorta. A comparison of patients with and without abdominal aortic aneurysms. Arch Surg. 115: 1373–1378.

[28] Minion DJ, Davis VA, Nejezchleb PA, et al (1994) Elastin is increased in abdominal aortic aneurysms. J Surg Res. 57: 443–446.

[29] Vine N, Powell JT (1991) Metalloproteinases in degenerative aortic disease. Clin Sci. 81: 233–239.

[30] Thompson RW, Holmes DR, Mertens RA et al (1995) Production and localization of 92-kilodalton gelatinase in abdominal aortic aneurysms. An elastolytic metalloproteinase expressed by aneurysm-infiltrating macrophages. J Clin Invest. 96: 318–326.

[31] Freestone T, Turner RJ, Coady A, et al (1995) Inflammation and matrix metalloproteinases in the enlarging abdominal aortic aneurysm. ArterioscThrombVasc Biol. 15: 1145–1151.

[32] Pyo R, Lee JK, Shipley JM, et al (2000) Targeted gene disruption of matrix metalloproteinase-9 (gelatinase B) suppresses development of experimental abdominal aortic aneurysms. J Clin Invest. 105: 1641–1649.

[33] Tamarina NA, McMillan WD, Shively VP, Pearce WH (1997) Expression of matrix metalloproteinases and their inhibitors in aneurysms and normal aorta. Surgery. 122: 264–272.

[34] Rizas KD, ippagunta N, Tilson MD (2009) Immune cells and molecular mediators in the pathogenesis of the abdominal aortic aneurysm. Cardiol Rev. 17: 201-210.

[35] Michel JB, Martin-Ventura JL, Egido J, et al (2011) Novel aspects of the pathogenesis of aneurysms of the abdominal aorta in humans. Cardiovasc Res. 90: 18-27.

[36] Yajima N, Masuda M, Miyazaki M, et al (2002) Oxidative stress is involved in the development of experimental abdominal aortic aneurysm: a study of the transcription profile with complementary DNA microarray. J Vasc Surg. 36: 379–385.

[37] Annambhotla S, Bourgeois S, Wang X, et al (2008) Recent advances in molecular mechanisms of abdominal aortic aneurysm formation. World J Surg. 32: 976-986.

[38] Sodeck G, Domanovits H, Khanakah G, et al (2004) The role of Chlamydia pneumoniae in human aortic disease-a hypothesis revisited. Eur J VascEndovasc Surg. 28: 547–552.

[39] Kilic A, Onguru O, Tugcu H, et AL (2006) Detection of cytomegalovirus and Helicobacter pylori DNA in arterial walls with grade III atherosclerosis by PCR. Pol J Microbiol. 55: 333–337.

[40] Sakalihasan N, Pincemail J, et al (1996) Decrease of plasma vitamin E (alpha-Tocopherol) levels in patients with abdominal aortic aneurysm. Ann NY Acad Sci. 800: 278-282.

[41] Leung JH, Wright AR, Cheshire N, Crane J, Thom SA, Hughes AD, Xu Y (2006) Fluid structure interaction of patient specific abdominal aortic aneurysms: a comparison with solid stress models. BioMedical Engineering OnLine. http://www.biomedical-engineering-online.com/content/5/1/33. Accessed: 2011 Dec 21.

[42] Vorp DA, VandeGeest JP (2005) Biomechanical determinants of abdominal aortic aneurysm rupture. Arteriosclerosis, Thrombosis, and Vascular Biology. 25: 1558-1566

[43] Kleinstreuer C, Li Z (2006) Analysis and computer program for rupture-risk prediction of abdominal aortic aneurysms. BioMedical Engineering OnLine.Available: http://www.biomedical-engineering-online.com/content/5/1/19. Accessed: 2010 April 15.

[44] Vilalta G, Nieto F, Vaquero C, Vilalta JA (2010) Quantitative Indicator of Abdominal Aortic Aneurysm Rupture Risk Based on its Geometric Parameters, World Academy of Science, Engineering and Technology: 70: 181-185.

[45] Shum J, Martufi G, DiMartino E et al (2011) Quantitative assessment of abdominal aortic aneurysm geometry. [45] Ann. Biomed Eng. 39: 277-286. doi:10.1007/s10439-010-0175-3.

[46] Scotti, CM, Shkolnik AD, Muluk SC, Finol EA (2005) Fluid-structure interaction in abdominal aortic aneurysms: Effects of asymmetry and wall thickness. Biomedical Engineering OnLine. http://www.biomedical-engineering-online.com/content/4/1/64.Accessed: 2012 Jan 21.

[47] Raghavan ML, Kratzberg J, de Tolosa EMC, et al (2006) Regional distribution of wall thickness and failure properties of human abdominal aortic aneurysm. J. Biomech. 39: 3010-3016.

[48] Frauenfelder T, Boutsianis E, Alkadhi H, Marincek B, Schertler T (2007) Simulation of blood flow within the abdominal aorta. Computational fluid dynamics in abdominal aortic aneurysms before and after interventions.Radiologe. 47: 1021-1028.

[49] M. Raghavan, D. Vorp, M. Federle, M. Makaroun, & M. Webster, Wall stress distribution on three-dimensionally reconstructed models of human abdominal aortic aneurysm. Journal of Vascular Surgery, 31, 2000, 760–769.

[50] D. Wang, M. Makaroun, M. Webster, & D. Vorp, Effect of intraluminal thrombus on wall stress in patient specific model of abdominal aortic aneurysm. Journal of Vascular Surgery, 3, 2002, 598–604.

[51] K. Wilson, A.J. Lee, P.R. Hoskins, F.G. Fowkers, C.V. Ruckley, & A.W. Bradbury, The relationship between aortic wall distensibility and rupture of infrarenal abdominal aortic aneurysm. Journal of Vascular Surgery, 37, 2003, 112–117.

[52] Vilalta G, Nieto F, Vilalta JA et al (2012) Predicción del riesgo de ruptura de aneurismas de aorta abdominal. Método basado en los biodeterminantes geométricos. DYNA Ingeniería e Industria. 87: 66-73. doi: http://dx.doi.org/10.6036/4145.

[53] Georgakaratos E, Ioannou CV, Kamarianakis Y, Papaharilaou Y, Kostas T, Manousaki E, Katsamouris AN (2010) The role of geometric parameters in the prediction of abdominal aortic aneurysm wall stress. Eur. J. VascEndovasc Surg. 39: 42-48.

[54] Antigua L. Patient-Specific Modeling of Geometry and Blood Flow in Large Arteries. Ph.D thesis.Politecnico di Milano 2002

[55] L. Antiga, B. Ene-Iordache, and A. Remuzzi (2003) Computational geometry for patient-specific reconstruction and meshing of blood vessels from MR and CT angiography. IEEE Transactions on Medical Imaging. 22: 674-684.

[56] Thomas JB, Antigua L, Che SL, Milner JS et al. Variation in the carotid bifurcation geometry of younger versus older adults. Stroke, 36: 2450-2456, 2005.

[56] Sacks MS, Vorp ML, RaghavanM;Federle MP, Webster MW (1999) In vivo three-dimensional surface geometry of abdominal aortic aneurysms. Ann. Biomed. Eng. 27:469-479.

[57] Doyle BJ, Eng AC, Burke PE, et al (2009) Vessel asymmetry as an additional diagnostic tool in the assessment of abdominal aortic aneurysm. J. Vasc Surg. 49: 443-454.

[58] Swedenborg J, Eriksson P (2006) The intraluminal thrombus as a source of proteolytic activity. Ann. NY Acad. Sci. 1085: 133-138. doi: 10.1196/annals.1383.044.

[59] Vorp DA, Lee PC, Wang DH, et al (2001) Association of intraluminal thrombus in abdominal aortic aneurysm with local hypoxia and wall weakening. J. Vasc. Surg. 34: 291-299. doi: 10.1067/mva.2001.114813.

[60] Biasetti J, Gasser TC, Auer M, et al (2009) hemodynamics conditions of the normal aorta compared to fusiform and saccular abdominal aortic aneurysm with emphasize on thrombus formation. Ann. Biomed. Eng. 38: 380-390. doi: 10.1007/s10439-009-9843-6.

[61] Georgakarakos E, Ioannou CV, Volanis S et al (2009) The influence of intraluminal thrombus on abdominal aortic aneurysm wall stress. Int. Angiol. 28: 325-333.

[62] Bluestein D, Dumont K, De Beule M et al (2009) Intraluminal thrombus and risk of rupture in patient specific abdominal aortic aneurysm-FSI modeling. Compt. Meth. Biomech Eng. 12: 73-81.

[63] Georgakarakos E, Ioannou CV, Papahaliraou Y et al (2011) Computational evaluation of aortic aneurysm rupture risk: What have we learned so far?. J. EndovascTher. 18: 214-225. doi: http://dx.doi.org/10.1583/10-3244.1.

[64] Doyle BJ, Corbett TJ, Callanan A (2009) An experimental and numerical comparison of the rupture locations of an abdominal aortic aneurysm. J. Endovasc. Ther. 16: 322-335.

[65] Darling RC, Messina CR, Brewster DC, et al (1977) Autopsy study of unoperated abdominal aortic aneurysm. The case for early resection.Circulation. 56 (3 suppl): II 161-164.

[66] Soudah E, Vilalta G, Vilalta JA et al (2012) Idealized abdominal aortic aneurysm (AAA) geometry as predictor of hemodynamic stresses. Accepted for oral presentation in 6thEuropean Congress on Computational Methods in Applied Sciences and Engineering (ECOMAS 2012). Vienna Sep 10-14, 2012.

[67] Raghavan ML, Harbaugh RE (2005) Quantified aneurysm shape and rupture risk. J. Neurosurg. 102: 355-362.

[68] McGloughlin TM Doyle BJ (2010) New approaches to abdominal aortic aneurysm rupture risk assessment: engineering insight with clinical gain. Aterioscler. Thromb. Vasc. Biol. 30: 1687-1694.

[69] VandeGeest JP, Wang DHJ, Bohra A, Marakoun MS, Vorp DA (2006) A biomechanics-based rupture potential index for abdominal aortic aneurysm risk assessment. Ann. N.Y. Acad. Sci. 1085: 11-21.

[70] Li Z, Kleinstreuer C (2005) A new wall stress equation for aneurysm rupture prediction. An. of Biomedical Eng. 33: 209-213.

[71] Inzoli F, Boschetti F, Zappa M, Longo T, Fumero R (1993) Biomechanical factors in abdominal aortic aneurysm rupture. Eur. J. of Vasc. Surg. 7: 732-739.

[72] Mower WR, Buraff LJ, Sneyd J (1993) Stress distribution in vascular aneurysm: factors affecting risk of aneurysm rupture. J. of Surgical Research. 55: 1556-161.

[73] Vorp DA, Raghavan ML, Webster MW (1998) Stress distribution in aortic abdominal aneurysm: influence of diameter and symmetry. J. of Vasc Surg. 27: 632-639.

[74] He CM, Roach MR (1994) The composition and mechanical properties of abdominal aortic aneurysms. J. of Biomech Eng. 109: 298-304.

[75] Raghavan ML, Webster MW, Vorp DA (1996) Ex-vivo biomechanical behavior of abdominal aortic aneurysm: assessment using a new mathematical model. Ann Biomed Eng. 24: 573-582.

[76] Heng MS, Fagan MJ, Collier JW, Desai G, McCollum PT, Chetter IC (2008) Peak wall stress measurement in elective and acute abdominal aortic aneurysms. J. of Vasc Surg. 47: 17-22.

[77] González A, García de la Figal J (2009) Analysis of mechanical behavior of aorta section (in Spanish). IngenieríaMecánica. 12: 9-18.

[78] De Putter S, Wolters BJBM, Rutten MCM, Breeuwer M, Gerritsen FA, Van de Vosse FN (2007) Patient-specific initial wall stress in abdominal aortic aneurysm with a backward incremental method. J. of Biomech. 40: 1081-1090.

[79] Volokh KY, Vorp DA (2008) A model of growth and rupture of abdominal aortic aneurysm. J. of Biomech; 41: 1015-1021.

[80] Tong P, Fung YC (1976) The Stress-Strain Relationship for the Skin. J. of Biomech. 9: 649-657.

[81] Rodríguez JF, Ruiz C, Doblaré M, Holzapfel GA (2008) Mechanical stresses in abdominal aortic aneurysm: influence of diameter, asymmetry, and material anisotropy. J. of Biomech Eng. 130: 256-267.

[82] Holzapfel GA, Gasser TC, Ogden RW (2000) A new constitutive framework for arterial wall mechanics and a comparative study of material models. J. of Elasticity. 61: 1-48.

[83] Papaharilaou Y, Ekaterinaris J A. Manousaki E, Katsamouris AN (2007) A decoupled fluid structure approach for estimating wall stress in abdominal aortic aneurysms. J. of Biomech. 40: 367-377.

[84] Vorp DA, VandeGeest JP (2005) Biomechanical determinants of abdominal aortic aneurysm rupture. Arteriosclerosis, Thrombosis and Vascular Biology. 25: 1558-1566.

[85] Vascops Vascular diagnostics. On-line survey: Clinical assessment of AAA rupture risk. Are biomechanical predictors needed? (2007). Last access: Sept-15-2010. Available in: http://www.vascops.com/files/survey2006.pdf. Accessed: 2011 March 24.

Chapter 6

Abdominal Aortic Aneurysm in Different Races Epidemiologic Features and Morphologic-Clinical Implications Evaluated by CT Aortography

Ana Mladenovic, Zeljko Markovic, Sandra Grujicic-Sipetic and Hideki Hyodoh

Additional information is available at the end of the chapter

http://dx.doi.org/10.5772/48379

1. Introduction

By definition AAA is dilatation in diameter of the main arterial vessel in abdomen-abdominal aorta for over 50% compared to expected normal diameter (1). This dilatation is caused by gradual decrease in elasticity and consistence of aortic wall, usually including weakness in middle layer of aortic wall (tunica media), which leads to extension of extern layer (tunica adventitia) and/or inner layer (tunica intima) (2,3). Blood that is pumped through aorta under pressure, gradually stretches this weakened wall and most often creates aneurysmatic dilatation.

The disease is most often found in elderly population (4). In 5% of population older than 65, presence of AAA is confirmed (4,5). It has been noticed that this disease is about 6 times more frequent in males than in female population (6).

Over time, most of AAA (around 80%) increases in diameter (2,6). It is not possible to foresee which aneurysm will increase and which one will remain stable. In most cases, the growth of aneurysm is slow. Aneurysms measuring 5 or more cm in diameter increase for 4-8mm annually (7). Aneurysms with greatest diameter of 4-5 cm grow 3-7mm annually, while those smaller than 4 cm in diameter grow 2-5 mm on average (7,8). This long-term disease presents with nonspecific symptoms and is often unpredictable. The most frequent complication and leading cause of mortality (over 80%) in patients with AAA is rupture.

In many epidemiologic studies it has been noticed that persons with positive family anamnesis for this disease, have significantly higher risk of developing the aneurysm and its rupture. Furthermore, other risk factors for aneurysm have been identified, such as obesity, hypertension, smoking and elevated blood cholesterol level (9-14). The role od diabetes mellitus, which is a well known risk factor in development of occlusive disease of blood vessels, in terms of aneurysm development remains controversial (15-20).

There are two current therapeutic approaches. The first one is surgery and the other is endovascular (Endovascular Aortic Repair – EVAR). In about half of the patients with intact aneurysm, as well as in those with ruptured one, endovascular approach can be applied. Advantages of endovasular treatment are avoiding general anesthesia, laparotomy and clamping the aorta. The procedure lasts shorter and recovery is fast. However, there are some disadvantages or technical limitations of this procedure. It is not possible to place the graft if proximal neck of the anuerysm is smaller than 15mm and conical in shape (21,22), because origins of renal arteries could be covered. Also, the neck of the aneurysm should be orientated at the angle no smaller than 60º towards the sagittal plane of the aorta, iliac arteries must not be tortuous and must measure at least 9 mm in diameter (23,24). During relatively short period of clinical application and development of EVAR (from 1991) the problem of frequently inadequate commercially available aortic stent-grafts for yellow race and patients with low BMI (21) has arised. The appliation of EVAR in yellow race patients showed that only 23-42% grafts, with fabrically defined dimensions, are adequate, in 23-46% they need certain corrections, while in about 30% of patients there is a contraindication for stent placement (25,26,27,28). Contemporary experience in the application of EVAR showed that overall number of complications is relatively high, even up to 30-40%. Also, one of the reasons is a not precise enough preprocedural morphologic evaluation of AAA and early diagnostics of postprocedural complications.

Modern generations od multidetector CT units (generation 16 slice, 2004 to 64 slice detectors-2007), offered a new visualisation quality and possibility to obtain more relevant diagnostic information compared to DSA. MDCT aortography reaffirmed the significance of preprocedural evaluation which ensures obtaining numerous and high quality information in each and every situation, considering the place of graft insertion, graft design and overall indication for EVAR, as well as relevant postprocedural evaluation and early diagnstics of possible complications.

During last 3 years, MDCT units with 10-times lower exponential doses per examination were constructed (29-35). At the same time, routine use of high-resolution ultrasonography as non-ionizing morphologic imaging enabled screening programmes for AAA in elderly and high-risk populaton, that are conducted and in progress in many countries (36,37,38).

2. Body

Main hypotheses of this multicentric study are:

1. Positive family anamnesis for AAA, as well as trauma, personal history of diabetes mellitus and hypertension, smoking, elevated LDL cholesterol, which are risk-factors for AAA
2. There are significant anatomic-morphologic differences in aneurysmatic infrarenal aorta between Caucasian and Asian patients

3. There are precise morphologic parameters based on MDCT aortography which determine indications and contraindications for EVAR, graft dimensions and the place of insertion
4. MDCT aortography enables early diagnostics of EVAR complications
5. The possibility of graft design in individual case is enabled by integrating measurements obtained by MDCT aortography in selective programme

The study was conducted in Clinical center of Serbia - Center for radiology and magnetic resonance and Institute for radiology, University Hospital Saporro (Japan), in period 2009-2011. In thiis study 31 Asian and 30 Caucasian patients with the infrarenal aortic aneurysm were included, as well as 130 Asian and 126 Caucasian patients with indication for CT aortography (CTA), which confirmed the absence of AAA. Election of patients of both races before referred to CT examination, was performed according to medical history, and definite indication for CT exam was set according to clinical findings and sonographic findings in distal aorta. Exclusion criteria were: rupture of aneurysm, aneurysm that exceeded infrarenal segment, discrete dilatation of aorta and finding of rough intramural and extraluminal calcifications in longer segment.

Data about risk factors for development of AAA (smoking, hypertension, elevated blood cholesterol level) were collected. One of the questions included the presence of diabetes mellitus in personal history. Questionnaire icluded demographic parameters (sex, age, race, education), antropometric data (body weight, body height, body surface, body mass index), personal history (diabetes, trauma, other) and family medical history (presence of AAA in relatives).

For classifying patients according to the level of nutrition, we used international classification recomended by World Health Organization (WHO) and US Institutes of Health: underweighted-BMI<18,4, normal weighted BMI between 18,5 and 24,9; overweighted BMI 25-29,9 and obese BMI>30. According to body height, all the patients were divided in 4 subgroups: shorter than 160 cm, between 160 cm and 170 cm, between 170-180 cm and taller than 180 cm.

Considering smoking, patients were divided into 3 subgroups according to duration of this habit: 10 years, between 10-20 years and over 20 years. Level of blood cholesterol over 3,4 mmol/l was considered elevated. For calculation of body surface (SA) we used Dubois & Dubois formula: SA= 0.20247 x height (m)0.725 x weight (kg)0.425. Considering that it is a complex logarithmic formula, we used software (calculator) for SA recommended by US National institutes of health (http://www.nih.gov). For the calculation of BMI we used established formula: BMI= body weight (kg) : body surface (m^2).

3. 64-slice MDCT protocol and measurements used in the study

CTA examination in both centers was performed on the same CT unit of the same generation, type and model of the machine. We performed examinations on 64-slice VCT

Lightspeed unit (GE, Milwaukee, IL, US). In all cases we used non-ionic contrast agent in concentration of 320-370 (1 ml – 370 mg iodine) applied by automatic injector in cubital vein reaching flow rate of 5 ml/sec.

Taking into account heterogeneity of selected population by constitution, sex, race and age, and expected heterogeneity in „delay time" of the examination start, we used programme mode „SmartPrep" for defining the appropriate time, by selecting the spot in aorta where appearance of contrast agent triggers the acquisition. Helical mode was used in SmartPrep protocol, 120 kV, 250-700 mAs, rotation speed of the tube 0,35 with slice thickness of 1,25 mm with 64 slice detector in 0.625mm reconstruction.

Postprocessing was performed with the same selected applications in both centers:

Volume Viwer Analysis-CTA Aorta and Advanced Vessel Analysis. Interobserver variability was avoided by the fact that examinations in both centers were performed by a single radiologist.

Number of global selected mathematic variables which define morphology at CTA examination usen in this study is 11. Overall number of methodologically defined transverse measurements is 36 (12 for infrarenal aorta and 24 for iliac arteries), overall number of linear measurements is 36 and volumetric measurements 3. All together, these measurements represent methodologic protocol used in the study for defining the morphology of aneurysmatic infrarenal aorta.

Linear, transverse and volumetric measurements were performed according to the protocol defined aforehead, which consisted of following parameters (Figure 1). All linear measurements were performed in 3 characteristic 2D and 3 characteristic 3D reconstructions (AP, PA and semi-oblique) and mean value was used as definite. We used software ruler tool which is a part of every Analysis-CTA Aorta. Proximal point for measuring aneurysmatic neck, linear distances of aorta, angle between AAA and all the other calculations were positioned in the orifice level of main renal artery. We performed following linear measurements:

- mean length of abdominal aorta (mm)(Figure 2)
- mean length of the neck of the aneurysm (mm)(Figure 3)
- mean linear distance from renal artery to aortic bifurcation (mm)(Figure 2)
- mean length of common iliac artery (mm)(Figure 4)
- AAA angle (degrees– ^{o})(Figure 2)

Calculations of aortic and iliac arteries volumes represent a part of the basic package of Analysis-CTA Aorta programme. Start and end point are defined (Figure 1). Computer calculates only the lumen of blood vessel that contains contrast agent with no calcium deposits, and without wall structures in cases of thrombosed extraluminal mass; if AAA contains only the dilated vessel wall, the lumen is calculated in total.

Transverse measurements were performed using Advanced Vessel CT Aorta Analysis programme which enables linear differentiating the lumen of contrast agent that fills the vessel from intramural and endoluminal calcifications, considering the similar attenuation values of calcium and contrast agent which cannot be differentiated visually (there is a possibility of misinterpreting calcified plaque as vessel lumen). We performed 6 typical measurements in the same plane, for the lumen of circulating blood (total of 12 "flow" diameters)(F.d.) and 6 measurements in the same plane for diameters of circulating blood together with thrombosed blood, aneurysm content and thickness of the vessel wall (total of 12 „real"diameters)(R.d)(Figure 5, Figure 7).

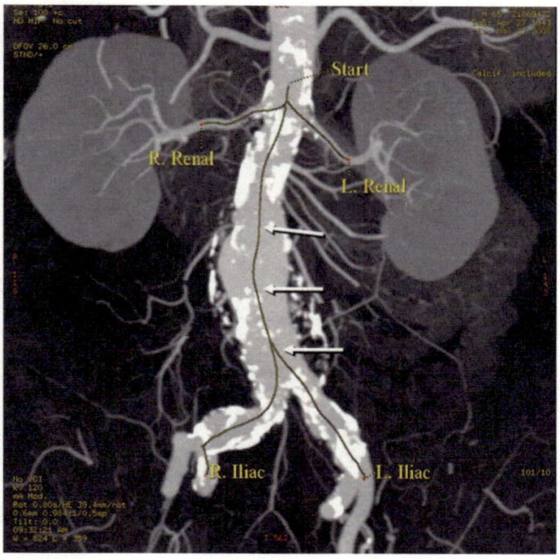

Figure 1. Characteristic points of interest to mark the CT angiographic analysis in Figure 2D.

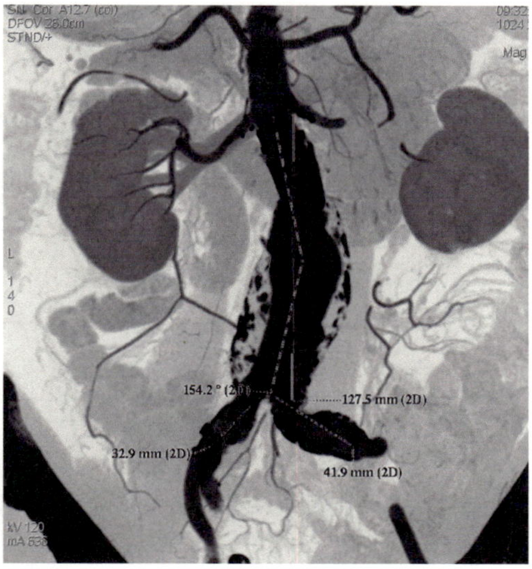

Figure 2. CT linear measurements of the aorta in the 2D image: mean length of abdominal aorta, mean linear distance from renal artery to aortic bifurcation and AAA angle

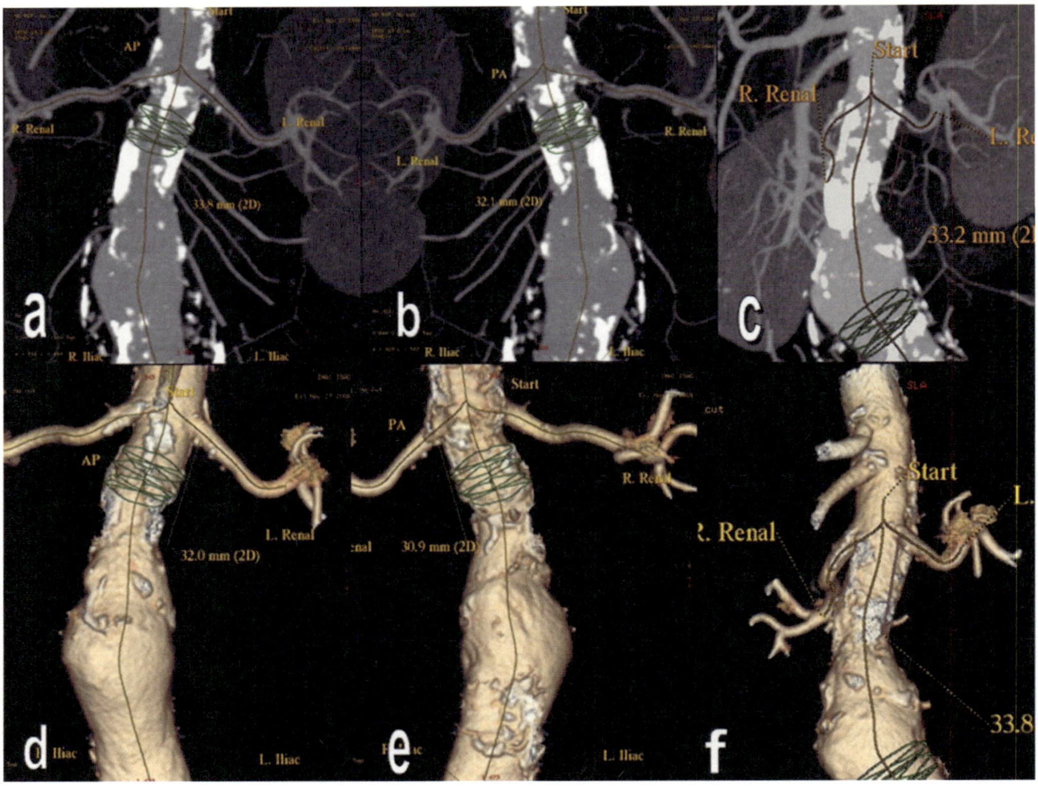

Figure 3. AAA neck length in 3 characteristic measurements in 2D (a-c) and 3D image (d-f).

The points of transverse measurements of abdominal aorta (a.a.) and common iliac artery (a.i.c.) performed in this study were following:

a. infrarenal, in the level of the neck of the aneurysm, the largest and the smallest F.d. and R.d. (F.d.a.a 1, F.d. a.a 2, R.d. a.a 1 and R.d. a.a. 2)
b. in the middle part of abdominal aorta, largest and the smallest F.d and R.d diameter (F.d. a.a 3, F.d. a.a 4, R.d. a.a 3 and R.d. a.a. 4)
c. just above the aortic bifurcation, the largest and the smallest F.d and R.d diameter (F.d. a.a 5, F.d. a.a 6, R.d. a.a 5 and R.d. a.a. 6);
d. proximal parts of both common iliac arteries distally from aortic bifurcation, the largest and the smallest F.d and R.d diameter (F.d. a.i.c 1, F.d. a.i.c 2, R.d. a.i.c 1 and R.d. a.i.c 2);
e. middle parts of both common iliac arteries below aortic bifurcation, the largest and the smallest F.d and R.d diameter (F.d. a.i.c 3, F.d. a.i.c 4, R.d. a.i.c 3 and R.d. a.i.c 4);
f. distal parts of both common iliac arteries above their bifurcations, the largest and the smallest F.d and R.d diameter (F.d. a.i.c 5, F.d. a.i.c 6, R.d. a.i.c 5 and R.d. a.i.c 6);

The precise localization of transverse measurements was defined according to the linear reconstruction of aorta and iliac arteries.

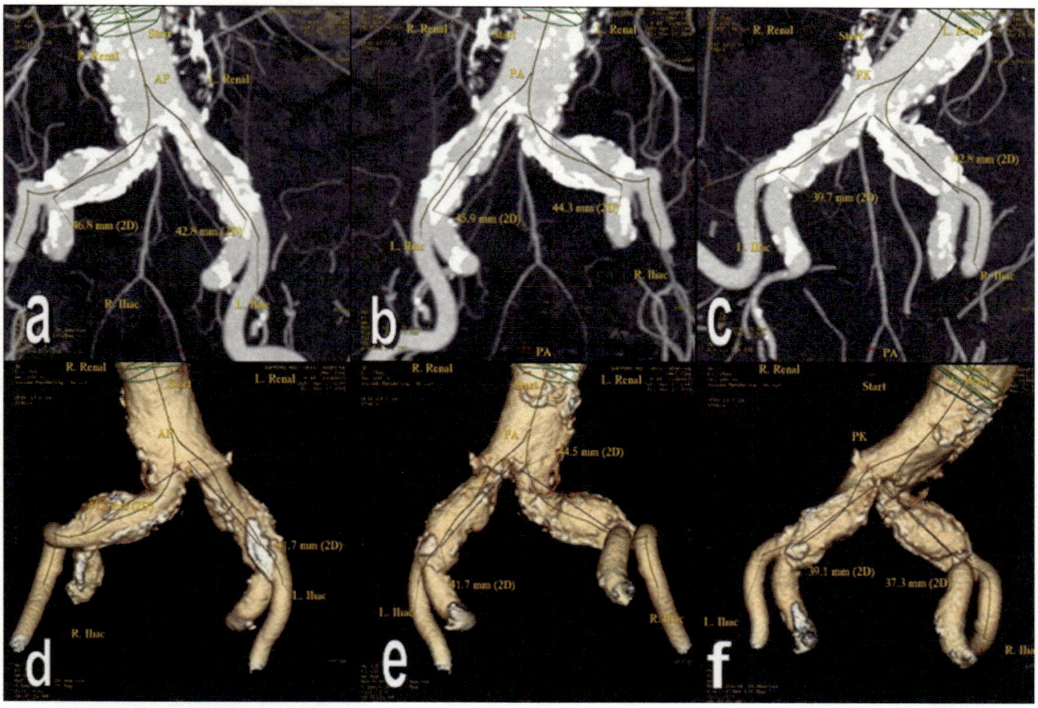

Figure 4. Measuring the length of the c.i.a in characteristic 3 position (AP, PA and oblique) in 2D (a-c) and 3D image (d-f)

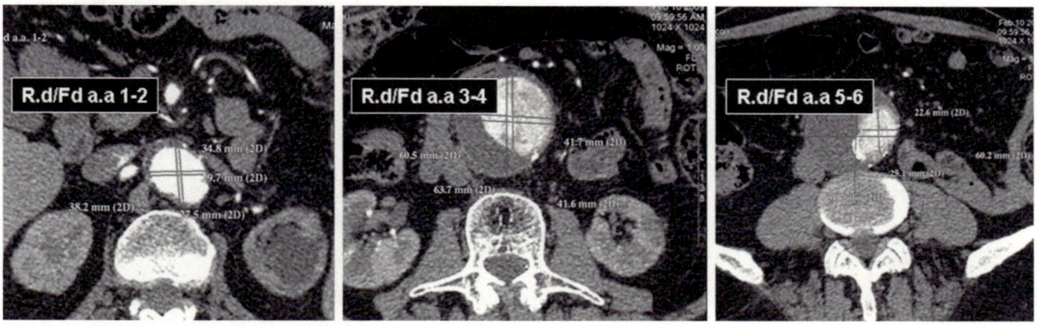

Figure 5. Transverse measurement of infrarenal aortic aneurysms (diameters Rd and Fd)

As a variable part of the protocol of morphologic measurements in this study, depending on the individual case, we performed other diagnostic explorations enabled by selected computer application, such as:

a. Defining tissue structure (attenuation) in the region of interest (Figure 8)
b. Defining the configuration of the blood vessel (Figure 9)
c. Defining calcifications (Figure 10)
d. Dynamic analysis of contrast agent flow
e. MDCT aortoscopy (Figure 11)
f. Coronal or sagittal 3D reconstruction (Figure 12)

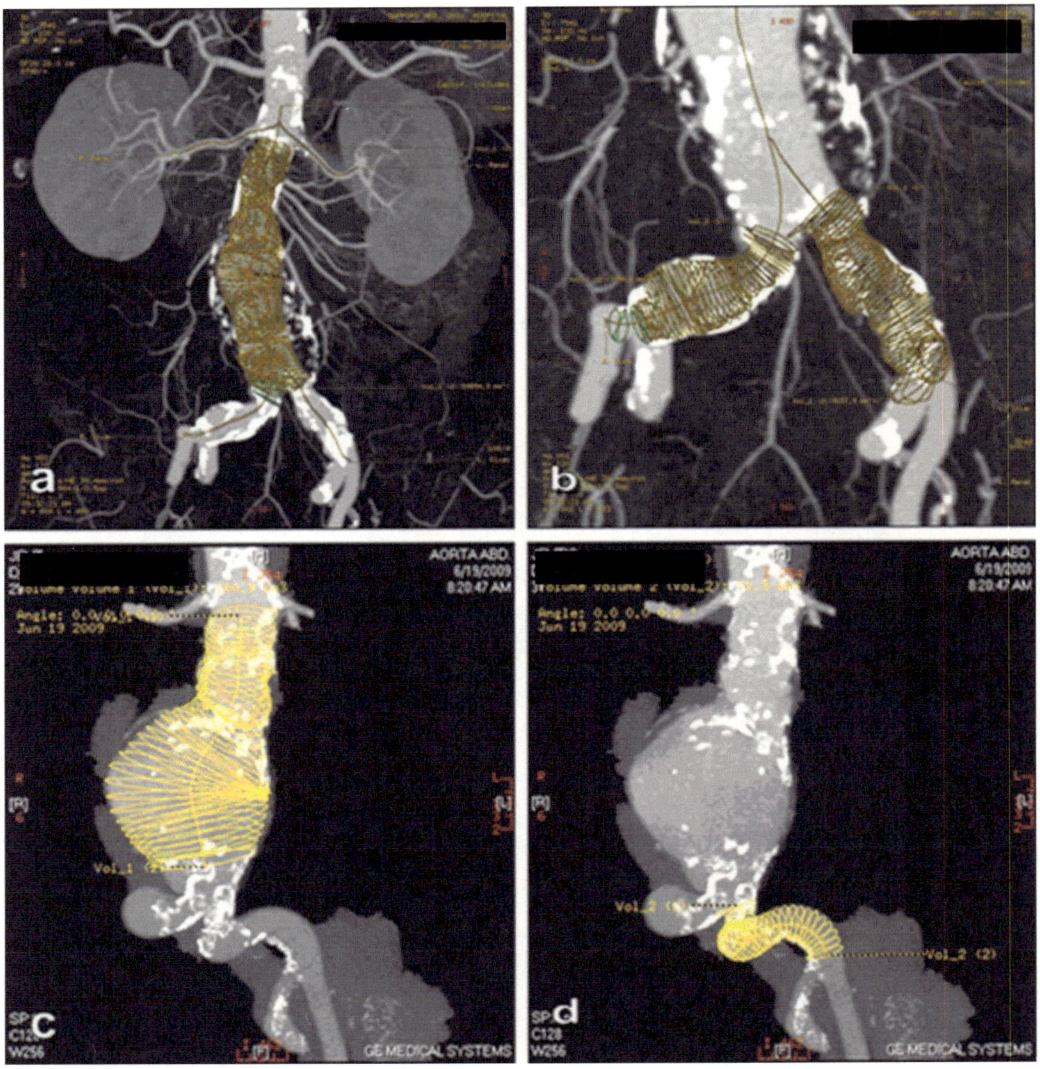

Figure 6. MD CT volumetric measurement of infrarenal aorta and aa.iliace comm bill in patients with calcium channel intraluminal nodular induration (a,b) patients with AAA and without calcium induration in the wall (c,d).

a) Defining tissue structure (attenuation) in the region of interest in different planes (most often transverse and sagittal). Using this exploration, known as „color mapping" it is possible to determine the density of the tissue in ROI or mean tissue density in the wider region. According to the attenuation distribution, it is possible to determine the structure or density of thrombotic aneurysmatic blood as well as differentiate contrast agent from calcified plaques which are pointed intraluminally. Every color represents a range of some interval of tissue density from 20-800 HU. Contrast agent is always represent by color green, low-density strustures (thrombus, blood, fat) by blue, atherosclerotic deposits by yellow and calcified indurations by red.

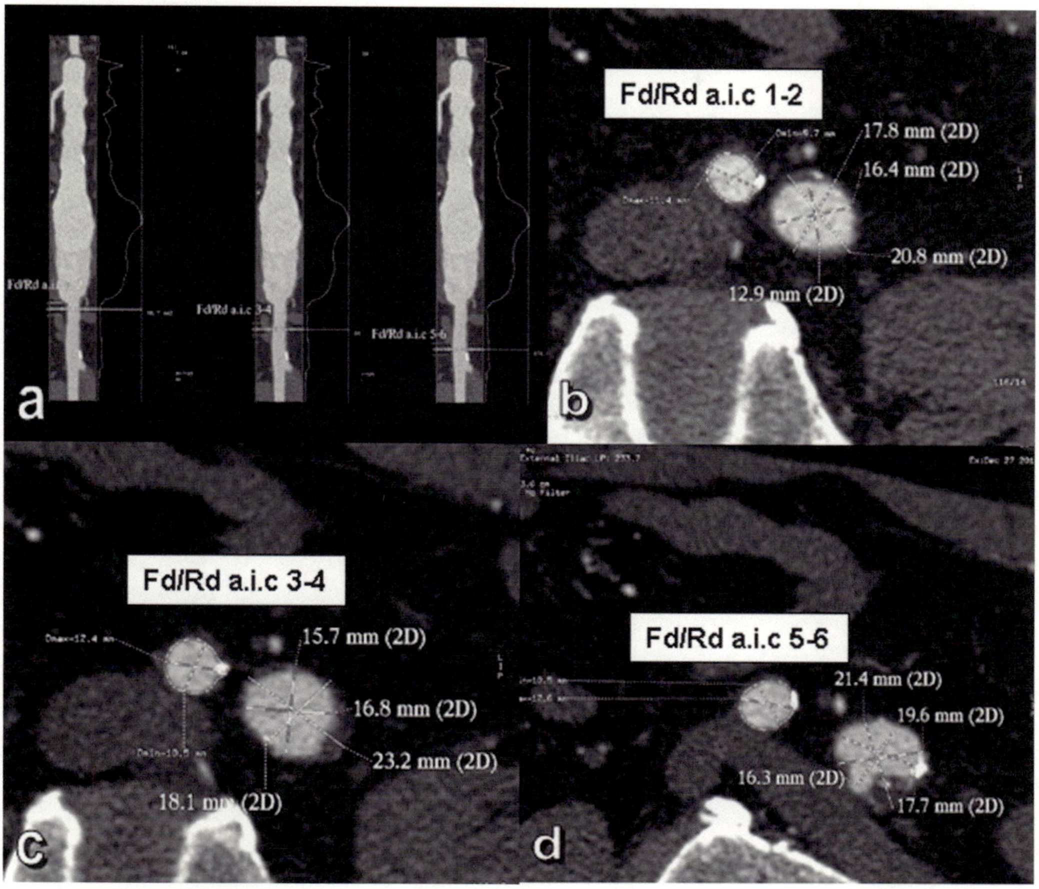

Figure 7. Transverse measurement of infrarenal aortic aneurysms (diameters Rd and Fd)(b-d) compared to the linear angiographic image (a) (a)

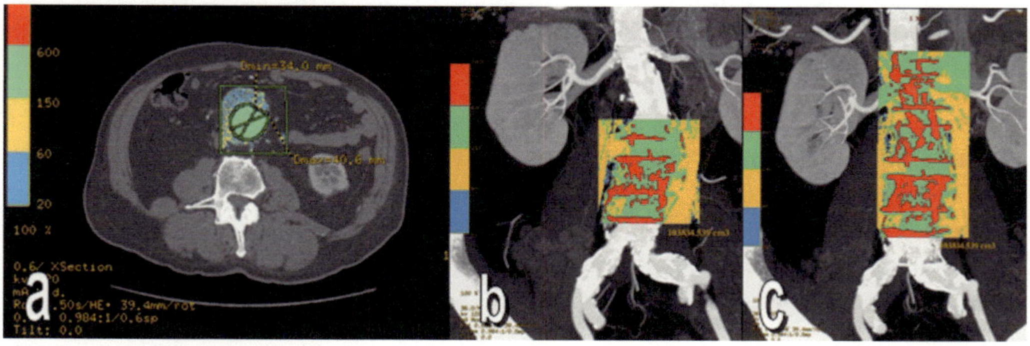

Figure 8. Defining tissue structure (attenuation) in the region of interest in the transverse (a) and coronary reconstruction (b,c)

b) Defining the configuration of the blood vessel enables precise visualization in cases of suspected dissection of the vessel wall and enables defining the wall thickness in all planes. Furthermore, it enables clear graphic demarcation of the lesions of aortic wall and differentiating from the extraluminal lesions. Additional option is definition of calcified indurations inside the „contoured" picture.

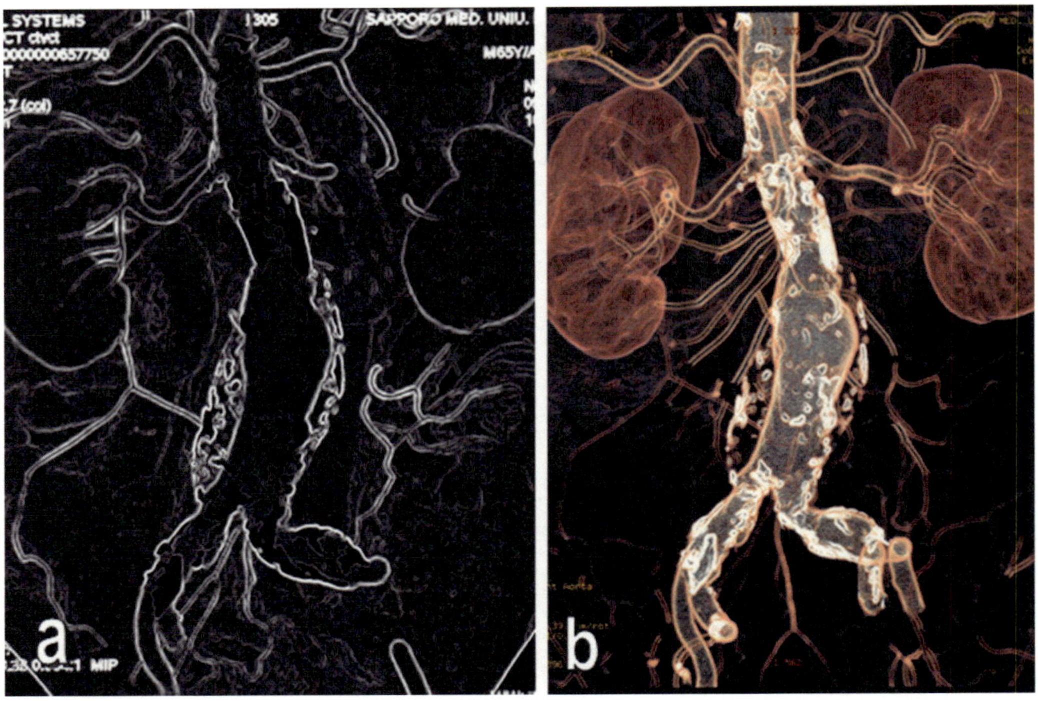

Figure 9. Contouring infrarenal aorta: linear (a) and with intramural calcifications (b)

c) Isolated defining extraluminal calcifications (Figure 3.21. a), intramural calcifications and altogether in frontal reconstruction along the aortic segment, in selected planes and positions. This exploration may imply on therapeutic approach in two projections at the level of c.i.a

d) Dynamic analysis of contrast agent flow represents the review of video-recording in selected plane, most often transverse or frontal, where dynamic of the contrast agent flow in aortic lumen can be analysed in real time mode.This exploration has a specific value in postprocedural evaluation and diagnostics of early complications of EVAR, most of all the proximal endoleak as a frequent complication. It is more sensitive than conventional digital aortography video -recording

e) MDCT aortoscopy, known also as „virtual aortography", is a special visualization option in „advanced" options of MD CT aortography, which is offered in standard postprocessing units of 16-64 slice MDCT units from the year 2007. It is a relatively simple, but powerful method of endoluminal examination in all planes, that enables optical presentation of the aortic wall inner surface, lesions of the aortic walls, the extent of anuerysmatic dilatation, endoluminal plaques and vessel arborization.

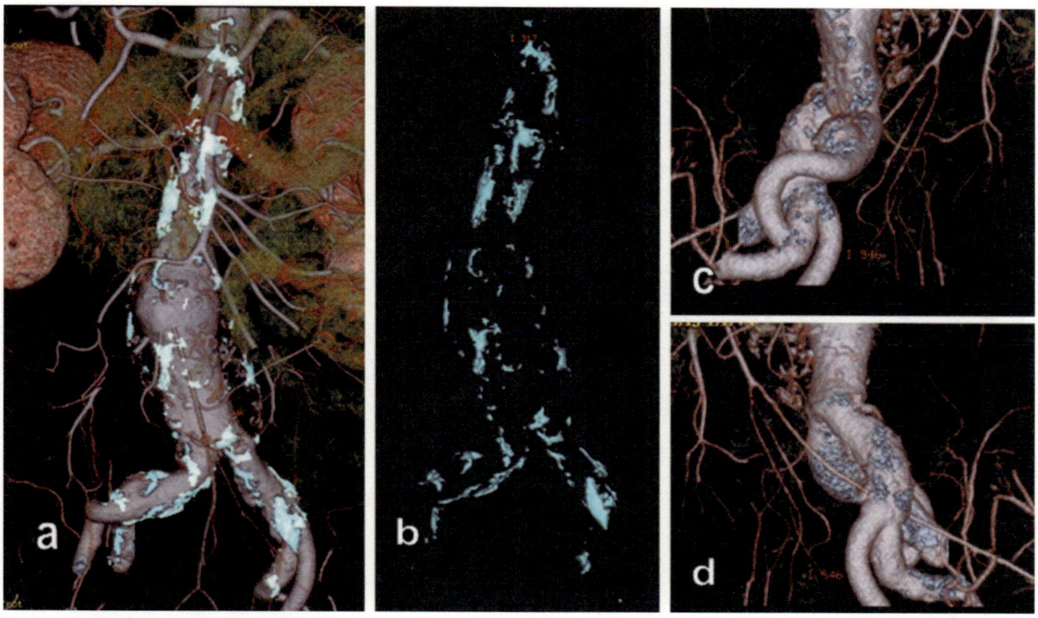

Figure 10. Defining calcifications of AAA - the level of the aortic extraluminarly (a) and intramural (b)

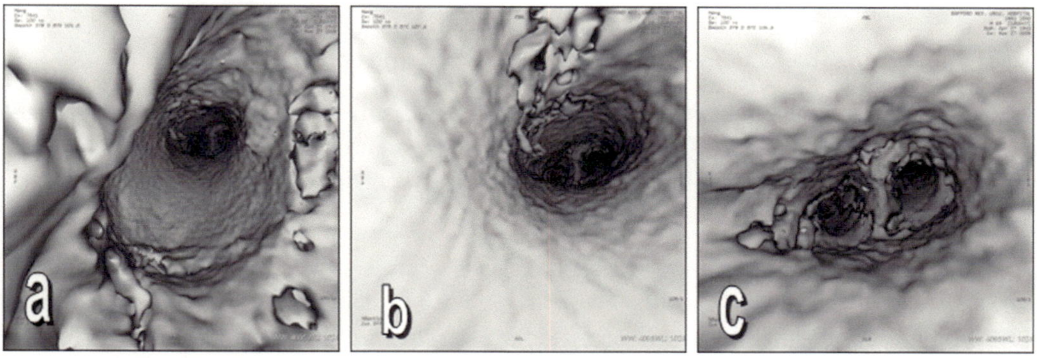

Figure 11. MDCT aortoscopy the level of renal arteries (a), middle third of a.a (b) and before the bifurcation (c)

f) Coronal or sagittal 3D reconstruction (VR 3D cut). It is a postprocessing option from the standard group which is more often used in diagnostics of parenchymatous organs and heart, and represents „listing" slices at selected distance (0,625 mm at least) in 3D presentation of the organ or lesion. In AAA, it can be used for visualization of thromobotic mass and its structure considering heterogeneity and the presence of calcified indurations. The analysis can be preformed in 6 standard planes: AP – anteroposterior; PA – posteroanterior; L –left lateral, R – right lateral, I – inferior-superior; S – superior-anterior, and additionally in every non-standard plane of rotated 3D image, which defines 4D visualization in terms of movement.

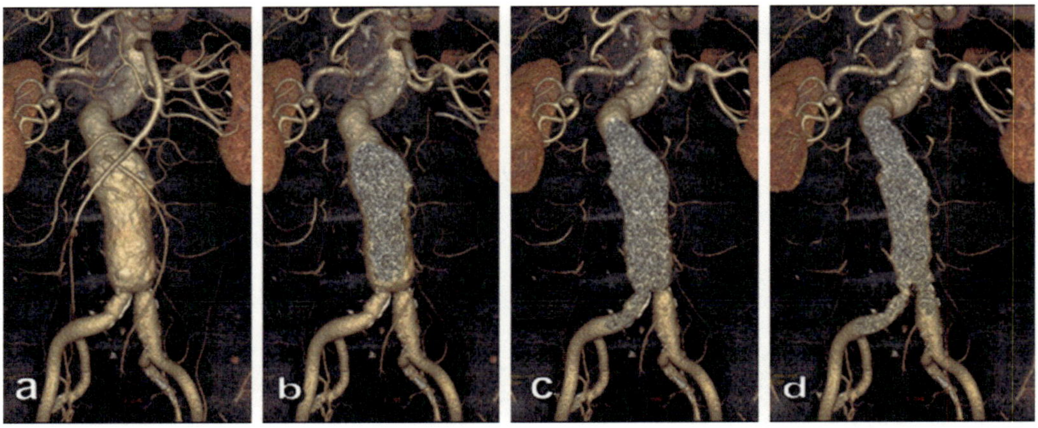

Figure 12. VR 3D cut option in coronary reconstuction in the antero-posterior direction (a) in 3 planes (b,c,d)

4. Statistic methodology

Considering the heterogeneity of the population included, as well as the number of analyzed variables, we used several statistical models for data analysis in this study:

Univariant and multivariant staistical methods – for testing statistic significance of difference between parameters for qualitative variables, as well as quantitative variables, univariant methods were used

χ^2 test –for testing the relationship between non-parametric variabes.

ANOVA - one-sample analysis of variance- univariant analysis of the effect of one selected factor on dependent variable. Comparing mean values, standard deviations in development of aneurysm between races and in the same race compared to control subjects, was performed using this method.

Median Test, Kolmogorov-Smirnov Z-test analysis of the mutual influence (of the selected variable among the groups), testing the compatibility of controls and patients in terms of developing the aneurysm, between races, and in the same race compared to the controls.

We determined the correlation coefficient (Pearson correlation) related to groups, smoking habit, and smoking history of all the subjects included, subjects according to sex (in males and females seperately).

According to univariant logistic regression analysis (ULRA) we tested the influence of selected variable (risk factors) and their correlation on the aneurysm development at the probability level $p \leq 0{,}01$.

Regression analysis (logistic model) In the model of MLRA we included all variables (risk factors) that were confirmed by univariant logistic regression analysis (ULRA) to be connected to the aneurysm development at the level of $p \leq 0{,}01$, so we determined the independent risk factors for development of aneurysm in all the subjects, and then seperately for male and female groups. All the variables were additionally tested in terms of age.

Odds Ratio (OR) or (expB) with confidence interval of 95%- chance ratio, or the possibility of the selected happening, the assessment of the correlation of risk factors (happening) and disease occurrence (development of aneurysm).

Statistic significance was determined at the level of probability of the null hypothesis $p \leq 0.05$ to $p<0.0001$. Statistical analysis was performed using SPSS ver.20, while graphs and tables were edited using MICROSOFT OFFICE (EXCEL and WORD).

5. Study results

Distribution of patients according to the site of aneurysm, mean values ± SD in demographic and anthropological criteria and CT measurements between two races of the respondents suffering from AAA is shown in Table 1. The other criteria did not find statistically significant differences in relation to race in patients with AAA.

Demographic / Anthropological variables, MD CT measurements	AP with AAA	EP with AAA	ANOVA, F	p
	Mean±Std.Dev.	Mean±Std.Dev.		
age	75,60±6,13	61,13±10,97	39,75	0,001***
hight (cm)	159,90±8,85	176,63±8,20	57,70	0,001***
body weight (kg)	56,46±11,55	80,00±11,99	59,94	0,001***
surface area (m2)	1,58±0,18	1,97±,189	70,50	0,001***
BMI (kg/m2)	22,04±3,77	25,38±3,19	13,64	0,001***
aneurysm neck length	22,73±6,9	38,72±11,92	3,176	0,013**
aver.c.i.a.length	47,41±12,99	59,68±15,25	11,25	0,001***
aver.distance a.a.	84,39±31,58	63,27±50,76	3,65	0,05*
Fd-a.a1	19,05±3,95	22,87±6,44	7,65	0,01**
Fd-a.a2	22,08±4,13	26,88±7,62	9,22	0,001***
Rd-a.a1	24,06±4,98	29,39±9,28	7,67	0,01**
Rd-a.a2	26,18±5,79	31,57±10,98	5,66	0,02*
Rd-a.a3	32,53±12,37	43,42±20,74	6,11	0,02*
Rd-a.a4	34,46±12,75	48,07±22,35	8,39	0,01**
Rd-a.a6	28,91±10,90	36,61±17,29	4,25	0,04*
volume c.i.a.	6405,86±2819,07	8560,63±5145,87	4,05	0,05*

Table 1. Distribution of patients according to the site of aneurysm, mean values ± SD of age, height, body weight, surface area, BMI index, aneurysm neck length, aver.c.i.a.length, aver.distance a.a., Fd-a.a1, Fd-a.a2, Rd-a.a1, Rd-a.a2, Rd-a.a3, Rd-a.a4, Rd-a.a6 and volume c.i.a. - where the parameters are found statistical differences (*, **) and the difference is highly statistically differences (***).

Distribution of respondents to the AP and EP aneurysm and control groups the same race by age, gender, BMI and body height is shown in Table 2.

Age / Gender BMI, Body height		patients with aneurysm				patients without aneurysm			
		AP		EP		AP		EP	
		No	%	No	%	No	%	No	%
Age	≤ 74	13	41,90	26	86,60	62	47,69	114	90.47
	≥74	18	58,10	4	13,40	68	52,31	12	9,53
Gender	Male	25	83,3	24	77,4	58	46,03	90	83,3
	Female	5	16,7	7	22,6	68	53,97	40	16,7
BMI (kg/m^2)	< 18,4	0	0,00	3	9,68	3	2,38	7	5,38
	18,5 -24,9	12	40,00	22	70,97	96	76,19	113	86,92
	25-29,9	15	50,00	6	19,35	24	19,05	7	5,38
	> 30	3	10,00	0	0,00	3	2,38	3	2,31
Body height (cm)	< 160	14	45,20	0	0,00	73	56,15	0	0,00
	160-170	12	38,70	7	23,3	50	38,46	24	19,05
	≥171	5	16,10	14	46,70	7	5,38	73	57,94
Total		31	100	30	100	126	100	130	100

Age χ^2=13,322; p=0,0001
Gender χ^2=0,337; p=0,561
BMI χ^2=12,785; p<0,005
Body height χ^2=28,57; p<0,0001

Table 2. Distribution of respondents to the AP and EP aneurysm and control groups the same race by age, gender, BMI and body height.

The presence of factors in patients and control subjects as well as univariant regression analysis (ULRA) for assessment risk-factors among patients and controls in AP and EP groups of patients is shown in Table 3a. The presence of risk-factors in patients and control subjects as well as multinivariant regression analysis (MLRA) for assessment risk-factors among patients and controls in AP and group of patients is shown in Table 3b and the presence of risk-factors in patients and control subjects as well as multinivariant regression analysis (MLRA) for assessment risk-factors among patients and controls in EP group of patients is shown in Table 3c.

PREDICTORS	AP patients with aneurysm		EP patients with aneurysm	
	Unst.B	*p	Unst.B	*p
(Constant)	9,549	0,000	27,901	0,000
Age (up to and over 75 years)	-0,096	0,848	0,912	0,591
Height (< 160, 160-170, ≥171 cm)	-0,050	0,896	0,657	0,382
BMI (< 18,4, 18,5-24,9, 25-29,9, > 30)	0,466	0,351	-3,386	0,000
Smoking (yes/no)	3,254	0,000	1,348	0,496
Smoking (to10,10-20, over 20 years)	-2,284	0,000	-2,969	0,001
BP (>140/90) (yes/no)	-1,695	0,003	-2,725	0,009
LDL- cholesterol (>3,4 mmol/l) (yes/no)	-4,677	0,000	-4,545	0,000
Diabetes Melitus (yes/no)	3,238	0,000	3,121	0,011

Tab 3a

* p value according to the results ULRA ($p \leq 0{,}01$)

PREDICTORS		OR	95% confidence interval	*p
Smoking	no yes	0,069	0,005-0,874	0,003
Length of smoking (years)	to 10 10-20 over 20	7,608	2,836-20,408	0,0001
Hypertension (> 140/90)	no yes	3,831	1,079-10,911	0,037
LDL- cholesterol (>3,4 mmol/l)	no yes	11,817	3,734-37,396	0,0001

Tab 3b

* p value according to the results of MLRA

PREDICTORS		OR	95% confidence interval	*p
BMI	< 18,4 18,5-24,9 25-29,9 > 30	4,923	1,873-12,941	0,001
Length of smoking (years)	to 10 10-20 over 20	2,784	1,743-4,446	0,0001
Hypertension (> 140/90)	no yes	3,421	1,089-10,767	0,036
LDL- cholesterol (>3,4 mmol/l)	no yes	6,696	2,092-21,430	0,001

Tab 3c

* p value according to the results of MLRA

Table 3. The presence of risk-factors in patients and control subjects as well as multinivariant regression analysis (MLRA) for assessment risk-factors among patients and controls in EP group of patients.

6. Evaluation of the metodology of imaging studies

Generation of spiral CT units enabled the examination of large blood vessels for the first time as a substitute for the invasive conventional angiography, most importantly for aorta, extracranial arteries of the neck and skull base, main trunks of visceral arteries of thorax and abdomen and ilio-popliteal vessels. There have been numerous attempts to affirm spiral angiography for the exploration of 2nd and 3rd order arteries of parenchymatous organs, but diagnostic sensitivity was disappointing (33,39). Development of CT technology from the year 2000, enabled the start of new epoch with multidetector CT units, that brought amazing possibilities of image acquisition and spatial to temporal resolution ratio (30,31). In the same terms, a new postprocessing editing of transverse CT images was developed, offering faster, more detailed and accurate reconstruction possibilities in all planes. Definitely, MDCT examination established itself as diagnostically most sensitive in postprocedural evaluation of AAA and became method of choice in this field. In year 2007, exponential dose for the examination of infrarenal aorta using standard protocol at 64-slice unit, was approximatelly 6-8 mSv for both sexes. In obese patients it was somewhat higher (29). During the following 3 years, introducing new pulse generators and faster rotating tubes in clinical practice, exponential dose for CT exam of infrarenal aorta was lowered for 8-10 times, remaining the preoccupation of inovators until now.

7. Evaluation of demographic, antropologic and epidemiologic results of the study

In the discussion of the results of this study, we used every available data base, but most of all US National Library of Medicine National Institutes of Health (www.ncbi.nlm.nih.gov/pubmed), as well as other browsers for medical papers in MEDLINE and other indexed publications. Browsing bibliographic data was performed using relevant key words (races, aorta, CT, aortography, MDCT, aneurysm etc.)

Sex distribution in both groups of patients and controls in this study showed three basic features: there is no statistically significant difference in terms of sex in patients, that in control Caucasian subjects predominant group consisted of females and that in analyzed groups of patients predomination of males was statistically significant. Compared to the most citated epidemiologic studies considering the sex of patients, showing 4-6 times more frequent development of aneurysms in men, in this study we showed slight predominance of male patients in Caucasian group (around 72%), while in Asian group the number of male patients was smaller (around 50%). According to available data on the frequency of AAA in different races, it is generally accepted that the disease is most frequent in Caucasian population (12,14). In USA, for example, the incidence of AAA is significantly higher in white males than Afro-americans, while in female population, there is no statistically significant difference in the occurrence of the disease. Asian population (yellow race) is the least frequently affected by AAA (10,12). In Africa, aneurysm of thoracic aorta is more frequent, as well as in Carribean population. African males are three times less affected than Europeans (40). Interesting epidemiologic fact might be that in Britain, the morbidity ratio of Asian population is insignificantly lower than Caucasians, which is not applicable for non-emigrants (9). In China, AAA is a rare disease, as well as in population of Indonesia (9).

It remains unclear why AAA predominantly affects male population. Almost all the studies that tangle this question, insist on the fact that male population has higher incidence of etiopathogenetic risk factors: arteriosclerosis, smoking, hypertension and elevated blood cholesterol level. Generally speaking, the cause of this fact remains unclear, and as predisposing factors arise hormones, genetic disposition, disposition to atherosclerosis, more frequent risk factors or the combination of aforementioned factors. Singh K and Bønaa KH from famous University Hospital of Tromsø, Norway, in their study including 6.386 subjest of both sexes, established the diagnosis of AAA using sonographic screening , in 263 (8.9%) males and 74 (2.2%) females (9,20). Bearing in mind that subjects ranged in age (form 24-85 years), they compared the diameter of infrarenal aorta in terms of age and concluded that in male population there was a progressive growth in diameter of infrarenal aorta during the process of ageing. The effect of elevated plasma fibrinogen level in male population also remained unclear (8,11,44).

In terms of age distribution, Caucasian patients are statistically significantly younger than Asian patients (for 15 years). Compared to other studies, European patients are shown to be significantly younger than in other Caucasian populations (21,40). This data becomes interesting if we analyze distribution by age subgroups, where dominant incidence in white race population is found in the subgroup of patients younger than 64 (66%), while almost half of these patients are even younger than 54. The same distribution is shown in the control group of this population. On the other hand, in the Asian group of patients, AAA occurs in much older population- dominant incidence was found in the subgroup of older than 75 (54,8%). In the light of these results, we can analyze AAA as a primary disease (in white race) or in the setting of generalized atherosclerotic pathologic changes in the process of ageing (yellow race). Special attention must be paid to EVAR procedure in the group of elderly population, patients with cardiopulmonary and cerebrovascular insufficiency.

Definite conclusion is that the incidence of AAA increases with age, which is explained by prolonged impact of risk factors, long period between latency of risk factors and aneurysm development, and increased sensitivity of aorta to risk factors in the process of ageing. Hypothetically, changes in elastin structure cause increased mechanic stress on collagen which forms a strong fiber network. Experiment models of aneurysmatic blood vessels showed that isolated destruction of elastin led to dilatation of the vessel for 25-65%; also, following dilatation and possible rupture occur due to the alteration of collagen (6). Half-life of elastin is considered to be 75 years, and aorta of adult does not have the ability to produce functional elastin (6,7,42).

In terms of correlation patient height in study population and control groups, we obtained expected results. There is a statistically significant difference in the average height (Caucasian population is 17 cm taller than Asian population, dominant group in Asian population are patients shorter than 160 cm, while in Caucasians dominant group consists of patients over 171 cm)(17,29).

Further, there is statistically significant difference in body weight in study populations-European patients weigh 25.6 kg more than the Asian population, on average. This might be explained by obesity as a modern social-medicine phenomenon in developed countries where there is an increase in AAA incidence. Body weight in this study arised as statistically significant risk factor for the development of AAA.

Considering the level of nutrition, in the yellow race the dominant group consisted of normal weighted (70,97%), while there was no obese subjects (with BMI over 30) in this population. On the other hand, in the white race population over 50% patients were overweighted and obese. BMI can be observed as a universal parameter nondependent of the race, and obtain valid results with the use of simple statistical models (21). This parameter excludes race constitutional features and heterogeneity of the subjects in terms of body weight and body height, since last two parameters in 20% of observed patients and control subjects showed no statistically significant difference. If we use BMI value of 23 (approximate height of 170cm and weight of 58kg-mean BMI value in both groups of patients BMI=22,04±3,77 for Asian group and BMI=25,38±3,19 for Caucasian group) as observation criterion, instead of race, and divide all the subjects in two subgroups, BMI-1 (BMI<23) and BMI-2 (BMI>23), a correlation of antropologic and morphologic parameters calculated by MDCT aortography can be obtained (21).

In this study, there was no statistically significant difference in the presence of risk factors in subjects of both groups. In the Asian population, only 3,2% showed no risk factors present, while in the Caucasian population this percentage was 3,3%. Since patients with no risk factors present represent statistically insignificant subgroup in both populations, we can consider the presence of risk factors as a leading impact factor on the pathogenesis of the development of AAA. Considering the number of present risk factors, in Caucasian population the dominant group consists of patient with 3 or 4 risk factors (40% + 30% = 70%), while in Asian population dominant group consists of patients with 2 or 3 risk facotrs present (45,2% + 19,4% = 64,6%). In terms of the presence and number of RF in patients of both races, there is statistically significant difference in development of the disease. In Asian population, AAA occurs most frequently in patients with 2 RF (with 1 or 2 RF: 64,6%) while in white race this percentage is almost 3 times lower, only 23,3%. As a conclusion, Asian population seems to be more prone to the development of this disease.

The number of associated risk factors in patients of Asian population is statistically significantly higher than in control subjects of the same population. Over 40% (41,54%) control subjects in this population showed no risk factors present, while 25,3% showed only 1 RF present. Number of subjects with 3 associated RF is insignificant (2,3%), while there were no subjects with all 4 RF present. In total, there was statistically significant difference in the presence of risk factors in the patients and controls of the Asian population. In the same term, there is a positive correlation in the presence of risk factors in the patients and controls in European population also, while it is especially applicable for the presence of 3 or 4 associated risk factors.

Tha analysis of the results considering smoking as risk factor in all the study subjects independently of race and smoking history, there was statistically significant number of smokers in both subgroups of patients compared to controls. The analysis of the results considering male and female populations showed that in patients of both populations smoking represents an extremely significant risk factor for the development of AAA. The results of multivariant logistic regresssion analysis were concordant.

On the contrary, hypertension as a risk factor in this study was proven to be controversial. In both races, the number of patients with hypertension was not significantly different than the number of normotensive patients. Epidemiologically significant finding was that in Asian population the number of normotensive patients was for 17% higher than hypertensive, while in European population there was 20% more hypertensive than normotensive patients. Generally speaking, in patients of both populations, hypertension is more commonly found than in control subjects, especially in the European population.

One of the referring studies considering pathogenesis of peripheral vascular diseases (McConathy, Oklahoma Medical Research Foundation) showed that in AAA, the level of cholesterol in plasma is lower than in patients with stenotic-occlusive arterial diseases, as well as VLDL level and apolipoprotein B, C-III and E. Total cholesterol is shown to be a stastically significant factor in the study of Reed-a et al. performed in integrated clinical-autopsy study in the 20-year period on 8000 men living in Hawaii (9). This study predominantly addressed the question of atherosclerosis as a risk risk factor in the development of AAA. The results concordant to this study were obtained in the Whitehall study of Strachan, published in British Journal of Surgery in 2005 considering younger population. Integrated epidemiologic study included 18.403 men, aged 40-64, working as accountants, in the period of 18 years. There were 99 lethal cases of ruptured AAA, and smoking and elevated systolic presure were isolated. Considering type of cholesterol, LDL and less importantly VLDL, are considered the dominant risk factor by many previous studies on this subject.

The analysis of results considering diabetes melitus (DM) as a risk factor in this study showed some unexpected results. The first „paradoxal" finding was extremely low number of patients in both groups with DM (3 patients in each group), with no significant difference between groups. In control groups of both populations, the incidence of DM is lower than 30%, with no statistically significant difference between controls and patients in both poulations. The unexpected result is that higher incidence of DM is found not in patient, but in control group of both populations. The most stunning result is the correlation of the presence of DM in patients and controls of the white race, where disease is significantly more frequent in the control subjects. These results raise the question: Does DM have etiopathogenetic correlation with the development of AAA, or closer to the results of this study- is DM some kind of protective factor in the AAA development? Meta analysis of 11 relevant studies considering correlation of DM and etiopathogenesis of AAA shed light to this „paradox". Out of 11, 4 studies were excluded for no existing or inadequate control group. The rest of the studies showed that there is a small possibility of associated DM in patients with AAA (OR=0.65, 0.60-0.70, p<0.001)(30). 3 referring studies found decreased prevalence of DM in patients with AAA (17,18,20).

8. Evaluation of morphologic measurements

European population showed statistically significantly longer neck of the aneurysm. With the premise that the length of the neck of 15 mm is the minimal infrarenal distance needed for graft insertion, this study showed that 31,7% patients in the Asian populaion had contraindication for EVAR, e. g. length of the neck of the AAA shorter than 15 mm. Furthermore, the mean length of the anuerysmatic neck in this population is 18,49 mm. Analyzing the subgroup of the Asian population with the neck length < 15 mm, we found that in 8 of 11 patients this length was < 10 mm, 9 mm on average.

The neck of AAA is the place of the proximal insertion of the graft, and in most cases there is a small distance between the normal and pathologic structures of aortic wall. The largest number of EVAR complications, of endoleak type, occur in this proximal part of graft insertion (43). CT aortography (CT fluoroscopy), as a dynamic analysis, enables monitoring of contrast agent flow along the aorta, or the region of interest established in examination protocol. More accurately, due to small slice thickness (0,625 mm), high spatial and temporal resolution, possibility of retroreconstruction in postprocessing at the distance of 0,2 mm and other technical features of this exam, it is possible to analyze CT exam as continuous video-recording in various visualization extensions. Also, „film" can be stoppped and paused in every moment to analyze the segment in 3D and 4D projetions, in all planes and projections.

Valuable advantage of these possibilities is that aorta, AAA and graft can be evaluated in all morphologic features, from the lateral aspects and also as ortogonally isolated transverse projections, a feature which cannot be performed using conventional aortography. These visualization possibilities favour MDCT over conventional aortography or catheter aortography. Beside the fact that it is a non-invasive procedure, additional advantage is that more diagnostic information on the early complications, such as proximal endoleak, can be obtained. Exceptional software features in standard postprocessing alow measuring of the contrast flow rate above the insertion place, inside the graft and distally, as well as different features of AAA before theraputic procedure. Critical moment for the development of proximal endoleak is physical contact of the contrast (blood) with graft contours. As it advances in cranio-caudal direction, contrast flow rate changes as a function of age, constitutional and hemodynamic cardiovascular parameters (stroke volume, width of aorta, degree of sclerotic changes, tortuosity, dilatation, etc.), but usually varies in range of 20-40 cm/sec. If the length of AAA neck is at the critical value (10-20 cm) this contact occurs in the place where vessel wall is already weakened, and its contractility, elasticity and histology are changed. Proximal endoleak can occur anywhere in the upper circumference of the graft, can be minimal, discrete and without clinical manifestations. Also, it can remain minimal in a long period of time, but usually there is a certain degree of progression, dilatation and degradation of the graft function.

Due to physical contact and strike of contrast flow onto the upper edge of the graft, the speed with which blood continues to flow, decreases gradually. Presumption is that the velocity gradient directly influences the possibility of proximal endoleak occurrence. Developing this hypothesis, in the sense of possible clinical implications and technical advances, study offered the idea that the first contact of contrast and graft occurs suprarenally, e. g. 2-3 cm cranially of the insertion place. As a consequence, in last 10 years, fenestrated grafts with suprarenal insertions have become comercially available (44,45). In this tudy, a new design of graft for AAA treatment is proposed, for patients with short aneurysmatic neck. Inovation is the annular extension of existing graft that is continuous with the basic graft on the back side, while it is opened on the front and lateral sides, where is also the orifice of renal arteries. If the force of contrast stroke at MDCT exam is marked as F1 in the common concept of insertion place, and as F2 in the proposed graft design with suprarenal insertion, we could say that F2>F1 and that blood, distally from the suprarenal insertion flows continuously with lower speed (29).

The angle between aneurysm and sagittal plane of aorta in Asian population was significantly larger than in Caucasian. Also, in Asian population there were no patients with contraindication for EVAR (considering mean angle and standard deviation), while in Caucasian population, this number was not statistically significant.

On the contrary to the length of infrarenal aorta, a.i.c. in control group of Caucasian population was statistically significantly longer than in Asian. The mean length of both femoral arteries in white race population was about 14 mm higher than in yellow race, which was statistically significant. There was no significant difference in the length of infrarenal aorta between Asian and Caucasian population, but the linear distance between lower renal artery and bifurcation was significantly higher in European patient group (mean value was about 20 mm longer). This result can be explained by variations in the angle of AAA. Compared to the Hong Kong authors, this study found that linear distance in the white race patients was twice longer (40).

Transverse CT measurements considering flow diameter were performed in advanced CT aortography postprocessing programme, after transverse visualizations in graphic tool „X-section". This software tool enables contouring flow diameter along complete length and is used for differentiating contrast agent from intraluminal and intramural calcifications, while it enables continuity and accuracy in measuring in each segment.

There was significant difference between the study populations at the level of largest and smallest flow diameter below main trunks of renal arteries (F.d. a.a. 1-2) as well as total diameter of aneurysm with the vessel wall structures at the level of maximum width of aneurysm (R.d. a.a. 3-4). Especially significant was the difference between diameters R.d. a.a. 3-4. To the best of our knowledge, there are no similar results published in literature, nor have these measurements been performed in populations of different races. CT aortographic measurements performed in this study were inspired by problems that doctors who perform EVAR encountered due to incompatibility of the comercially available grafts for the patients of yellow race.

Infrarenal segment of aorta in patients with AAA is a nondilated part. However, the fact that infrarenal segment of aorta in all the subject of Asian population was significantly wider than transverse diameter of control subjects, and additionally, that it is related to the neck which is not dialated in transverse diameter, leads to conclusion that AAA patients in general have wider aneurysmatic neck than infarenal segment of control subjects (with discrete aortic dilatation or normal findings). Furthermore, the width of this segment may be disposing factor for the development of AAA or/and vice versa, that the development of AAA leads to dilatation of the aneurysmatic neck.

Most of the studies showed that the diameter of abominal aorta aneurysm grows for 0,08 cm annually, so the most accurate conclusions could be obtained by comparing subjects of the same age (29,40).

Asian population with the presence of aneurysm had significanty higher following diameters F.d. a.i.c. 2-6 i R-d. a.i.c. 1-6. compared to controls, while in F.d. a.i.c 1 there was no significant difference. The most prominent result was found in the transverse diameters F.d. a.c.i 1 of patients and controls. This was the only parameter where there was no difference in patients and controls of the Asian population, while in Caucasian there was a border-line difference. The exact place is just above the bifurcation, where depending on the bifurcation angle, there is a different flow gradient that correlates with the angle of bifurcation, which is lower in the population of yellow race. Additionally, there is a subtle difference between the blood flow velocity of the aorta and proximal parts of iliac arteries. The changes in the vessel wall, as well as propagation of the aneurysm from aorta to iliac arteries, have no direct impact on Fd diameter.

9. Possibilities of computer integration in postprocedural evaluation of AAA

In the preprocedural evaluation of EVAR method, nowadays the use of separate workstation is common. It is often used by vascular surgeons in order to obtain 3D visualization and measuring in individual case, for precise planning and choice of suitable type and dimensions of the graft. Actually, they use specially developed software applications on Windows platform, which are suitable for personal computers; widely spread are „3Mensio surgery", "TeraRecon" and "OsiriX".

This study showed that there is clearly defined user's need to upgrade MDCT aortography postprocessing and integrate it with softwares alowing typization and individualization of stent grafts in each case, as a definite preprocedural finding, similar to stenting procedures in non-vascular interventional radiology.

10. Conclusion

This study showed that modern imaging techniques, particularly high-resolution MDCT diagnositcs, discovered fresh and unexpected possibilities to obtain new knowledge on anatomy and morphology of the human body, as well as numerous clinical implications, applicable to all organs, organic systems, pathologic and pathophysiologic features, and studies in the field of anatomy.

The use of modern low-dose MDCT diagnostics will allow the development of screening programmes for many diseases of enormous diagnostic significance, related to blood vessels, such as coronary disease, cerebrovascular insuficiency, arteriosclerosis etc. In conclusion, the possibilities of correlating anatomy and morphology of different races in the context of a particular disease or planned study are limitless with use of CT diagnostics.

Author details

Ana Mladenovic* and Zeljko Markovic
Faculty of Medicine Belgrade University, Clinical Center of Serbia, Center of Radiology and Magnetic Resonance, Serbia

Sandra Grujicic-Sipetic
Institute of Epidemiology Faculty of Medicine Belgrade University, Serbia

Hideki Hyodoh
Department of Radiology, Sapporo Medical University, Sapporo, Japan

Acknowledgments

Edition of this chapter is supported by GE Healthcare - Technopharm, Belgrade, Serbia.

11. References

[1] Ernst CB (1993) Abdominal aortic aneurysm. N Engl J Med. 328:1167–1172
[2] Dalen JE. (1983) Diseases of the aorta. In: Petersdorf RG, Adams RD, Braunwald E, et al., eds. Harrison's principles of internal medicine. 10th ed. New York, NY: McGraw-Hill Book Company. pp.1488-91.
[3] Thompson RW, Geraghty PJ, Lee JK (2002) Abdominal aortic aneurysms: Basic mechanisms and clinical implications. Curr Probl Surg. 39(2):110–230.
[4] Beckman JA (2006) Aortic aneurysms: pathophysiology, epidemiology, and prognosis .In: Creager MA , Dzau VJ , Loscalzo J , eds. Vascular Medicine . Philadelphia:Saunders Elsevier, Inc . pp. 543 – 559.
[5] Tilson MD, Gandhi RH (1995) Arterial aneurysms: etiological considerations. In: Rutherford RB, ed. Vascular surgery. 4th ed. Philadelphia, PA: WB Saunders Company. pp. 253-64.
[6] Anidjar S, Kieffer E. (1992) Pathogenesis of acquired aneurysms of the abdominal aorta. Ann Vase Surg. 6:298-305.
[7] Patel MI, Hardman DT, Fisher CM, et al. 1995) Current views on the pathogenesis of abdominal aortic aneurysms. J Am Coll, Surg. 181:371-82.

* Corresponding Author

[8] Dobrin PB. (1989) Pathophysiology and pathogenesis of aortic aneurysms: current concepts. Surg Clin North Am 69: 687-703.

[9] James F. Blanchard (1999) Epidemiology of Abdominal Aortic Aneurysms, Epidemiologic Reviews by The Johns Hopkins University School of Hygiene and Public Health. Vol. 21, No. 2

[10] Stephen W.K. Cheng, Albert C.W. Ting and Simon H.Y. Tsang (2003) Epidemiology and Outcome of Aortic Aneurysms in Hong Kong, World Journal of Surgery. 2, 241-245.

[11] Yii MK. (2003) Epidemiology of abdominal aortic aneurysm in an Asian population. Source, ANZ J Surgery 73(6):393-5.

[12] Spark JI, Baker JL, Vowden P, Wilkinson D. Source (2001) Epidemiology of abdominal aortic aneurysms in the Asian community. Br J Surg. 88(3):382-4.

[13] Vowden P, Wilkinson D. (2001) Epidemiology of abdominal aortic aneurysms in the Asian community. Br J Surg. 88(3):382-4.

[14] Wei WI, Siu KF, Wong J. (1985) Abdominal aortic aneurysm in Chinese patients. Br J Surg. 72(11):900-2.

[15] Oxlund H, Rasmussen LM, Andreassen TT. (1989) Increased aortic stiffness in patients with type 1 (insulin-dependent) diabetes mellitus. Diabetologia 32:748-52.

[16] Forouhi NG, Merrick D, Goyder E, Ferguson BA, Abbas J,Lachowycz K. (2006) Diabetes prevalence in England, 2001 estimates from an epidemiological model. Diabet Med. 23(2):189-97.

[17] Wild S, Roglic G, Green A, Sicree R, King H. (2004)Global prevalence of diabetes: estimates for the year 2000 and projections for 2030. Diabetes Care. 27(5):1047-53.

[18] Ubink-Veltmaat LJ, Bilo HJ, Groenier KH, Houweling ST, Rischen RO, Meyboom-de Jong B. (2003) Prevalence, incidence and mortality of type 2 diabetes mellitus revisited: a prospective population-based study in The Netherlands (ZODIAC-1). Eur J Epidemiol. 18(8):793-800

[19] Kang SS, Littooy FN, Gupta SR. (1999) Higher prevalence of abdominal aortic aneurysms in patients with carotid stenosis but without diabetes. Surg. 126:687–692.

[20] Popov Petar, Ružićić Dušan, Babić Srđan, Tanasković Slobodan, Gajin Predrag. Lozuk Branko, Radak Đorđe. (2011) Učestalost pojave aneurizme abdominalne aorte u bolesnika sa diabetes mellitusom, Medicinska istraživanja. 45:23-34.

[21] Ana S. Mladenovic, Zeljko Markovic, Hideki H Hyodoh, and Tatjana Stosic-Opincal. (2012) Correlation of CT Aortography Measurements of Infrarenal Aortic Aneurysms and Body Mass Index in Preprocedural Evaluation for Endovascular Repair, Clinical Anatomy. DOI 10.1002/ca.22027

[22] Stephen WK, Cheng, Albert CW, Ting, Pei Ho, Jensen T. P. (2004) Poon Aortic Aneurysm Morphology in Asians: Features Affecting Stent-Graft Application and Design. Journal of Endovascular Therapy. 6: 605-612.

[23] Cambria Richard P., LaMuraglie Glenn M., Gertler Jonathan P., Abbott William M., Waltman Arthur C. (2000) Endovascular Repair of Abdominal Aortic Aneurysm: Current Status and Future Directions, AJR: 175:332-343

[24] Ahn SS, Rutherford RB, Johnston KW. Reporting standards for infrarenal endovascular abdominal aortic aneurysm repair. J Vasc Surg. 1997;25:405-410.

[25] Carpenter JP, Baum RA, Barker CF, Golden MA, Mitchell ME, Velazquez OC, Fairman RM. (2001) Impact of exclusion criteria on patient selection for endovascular abdominal aortic anerysm repair. J Vasc Surg. 34:150-4.

[26] Parody JC, Palmaz JC, Barone HD. (1991) Transfemoral intraluminal graft implantation for abdominal aortic aneurysms. Ann Vasc Surg 5(6):491-499.

[27] MacSweeney ST, Powell JT, Greenhalgh RM. (1994) Pathogenesis of abdominal aortic aneurysm. Br J Surg 81:935-41.

[28] Lazar Davidović, Miroslav Marković, Dušan Kostić, Ilijas Činara, Dragan Marković, Živan Maksimović, Slobodan D. Cvetković, Radomor B. Sinđelić, Tanja Illc. Ruptured Abdominal Aortic Aneurysms: Factors Infl uencing Early Survival. Ann Vasc Surg. (2005) 19(1): 29-34.

[29] Ana S. Mladenovc, Zeljko Z. Markovic, Hideki H. Hyodoh, Sandra Grujicic-Sipetic, NakajimaYasuo. (2011) Quantification of Dilated InfrarenalAorta by 64 Multidetector Computed Tomographic Evaluationin Preventing EVAR Complications in Patients of Different Races, Journal of Computer Assisted Tomography. 35 462-467

[30] Hirose Y, Hamada S, Takamiya M. (1992) Aortic aneurysms: growth rates measured with CT. Radiology 185:249-52.

[31] Bellon EM, Miraldi FD, Wiesen EJ. (2004) Performance evaluation of computed tomography scanners using a phantom model. Am J Roentgenol;132:345-352.

[32] Rubin GD. (2001) Techniques for performing multidetector-row computed tomographic angiography. Tech Vasc Interv Radiol. 4: 2-14.

[33] Pamela T. Johnson, Jennifer K. Chen, Bart L Loeys, Harry C. Dietz, Elliot K. Fishman. (2007) MDCT Angiography Findings, AJR 2007;189:226.

[34] Flohr TG, Schaller S, Stierstorfer K, Bruder H, Ohnesorge BM, Schoepf UJ. (2005) Multi-Detector Row CT Systems and Image-Reconstruction Techniques, Radiology 235:756-773.

[35] Saini S. (2004) Multi-Detector Row CT: Principles and Practice for Abdominal Applications Radiology. 233:323-327.

[36] Lederle FA, Walker JM, Reinke DB. (1988) Selective screening for abdominal aortic aneurysms with physical examination and ultrasound. Arch Intern Med. 148:1753-6.

[37] Collin J, Araujo L, Walton J. (1988) Oxford screening programme for abdominal aortic aneurysm in men aged 65 to 74 years. Lancet. 2:613-15.

[38] Arko FR, Filis KA, Seidel SA. How many patients with infrarenal aneurysms are candidates for endovascular repair? (2004) The Northern California experience. J Endovasc Ther. 11:33–40.

[39] Brewster DC , Cronenwett JL. (2003) Guidelines for the treatment of abdominal aortic aneurysms. Report of a subcommittee of the Joint Council of the American Association for Vascular Surgery and Society for Vascular Surgery . J Vasc Surg. 37(5) :1106 – 17

[40] Ana S Mladenović, Zeljko Z Markovic, Hideki H Hyodoh. (2011) Anatomic differences of the distal aorta with dilatation or aneurysm between patients from Asia and Europe as seen on CT imaging. European Journal of Radiology, doi:10.1016/j.ejrad.2011.05.014

[41] Brewster DC, Cronenwett JL, Haller, Jr JW, Johnston KW, Krupski WC, Matsumura JS. (2003) Guidelines for the treatment of abdominal aortic aneurysm: report of a subcommittee of the Joint Council of the American Association for Vascular Surgery and Society for Vascular Surgery. J Vasc Surg 37:1106-1117

[42] Alcorn HG, Wolfson SK Jr, Sutton-Tyrrell K. (1996) Risk factors for abdominal aortic aneurysms in older adults enrolled in the Cardiovascular Health Study. Arterioscler Thromb Vase Biol. 16:963-70.

[43] Brewster DC , Cronenwett JL. (2003) Guidelines for the treatment of abdominal aortic aneurysms. Report of a subcommittee of the Joint Council of the American Association for Vascular Surgery and Society for Vascular Surgery . J Vasc Surg. 37 (5) :1106-17.

[44] Greenhalgh RM , Brown LC , Kwong GP , Powell JT , Thompson SG. (2004) EVAR trial participants. Comparison of endovascular aneurysm repair with open repair in patients with abdominal aortic aneurysm (EVAR trial 1), 30-day operative mortality results: randomised controlled trial . Lancet . 364: 843-8.

[45] Lazarus HM. (1992) Endovascular grafting for the treatment of abdominal aortic aneurysms. Surg Clin North Am 72:959–968.

Chapter 7

Splenic Artery Aneurysms

Ahmad Alsheikhly

Additional information is available at the end of the chapter

http://dx.doi.org/10.5772/46031

1. Introduction

The spleen is a wedge-shaped organ that lies in relation to the 9th and 11th ribs, located in the left upper quadrant of the abdomen (left hypochondrium), and partly in the epigastrium; thus, it is situated between the fundus of the stomach and the diaphragm (see the following image). The spleen is highly vascular and reddish purple; its size and weight are variable. Normally spleen is not palpable.

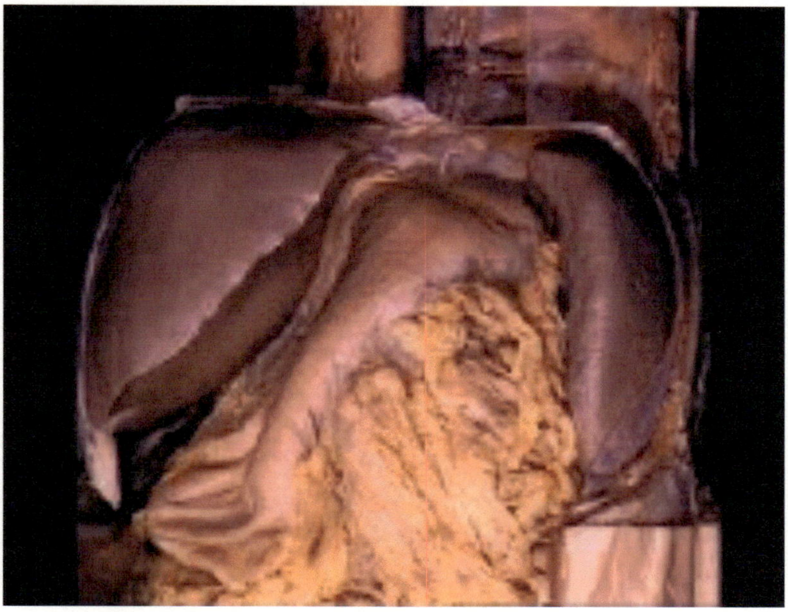

Figure 1.

The spleen develops in the cephalic part of dorsal mesogastrium (from its left layer; during the sixth week of intrauterine life) into a number of nodules that soon fuse to form a lobulated spleen. Notching of the superior border of the adult spleen is evidence of its multiple origins.[1]

The spleen has 2 ends, 3 borders, and 4 surfaces, as follows:

The 2 ends

The anterior end of the spleen is expanded and more like a border; it is directed forward and downward to reach the midaxillary line. The posterior end is rounded; it is directed upward and backward and rests on the upper pole of the left kidney.

The 3 borders

The superior border of the spleen is notched near the anterior end, the inferior border is rounded, and the intermediate border is directed toward the right.

The 2 surfaces

There are 2 surfaces: diaphragmatic and visceral. The diaphragmatic surface is smooth and convex. The visceral surface is irregular and concave and has impressions. The gastric impression is for the fundus of the stomach; this is the largest and most concave impression on the spleen. The renal impression is for the left kidney and lies between the inferior and intermediate borders. The colic impression is for the splenic flexure of the colon; its lower part is related to the phrenicocolic ligament. The pancreatic impression for the tail of the pancreas lies between the hilum and colic impression (see the image below).

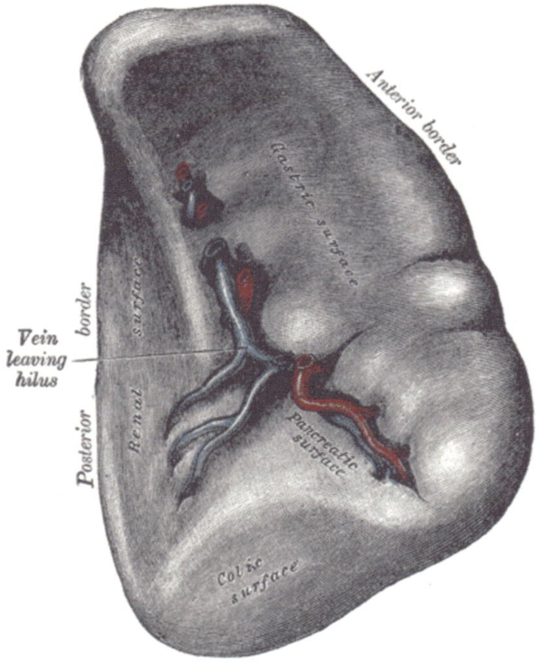

Figure 2. Spleen showing the different surfaces and impressions caused by different organs with relation to the hilum of the spleen.

1.1. Hilum

The hilum lies on the inferomedial part of the gastric impression. It transmits the splenic vessels and nerves and provides attachment to the gastrosplenic and splenorenal (lienorenal) ligaments.

1.2. Peritoneal relations

The spleen is surrounded by peritoneum and is suspended by multiple ligaments, as follows:

The gastrosplenic ligament: This ligament extends from the hilum of the spleen to the greater curvature of the stomach; it contains short gastric vessels and associated lymphatics and sympathetic nerves

The splenorenal ligament: This ligament extends from the hilum of the spleen to the anterior surface of the left kidney; it contains the tail of the pancreas and splenic vessels

The phrenicocolic ligament: This ligament is a horizontal fold of peritoneum extending from the splenic flexure of the colon to the diaphragm in the midaxillary line; it forms the upper end of the left paracolic gutter.

1.3. Visceral relations

The visceral surface of the spleen is related to the following organs:

- The fundus of the stomach
- Anterior surface of the left kidney
- Splenic flexure of the colon
- Tail of the pancreas

The diaphragmatic surface is related to the diaphragm, which separates the spleen from the pleura and the lung.

1.4. Blood supply

The blood supply of the spleen is by the splenic artery (in the past called the lienal artery), which is the largest branch of the celiac trunk. The artery passes through the splenorenal ligament to reach the hilum of the spleen. At the hilum, it divides into multiple branches. Within the spleen, it divides into straight vessels called penicillin, ellipsoids, and arterial capillaries.

The splenic circulation is adapted for the mechanism of separation and storage of the red blood cells. On the basis of the blood supply, the spleen has superior and inferior vascular segments. The 2 segments are separated by an avascular plane.

Apart from its terminal branches, the splenic artery gives off branches to the pancreas, 5-7 short gastric branches, and the left gastro-omental (gastroepiploic) artery (see the image below).

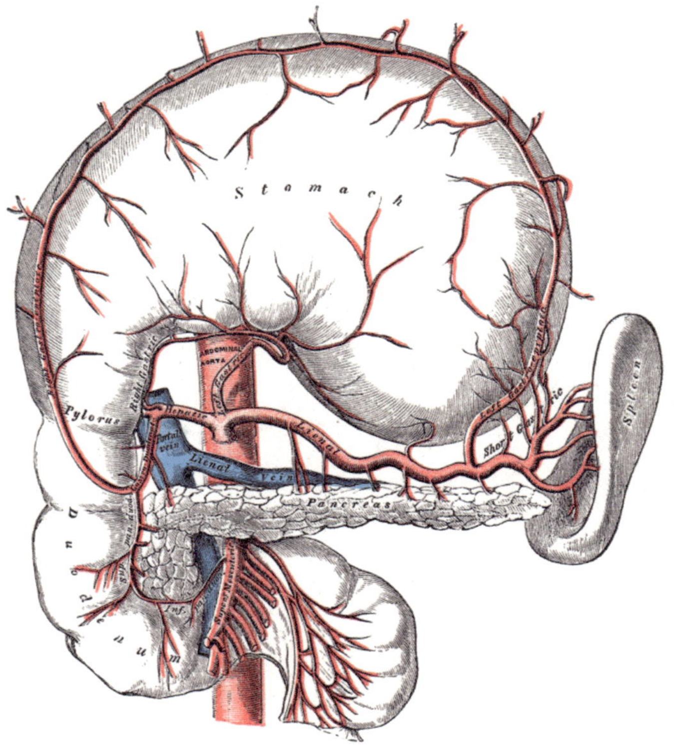

Figure 3.

1.5. Venous drainage

The principal venous drainage of the spleen is through the splenic vein. It is formed at the hilum and runs behind the pancreas then joins the superior mesenteric vein behind the neck of the pancreas to form the portal vein. Its tributaries are the short gastric, left gastro-omental, pancreatic, and inferior mesenteric veins.

1.6. Lymphatic drainage

Splenic tissue proper has no lymphatics. However, a few arise from the capsule and trabeculae and drain to the pancreaticosplenic lymph nodes.

1.7. Nerve supply

Sympathetic fibers are derived from the celiac plexus.[2, 3, 4]

1.8. Surface marking

The spleen is marked on the left side of the back with the long axis of the 10th rib. The upper border is marked along the upper border of the 9th rib; the lower border, along the 11th rib. The medial end lies 5 cm from the midline, and the lateral extension is to the midaxillary line.[5]

Microscopically, the spleen is made up of 4 components: (1) supporting tissue, (2) white pulp, (3) red pulp, and (4) vascular system.

Supporting tissue is fibroelastic and forms the capsule, coarse trabeculae, and a fine reticulum.

The white pulp consists of lymphatic nodules arranged around an eccentric arteriole called the Malpighian corpuscle.

The red pulp is formed by a collection of cells in the interstices of the reticulum, in between the sinusoids. The cell population includes all types of lymphocytes, blood cells, and fixed and free macrophages. The lymphocytes are freely transformed into plasma cells, which can produce large amounts of antibodies and immunoglobulins. The vascular system traverses the spleen and permeates it.[3]

2. Physiologyof the spleen

The spleen is a major hematopoietic organ containing approximately 25 percent of the total lymphoid mass of the body; and it is capable of supporting elements of the erythroid, myeloid, megakaryocytic, lymphoid, monocytic, and macrophagic (reticuloendothelial) systems. As such, it is important in the following situations:

2.1. Phagocytosis

Phagocytosis is one of the most important functions of the spleen. The spleen forms a component of the reticuloendothelial system. The splenic phagocytes include reticular cells, free macrophages of the red pulp, and modified reticular cells of the ellipsoids. The phagocytes present in the organ remove debris, old and effete red blood cells (RBCs), other blood cells, and microorganisms; thus, the splenic phagocytes filter the blood. Phagocytosis of circulating antigens initiates the humoral and cellular immune responses.

This function is most apparent when the spleen has been removed, since splenectomized patients are susceptible to bacterial sepsis, especially with encapsulated organisms.

2.2. Hematopoiesis

The spleen is an important hematopoietic organ during fetal life; lymphopoiesis continues throughout life. The manufactured lymphocytes take part in immune responses of the body. In the adult spleen, hematopoiesis can restart in certain diseases such as chronic myeloid leukemia and myelosclerosis.

2.3. Active immune responses

Following antigenic stimulation, increased lymphopoiesis for cellular responses and increased formation of plasma cells for humoral responses occurs.

2.4. Storage of erythrocytes

The RBCs are stored in the spleen. Approximately 8% of the circulating RBCs are present within the spleen. However, this function is seen well in animals than humans.[6]

3. Splenic Artery Aneurysms (SAAs)

3.1. General considerations

An arterial aneurysm is one of the most common vascular disorders causing morbidity and mortality in humans. It occurs in most arteries of the body and is especially common in the elderly. They have a variable sizes, shapes, and locations.

An aneurysm is defined as a permanent localized dilatation of an artery having at least a 50% increase in diameter compared to the expected normal arterial diameter, so clinicians should know the normal arterial diameters throughout the body to decide the presence or absence of an aneurysm. [7]

Splenic artery aneurysms are a type of splanchnic arteries aneurysm, although the later are rare but clinically very important vascular conditions. These interesting lesions have been recognized since more than 200 years. [8, 9]

Splanchnic artery aneurysms represent intra-abdominal aneurysms that are not part of the aorto-iliac system and include aneurysms of the celiac, superior and inferior mesenteric arteries with their branches.

Of all intra-abdominal aneurysms, only approximately 5% affect the splanchnic arteries. (10) In general population, their prevalence has been estimated to be varying from 0.1% to 2 %. [11]

The frequency of the anatomic distribution of the splanchnic arteries aneurysms is estimated to be the following:

1. Splenic artery aneurysms (SAAs), 60% (see the image below).
2. Hepatic artery, 20%
3. Superior mesenteric artery, 6%
4. Celiac artery, 4%
5. Gastric and gasrtoepiploic arteries, 4%
6. Jejunal, ileal, and colic arteries, 3%
7. Pancreaticoduodenal and pancreatic arteries, 2%
8. Gastroduodenal artery, less than 1.5%
9. Inferior mesenteric artery, less than 1%. (11)

3.2. Prevalence and epidemiology

SAAs are the most common of the splanchnic artery aneurysms and account for as many as 60% of all reported splanchnic aneurysms. They are recognized for their significant potential

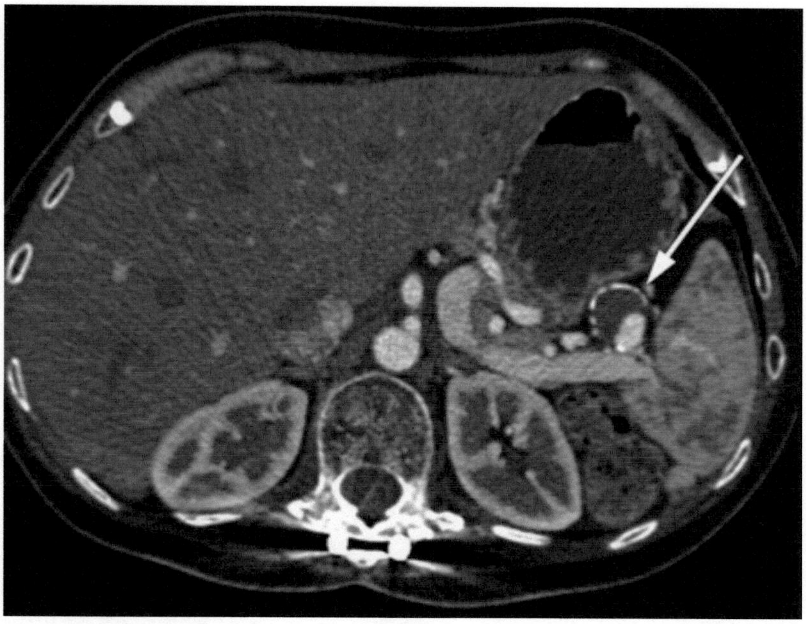

Figure 4. A Peripherally calcified, and thrombosed splenic artery aneurysm, (CT view)

to rupture. In spite of their relatively high prevalence in comparison to other splanchnic aneurysms, there are few large series in the literature. The prevalence of the lesion in the general population is low. A large general autopsy study estimated their all incidence to be 0.01 %(12), whereas more specific examination of the splenic arteries in an autopsy study of patients older than 60 years revealed an incidence of 10 %(13).

The prevalence of incidentally noted aneurysmal changes in the splenic artery on arteriographic studies was reported to be 0.78%, and such changes have been found incidentally in 0.1% to 10% of autopsies. (11).

In contrast to routine atherosclerotic or degenerative aneurismal diseases, SAAs are found much more commonly in women than in men with an approximate ratio of 4:1. (11), they are also noted to occur in younger patients at a mean age of 52 years. (14)

SAAs are usually saccular and less than 2 cm in diameter, with the majority being in the mid or distal portion of the splenic artery or at its bifurcation points. (14)

Giant SAAs with diameter larger than 10 cm have been reported, and in contrast to smaller SAAs, these lesions appear to be more common in men. (15)

3.3. Pathogenesis and aetiology

The most clinical risk factors are the following:

1. Female gender.
2. Multiple pregnancies.

3. Portal hypertension.
4. Systemic hypertension.
5. Arterial fibrodysplasia.
6. chronic inflammatory processes
7. Arteriosclerosis.
8. Less commonly, polyarteritis nodosa, systemic lupus erythematosus, and anomalous splenic artery origin. (16).

In one reported series, it was noted that 80% of the patients with SAAs were females who had an average of 4.5 pregnancies and 50% of females with SAAs had more than 6 pregnancies. (17, 18).

Portal hypertension may be present in 25% of patients with SAAs, while about 10% are awaiting liver transplantation. (19).

Blunt splenic trauma and pancreatitis frequently noted in association with SAAs. Local hemodynamic aspects, hormonal factors, and medial degeneration have all been considered as causative factors in the development of SAAs. (20).

Increased blood volume which results into increased cardiac output, and portal congestion are thought to be related to an increased splenic artery blood flow and SAAs formation. (21).

Impaired elastin formation and degeneration of the internal elastic lamina could be added as hormonal factors which contribute to SAAs formation during pregnancy; It seems that splenic artery is more susceptible to these changes than other vessels. (22).

Histological changes which are noted microscopically during SAAs formation include calcifications, intimal hyperplasia, arterial dysplasia, fibromuscular dysplasia, and medial degeneration. (23).

3.4. Clinical and diagnostic aspects of splenic artery aneurysms

Most SAAs are found incidentally at the time of first presentation during abdominal imaging examination for unrelated disorders. A classic calcified ring may be noted in the left upper abdominal quadrant on a plain x—ray film of the abdomen. (see the image below):

There may be an abdominal bruit, but the majority of cases are showing normal physical examinations especially with asymptomatic patients.

Symptoms are including the following:

1. Vague abdominal pain, nausea and vomiting.(24).
2. Symptoms related to compression of adjacent organs.
3. Sever left-sided pain due to rupture or acute aneurysm expansion.
4. Shock, abdominal distension, and death due to intraperitoneal rupture.
5. Double-rupture phenomenon which may occur in bout 20% to 30% of cases provides a proper diagnosis of rupture into the lesser sac, before free intraperitoneal rupture diagnosed.(25,26).
6. Gastrointestinal tract, pancreatic ducts, or splenic vein rupture.(27).

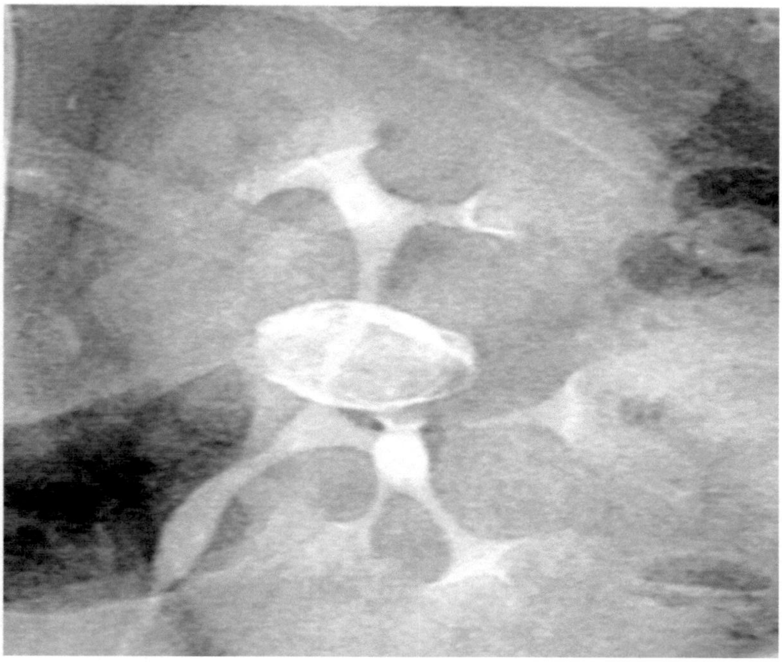

Figure 5.

The overall mortality of ruptured SAAs is about 25%.(26). Pregnancy may be associated with a rate of 20% to 50% of all ruptures.(28).

The association of SAAs and pregnancy is very well documented, in addition to that rupture during pregnancy usually occurs at the third trimester which can lead to maternal and fetal death of 80% to 90%, respectively.(29). Actually this can lead to understand the misdiagnosis of the situation as an obstetric emergency.

Rupture due to portal hypertension is associated with a rate of about 20% .(30).

3.5. Treatment of splenic artery aneurysms

Ruptured , symptomatic SAAs, and those in pregnant women require urgent treatment. Enlarging or those greater than 2 cm in diameter SAAs have less stringent indications, although these criteria are not absolute. Patients with portal hypertension or waiting for liver transplantation should be treated as well.(31). Patient's medical condition and age could play a role the treatment option. Most vascular surgeons would consider suitable elective intervention for asymptomatic patients with lesions those diameter is greater than 2 cm when the surgical risk is thought to be low. If one estimates the incidence of rupture to be 2% with a death rate of at least 25% when rupture has occurred, operative mortality rates should be less than 0.5% to justify elective surgical treatment, in one author's study.(31).

Traditional operative therapy of SAAs includes proximal and distal ligation or aneurysmectomy or both modalities for lesions in the proximal or middle part of the splenic artery.(see the images below).

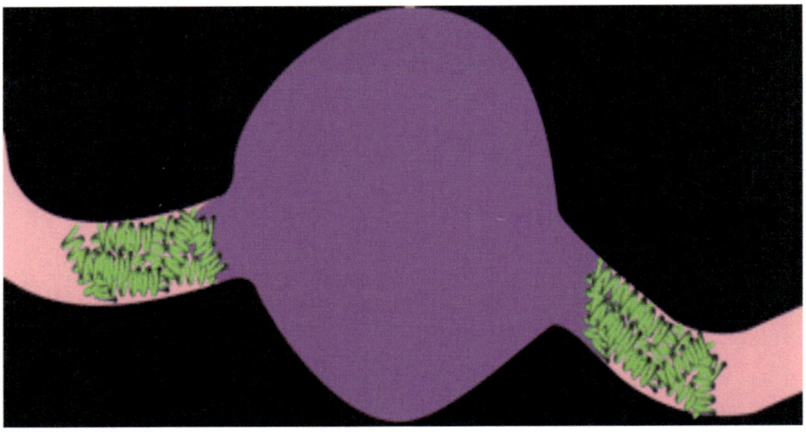

Figure 6. Drawing illustrates how coils are placed distal and then proximal to the aneurysm, thereby trapping the aneurysm and isolating it from the circulation, with resultant thrombosis of the aneurysm.

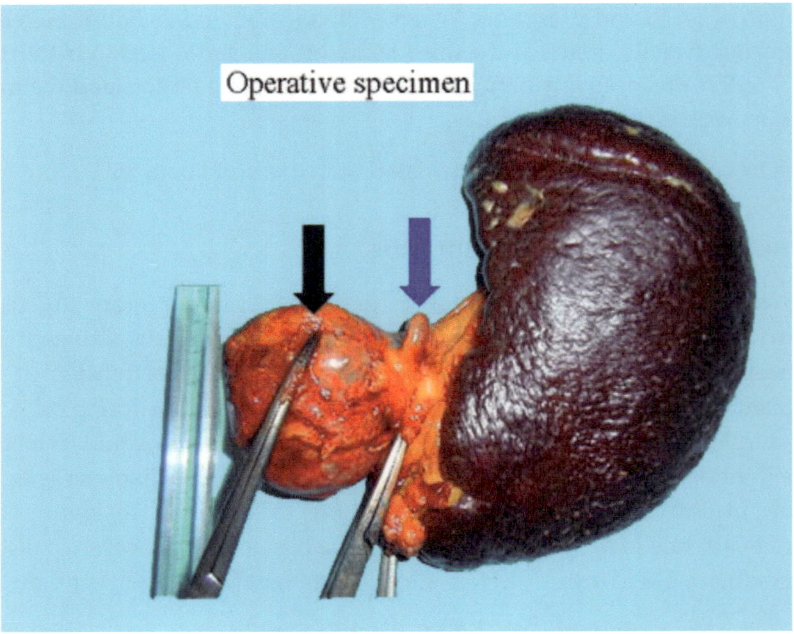

Figure 7.

Revascularization of the distal splenic artery in not generally warranted due to that collateral flow to the spleen in maintained by the short gastric arteries. For those lesions near to the splenic hilum, splenectomy is the most common procedure. Distal pancreatectomy may occasionally be needed for the treatment of these distal lesions as well. (24, 31, 32 and 33).

Laparoscopic repair of SAAs by clipping or exclusion has been reported; intraoperative ultrasonography is believed to be an important adjunct to this procedure.(34). Laparoscopic occlusion combined with coil embolization has been proposed as a treatment for aberrant SAAs located in the retropancreatic position, for which traditional procedures would be exceptionally difficult.(24,35).

Endovascular exclusion of SAAs has been used more recently with good success. Treatment options include coil embolization of the splenic artery both proximal and distal to the aneurysm itself, thereby effectively trapping the lesion. Other options include embolization of the aneurysm sac with coils or cyanoacrylate glue or both modalities simultaneously or occlusion of the lesion with percutaneous or open thrombin injection.(24,36). In addition, stent-grafting has been performed, especially for saccular lesions of the mid splenic artery. There has been some concern regarding splenic infarction and pancreatitis when embolization of very distal splenic artery lesions has been performed. (24, 37 and 38).

The objective of splenic arterial embolization is to improve the results of nonsurgical management. Indications for splenic arterial embolization vary, depending on local management protocols. embolization is performed with microcoils as distally as possible, to preserve perfusion to the splenic parenchyma. Patients with a high risk for secondary rupture of the aneurysm should undergo embolization with coils in a more proximal segment of the splenic artery to reduce the pressure in the splenic parenchyma and help the reservation of the spleen. The placement of coils in a middle segment of the splenic artery allows reconstitution of the blood supply through collateral vessels, principally via the short gastric and gastroepiploic arteries, to the patent distal splenic, transgastric, and transpancreatic arteries. Proximal embolization performed exclusively with coils decreases the volume of splenic arterial blood flow and thereby produces relative hypotension in the splenic bed, which allows the spleen to repair itself without infarction (39)

In a review of 48 endovascular procedures for splanchnic artery pseudoaneurysms, 20 interventions on the splenic artery were performed. Six end-organ infarcts were noticed, all were within the splenic bed. Two additional patients developed splenic atrophy diagnosed on CT scanning after previous embolization of the splenic artery, without clear clinical evidence of initial splenic infarction. (40). In another study, one episode of splenic infarction associated with sever pancreatitis was noted after embolization of a distal splenic artery aneurysm. (37). (see the image below).

Post-embolization transverse contrast-enhanced CT scan obtained at follow-up shows a coil within the splenic artery (arrow), as well as complete infarction of the spleen, which is not contrast enhanced.

However, other authors have reported splenic infarction after embolization of even more proximal SAAs as well. (41).

3.6. Results of different treatment options for splenic artery aneurysms:

The results of open operative therapy are dependent on whether the procedure is an elective or emergency one, in addition to the anatomical complexity of the lesion and the nature of the required repair. Elective procedures have significantly lower perioperative morbidity and mortality compared to the emergency techniques for ruptured aneurysms which carries death rate greater than 50% in many reported series. (42).

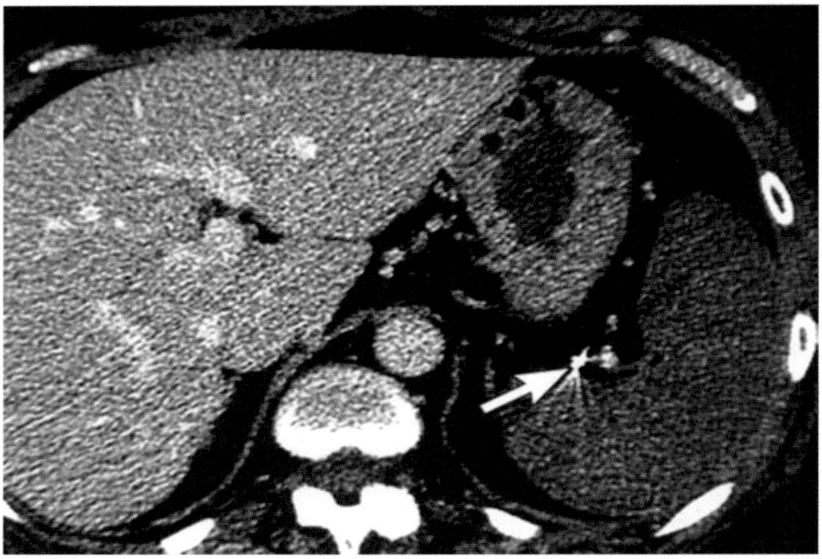

Figure 8.

Technical success after percutaneous coil embolization of SAAs is acceptable and ranges from 81% to 98%, although some studies showed that the presence of hemodynamic instability should not preclude endovascular management. (43,44).

End-organ ischaemia is an especial concern with regard to endovascular repair. Direct complications can result from this option of treatment such as arterial dissection, acute thrombosis, or embolization to nontarget tissues, or inadequate collateral circulation after deliberate vessel occlusion. It has been concluded that cases with aneurysmal lesion at the splenic hilum may be better managed by open repair and splenectomy.(45).

Although initial technical success rates with an endovascular procedure for treating SAAs approach 100%, the long-term success is less well defined.(46).

Ultrasound-guided percutaneous thrombin injection appears to be a viable method for treating failed endovascular interventions or even an alternative to initial endovascular treatment.(47). Actually, this technique is similar to thrombin injections for femoral artery pseudoaneurysms, were ultrasound or CT guidance or both are used to help delivering thrombin to the nidus of an aneurysm, thus facilitating thrombosis. This is particularly applicable to saccular aneurysms with a narrow neck arising from the parent vessel. Continued studies, even after secondary technical success, are imperative due to the natural history of SAAs after endovascular treatment remains unclear. This is true for saccular aneurysms treated by coil or thrombin embolization. Reports of reperfusion and even rupture after successful embolization support that a thrombosed aneurysm may not represent the definitive treatment in all cases.(47,48).

Author details

Ahmad Alsheikhly
Hamad Medical Corporation, Doha, Qatar

4. References

[1] Sadler TW. Chapter 14: Digestive system. In: *Langman's Medical Embryology*. 11th ed. Philadelphia, Pa: Lippincott Williams & Wilkins; 2009:215-6.

[2] Gray H. Chapter 88: The spleen. In: Standring S, ed. *Gray's Anatomy: The Anatomical Basis of Clinical Practice*. 39th ed. Edinburgh, UK: Churchill Livingstone Elsevier; 1239-44.

[3] Snell RS. Chapter 5: The abdomen: part II. The abdominal cavity. *Clinical Anatomy by Regions*. 8th ed. Baltimore, Md: Lippincott, Williams & Wilkins; 2007:259-60.

[4] Lee McGregor A, Decker GAG, du Plessis DJ. Chapter 8: The spleen. *Lee McGregor's Synopsis of Surgical Anatomy*. 12th ed. Oxford, UK: Butterworth-Heinemann; 1986:106-13.

[5] Romanes GJ. Abdomen: spleen. In: *Cunningham's Manual of Practical Anatomy. Vol II: Thorax and Abdomen*. Vol 2. 15th ed. New York, NY: Oxford Medical Publications, Oxford University Press; 1986.

[6] Guyton AC, Hall JE. Chapter 15: Vascular distensibility and functions of arterial and venous systems. *Guyton and Hall Textbook of Medical Physiology*. 11th ed. Philadelphia, Pa: Saunders; 2005:179-80.

[7] Johnston KW, Tilson MD, Stanley JC. The subcommittee on reporting standards for arterial aneurysm, International society for cardiovascular surgery. Suggested standards for reporting on arterial aneurysm. *J Vass Surg*, 1991; 13:452-458.

[8] Abbas MA, Stone WM, Bower TC, Panneton Jm, Cherry KJ. Splenic artery aneurysms: two decades experience at Mayo clinic. *Ann Vass Surg*. 2002; 16: 442-449.

[9] Carr SC Nemcek AA Jr, Yao JS. Current management of visceral artery aneurysms. *Surgery*. 1996; 120:627-634.

[10] Graham LM, Lindenauer SM. Celiac artery aneurysms: historic (1745- 1949) versus contemporary (1950-1984) differences in etiology and clinical importance. *J Vass Surg*. 1985; 2: 757- 764.

[11] Messina LM, Shanley CJ. Visceral artery aneurysms. *Surg Clin North AM*. 1997; 77:425-442.

[12] Moore SW, Guida PM, Schumacher HW: Splenic artery aneurysm. *Bull Soc Int Chir* 1970; 29:210-218.

[13] Bedford PD, Lodge B: Aneurysm of the splenic artery. *Gut* 1960; 1: 312-320.

[14] Dave SP, Reis ED, Hossain A, et al: Splenic artery aneurysm in the 1990s. *Ann Vasc Surg* 2000; 14:223-229.

[15] Pescarus R, Montreuil B, Bendavid Y: Giant splenic artery aneurysms: case report and review of the literature. *J Vasc Surg* 2005; 42:344-347.

[16] Lee PC, Rhee RY, et al. Management of splenic artery aneurysms: The significance of portal and essential hypertension. *J Am Cool Surg* 1999; 189: 483-490.

[17] Stanley JC, Wakefield TW, Graham LM, et al: Clinical importance and management of splanchnic artery aneurysms. *J Vasc Sur* 1986; 3:836-840.

[18] Sellke FW, Williams GB, Donovan DL, Clarke RE: Management of intra-abdominal aneurysms associated with periarteritis nodosa. *J Vasc Surg* 1986; 4:294-298.

[19] Ayalon A, Wiesner RH, Perkins JD, et al: Splenic artery aneurysms in liver transplant patients. *Transplantation* 1988; 45:386-389.

[20] Trastek VF, Pairolero PC, Joyce JW, et al: Splenic artery aneurysms. *Surgery* 1982; 91:694-699.

[21] Sadat U, Noor N, Tang T, Varty K: Emergency endovascular repair of ruptured visceral artery aneurysms. *World J Emerg Surg* 2007; 2:17.

[22] Hallett Jr JW: Splenic artery aneurysms. *Semin Vasc Surg* 1995; 8:321-326.

[23] Mattar SG, Lumsden AB: The management of splenic artery aneurysms: experience with 23 cases. *Am J Surg* 1995; 169:580-584.

[24] Alsheikhly A.S.: Ruptured True Aneurysm of the Splenic Artery: A Rare Cause of Haemoperitoneum: *The Middle East Journal of Trauma and Emergency medicine* 2008;8:197-199.

[25] Mattar SG, Lumsden AB: The management of splenic artery aneurysms: experience with 23 cases. *Am J Surg* 1995; 169:580-584.

[26] de Vries JE, Schattenkerk ME, Malt RA: Complications of splenic artery aneurysm other than intraperitonealrupture. *Surgery* 1982; 91:200-204.

[27] Wagner WH, Allins AD, Treiman RL, et al: Ruptured visceral artery aneurysms. *Ann Vasc Surg* 1997; 11:342-347.

[28] Trastek VF, Pairolero PC, Joyce JW, et al: Splenic artery aneurysm. *Surgery* 1982; 91:694-699.

[29] Barrett JM, Van Hooydonk JE, Boehm FH: Pregnancy-related rupture of arterial aneurysms. *Obstet Gynecol Surv* 1982; 37:557-566.

[30] Stanley JC, Fry WJ: Pathogenesis and clinical significance of splenic artery aneurysms. *Surgery* 1974; 76:898-909.

[31] Nosher JL, Chung J, Brevetti LS, et al: Visceral and renal artery aneurysms: a pictorial essay on endovascular therapy. *Radiographics* 2006; 26:1687-1704.

[32] Messina LM, Shanley CJ: Visceral artery aneurysms. *Surg Clin North Am* 1997; 77:425-442.

[33] Abbas MA, Stone WM, Fowl RJ, et al: Splenic artery aneurysms: two decades experience at Mayo Clinic. *Ann Vasc Surg* 2002; 16:442-449.

[34] Arca MJ, Gagner M, Heniford BT, et al: Splenic artery aneurysms: methods of laparoscopic repair. *J Vasc Surg* 1999; 30:184-188.

[35] Mastracci TM, Cadeddu M, Colopinto RF, Cina C: A minimally invasive approach to the treatment of aberrant splenic artery aneurysms: a report of two cases. *J Vasc Surg* 2005; 41:1053-1057.

[36] Huang IH, Zuckerman DA, Matthews JB: Occlusion of a giant splenic artery pseudoaneurysm with percutaneous thrombin-collagen injection. *J Vasc Surg* 2004; 40:574-577.

[37] Saltzberg SS, Maldonado TS, Lamparello PJ, et al: Is endovascular therapy the preferred treatment for all visceral artery aneurysms?. *Ann Vasc Surg* 2005; 19:507-515.

[38] Carroccio A, Jacobs TS, Faries P, et al: Endovascular treatment of visceral artery aneurysms. *Vasc Endovasc Surg* 2007; 41:373-382.

[39] LinkDP, Seibert JA, Gould J, Lantz BM. On-line monitoring of sequential blood flow reduction during splenic embolization. *Acta Radio* 1989; 30: 101–*103.*

[40] Tulsyan N, Kashyap VS, Greenberg RK, et al: The endovascular management of visceral artery aneurysms and pseudoaneurysms. *J Vasc Surg* 2007; 45:276-283.

[41] Sachdev U, Baril DT, Ellozy SH, et al: Management of aneurysms involving branches of the celiac and superior mesenteric arteries: a comparison of surgical and endovascular therapy. *J Vas Surg* 2006; 44:718-724.

[42] Pulli R, Dorigo W, Troisi N, et al: Surgical treatment of visceral artery aneurysms: a 25-year experience. *J Vasc Surg 2008*; 48:334-342.

[43] Gabelmann A, Gorich J, Merkle EM: Endovascular treatment of visceral artery aneurysms. *J Endovasc Ther* 2002; 9:38-47.

[44] Salam TA, Lumsden AB, Martin LG, Smith 3rd RB: Nonoperative management of visceral aneurysms and pseudoaneurysms. *Am J Surg* 1992; 164:215-219.

[45] Saltzberg SS, Maldonado TS, Lamparello PJ, et al: Is endovascular therapy the preferred treatment for all visceral artery aneurysms?. *Ann Vasc Surg* 2005; 19:507-515.

[46] Sachdev U, Baril DT, Ellozy SH, et al: Management of aneurysms involving branches of the celiac and superior mesenteric arteries: a comparison of surgical and endovascular therapy. *J Vasc Surg* 2006; 44:718-724.

[47] Szopinski P, Ciostek P, Pleban E, et al: Percutaneous thrombin injection to complete SMA pseudoaneurysm exclusion after failing of endograft placement. *Cardiovasc Intervent Radiol* 2005; 28:509-514.

[48] Carr SC, Pearce WH, Vogelzang RL, et al: Current management of visceral artery aneurysms. *Surgery* 1996; 120:627-633.

[49] Onohara T, Okadome K, Mii S, et al: Rupture of embolized coeliac artery pseudoaneurysm into the stomach: is coil embolization an effective treatment for coeliac anastomotic pseudoaneurysm?. *Eur J Vasc Surg* 1992; 6:330-332.

Chapter 8

Studying the Flow Dynamics Within Endografts in Abdominal Aortic Aneurysms

Efstratios Georgakarakos, Antonios Xenakis, George S. Georgiadis, Konstantinos C. Kapoulas, Evagelos Nikolopoulos and Miltos Lazarides

Additional information is available at the end of the chapter

http://dx.doi.org/10.5772/46034

1. Introduction

Endovascular Treatment (EVAR) is considered the treatment of choice for the majority of Abdominal Aortic Aneurysms (AAA) nowadays, since it demonstrates improved perioperative morbidity and aneurysm-related mortality, comparing to conventional open repair. However, despite the initial technical success and early discharge of the patient, this technique is amenable to early and late complications, the most important of which are the endoleaks (ie. recurrence of blood flow detection within the aneurysm sac) accompanied sometimes with variable degrees of intrasac pressurization (Georgakarakos et al, 2012a). Furthermore, the hemodynamic changes that the endograft sustains during the follow-up period make it prone to positional changes with subsequent risk for endograft migration and loss of sealing between the endograft and either the aneurysm neck or the iliac fixation sites.

Computer-enhanced geometric modeling and Finite Volume Analysis have been used to study the biomechanical behavior of the aortic aneurysms before and after the insertion of the endograft device (Georgakarakos et al, 2012b). Numerical modeling of endovascular-treated AAA is used to determine the stresses and forces developed on AAA sac and stent-graft materials in-vivo, estimating hemodynamic parameters, such as the pressure and stress distribution over the main body, the bifurcation, the limbs of a stent-graft or the drag and displacement forces predisposing to graft migration. Consequently, the study of flow dynamics within aortic endografts holds a fundamental role in the delineation of the endograft behavior under pulsatile flow, providing useful information for developing and modifying the endograft design and surgical techniques. This chapter discusses the aforementioned changes, by using three-dimensional (3D) reconstructed endograft model.

2. Reconstruction of the AAA endograft model

Finite Volume Analysis technique has a crucial role in the computational research of hemodynamic systems, utilizing small subsections (elements) of 3-dimentional structures created by segmentation and meshing. By solving Navier-Stokes equations for all finite volumes of the model, Computational flow dynamics (CFD) techniques utilize numerical methods and algorithms to analyze problems that involve fluid flows. Furthermore, Fluid Structure Interaction (FSI) methods combine fluid and structural equations, solved either simultaneously or separately (partitioned approach), in order to determine the flow fields and solid body stresses on a deformable model. Most researchers acquire information on the 3D AAA realistic, complex geometry using patient-specific DICOM data derived from high-resolution spiral CT or MR angiography (Georgakarakos et al, 2012b).

Our study group used a reconstructed 3D model of a AAA endograft using commercially available appropriate, validated software (MIMICS 13.0, Materialise NV, Leuven, Belgium), based on the DICOM images derived from contrast-enhanced high-resolution computed tomography. The computational model (**Figure1**) includes the aortic neck proximal to the endograft and the iliac arteries distal to the endograft limbs. A validated Finite Volume analysis software ANSYS v 12.1 (Ansys Inc., Canonsburg, PA, USA) was used for Computational Fluid Dynamics (CFD). The velocity and pressure waveforms during a period of 1.2 s as previously described in a one-dimensional fluid-dynamics model for the abdominal aorta (Olufsen et al, 2000 and Li et al, 2005) were used for both models as inlet and outlet boundary conditions. Blood was assumed to be non-Newtonian fluid, according to the Carreau-Yasuda model, with a density of 1050 kg/m^3.

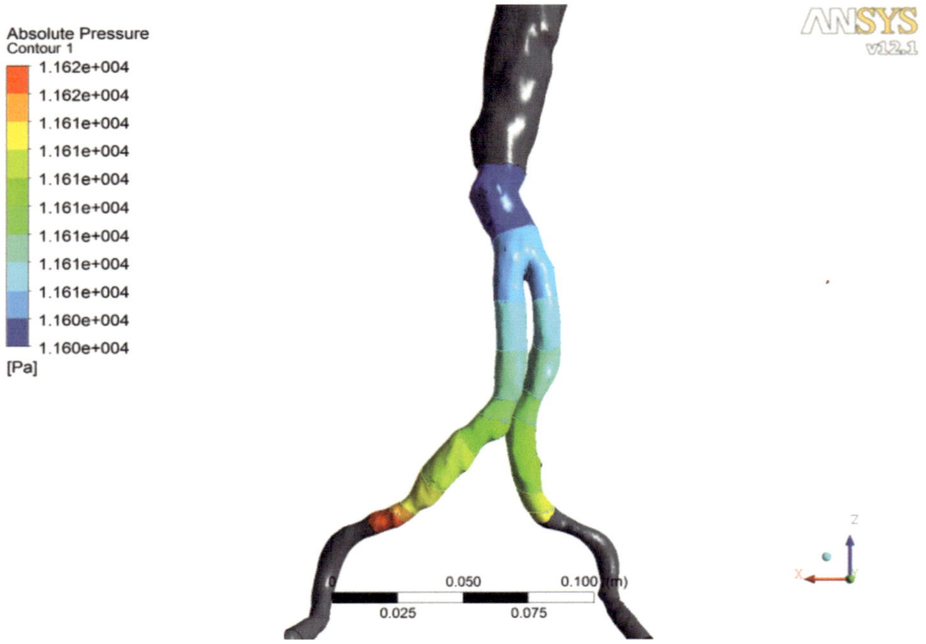

Figure 1. Reconstructed images of the aortic endograft using purpose-developed software.

Accordingly, the velocity streamlines and the pressure distribution were calculated over the entire surface of the endograft and are demonstrated in 6 distinct time-phases through the cardiac cycle (**Figure2**). For study reasons, the cardiac cycle was dived in six distinct phases, namely the late diastole (t_1), the accelerating systolic phase (t_2), the peak systolic phase (t_3), the late deceleration (t_4), the end-systolic (t_5) and the early diastolic phase (t_6).

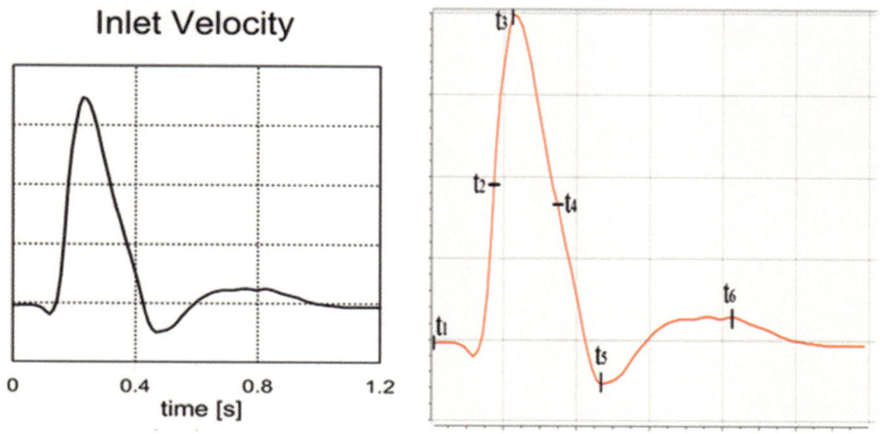

Figure 2. Plot of the flow waveform used for the calculations in our endograft model (left panel). Six distinct phases are depicted in each cardiac cycle. t_1 depicts the late diastole, t_2 the accelerating phase, t_3 represents the peak systolic phase, t_4 the late deceleration, t_5 depicts the end-systole and t_6 the early diastolic phase (right panel).

3. Changes in flow patterns and pressure distribution

Figures 3-8 depict the flow patterns in the endograft throughout the cardiac cycle. A flow disturbance is seen near the inlet zone (panel top-left) during the late diastole, t_1 (Figure 3). The flow pattern is normalized during the entire systolic phase, ie. t_2 to t_4 (Figures 4-6) and exhibits disturbance again, from the the end-systole t_5 early diastole t_6 (Figures 7,8). Interestingly, there is disturbed flow in the iliac limb unilaterally (left) during the decelerating systolic phase (Figure 6), whereas the irregular flow is also transmitted in the contralateral (right) iliac limb, during the next time-step (end-systolic phase, t_5, Figure 7).

	t_1	t_2	t_3	t_4	t_5	t_6
Pressure values (mmHg)						
Max	87	167	147	120	104	97
Min	87	136	136	115	102	96

Table 1. Maximum and minimum values of pressure in the endograft surface, for the different phases of the cardiac cycle. Excessively high values of pressure due to alteration in the iliac limbs geometry were excluded (outlier values).

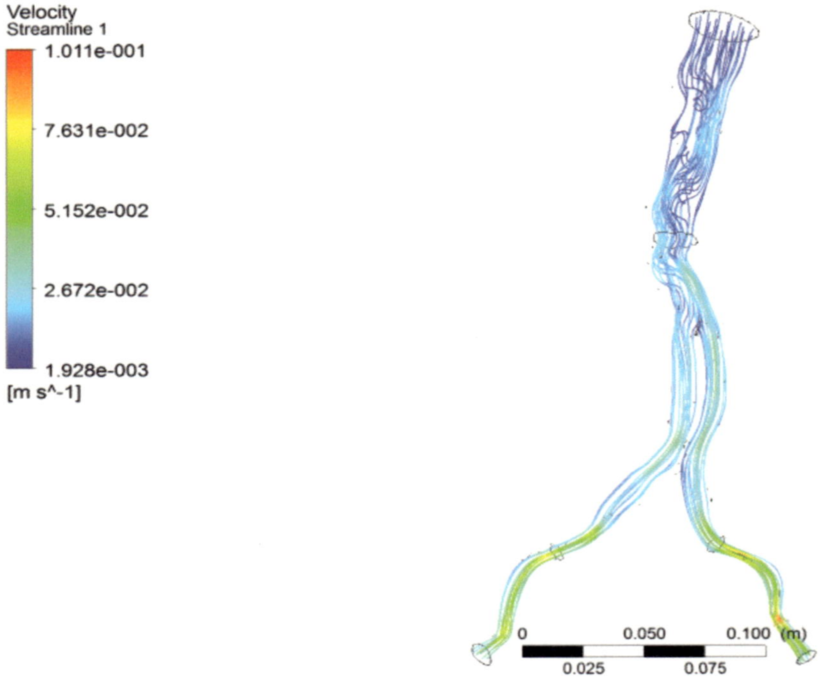

Figure 3. The velocity streamlines, as demonstrated for the late diastolic phase (t_1).

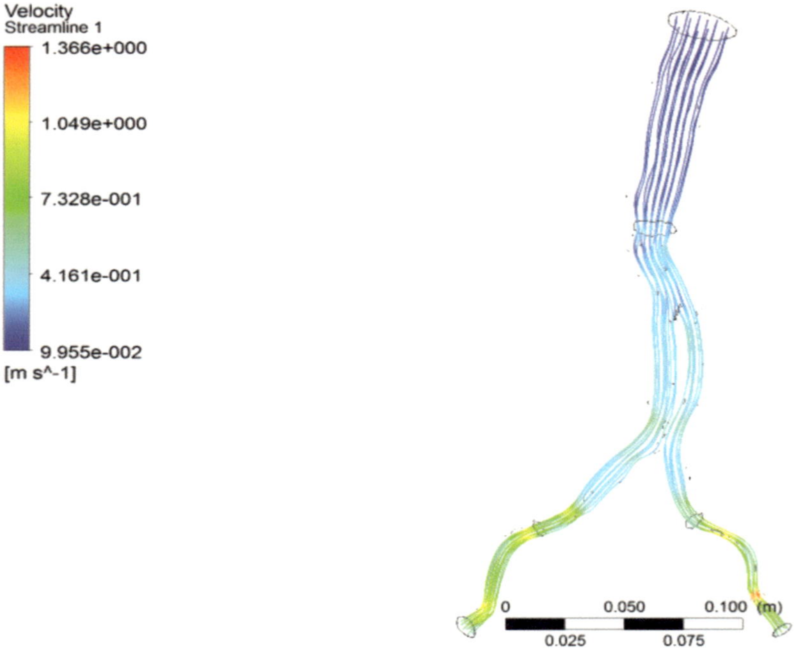

Figure 4. The velocity streamlines, as demonstrated for the accelerating systolic phase (t_2).

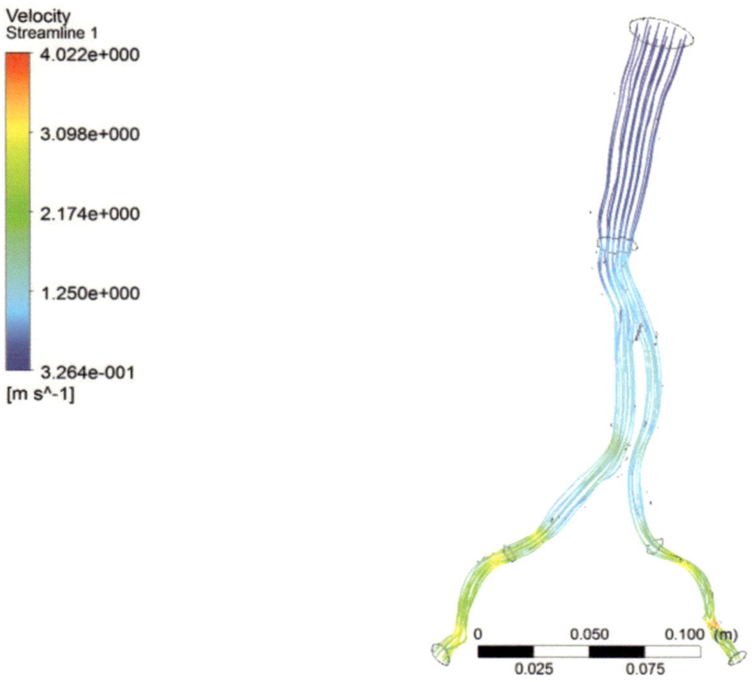

Figure 5. The velocity streamlines, as demonstrated for the peak systolic phase (t_3).

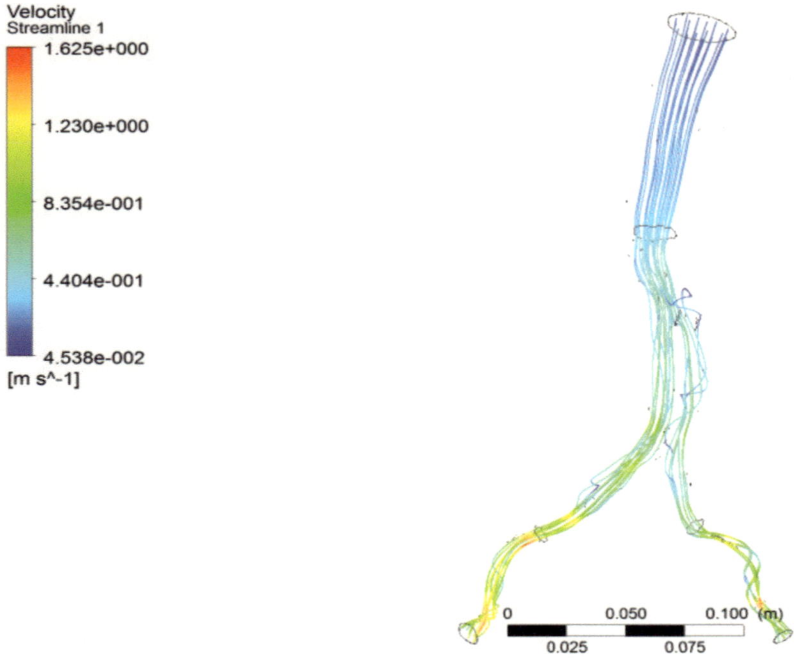

Figure 6. The velocity streamlines, as demonstrated for the decelerating systolic phase (t_4).

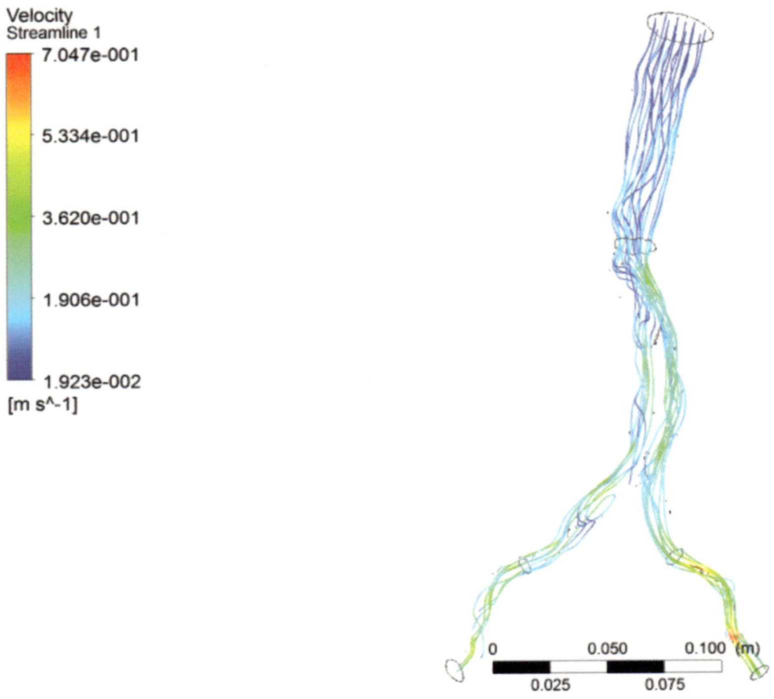

Figure 7. The velocity streamlines, as demonstrated for the end-systolic phase (t_5).

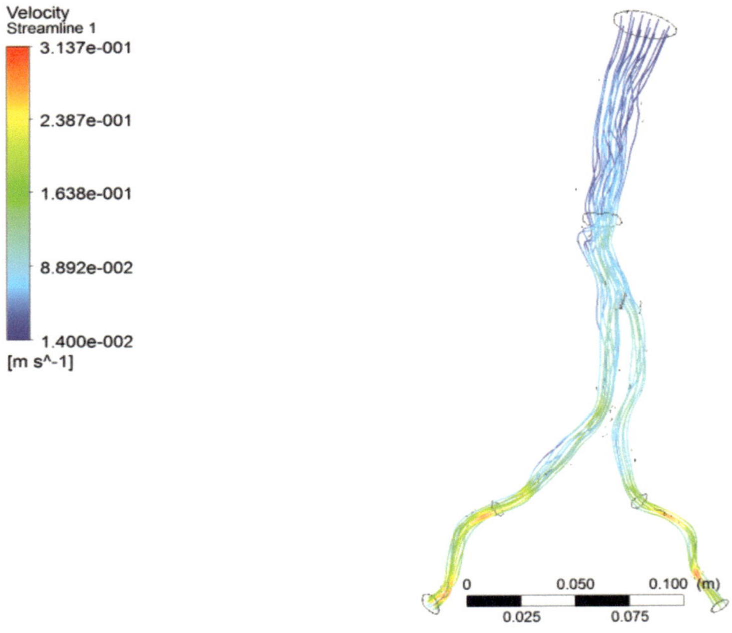

Figure 8. The velocity streamlines, as demonstrated for the early diastolic phase (t_6).

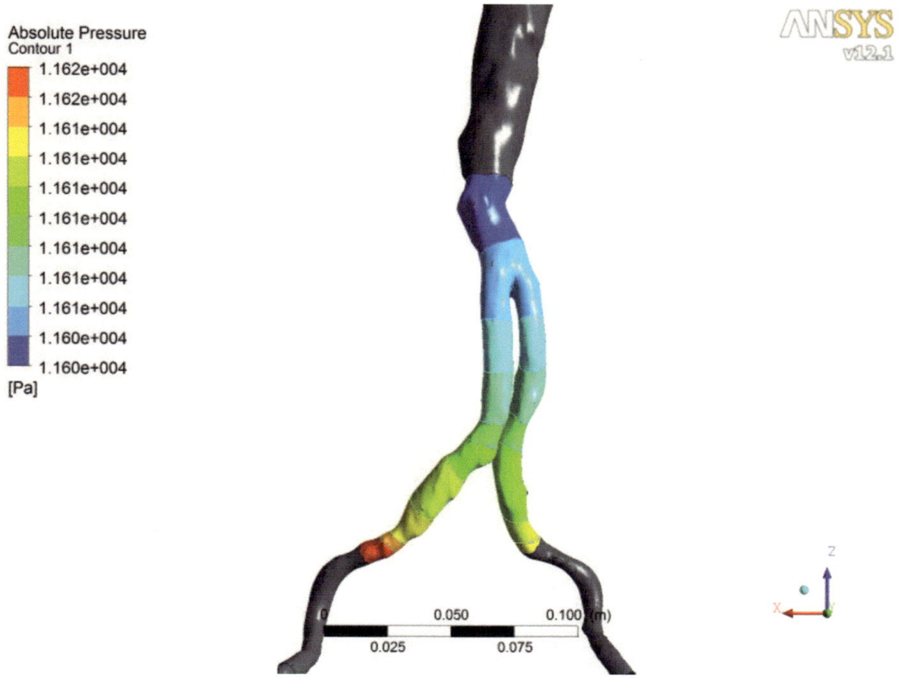

Figure 9. The distribution of pressures across the endograft, as demonstrated for the late diastolic phase (t_1).

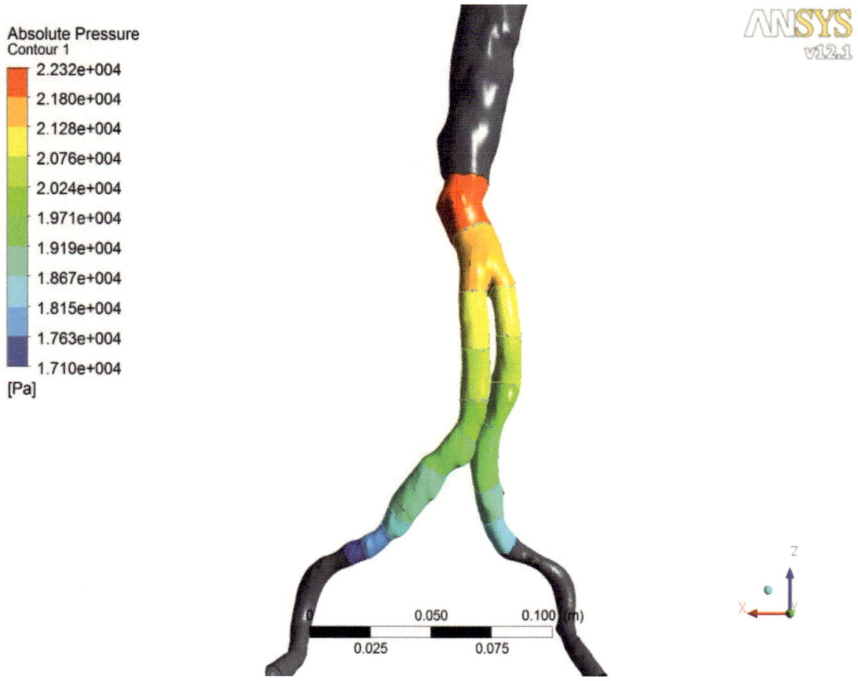

Figure 10. The distribution of pressures across the endograft, as demonstrated for the accelerating systolic phase (t_2).

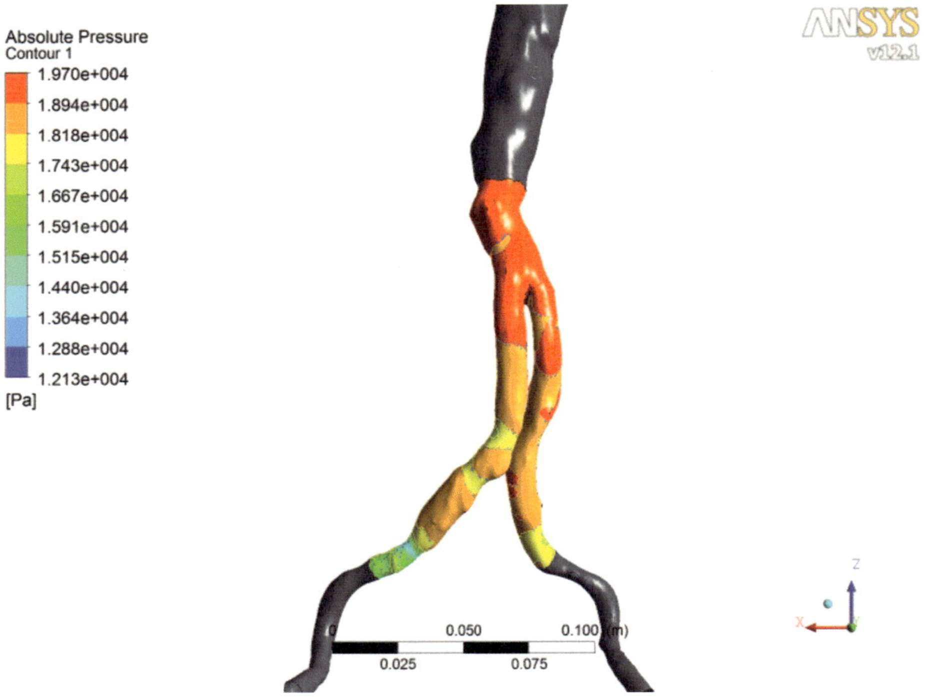

Figure 11. The distribution of pressures across the endograft, as demonstrated for the peak systolic phase (t_3).

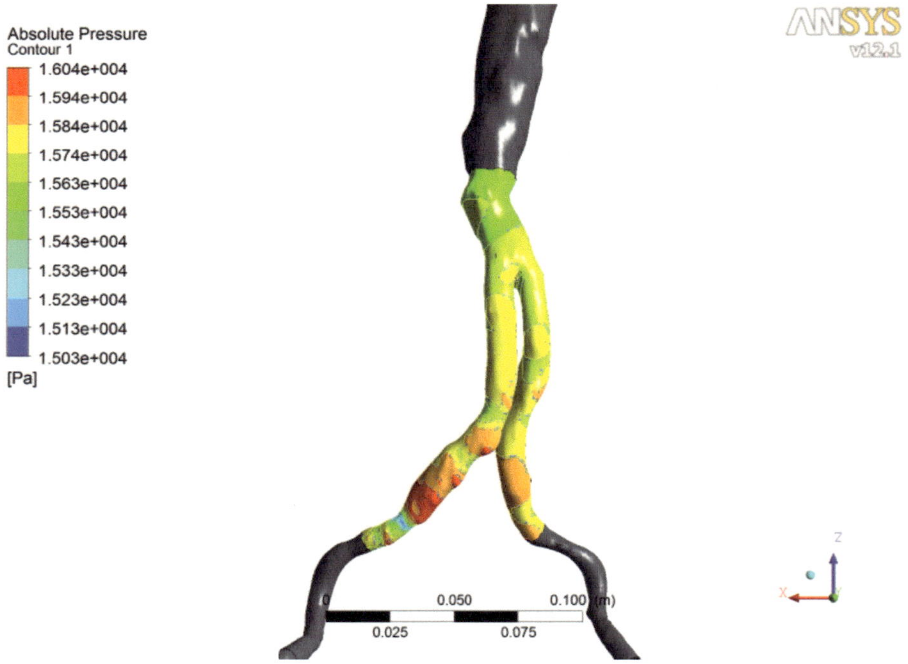

Figure 12. The distribution of pressures across the endograft, as demonstrated for the decelerating systolic phase (t_4).

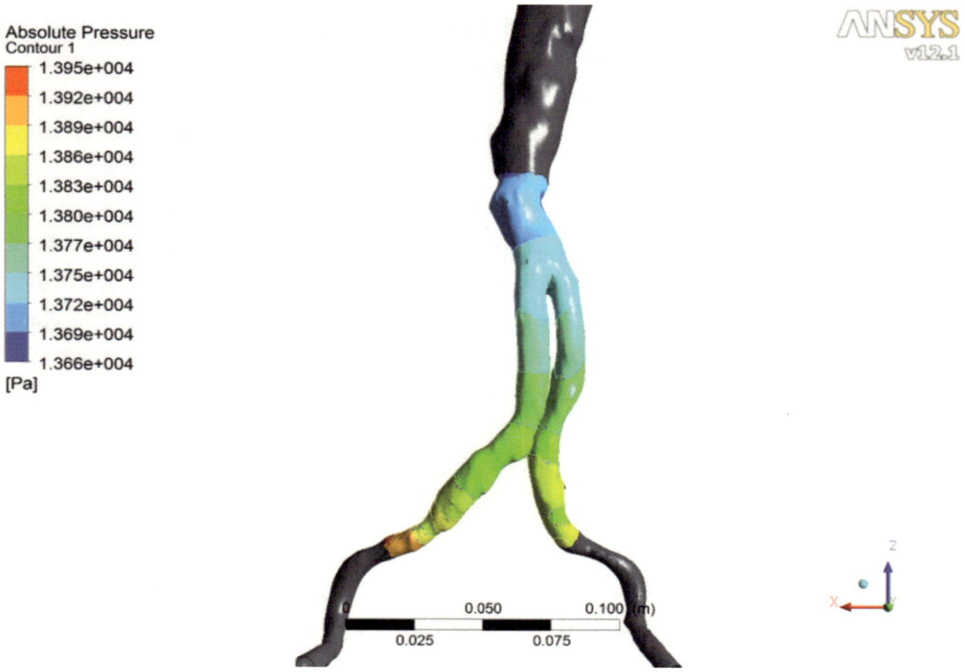

4.

Figure 13. The distribution of pressures across the endograft, as demonstrated for the end-systolic phase (t_5).

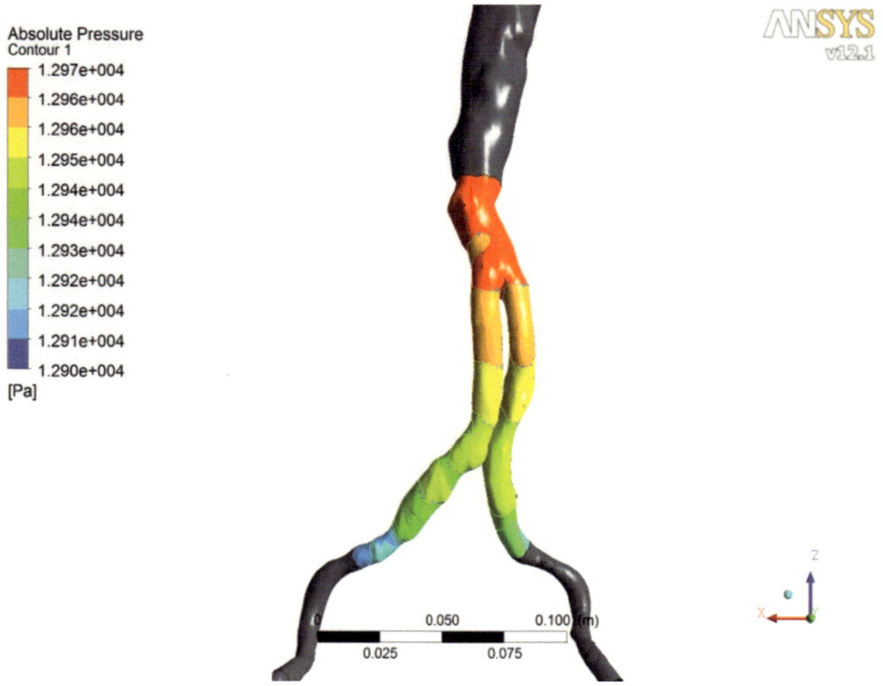

Figure 14. The distribution of pressures across the endograft, as demonstrated for the early diastolic phase (t_6).

Table 1 depicts the minimum and maximum pressure values along the endograft surface, for the different phases of the cardiac cycle (as described above). As depicted in Figures 9-14 and Table 1, there is a similar, homogenous distribution of the pressure values along the different parts of the endograft during the diastolic phase (t_6 and t_1). However, when it comes to the systolic phase (t_2 and t_4), there is a marked linear decrease of the pressure values from the endograft inlet to the iliac limbs (outlet). The greatest pressure value difference is marked in the accelerating systolic phase (t_2). Interestingly, the highest and lowest pressure values are demonstrated in the inlet-main body area and the iliac limbs of the endograft, respectively, during the accelerating and peak systolic phase, whereas this pressure relation is reversed in the decelerating systolic phase (t_4), where the highest values are located distally (outflow). Moreover, there seems to be a narrower range of pressure distribution in the peak systolic phase (t_3). Finally, in the early diastolic phase (t_6) there is again a reverse in the pressure distribution compared to the early systolic phase, with the highest pressure being located in the inflow area of the endograft.

Figures 15-17 demonstrate the vertical velocity patterns and the secondary flow fields in the different parts of the endograft, during the peak systolic and the diastolic phase. The bifurcation of the endograft in two distinct outflow tracts (iliac limbs) causes a disturbance of flow especially in the secondary flow fields and generation of local vortices mainly in the proximal iliac parts (Figure 16), before this marked difference is subsided in the most distal iliac outflow parts (Figure 17). This pattern is also met in the diastolic phase, but with a greater discrepancy being present in this phase (Figures 15-17). In both iliac limbs there was a skewing of the flow towards the inner wall and significant flow separation towards the outer wall.

4. The forces exerted on the endograft surface

The forces applied on the surface of the endograft are demonstrated in Figures 18-20. The forces generated by the pressure are directed mainly vertical to the endograft surface (Figure 18) throughout the cardiac cycle. The tangential forces are mainly caused by the flow of blood and the boundary layer that is formed near the aortic wall, while their direction is depended on the cardiac phase. So, their vector heads forward during the early, peak (Figure 19) and late systolic phase, whereas the direction is reversed during the end systole (Figures 2 and 20) and late diastole. Notably, the values of the tangential forces are lower than the pressure ones by many orders of magnitude. The total sum of the pressure and viscous forces acting on the surface of the graft resolving into the x, y and z components, determines the drag forces that the endograft is subjected to, making it prone to migration.

5. Discussion

(CFD) techniques provide a valuable and reliable tool in the study of the hemodynamic behavior of the cardiovascular system after therapeutic interventions (Frauenfelder, 2006).

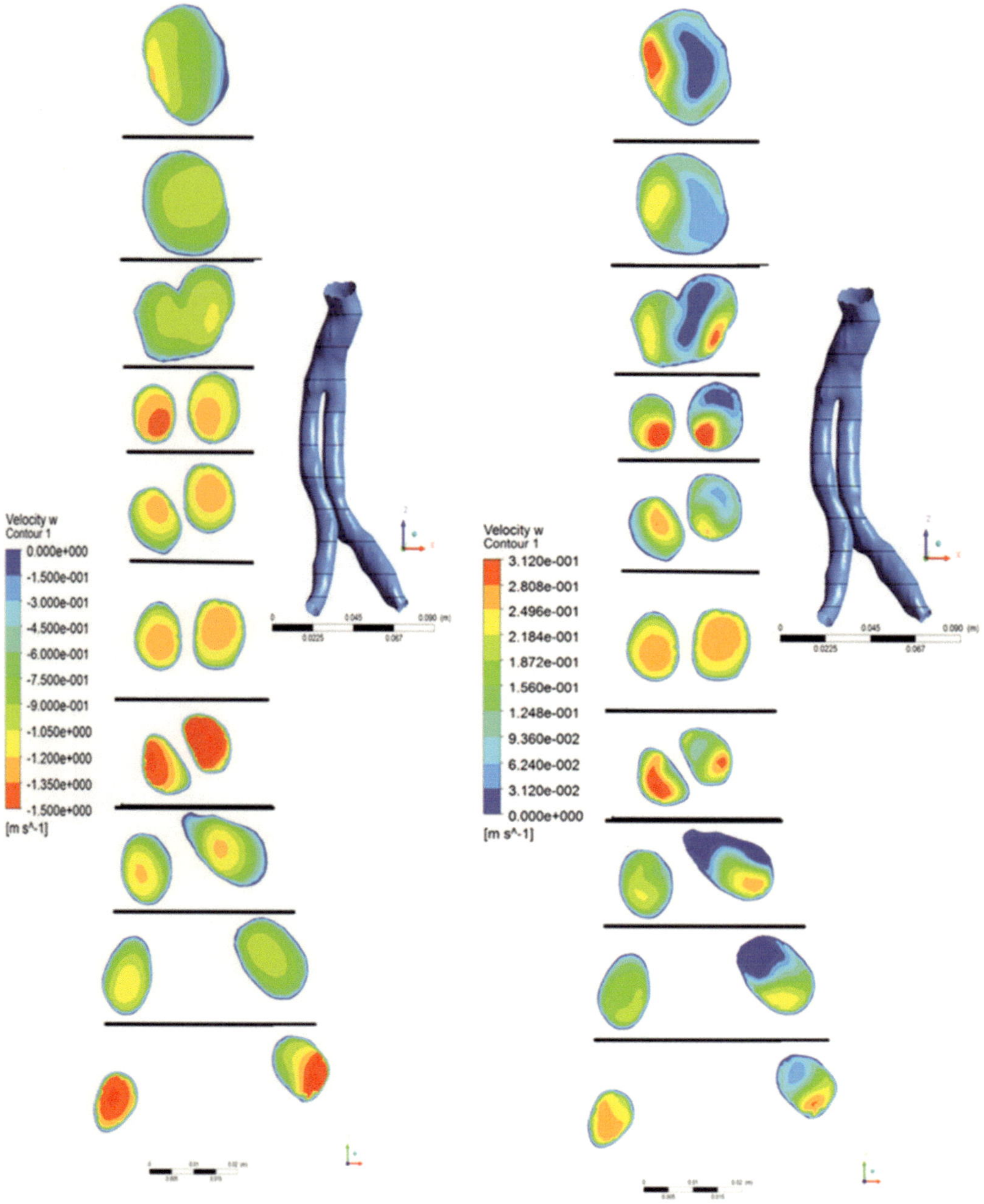

Figure 15. Distribution of velocity values in the transverse axis (-z) along ten cross-section of the endograft, during the peak systolic phase (left panel) and the diastolic phase (right panel).

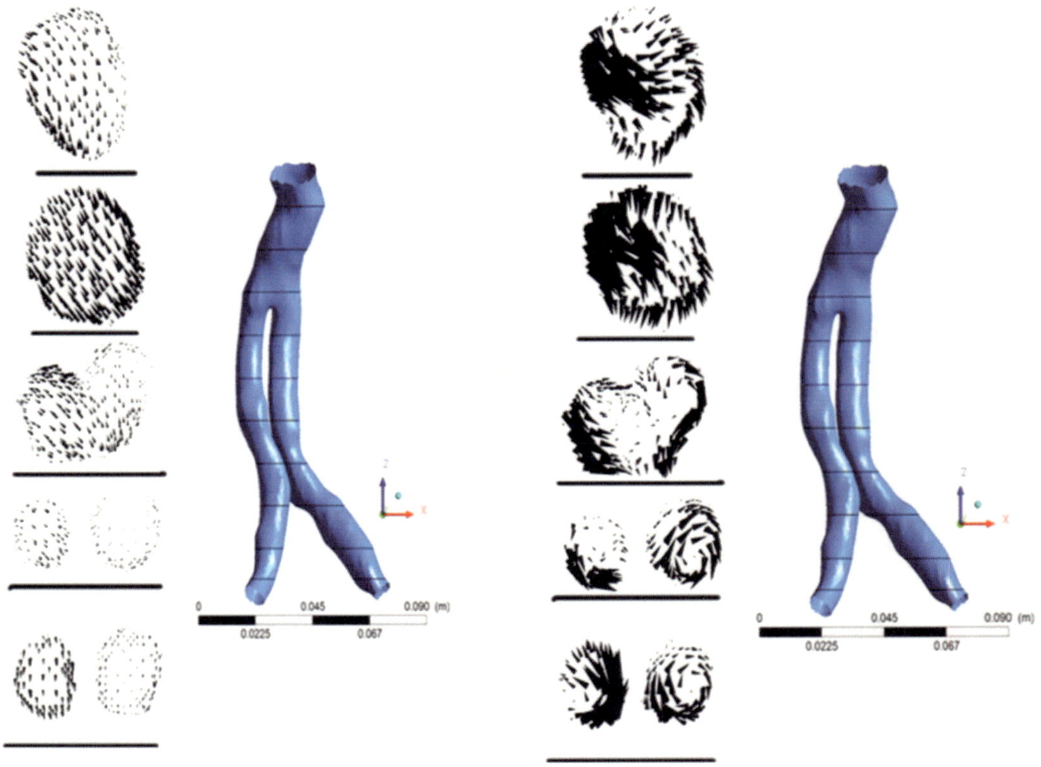

Figure 16. Distribution of velocity profiles in the secondary flow fields along the transverse axis (-z) in the 5 cephalad cross-sections (endograft inlet to proximal thirds of the iliac limbs) of the endograft, during the peak systolic (left panel) and the diastolic (right panel) phase.

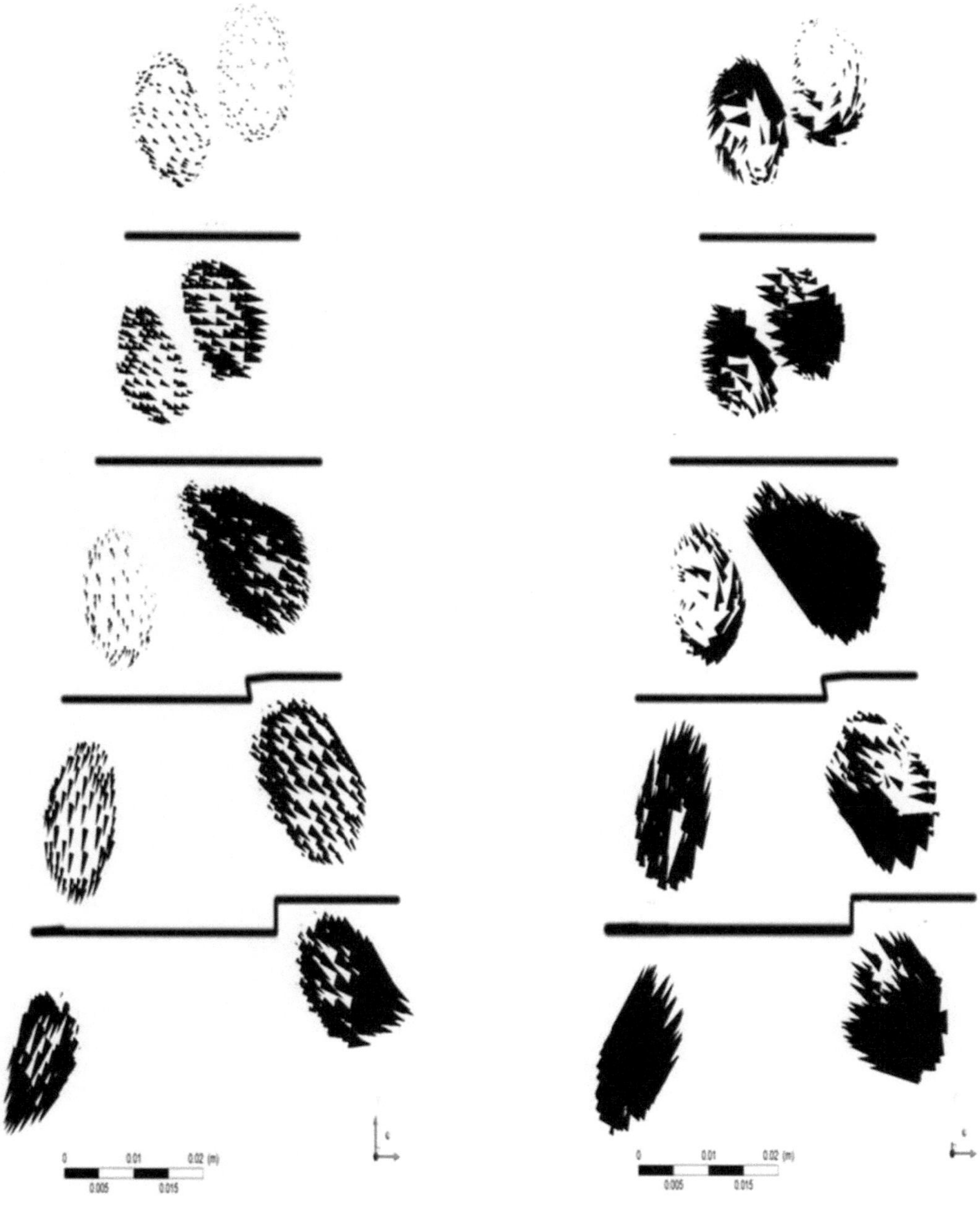

Figure 17. Distribution of velocity profiles in the secondary flow fields along the transverse axis (-z) in the 5 caudal cross-sections (proximal to distal thirds of the iliac limbs) of the endograft, during the peak systolic (left panel) and the diastolic (right panel) phase.

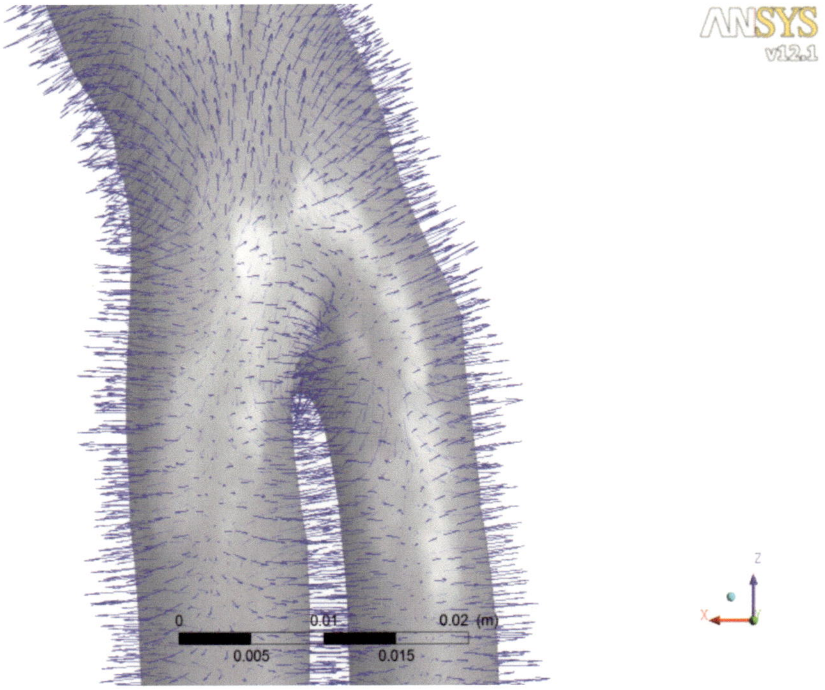

Figure 18. The pressure forces on the endograft bifurcation area (peak systolic phase).

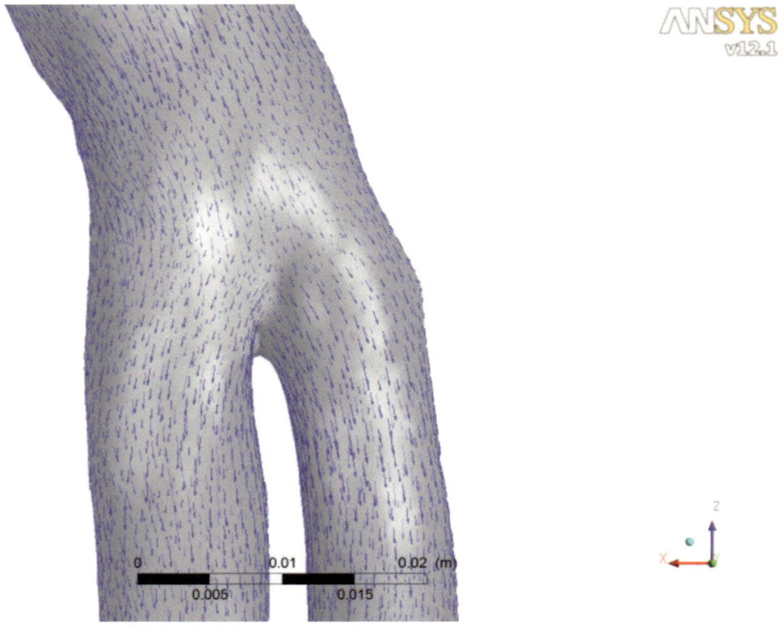

Figure 19. The tangential forces on the endograft bifurcation area (peak systolic phase).

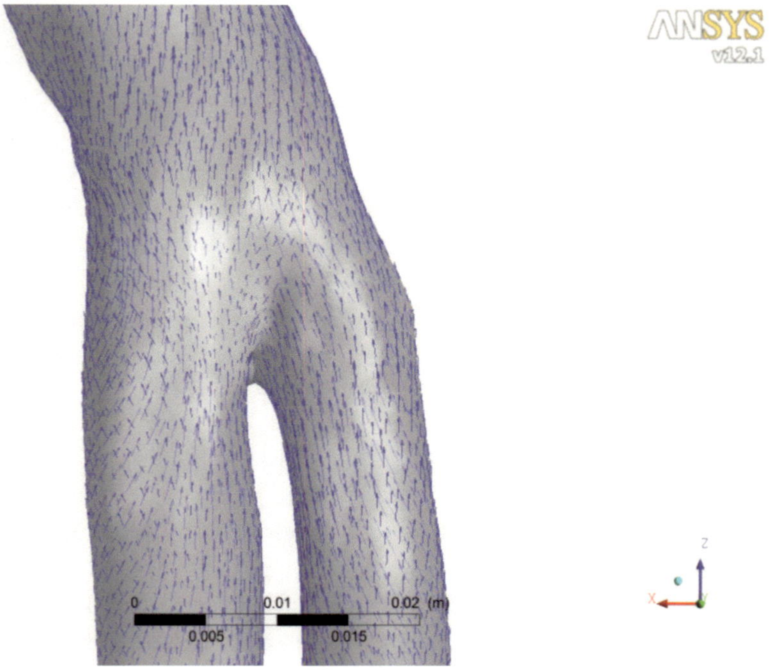

Figure 20. The tangential forces on the endograft bifurcation area during the end systolic phase, t_5).

The insertion of an endograft causes alterations in the hemodynamic environment of the AAA, regarding the pressures and stresses exerted on the AAA sac as well as the flow patterns inside the endograft lumen (Molony et al, 2009). There is a reduction in the intrasac pressure and the stress values on the sac of the stented AAA, leading to sac shrinkage. Chong and How (2004) used flow visualization and laser Doppler anemometry to study in vitro the flow patterns within a stent graft in different phases of the cardiac cycle. According to their study, the main trunk of the endograft is characterized by complex flow patterns with evidence of instability in systolic acceleration phase, developing into a number of vortical structures during systolic deceleration. The flow phenomena in the iliac limbs are strongly influenced by the geometry and the configuration of the limbs (Morris 2006 and Molony, 2008) and any degree of existing constriction caused in the iliac limbs. Basically, the flow in both limbs is triphasic, with a large retrograde component in end-systole (Chong and How, 2004) and formation of recirculating zones. The profiles are significantly more disturbed in the deceleration phase than at maximum velocity (Chong and How, 2004).

Finally, local geometric factors play a role in the determination of velocity values and flow patterns (recirculating zones, flow separation, skewed flow, vortices and Dean flows) with the out-of-plane endograft geometry determining greatly the outlet flow rates, flow patterns and drag forces (Morris 2006). Extrinsic constriction (due to calcified or stenosed iliac vessels) or excessive kinking in the iliac limbs can lead either to thrombosis of the graft limbs or altered flow patterns that induce excessive disturbances in shear stresses (not shown in our model), leading also to recirculating zones and prolonged transit times of platelets with consequent apposition and formation of thrombus in the endografts. The latter constitutes a rather common incidental finding, occurring more frequently that previously assumed (Wu et al, 2009). Finally, the study and understanding of the hemodynamic alterations and the parameters that influence them, could lead to better designs of endovascular grafts, in order to eliminate the factors that predispose to endograft migration as well as to generation of endoleaks (Figueroa 2009 and 2010, Liffman 2001, Mohan 2002).

6. Conclusion

Aortic endografts are subject to hemodynamic alterations that determine the flow patterns within the different parts of the endografts and influence the values and distribution of pressures and stresses onto their surface during the different phases of the cardiac cycle. Certain geometric factors such as the inlet-to-outlet ratio of the graft as well as the out-of-plane configuration of the main body and iliac limbs have been implicated as major determinants of the aforementioned hemodynamic alterations. Computational simulation techniques can help towards the understanding of these interactions and help us further design better endografts with greater resistance to migration, endoleaks and dislocation of modular stent-grafts, all of which are influenced by the hemodynamic environment that endografts are exposed to.

Author details

Efstratios Georgakarakos, George S. Georgiadis,
Konstantinos C. Kapoulas, Evagelos Nikolopoulos and Miltos Lazarides
"Democritus" University of Thrace Medical School, Alexandroupolis, Greece

Antonios Xenakis
Fluids Section, School of Mechanical Engineering, National Technical University of Athens, Athens, Greece

7. References

Georgakarakos E, Georgiadis GS, Ioannou CV, Kapoulas KC, Trellopoulos G, Lazarides M. (2012a). Aneurysm sac shrinkage after endovascular treatment of the aorta: beyond sac pressure and endoleaks. *Vasc Med.*;17:168-73.

Georgakarakos E, Georgiadis GS, Xenakis A, Kapoulas KC, Lazarides MK, Tsangaris AS, Ioannou CV. (2012b). Application of bioengineering modalities in vascular research: evaluating the clinical gain. *Vasc Endovascular Surg.*;46:101-8.

Chong CK, How TV, Gilling-Smith GL, Harris PL. (2003). Modeling endoleaks and collateral reperfusion following endovascular AAA exclusion. *J Endovasc Ther.*;10:424-32.

Chong CK, How TV. (2004). Flow patterns in an endovascular stent-graft for abdominal aortic aneurysm repair. *J Biomech.*;37:89-97.

Figueroa CA, Taylor CA, Yeh V, Chiou AJ, Zarins CK. (2009). Effect of curvature on displacement forces acting on aortic endografts: a 3-dimensional computational analysis. *J Endovasc Ther.*;16:284-94.

Figueroa CA, Taylor CA, Yeh V, Chiou AJ, Gorrepati ML, Zarins CK (2010). Preliminary 3D computational analysis of the relationship between aortic displacement force and direction of endograft movement. J Vasc Surg.;51:1488-97.

Frauenfelder T, Lotfey M, Boehm T, Wildermuth S. (2006). Computational fluid dynamics: hemodynamic changes in abdominal aortic aneurysm after stent-graft implantation. Cardiovasc Intervent Radiol.;29:613-23.

Li Z, Kleinstreuer C, Farber M. (2005). Computational analysis of biomechanical contributors to possible endovascular graft failure. *Biomech Model Mechanobiol.*;4:221-34.

Liffman K, Lawrence-Brown MM, Semmens JB, Bui A, Rudman M, Hartley DE. (2001). Analytical modeling and numerical simulation of forces in an endoluminal graft. *J Endovasc Ther.*;8:358-71.

Mohan IV, Harris PL, Van Marrewijk CJ, Laheij RJ, How TV. (2002). Factors and forces influencing stent-graft migration after endovascular aortic aneurysm repair. *J Endovasc Ther.*;9:748-55

Molony DS, Callanan A, Morris LG, Doyle BJ, Walsh MT, McGloughlin TM. (2008). Geometrical enhancements for abdominal aortic stent-grafts. *J Endovasc Th*er.;15:518-29.

Molony DS, Callanan A, Kavanagh EG, Walsh MT, McGloughlin TM. (2009). Fluid-structure interaction of a patient-specific abdominal aortic aneurysm treated with an endovascular stent-graft. *Biomed Eng Online*.6;8:24.

Morris L, Delassus P, Grace P, Wallis F, Walsh M, McGloughlin T. (2006). Effects of flat, parabolic and realistic steady flow inlet profiles on idealised and realistic stent graft fits through Abdominal Aortic Aneurysms (AAA). *Med Eng Phys.*;28:19-26.

Olufsen MS, Peskin CS, Kim WY, Pedersen EM, Nadim A, Larsen J. (2000). Numerical simulation and experimental validation of blood flow in arteries with structured-tree outflow conditions. *Ann Biomed Eng.*; 28:1281-99.

Wu IH, Liang PC, Huang SC, Chi NS, Lin FY, Wang SS. (2009). The significance of endograft geometry on the incidence of intraprosthetic thrombus deposits after abdominal endovascular grafting. *Eur J Vasc Endovasc Surg.*;38:741-7.

Chapter 9

Abdominal Aortic Aneurysms – Actual Therapeutic Strategies

Ionel Droc, Dieter Raithel and Blanca Calinescu

Additional information is available at the end of the chapter

http://dx.doi.org/10.5772/48596

1. Introduction

AAA is the thirteenth cause of death in UK accounting for 1.2% of male and 0.6 of female mortality, and the third cause of sudden death after coronary artery disease and stroke. [1-3]

Abdominal aortic aneurysms are identified in the elderly population; only a few patients die because of AAA rupture prior to the age of 60. The incidence of the disease in the general population is 60/1000 inhabitants [4] and between 1.8% and 6.6% in autopsies studies. In studies of natural history of AAA the rate of aneurysm rupture and death could exceed 60% within 3 years of the initial diagnosis. [5]

2. Pathogenesis

The pathogenesis of aortic aneurismal disease is multifactorial. There is no consensus as to the cause of aortic aneurysms. Hypertension exists in about half of patients and is obviously an aggravating condition. Tertiary syphilis was once an important cause of aneurysms, particularly of the ascending thoracic aorta, but is a less common cause now.

Genetic components have been identified in Marfan's syndrome and Ehlers Danlos disease. Even in the most common, degenerative, form of aortic aneurysms there is a genetic component. Familial clustering of aortic aneurysms is evident as up to 20% of patients have one or more first-degree relatives who have also suffered from the disease.[6] More studies are clearly needed to establish details of the genetic interplay in aortic aneurysms.

At times, an aneurysm may be caused by an extrinsic factor, such as an infection (micotic aneurysm) or trauma (pseudoaneurysm).

Traditional views states that most aneurysms were caused by degenerative atherosclerotic disease but it affects different layers of the aortic wall. Atherosclerosis mainly affects the intima, causing occlusive disease, while aortic aneurysm is a disease of the media and adventitia. They are distinct conditions that nonetheless often occur together.

Histologically, AAAs are characterized by chronic inflammation with destruction of the extracellular matrix, remodelling of the wall layers, and reduction in number of smooth muscle cells. The effectors of destruction are a group of enzymes capable of degrading the major connective tissue components: collagen, elastin, fibronectin, laminin and the proteoglycans.[7] The inflammatory infiltrate consists of macrophages as well as T and B lymphocytes, which excrete proteases and elastases causing wall degradation.[8] The reason for this migration is unclear.

Degradation of elastin has been associated with dilatation while rupture of the wall is related to collagen degradation. Experimental studies of elastase induced aneurysms indicate that an inflammatory reaction within the aortic media is crucial for aortic dilatation.

In both clinical and experimental studies, metalloproteinases (MMP), one of the most prominent group of elastases, have emerged as playing a role in the development of aortic aneurysms. [9,10] The MMPs are inhibited by the family of tissue inhibitors of metalloproteinases (TIMPs), including TIMP-1 and TIMP-2. An imbalance between the activated MMPs and their natural inhibitors may be responsible for the destruction of the aortic wall. Therapeutic trials with doxycycline, a MMP inhibitor, are ongoing and preliminary results are encouraging with less progression of aneurysmal size in treated patients.[11]

Commonly assessed in AAA are also proteins involved in, stimulated by or associated with thrombosis, for example, fibrinogen and D-dimer.[12]

A human biopsy study has confirmed the association between the extent of inflammation of the aortic wall and aortic diameter.[13] Interleukin-6 (IL-6), metalloproteinase-9 (MMP-9-gelatinase B) and C-reactive protein (CRP) are markers of inflammatory processes and have all been associated with AAA pathogenesis [13,14,15] as well as collagen type IV, fibronectin and other matrix proteins. High levels of MMP-9 and MMP-3 have been found in abdominal aortic aneurysmal tissue. Levels of MMP-9 are associated with aneurysmal size. [14,16,17] Hovsepian et al. Reported that MMP-9 plasma levels appeared to directly reflect the amount of MMP-9 produced within aneurysm tissue. MMP-9 plasma levels also decreased substantially after surgical AAA repair.[18]

Circulating concentrations of many kinds of biomarkers have been measured and compared in patients with abdominal aortic aneurysm (AAA) and subjects without AAA to assess their possible role in the pathogenesis or progression of AAA (Table 1). Circulating biomarkers could play a role in the diagnosis of AAA reflecting also the AAA activity in asymptomatic phases and may have a role in predicting subsequent progression and thus the prognosis of AAA.

Most investigated potential biomarkers show either no correlation or a weak correlation with the clinical course of AAA. Few have any potential for clinical use. Another limitation is related to the fact that many biomarkers for AAA are not disease specific; most of them also are markers for atherosclerosis.

Biomarker	Number of patients	Summary of findings	Author, year
MMP-9	36	Plasma MMP-9 may predict the natural history of AAA	Lindholt J. et al. 2000
MMP-9, MMP-2 TIMP-1, TIMP-2	76	Both MMP-2 and 9 failed to show relevance as serum markers for aortic dilatation.	Eugster T et al. 2005
	30 medium-sized ruptured AAA 30 large asymptomatic AAA (aAAA)	AAA rupture is associated with higher levels of MMP-9 in the aortic wall. There is no association to TIMP-1 or TIMP-2 levels. MMP-2 levels are positively, whereas MMP-9 levels are negatively correlated to aAAA. This may indicate that MMP-9 may have a determinant role in the AAA wall for the progression towards rupture, whereas MMP-2 pay a role for expansion.	E. Petersen et al. 2002 [19]
	37	Plasma levels of MMP-9 can accurately discriminate between patients with and without an endoleak with both high sensitivity and specificity. Anterior-postreior aneurysmal diameter (Dmax) was significantly larger in the endoleak group, however, plasma MMP-9 levels were not associated with Dmax or intraluminal thrombus volume.	F.A.M.V.I. Hellenthal et al.2012 [20]
MMP-9, MMP-1	52 non-ruptured AAA 16 ruptured AAA	The concentrations of MMP1 and MMP9 were significantly elevated in the plasma of ruptured AAA compared with non-ruptured AAA. There was no significant correlation between AAA diameter and enzyme concentration within the ruptured and non-ruptured cohorts.	W.R.W Wilson et al. 2008 [21]
P-Elastase	79	P-elastase was positively correlated with the mean annual AAA expansion rate.	Lindholt J. Et al. 2003
IFN-gamma	50	Elevated IFN-gamma concentrations seem to predict an increased rate of expansion in AAA.	Junoven J et al. 1997
TNF-alpha, IL-8	90	IL-8 and TNF-alpha can be used as endogenous markers of the process of AAA development.	Treska V et al. 2000
IL-6	7	In multivariate analysis the level of IL-6 was independently correlated with aortic diameter	Rodhe LE et al 1999
IL-6, MMP-9, CRP	213	No correlation was found between levels of circulating IL-6, MMP-9, CRP and the expansion of small-diameter AAAs, indicating no clinical use of these markers in AAA surveillance.	Karlsson L. Et al.2009 [22]

Biomarker	Number of patients	Summary of findings	Author, year
C-reactive Protein (CRP)	Sympt 52 Ruptured 62	No correlation. A significant elevation of CRP could be found in patients who presented symptoms or rupture of an AAA.	Domanivits H et al.2002
	545	CRP levels are elevated in larger aneurysms but do not appear to be associated with rapid expansion.	Norman P et al. 2004
	151	CRP did not correlate with size or expansion rate of AAA	Lindholt J et al 2001
Serum highly sensitive CRP	39	Serum hsCRP is associated with aneurysmal size.	Vainas T et al. 2003
CRP, alpha 1-antitripsin	35 AAA patients 35 controls	A positive correlation was found between CRP and AAA diameter and alpha 1-antitripsin and AAA growth. Alpha 1-antitripsin may be a promising biomarker of AAA growth.	M. Vega de Ceniga et al.2009 [23]
D-dimer, fibrinogen/fibrin	36	The largest diameter of AAA is correlated with the preoperative levels of D-dimer and FDP	Yamazuni K et al.1998
	834 cases with AAA and 6971 controls for fibrinogen 264 cases with AAA and 403 controls for D-dimer.	Plasma fibrinogen and D-dimer concentrations are likely to be higher in cases with AAA than control subjects. Higher plasma fibrinogen and D-dimer concentrations may be associated with the presence of AAA.	Takagi H. Et al. 2009 [12]
	110 patients with AAA 110- controls	Fibrinogen was positively correlated with AAA size ($r = 0.323$; $p < 0.01$) and the percentage of intra-luminal thrombus occupying the lumen ($r = 0.358$; $p < 0.05$).	Al-Barjas et al. 2006 [24]
Insulin-like Growth Factor 1 (IGF-I)	115 small AAAs	Serum IGF-I, but not IGF-II, correlated positively with AAA size and AAA growth. IGF-I levels may serve as a novel biomarker for the natural history of AAA.	J.S. Lindholt et al. 2011 [25]

Table 1. Summary of published studies reporting the role of circulating biomarkers in the growth and rupture of AAA

Active investigations continue to identify markers other than size that would predict a risk of rupture. Circulating biomarkers could also indicate optimal intervals between the surveillance intervals. Finally, the identification of biomarkers also may identify potential pathogenic pathways, and thus may open possibilities for pharmacological inhibition of growth, and provide a tool for monitoring this inhibition.[26]

In the future, extended longitudinal studies will be necessary to assess the true potential of matrix-turnover and other biomarkers. New methods, including proteomics and genome wide association studies, may identify new pathways and new potential biomarkers.

3. Treatment

Surgical repair was first reported in 1962 and still remains the treatment with the best long-term results. The surgical technique is illustrated in **Figure 1**. It is a major surgical procedure done under general anaesthesia, usually consisting of a midline laparotomy and cross clamping of the aorta and iliac vessels.

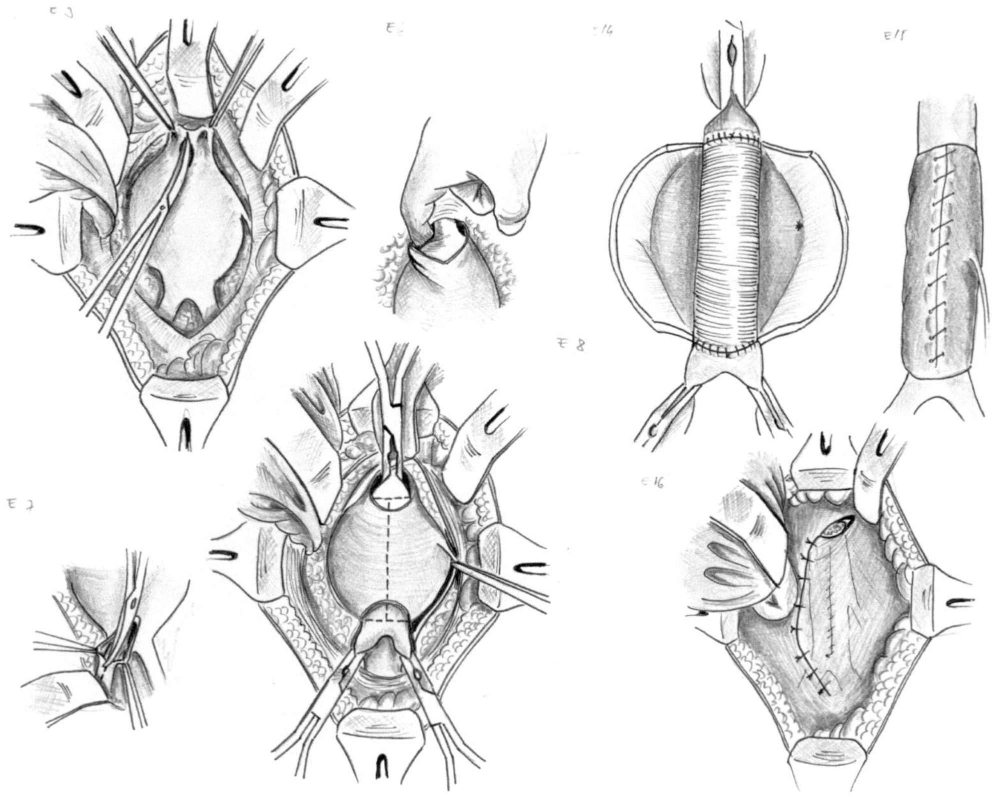

Figure 1. Open surgery technique for AAA

The mortality of elective surgery is between 3 and 7%. These rates increase significantly in patients with comorbidities, particularly with coronary artery disease and carotid artery disease. Surgical results are impaired by chronic renal failure and COPD.

Increasing age is an important adverse determinant of mortality in both ruptured and intact aneurysms.

In the USA statistics indicate that more than 15000 deaths/year are caused by aneurysm rupture.

This is the reason why there are screening studies among the target population in order to save lives and decrease health costs. The great interest is to detect and treat the AAA before rupture but the problem is that most of them are asymptomatic.

Because open surgery has non-negligible mortality and postoperative complications associated with a long hospital stay (10.8 days average) scientists tried to develop alternative methods to treat this disease addressing those cases with surgical high risk.

Minimally invasive techniques were developed in order to exclude the aneurysm from the circulation and to provide a new circulator channel towards the legs. Potential applications of endovascular grafts have been found in all areas of vascular surgery but their use for aortic aneurysms was the first to be explored. Endovascular aneurysm repair (EVAR) is an alternative to open surgery in the management of AAA. Juan Parodi and colleagues performed the first endovascular aneurysm repair in Argentina in 1991 [27,28]. Two decades after, the technique has evolved immensely and new devices developed allowing to a greater number of patients to be treated with EVAR. Repair of aortic abdominal aneurysm (AAA) is performed to prevent progressive expansion and rupture. [27, 29 30]

EVAR is progressively replacing open surgery and now accounts for more than half AAA repairs [31] as for example endovascular repair of AAA in Kaiser Hawaii Hospital (USA) was 50% in 2004 of the surgical activity.

A study published in November 2011 identifies the rate of endovascular treatment for AAA in different countries during 2005-2009 (**Figure 2**), whose prospective data were included in

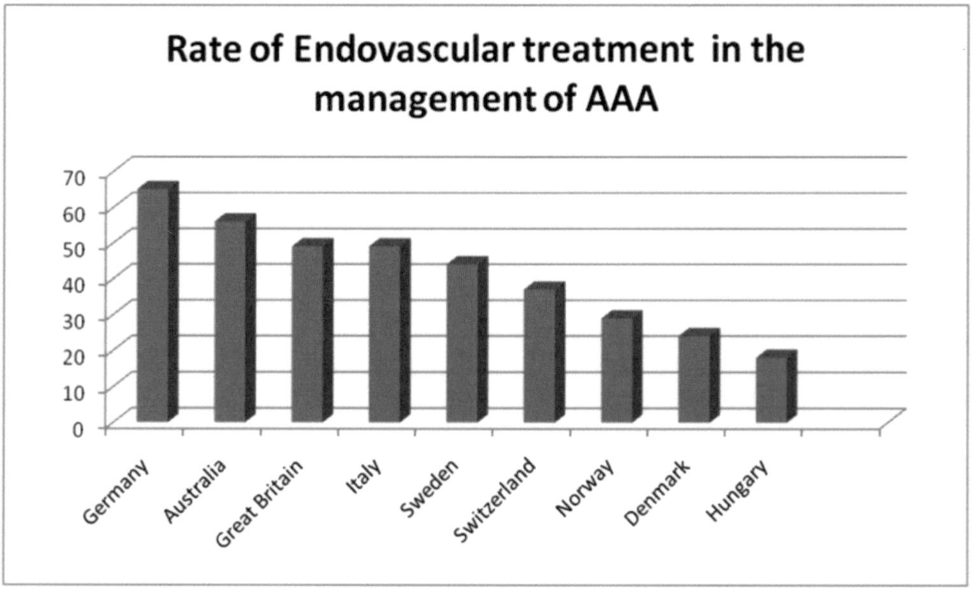

Figure 2. Rate of EVAR in the management of AAA in different countries

the VASCUNET database [32]. The study shows a rapid and extensive implementation of the endovascular treatment, with the advent of studies with favourable results in this direction.

EVAR in addition to the advantage of being a minimally invasive method and as such preferred by the patients, has many proven benefits compared with traditional open surgery: low rate of peri- and postoperative mortality and morbidity, shorter hospital stay, significantly reduced intraoperative blood loss and faster recovery. [33, 34, 35] One drawback is the significantly higher reintervention rate compared to open repair.

4. Evidence base for EVAR

In order to evaluate this new method there are registries [36] (retrospective studies) as: RETA (registry of endovascular treatment for aneurysms) in the UK, started in 1996 [37], EUROSTAR also started in 1996 [38], the Lifeline registry in the USA started in 1998 [39]. There are also randomized, controlled, multicenter trials: EVAR 1 and 2 initiated in 1999 and DREAM (Dutch randomized endovascular aneurysm management) started in 2000.

In RETA, 31 UK centers submitted data. From January 1996 to December 1998 611 cases were enrolled. Four percent received an aortic tube device, 60% an aorto-iliac device and 36% an aorto uni-iliac device with femoro-femoral crossover graft. The objectives were to assess early morbidity and mortality. Conversion to open repair was in 5% of cases. The overall mortality was 7% vs. 12% for open surgery. Endoleaks were more common in larger aneurysms (2% if aneurysm diameter was < 6 cm and 10% if it was > 6 cm) [37].

EUROSTAR (European collaboration on stent graft techniques for aortic aneurysm repair) Registry was established in 1996. The results were published in JVS in October 2000, 88 European centers have contributed, enrolling 2464 patients with a main follow up of 12.19 months. The 30 days mortality was 3.1%. The cumulative risk of late conversion was 2.1%/year and of rupture 1%/year. The significant factors for rupture were: type I endoleak, type III endoleak, graft migration and postoperative kinking of the endograft. The feasibility rate of the procedure was 97% of patients using first and second generation devices. The rate of late failure of the devices was 3%/year.[38,40]

The Lifeline registry was established in 1998 in the USA and the results were published in JVS in July 2005. The end point was to evaluate the long-term outcome of patients treated with EVAR using 5 devices who had FDA approval (Guidant Ancure, Medtronic AneuRx, Gore Excluder, Endologix PowerLink, Cook Zenith). It enrolled 2664 patients with EVAR vs. 334 open repair control patients. The 30 day mortality of EVAR was 1.7% which was not different from surgical control (1.4%), this in spite of the EVAR patients who were significantly older and sicker (more comorbidities). The risk of rupture of the aneurysm after EVAR was 3 times higher (2.1%) in women than in men (0.7%). The risk of rupture of the AAA remained stable over a 6 year period at a level of 1%/year. The surgical conversion rate was 3% at a year and 5% at 6 years (low). All this shows that EVAR is safe and effective in preventing aneurysm rupture and avoiding AAA related death. [39]

The most known and discussed randomized, controlled, multicentre trials are the UK EVAR1 and 2 which were initiated in 1999 and published in "The Lancet" in 2004 [41] and 2005 [42]. EVAR 1 compares endovascular procedures vs. open repair. A great number of patients (2068) were enrolled, aged over 60 years with a non ruptured AAA and who had an aneurysm of more than 5.5 cm in CT scan diameter. Morphological suitability for EVAR [43] and choice of the stent graft was decided by each center (41 centers enrolled). The 30-day mortality rate was 1.7% compared with 4.7% for open surgery. The secondary interventions were 9.8 for EVAR and 5.8 for open repair. Patients unfit for open repair because of significant comorbidities were randomized for EVAR or best medical treatment in the EVAR 2 trial. 338 patients aged 60 years or older with an AAA >5.5 cm in diameter were enrolled. The primary end point was aneurysm related mortality, postoperative complications and hospital costs. The risk of rupture is 25%/year for aneurysms with diameters greater than 6 cm. The 30-day mortality was 9% in EVAR group and in the non intervention group was 9.0 / 100 pers / year. There was no significant difference between the EVAR group and non intervention group for all cause mortality.

The DREAM trial initiated in 2000 enrolled 345 patients considered suitable for both types of treatment. The 30-day mortality after EVAR was 1.2% compared with 4.6% for open surgery. The results were published in 2002 in Journal of Cardiovascular Surgery [44, 45].

The Veteran open vs. endovascular repair (OVER) trial started enrollment in October 2002 in the US. It was design to enroll 5 years followed by a 4 year follow up. In total a 9 years survey. The primary outcome is long-term survival and secondary outcomes included morbidity, procedure failures and need for secondary procedures and costs. 33 centers are participating, 684 patients were enrolled in September 2006 and the investigators expect 900 by the end of the study. Patients enrolled had aneurysms of more than 5cm and were candidates for both procedural types. [46]

The French trial *"Anevrisme Chirurgie vs Endoprothese"* (ACE) also had the same enrollment conditions and primary and secondary end points.

In OVER and ACE trials were used newer devices for treating AAA than those used in EVAR 1 and DREAM (procedures performed between 1999-2003)[46]. The Gore Excluder and Medtronic AneuRx represent 2/3 from the devices used in OVER compared with only 11% used in EVAR 1.

Speaking about costs the shorter ITU and hospital stay in the EVAR group, with initial comparable costs, the cost per patient over 4 years is higher in EVAR because the cost of the endograft and subsequent of secondary interventions **(Figure 3)**[43].

In summary, EVAR has lower perioperative mortality but there is no difference in long term overall mortality. This procedure is associated with 10% risk of aneurysm related complications/ year, but they can be solved by further endovascular reinterventions [43].

EVAR is a safe, effective and durable treatment for infrarenal aortic aneurysms with suitable anatomy.

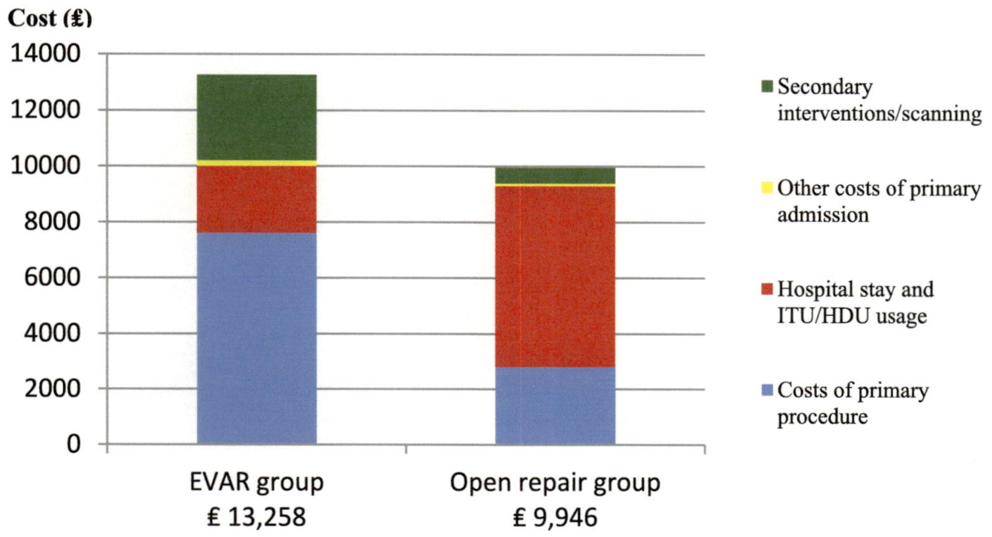

Figure 3. EVAR costs per patient (modified after [43])

5. Indications and anatomical suitability

Patient selection is an important element of successful EVAR. We should carefully investigate and consider the anatomy of the abdominal aorta, the relationship with the emergence of the renal arteries, the calibre, tortuosity and calcifications of the iliac arteries. The misevaluation of morphological aspects can lead to immediate or late failure of the procedure. With the refinement of medical devices (multislice CT scan with 3D reconstruction, substraction angiography, sophisticated computer data analysis), we can detect all the morphological modifications in the aneurismal area in segments immediately adjacent.

The Clinical Practice Guidelines of the European Society for Vascular Surgery on the management of AAA, published in April 2011, sets out a series of recommendations in all aspects of diagnosis and management strategies of AAA (Figure 4,5) [47].

There is a consensus that in the case of small aneurysms, with a diameter between 3.0-3.9 cm, the risk of rupture in negligible. Therefore, these aneurysms do not require surgery, supervision by Doppler Ultrasound at regular intervals being sufficient. The management of the AAA with a diameter between 4.0 – 5.5 was determined by two multicenter, randomised, controlled studies, that compared the natural evolution of these aneurysms versus early intervention: UK Small Aneurysm Trial (UKSAT) and American Aneurysm Detection and Management Study (ADAM) respectively [48, 49] and a smaller study, that compared endovascular treatment versus surveillance, the CAESAR study [50]. The PIVOTAL study including aneurysms with diameters between 4.0- 5.0 cm compared the endovascular treatment versus Doppler Ultrasound surveillance [51].

Medium-term results of these studies did not indicate a statistically significant difference in terms of overall mortality at 5 years, the results being similar in the long-term, at 12 years

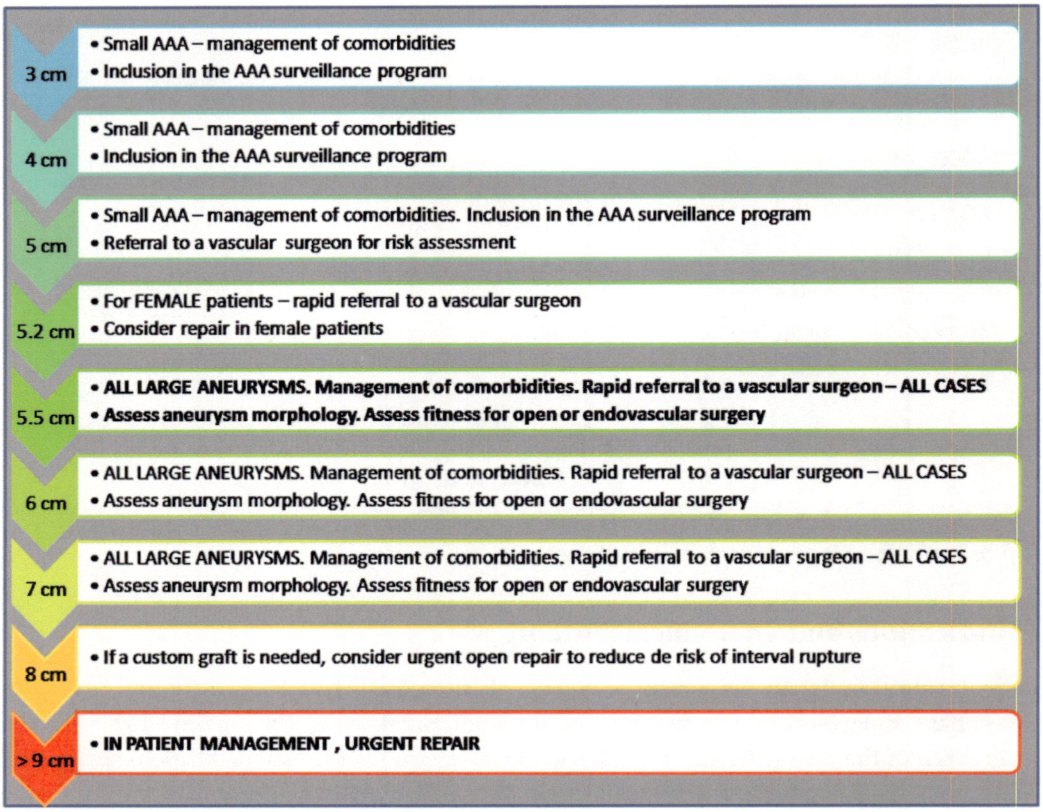

Figure 4. Management strategy of AAA according to the size of the aneurysm (modified after [47])

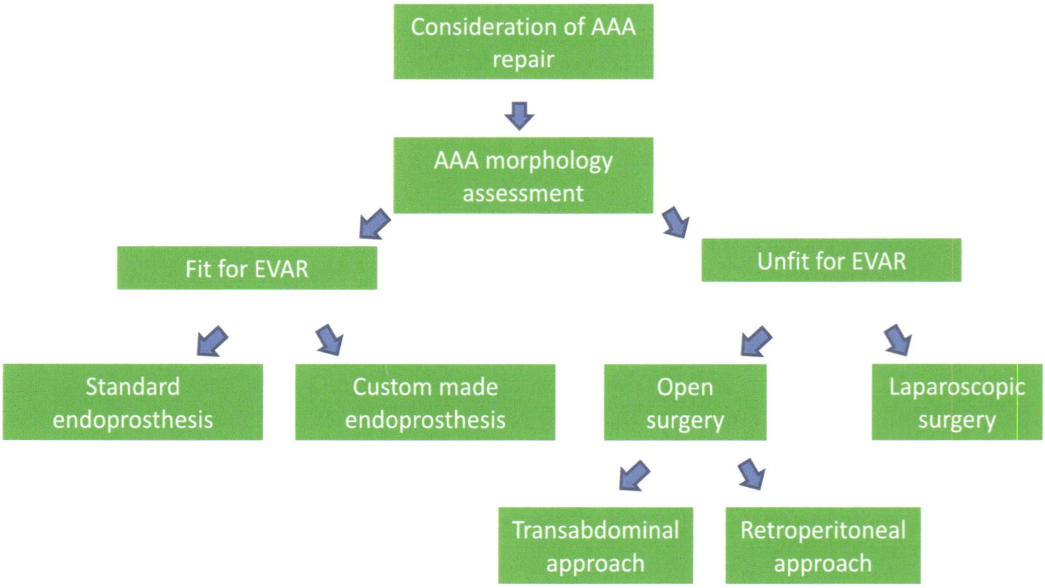

Figure 5. Management of large aneurysms, with a diameter ≥5,5 cm (modified after [47])

[48, 52]. The rupture rate of the aneurysms was 1% in the surveillance group and the overall mortality rate was 5,6% in the early intervention group.

The results of the above mentioned large studies, UKSAT and ADAM were recently included in the COCHRANE study, that underlines the safety and through this the benefits of the Doppler ultrasound surveillance of the AAA with a diameter between 4.0 and 5.5 cm [53].

Performing Doppler Ultrasound surveillance of small aneurysms (4.0-5.5 cm) is safe and recommended for asymptomatic aneurysms. If the aneurysm reaches the 5.5 cm diameter limit, measured by Doppler ultrasound (in male patients), it becomes symptomatic or there is an annual diameter increase of >1cm/year, the patient must be immediately referred for further investigation to the specialised vascular surgery department.

As highlighted, the diameter of the AAA establishes the moment for intervention, but this criteria alone is not enough to establish the indication for the endovascular treatment of the AAA. With new treatment methods new complications occur, requiring further investigations in order to assess the feasibility of the AAA for EVAR. The morphological criteria of the AAA are the ones that can establish or exclude the indication of EVAR. The failure to comply with these criteria, requested also in the instruction manuals of the endoprostheses currently on the market may lead to the increase of the peri- and postoperative complication, reintervention and post-EVAR mortality rate.

An average 34% of AAA is not eligible for EVAR, most of them because of an adverse morphology. [54]

The universal classification system defines the aneurysm in relation with the origin of renal arteries:

- infrarenal, with a segment of normal (undilated) aorta named neck
- pararenal or juxtarenal, when aneurysm originate just after the renals
- suprarenal, the aneurysm includes the origin of renals or above without involvement of the superior mesenteric artery

Another classification employed for EUROSTAR and DREAM trials is shown in **figure 6,** taking into account the distance from the renals and the bifurcation of the aorta as well as the involvement of iliac arteries (the common iliac artery, arriving or not to the bifurcation of iliac arteries, occlusion or stenosis of the common iliac arteries).

The French system proposed by Kieffer & Chiche (2005) is also based on the distal extension of the aneurysm and is comparable with the EUROSTAR classification (Type I-V).

The proximal neck is by far one of the most important anatomic finding in planning an endovascular procedure. It can be classified as shown in **figure 7.**

The diameter of the neck, its length, shape and angulation are to be considered. Aortic neck angulation is defined as the angle between the axes of the proximal infrarenal aorta and the longitudinal axis of the aneurysm. It is classified as: mild < 40 degrees, moderate < 60dgr, and severe > 60dgr.

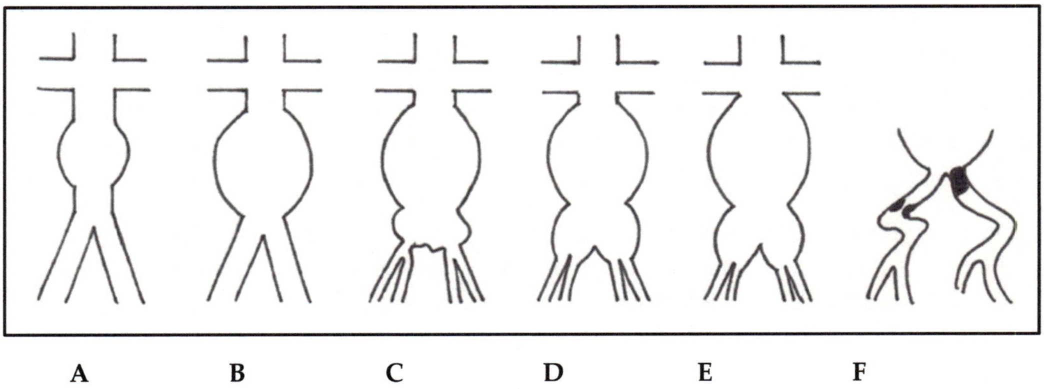

Figure 6. Classification of AAA (modified after [40])

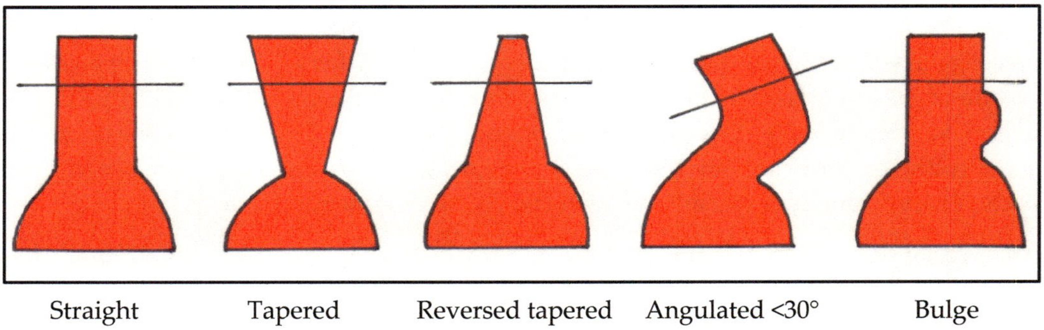

Figure 7. Morphology of the aortic neck (modified after [40])

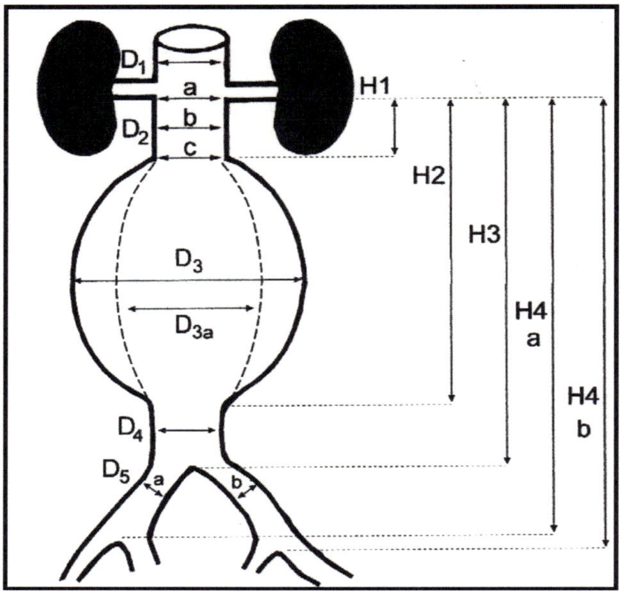

Figure 8. Preoperative measurements (EUROSTAR)

The neck is the place where the endoprotheses are fixed and sealed. Seal is the apposition of the outer surface of the endograft to the luminal surface of the aorta in order to exclude the aneurysm sac from the systemic pressure. Fixation is the counterforce that prevents migration and helps to maintain seal.

Concerning the iliac arteries, the landing zone of the majority of grafts, we are interested in patency and diameter, length of the common iliac artery, shape or aneurismal, angulation or tortuosity and calcifications.

Figure 8 shows a preoperative scheme for planning an endovascular repair showing all the anatomical features discussed above.(after [40])

5. Types of endoprostheses in use

The grafts are classified in different manners. From the anatomic point of view, they can be: bifurcated (Ao bi-iliac), Ao – uni-iliac and tube (for Ao – Aortic – these were the most used, but now they are out of the market). They can be modular (most of them) or unibody (Powerlink).

Figure 9 shows the images of some endoprosthesis in use today: modular (a,b,c) and unibody (d).

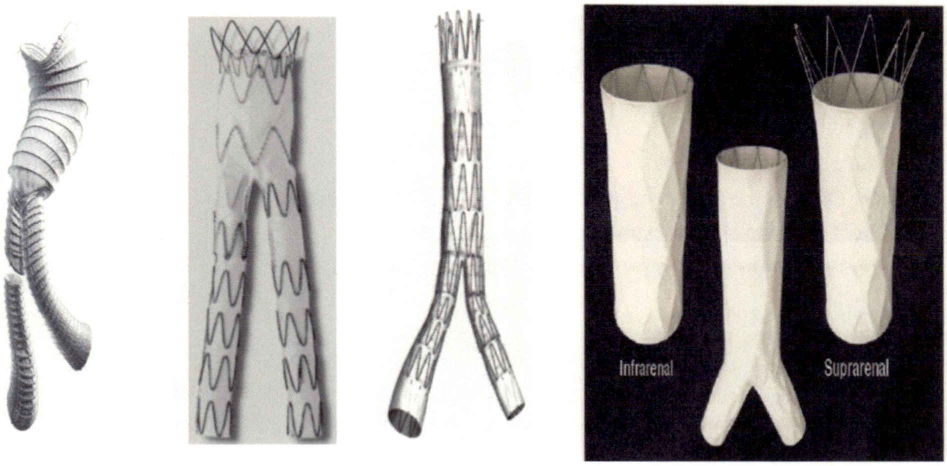

a) Anaconda *b) Talent* *c) Zenith* *d) Powerlink*

Figure 9. Most used endoprosthesis

The modular devices have at least two component grafts. The main body deployed on the neck of the aneurysm *("hanging from the Aorta")* and the two legs that arrives on the common iliac arteries. The unibody prostheses build up the endoluminal channel from the bottom to the top, sitting on the aortic bifurcation (concept of anatomical fixation) [55]. This prevents distal migration of the endoprostheses.

The characteristics of the most used endografts [56, 57] are shown in the **table 2:**

Endograft characteristics							
Device	**Material**	**Confi-guration**	**Deployment**	**Fixation**	**Aortic graft diam.**	**Iliac graft diam.**	**Supra-renal stent**
Zenith (Cook)	Polyester	Modular	Self-expanding	Compression-fit and barbs	22-36	8-24	Yes
Talent (Medtronic)	Polyester	Modular	Self-expanding	Compression-fit	24-34	8-24	Yes
Excluder (Gore)	ePTFE	Modular	Self-expanding	Compression-fit and anchors	23/26/28.5	12-14.5	No
Anaconda (Terumo)	Twilleave	Modular	Self-expanding	Compression-fit and hooks	19.5-34	9-18	No
Powerlink (Endologix)	ePTFE	One-piece	Self-expanding	Compression-fit	25/28	16	Optional
E-Vita (Jotec)	Polyester	Modular	Self-expanding	Compression-fit	24/34	14-26	yes

Table 2. The characteristics of the most used endografts [56, 57]

The characteristics of an ideal stent graft are:

- Low overall cost,
- Stent-graft size ranging,
- Long durability (metallic ultrastructure + graft material),
- Good biocompatibility and sealing capacity,
- Delivery device flexibility, lowest delivery device size,
- Radial force stability,
- Customization

The new results of the endovascular management of AAA (by type of endograft) are shown in **table 3** (retrospective or prospective studies) published in 2010 [58-63].

EVAR is not a procedure without complications[64-66]. One of the most redoubtable are the *endoleak* [67]. They are defined as persistence of the blood flow outside the lumen of the endograft, but within the aneurismal sac [68]. An endoleak may perfuse the aneurysm sac leading to aneurysm expansion and may be rupture. It represents the inability to obtain or maintain secure seal between the aortic wall and the graft [1]. The incidence of endoleaks is in range of 14%. They are classified in four types (from I to IV) [see the **table 4** [1] modified].

The technique of introduction and deployment of the endograft is shown in **figure 10**. The access sites are the two femoral arteries. The anaesthesia required is general anaesthesia or loco-regional (peridural) [69].

Device	Author	Study Type	Nº cases	Period	Outcome		Clinical success
					Peri OP mortality	Limb patency 24months	
Anaconda (Terumo)	Freyrie [58]	Prospective single center	127	2005-2009	0	96,7	100
Excluder (Gore)	Ghotbi [59]	Retro-spective	100	2006-2009	0	100	100
Endourant (Medtronic)	Bockler [60]	"Engage" prospective	180	2008-2009	1,7	100	99,4
Zenith (Cook)	Bequemin [61]	Prospective single center	212	2000-2004	0,9		99,5
Powerlink (Endologix)	Krajcer [62]	Prospective single center	50	2008-2010	0	100	98
Evita (Jotec)	Moula-kakis [63]	Retro-spective single center	30	2008-2009	0	100	100

Table 3.

I. Attachment site leaks
- Proximal end of endograft
- Distal end of endograft
- Iliac occlude [plug]
II. Branch leaks (collateral back bleeding)
- simple (one)
- complex (two or more branches)
III. Graft defect (modular dissociation)
- minor < 2mm
- major ≥ 2 mm
IV. Graft material porosity

Table 4. Classification of Endoleaks [1]
Both types I and III are significant risk factors for late aneurysm rupture and should be treated. Types II are considered benign and type IV usually resolves spontaneously during the post procedure period.

With this procedure, we can reduce blood lost (using also devices like the cell-saver) and consequent transfusion requirement, ITU and hospital stay. More patients can be treated where comorbidity previously excluded them. The follow-up is done by using CT scan exams at 1, 3, 6 and 12 months after the procedure. There are changes in the aneurysm volume after endovascular repair in terms of shrinking [61,70,71].

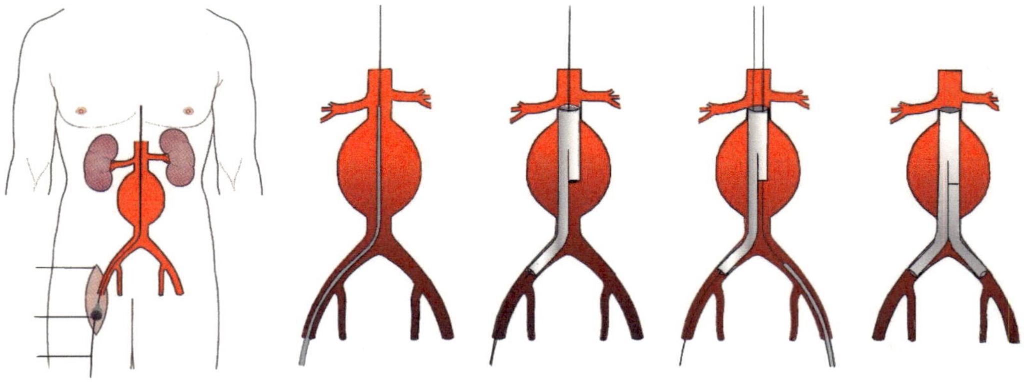

Figure 10. Schema of modular endograft deployment

6. Operative data and results (Nürnberg experience and Army's Clinic Center for Cardiovascular Diseases, Bucharest)

We have conducted a prospective, randomized study starting from 1994, including patients diagnosed with infrarenal aortic aneurysm with a diameter ≥ 5.5 cm. The purpose of this study was to assess the results of abdominal aortic aneurysm repair of two large volume centers, in terms of perioperative, early and midterm complications, reintervention rate and mortality.

Exclusion criteria were: Presence of comorbidities that could affect the postoperative surveillance: Renal insufficiency with serum creatinine level > 1.5 mg/dl, serum urea > 50 mg/dl, mental illnesses, hypersensitivity to the contrast agent, unable to be followed as an outpatient, claustrophobia, the presence of previously implanted metal devices: pace makers, mechanical heart valves etc.

Collected data: The collected data was entered in an excel database. Patient demographics and other variables were introduced, like:

- Qualitative variables: endovascular treatment indication, name and type of prosthesis used, vascular access method (percutaneous puncture of the femoral artery, surgical incision, temporary iliac conduit), type of anaesthesia, postoperative complications occurred (endoleak, endograft migration, kinking)
- Continuous quantitative variables: pre- and postoperative data on aneurysm morphology determined by CTA preoperatively and by DUS and CTA postoperatively (maximal anterior-posterior and transverse dimension of the aneurysm sac, length of the aneurysm, size and morphological changes of the aneurysm neck, the distance between the aneurysm and the emergence of the renal arteries, common iliac artery length and diameter) duration of intervention, the amount of blood loss, reinterventions.

In Nürnberg, we started endovascular treatment in 1994 with Ancure stent-graft. In our 14–years experience of 1502 cases (ending dec. 2007) we have used 13 different endografts.

From them, 1391 were men and 111 women, with a mean age of 71.5 years (41-98). The median follow up was 41 months (1.0-98) and the AAA had a mean diameter of 52.4 cm. For short and angulated necks we prefer now the Powerlink (Irvine, CA, USA) device, which we have started in 1999 [72]. Ending Dec. 2007, 519 cases were done using Powerlink grafts.

The 30 day mortality was 1.7%. The total reintervention rate was 5.3%, while no distal migration, conversion or post Evar rupture occurred. Using this device we arrive to treat endovascularly 85-90% of the infrarenal AAAs in our hospital.

At the **Army's Clinic Center for Cardiovascular Diseases,** Bucharest, between July 2008 - December 2010, 17 patients underwent EVAR for Abdominal Aortic Aneurysm (AAA), with age range between 49-82 years and aneurysm mean diameter 7.1 ± 0,5 cm (range: 5.4 – 8.2 cm) [73].

The preoperative assessment was achieved using Doppler Ultrasound (DUS), Multislice CT, and sometimes DSA (Digital Substraction Angiography). The measurements for the graft type and dimensions were done according to the Multislice CT analyzing. (**Figure 11 a, b and c**).

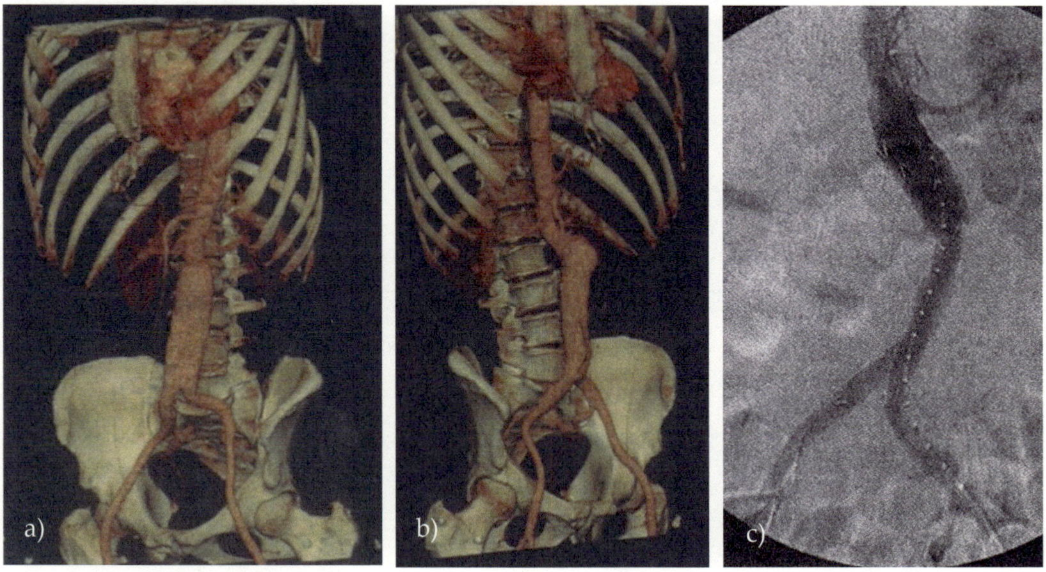

Figure 11. a), b) Preoperative multislice CT of a infrarenal AAA, with a suitable anatomy (2.2 cm neck length, no involvement of iliac arteries, 5.3 cm transversal diameter. **c)** Preoperative substraction angiography – with a catheter measuring the real length of the Aorta

The EVAR devices used for these patients were:

- Anaconda (Vascutek, Terumo, Inchinnan, Scotland)-1 patient
- Talent (Medtronic, Santa Rosa, CA, USA) -3 patients
- Powerlink (Endologix, Irvine,CA, USA) – 7 patients
- EVITA (Iotec, Hechingen, Germany)- 6 patients.

The access was bifemoral, through open femoral incision, with peridural anaesthesia.

Until present they followed our institutions surveillance protocol, that consisted of both DUS and CTA examination at 1,3,6,12 months and yearly after EVAR. None of them went through all of the surveillance dates (due to high examination costs) but each has at least 3 sets of examinations, one set consisting of both DUS and CTA.

The technical success rate was 100%, with no perioperative and postoperative complications regarding endoleaks, graft migration and graft component failure. 4 patients had access site complications, 3 had groin haematomas that reabsorbed after approximately 1 week and 1 returned with an infection at the level of the inguinal incision, which resolved also with wound care. There were no conversions to open repair up to present. The stent-graft patency rate at this point at these patients is 100%.

Figures 12 and **13** show two cases of AAAs treated with two different devices and two different strategies: Anaconda (Terumo) device and Powerlink (Endologix) stent graft.

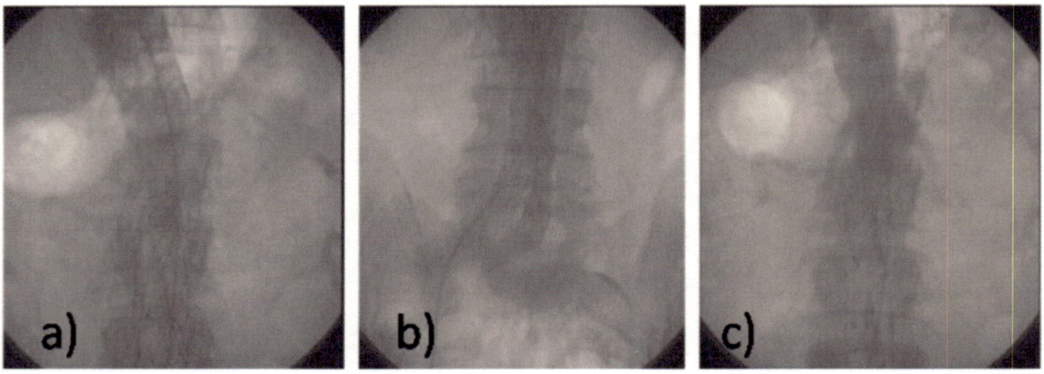

Figure 12. AAA treated with Powerlink Endograft **a)** Proximal extension; **b)** Main body of the stent-graft; **c)** The two iliac segments of Powerlink® system

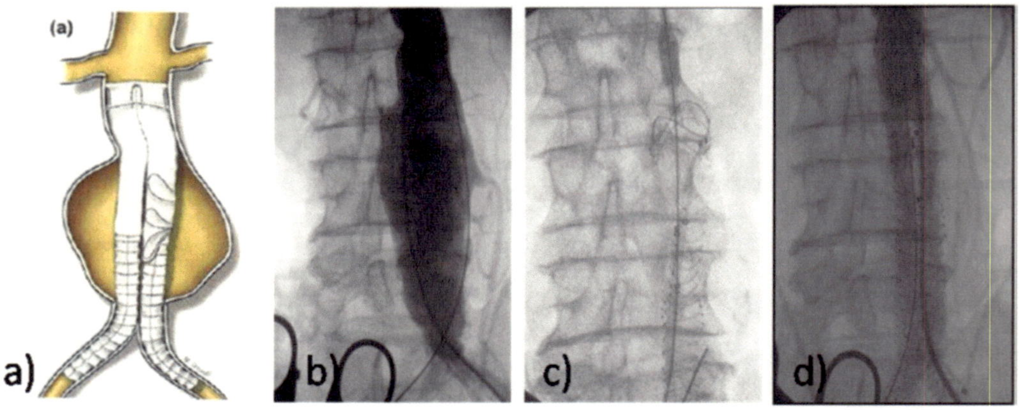

Figure 13. **a)** Anaconda endograft for infrarenal abdominal aortic aneurysm therapy; **b)** Angiography at the beginning of the procedure; **c)** The main body of the stent; **d)** The two iliac Anaconda system

7. Particular situations

7.1. Ruptured AAA

In open repair of ruptured AAAs the perioperative mortality ranges between 30% and 65%[74,75].Emergency EVAR is an alternative in selected patients with RAAA. The first report of emergency repair of an AAA was in 1994. Possible advantages are avoiding general anesthesia and laparotomy. Though a major inconvenient is the need of an endovascular team to be available at all times and to assess the preoperative CT scan in order to choose the size of the device. Following the emergent CT scan the anatomical suitability for EVAR was evaluated, including the access vessels [76].Several modular or unibody devices can be used but aorto-uni-iliac devices with subsequent fem-fem crossover bypass and occlusion of contralateral iliac artery could also be used. Veith [77] reported in 2009 a series of 57 patients with R-AAA treated endovascularly. 25 of these patients received the **VI graft (**distributed in Europe by Datascope-Maquet), made of a large Palmaz stent attached to a PTFE graft. This graft is used in aortofemoral configuration. This graft is "a one size fits most "because the proximal diameter can vary from 20 to27mm depending on the balloon inflation pressure. The periprocedural mortality was only 12,3%,inspite of serious medical comorbidities of the patients.

In the series reported by Kapma in 2005 on 253 patients treated with E-EVAR vs open surgery the perioperative mortality was lower (13%) in the Evar group compared with OR (30% p=0,021).According to the SVS practical guidelines [31] E-EVAR should be considered for treatment of a R-AAA, if anatomically feasible, with a **strong** level of recommendation and a **moderate** quality of evidence.

7.2. Juxtarenal AAA

Juxtarenal AAA have short (11-15mm), or very short (< 10mm) necks. The anatomically unsuitable AAAs has short and/or angulated necks. They have a high risk of stent graft distal migration and proximal type I endoleak, because the inability to provide a sufficient proximal landing zone to secure fixation and seal. The strategy for treating this challenging AAAs is to build up the endoluminal exclusion system from the aortic bifurcation to the renal artery level with suprarenal fixation. At Nürnberg Hospital we used the Powerlink unibody bifurcated stent graft with a long suprarenal cuff. A Palmaz stent can be used for proximal fixation in hostile necks (short necks with severe angulation).

Suprarenal fixation does not lead to a significant increase of acute renal events (renal insufficiency, high blood pressure) compared with infrarenal fixation [72]

Figure 14 shows an angiography of AAA treated with a Powerlink graft with suprarenal fixation; for better sealing a proximal ballooning at the end of the procedure was performed.

7.3. AAA with iliac extension

The iliac extension of the AAAs can put technical problems in choosing the graft, especially if the iliac aneurysm reaches the bifurcation of the iliac artery (fig.11a). In this situation, the

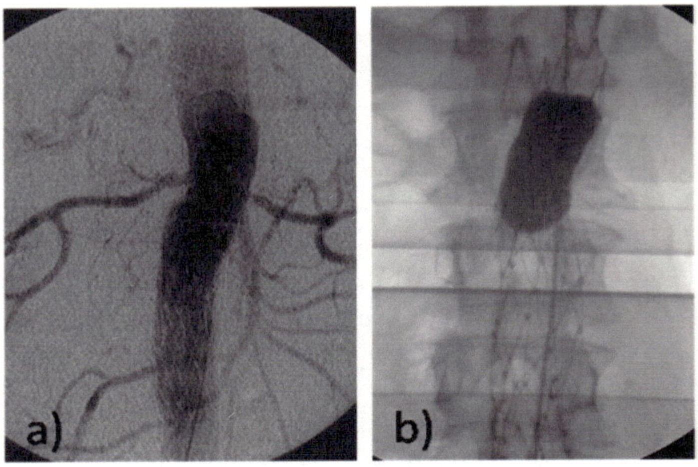

Figure 14. **a)** After suprarenal prox. Cuff; **b)** Proximal balloning. Fenestrated grafts are now available to treat juxtarenal AAA [78-80]

leg of the graft should land on the external iliac artery, covering the hypogastric artery (post-operation complications can occur like buttock claudication). In the case of planning to cover one hypogastric artery, we should close the artery (by coiling for ex.) a few days before implanting the endograft, in order to prevent distal type II endoleak.

Figure 15 shows a 72 year old patient treated at the Army's Center for Cardiovascular Diseases, using a Powerlink graft with left iliac graft extension - left hypogastric artery was occluded with coils 24h before the intervention.

In order to preserve the hypogastric artery, custom made, fenestrated or branched endografts can be used. Although this procedure was performed to prevent pelvic ischemia, this is not always the case. **Figure 16** presents a case of a 75 year old male patient with AAA

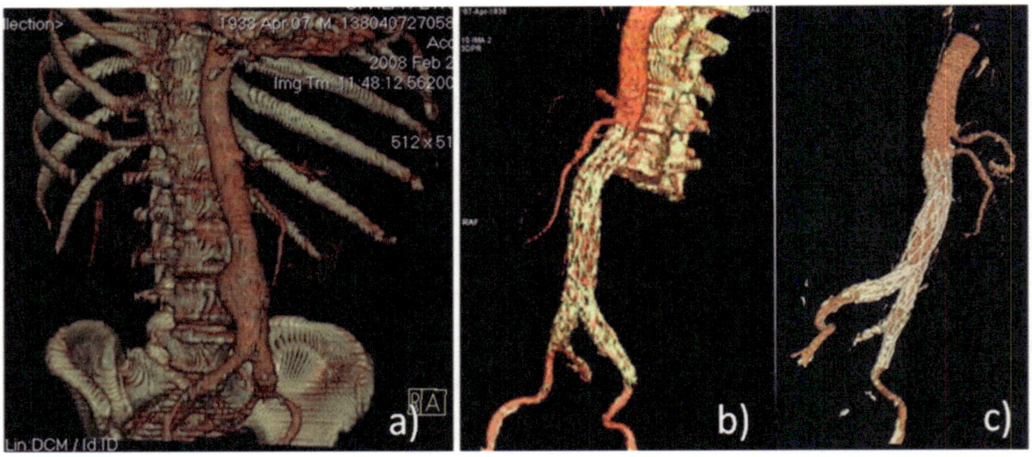

Figure 15. Patient O.P., 72 years old, preoperative multislice CT; **a)** AAA with left iliac extension; **b)** multislice CT-Scan at 3 months after EVAR with PowerLink endoprosthesis; **c)** multislice CT-Scan 2 years after EVAR with PowerLink endoprosthesis.

treated by EVAR with a fenestrated endograft that presented to our department with buttock claudication 6 months after EVAR. The performed angiography evidentiated an occluded right hypogastric artery. Conservative treatment with Vasaprostan 20μg was instituted with good results.

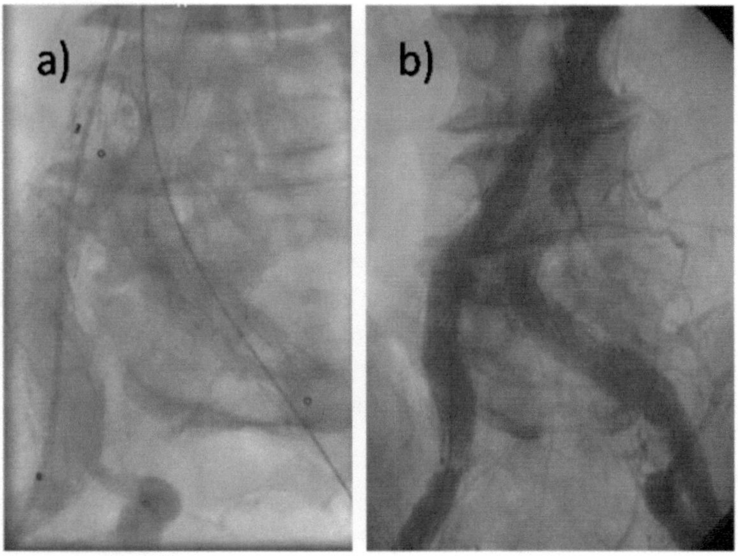

Figure 16. 75 year old male patient with AAA treated by EVAR Completion angiography after EVAR using a fenestrated endograft for the right hypogastric artery. **b)** Angiography performed 6 months after the intervention showing an occluded right hypogastric artery.

7.4. AAA and comorbidities: Coronary artery disease, carotid stenosis.

It is well known today that cardiac complications of patients with AAAs treated endovascularly is between 3 to 7%[31]. In order to avoid useless coronarographic investigations , we have to identify clinical parameters to indicate prior myocardial revascularization (surgery or stenting). Kieffer and Coriat, in a study published in 1999, on 270 patients operated for terminal Aorta pathology (aneurismal or stenotic) show an incidence of 55% of coronary stenosis in the AAA population which requires in 25% of cases myocardial revascularization. The risk factors which were identified were age >65 years and history of myocardial infarction. Stable angina with left main disease, or triple-vessel disease, as well as patients with two vessel disease that includes proximal LAD are candidates for preoperative coronary revascularization. The coronary intervention should be done prior to AAA treatment in one month interval. However the perioperative mortality can arrive to 25% (with extracorporeal circulation and cardiac arrest)

The carotid stenosis with a hemodynamic impact has a prevalence of 10.5%in the AAA patients.

Coronary and/or carotid lesions, treated or not, represent a significant risk factor for postoperative death. For this, systematic preoperative screening is mandatory [81,82].

Steinmetz published in 2008 an analysis of outcome after using high risk criteria selection to surgery vs. EVAR [83].The conclusion was that high risk criteria cannot be decisive in the choice of treatment.

8. Future developments

8.1. Totally percutaneous procedures

Because local groin wound complications as a result of the exposure of the two common femoral arteries are not negligible [84], surgeons and engineers tried to develop alternative access techniques. One of them is the fully percutaneous procedure. The main device available is Perclose ProstarXL(Abbott). For technical success patient and device selection should be done. Severe femoral artery calcification, scarred groins, femoral artery aneurysms are contraindications for the use of these devices. The overall related complications were 4.4%. Among them infection and artery trombose are the most redoubtable. The hospital stay is shorter in patients undergoing P-EVAR (2.7 days vs. 3.5 days) compared with EVAR. In conclusion, P-EVAR appears safe and effective in selected patients.

8.2. MRI devices

A new research field in our days is based on the hypotheses that the endografts can be visualized and navigated in vivo solely under Rt-MRI(real time magnetic resonance imaging). MRI can provide immediate assessment of endograft apposition and aneurysm exclusion. MRI offers also better soft tissue visualization, detecting type I endoleaks by depiction of complex 3D anatomy.

The technique is now applicable on murine models of AAA [85]. They have used a passive commercial endograft, image based on metal MRI artefacts, and active homemade endografts incorporating MRI receiver coils (antennae). Active devices proved to be most useful. The MRI images proved graft apposition and aneurysm exclusion. MRI imaging also permits immediate post-procedural anatomical and functional evaluation of the successful procedure.

In conclusion, MRI may be equivalent or superior to computed tomography for procedure planning and surveillance of the endografts. Future development of active devices is required, in order to have a commercial graft that can be used in clinical testing and practice.

9. Conclusions

Our results show that in the modern era of abdominal aortic aneurysm treatment EVAR is an appropriate treatment for selected patients, especially those at high risk for open surgical repair.

The future of EVAR as the potential gold standard for aortic aneurysm therapy rests upon the vision and creativity of both surgeons and technology innovators to realize the potential of endovascular interventions, and take them toward a broader and more effective portfolio of techniques and devices that will define the XXI-st Century Endovascular Aortic Surgery.

Author details

Ionel Droc* and Blanca Calinescu
Cardiovascular Surgery Department, Army's Clinic Center for Cardiovascular Diseases, Bucharest, Romania

Dieter Raithel
Klinikum Nürnberg Sud, Nürnberg, Germany

10. References

[1] Jaunoo S (2008) Endovascular aneurysm repair (EVAR). International Journal of Surgery. 6:266-269.
[2] Wyatt M.G (1999) Aneurysmal disease. In: Davies A.H, editor. Vascular Surgery Highlights 1998-1999. Oxford: Health Press. pp. 41-48.
[3] Garcia-Madric C, Josa M, Riambau V, Mestres C.A, Muntana J, Mulet J (2004) Endovascular versus open surgical repair of abdominal aortic aneurysm: a comparison of early and intermediate results in patients suitable for both techniques. Eur J Vasc Endovasc Surg. 28:365-372.
[4] Melton L, Bickerstaff L, Hollier L et al. (1984) Changing incidence of abdominal aortic aneurysms: A population-based study. Am J Epidemiol. 120:379-386.
[5] Reilly J.M, Tilson M.D (1989) Incidence and etiology of abdominal aortic aneurysms. Surg Clin North Am. 69:705-711.
[6] Pannu H, Fadulu V.T, Chang J et al. (2005) Mutations in transforming growth factor-beta receptor type II cause familial thoracic aortic aneurysms and dissections. Circulation.112:513-520.
[7] Busuttil R.W, Rinderbriecht H, Flesher A et al. (1982) Elastase activity: the role of elastase in aortic aneurysm formation. J Surg Res. 32:214-217.
[8] Safi H.J (2007) Thoracic aortic aneurysms: classification, incidence, etiology, natrural history and results. In: Lumsden A.B, Lin P.H, Changyi Chen, Parodi J.C, editors. Advanced Endovascular Therapy of Aortic Disease. Malden: Blackwell Publishing. pp. 25-30
[9] Ailawadi G, Eliason J.L, Upchurch G.R Jr. (2003) Current concepts in the pathogenesis of abdominal aortic aneurysm. J.Vasc Surg. 38:584-588.
[10] Grootenboer N, Bosch J.L, Hendriks J.M, van Sambeek M.R.H.M (2009) Epidemiology, Aetiology, Risk of Rupture and Treatment of Abdominal Aortic Aneurysms: Does Sex Matter?. Eur J Vasc Endovasc Surg. 38:278-284.
[11] Mosorin M, Junoven J, Biancari F, Satta J, Surcel H.M, Leinonen M et al. (2001) Use of doxycycline to decrease the growth rate of abdominal aortic aneurysms: A randomized, double-blind, placebo-controlled pilot study. J Vasc Surg. 34:606-610.
[12] Takagi H, Manabe H, Kawai N, Goto S, Umemoto T (2009) Plasma Fibrinogen and D-dimer Concentrations are Associated with the presence of Abdominal Aortic Aneurysm: A Systematic Review and Meta-analysis. Eur J Vasc Endovasc Surg. 38:273-277

* Corresponding Author

[13] Freestone T, Turner R.J, Coady A, Higman D.J, Greenhalgh R.M, Powell J.T (1995) Inflammation and matrix metalloproteinases in the enlarging abdominal aortic aneurysm. Arterioscler Thromb Vasc Biol. 15(8):1145-51.
[14] McMillan W.D, Tamarina N.A, Cipollone M, Johnson D.A, Parker M.A, Pearce M.A, Pearce W.H (1997) Size matters: the relationship between MMP-9 expression and aortic diameter. Circulation. 96(7):2228-32.
[15] Pyo R, Jason L.K, Shipley M, Curci J.A, Mao D, Ziporin S.J et al. (2000) Targeted disruption of matrix-metalloproteinase-9 (gelatinase B) suppresses development of experimental abdominal aoric aneurysms. J Clin Invest. 105:1641-9.
[16] Thompson R.W, Parks W.C. (1996) Role of matrix metalloproteinases in abdominal aortic aneurysms. Ann NY Acad Sci. 800:157-174.
[17] Newman K.M et al. (1994) Identification of matrix metalloproteinases 3 (stomelysin-1) and 9 (gelatinase B) in abdominal aortic aneurysms. Arterioscler Thromb. 14: 1315-1320.
[18] Hovsepian D.M, Ziporin S.J, Sakurai M.K, Lee J.K, Curci J.A, Thompson R.W (2000) Elevated plasma levels of matrix metalloproteinase-9 in patients with abdominal aortic aneurysms: a circulating marker of degenerative aneurysm disease. J Vasc Interv Radiol. 11(10):1345-52
[19] Petersen E, Wagberg F, Angquist K.A (2002) Proteolysis of the Abdominal Aortic Aneurysm Wall and the Association with Rupture. Eur J Vasc Endovasc Surg. 23:153-157.
[20] Hellenthal F.A.M.V.I et al. (2012) Plasma Levels of Matrix Metalloproteinase-9: A Possible Diagnostic Marker of Successful Endovascular Aneurysm Repair. Eur J Vasc Endovasc Surg. 43:171-172.
[21] Wilson W.R.W, Anderton M, Choke E.C, Dawson J, Loftus I.M, Thompson M.M (2008) Elevated Plasma MMP1 and MMP9 are Associated with Abdominal Aortic Aneurysm Rupture. Eur J Vasc Endovasc Surg. 35:580-584.
[22] Karlsson L, Bergqvist D, Lindback J, Parsson H (2009) Expansion of Small-diameter Abdominal Aortic Aneurysms is Not Reflected by the Release of Inflammatory Mediators IL-6, MMP-9 and CRP in Plasma. Eur J Vasc Endovasc Surg. 37:420-424.
[23] Vega de Ceniga M, Esteban M, Quintana J.M, Barba A, Estallo L, De la Fuente N, Viviens B, Martin-Ventura J.L (2009) Search for Serum Biomarkers Associated with Abdominal Aortic Aneurysm Growth- A Pilot Study. Eur J Vasc Endovasc Surg. 37:297-299.
[24] Al-Barjas H.S, Ariens R, Grant P, Scott J.A (2006) Raised plasma fibrinogen concentration in patients with abdominal aortic aneurysm. Angiology. 57:607-14.
[25] Lindholt J.S et al. (2011) Insulin-like Growth Factor I- A Novel Biomarker of Abdominal Aortic Aneurysms. Eur J Vasc Endovasc Surg. 42:560-562.
[26] Urbonavicius S, Urbonaviciene G, Honore B, Henneberg E.W, Vorum H, Lindholt J.S (2008) Potential Circulating Biomarkers for Abdominal Aortic Aneurysm Expansion and Rupture – a Systematic Review. Eur J Vasc Endovasc Surg. 36:273-280.
[27] Parodi J.C, Palmaz J.C, Barone H.D (1991) Transfemoral intraluminal graft implantation for abdominal aortic aneurysms. Ann Vasc Surg. 5:496.
[28] Parodi J.C (1995) Endovascular repair of abdominal aortic aneurysms. In: Chuter T, Donayre C.E, White R.A, editors. Endoluminal Vascular Prostheses. Brown and Company. pp.37-55.

[29] Matsumura J.S, Brewster D.C, Makaroun M, Naftel D.C (2003) A multicenter controlled clinical trial of open versus endovascular treatment of abdominal aortic aneurysm. Journal of Vascular Surgery. 37:262-271.

[30] Goncalves F.B, Rouwet E.V, Metz R, Hendriks J.M, Vrancken Peeters M.P, Muhs B.E, Verhagen H.J (2010) Device-specific outcomes after endovascular abdominal aortic aneurysm repair. J Cardiovasc Surg. 51:515-531.

[31] Chaikof E.L, Brewster D.C, Dalman R.L, Makaroun M, Illig K.A, Sicard G.A, Timaran C.H, Upchurch Jr G.R, Veith F.J (2009) SVS practice guidelines for the care of patients with abdominal aortic aneurysm: Executive summary. Journal of Vascular Surgery. 50:880-896.

[32] Mani K, Lees T, Beiles B, Jensen L.P, Venermo M, Simo G, Palombo D et al. (2011) Treatment of Abdominal Aortic Aneurysm in Nine Countries 2005-2009: A Vascunet Report. . Eur J Vasc Endovasc Surg. 42; 598-607.

[33] EVAR Trial Participants (2005) Endovascular aneurysm repair versus open repair in patients with abdominal aortic aneurysm (EVAR trial 1): randomised controlled trial. The Lancet. 365: 2179-86.

[34] Prinssen M, Verhoeven E.L, Buth J, Cuypers P.W, van Sambeek M.R, Balm R et al. (2004) A randomised trial comparing conventional and endovascular repair of abdominal aortic aneurysms. N Engl J Med. 351:1607-18.

[35] Aljabri B, Al Wahaibi K, Abner D, Mackenzie K.S, Corriveau M.M, Obrand D.I et al. (2006) Patient-reported quality of life after abdominal aortic aneurysm surgery: a prospective comparison of endovascular and open repair. J Vasc Surg. 44(6):1182-7.

[36] Schroeder T.V (2006) Registries on endovascular aortic aneurysm repair. Pitfalls and benefits. J Cardiovasc Surg. 47:55-59.

[37] Thomas S.M, Gaines P.A, Beard J.D (2001) Short-term (30 day) outcome of endovascular treatment of abdominal aortic aneurysm: results from the prospective Registry of Endovascular Treatment of Abdominal Aortic Aneurysm (RETA). Eur J Vasc Endovasc Surg. 21:57-64.

[38] Harris P.L, Vallabhanemi R, Desgranges P, Becquemin J.P, van Marrewijk C, Laheij R (2000) Incidence and risk factors of late rupture, conversion, and death after endovascular repair of infrarenal aortic aneurysms: The EUROSTAR experience. Journal of Vascular Surgery. 32:739-749.

[39] Lifeline Registry of EVAR Publications Committee (2005) Lifeline registry of endovascular aneurysm repair: Long-term primary outcome measures. Journal of Vascular Surgery. 42:1-10.

[40] Hobo R, Sybrandy J, Harris P.L, Buth J (2008) Endovascular repair of abdominal aortic aneurysms with concomitant common iliac artery aneurysm: outcome analysis of the EUROSTAR experience. Journal of Endovascular Therapy. 15:12-22.

[41] The EVAR trial participants (2004) Comparison of endovascular aneurysm repair with open repair in patients with abdominal aortic aneurysm (EVAR trial 1), 30-day operative mortality results: randomised controlled trial. The Lancet. 364:843-848.

[42] The EVAR trial participants (2005) Endovascular aneurysm repair and outcome in patients unfit for open repair of abdominal aortic aneurysm (EVAR trial 2): randomised controlled trial. The Lancet. 365:2187-2192.

[43] Beard J.D (2006) EVAR for fit patients: evidence from the randomised trials. In: Wyatt M.G, Watkinson A.F, editors. Endovascular Therapies- Current Evidence. United Kingdom: Shrewsbury.pp.29-36.
[44] Prinssen M, Buskens E, Blankensteijn J.D (2002) The Dutch Randomized Endovascular Aneurysm Management (DREAM) trial background, design and methods. J Cardiovasc Surg. 43:379-384.
[45] Blankensteijn J.D, de Jong S.E, Prinssen M, van der Ham A.C, Buth J (2005) Dutch Randomized Endovascular Aneurysm Management (DREAM) trial group: two-year results of a randomized trial comparing conventional and endovascular repair of abdominal aortic aneurysms. N Engl J Med. 352:2398-2405.
[46] Lederle F.A (2007) The veterans open versus endovascular repair (OVER) trial for AAA - what will it add to EVAR 1 and DREAM? In: Becquemin J.P, Alimi Y.S, editors. Controversies and Updates in Vascular Surgery 2007. Minerva Medica. pp.101-102.
[47] Moll F.L, Powell J.T, Fraedrich G, Verzini F, Haulon S, Waltham M , van Herwaarden J.A, Holt P.J.E, van Keulen J.W, Rantner B, Schlosser F.J.V, Setacci F, Ricco J.B (2011) Management of Abdominal Aortic Aneurysms Clinical Practice Guidelines of the European Society for Vascular Surgery. Eur J Vasc Endovasc Surg. 41; S1-S58.
[48] The UK Small Aneurysm Trial Participants (1998) Mortality results for randomised controlled trial of early elective surgery or ultrasonographic surveillance for small abdominal aortic aneurysms. The Lancet. 352:1649-55.
[49] Lederle F.A, Wilson S.E, Johnson G.R, Reinke D.B, Littooy F.N, Acher C.W et al. (2002) Aneurysm Detection and Management Veterans Affairs Cooperative Study Group. Immediate repair compared with surveillance of small abdominal aortic aneurysms.N Engl J Med. 346:1437-44.
[50] Cao P (2005) Comparison of surveillance vs aortic endografting for small aneurysm repair (CAESAR) trial: study design and progress. Eur J Vasc Endovasc Surg. 30:245-51.
[51] Ouriel K (2009) The pivotal study: a randomised comparison of endovascular repair versus surveillance in patients with smaller abdominal aortic aneurysms. J Vasc Surg. 49: 266-9.
[52] Powell J.T, Brown L.C, Forbes J.F, Fowkes F.G, Greenhalgh R.M, Ruckley C.V et al. (2007) Final 12-year follow-up of surgery versus surveillance in the uk small aneurysm trial. Br J Surg. 94: 702-8.
[53] Ballard D.J, Filardo G, Fowkes G, Powell J.T (2008) Surgery for small asymptomatic abdominal aortic aneurysms. Cochrane Database Syst Rev. CD001835.
[54] Argenteri A, Curci R, Bianchi G, Orlandi M, de Amicis P (2009) Morphology and classifications of abdominal aortic aneurysms. In: Setacci C, Gasparini D, Reimers B, Cremonesi A, Rossi P.T, editors. Aortic Surgery New Developments and Perspectives. Minerva Medica. pp. 215-225.
[55] Raithel D, Qu L, Hetzel G (2007) Adapting the graft to the patient's anatomy: is this a way of solving all the problems? In: Becquemin J.P, Alimi Y.S, editors. Controversies and Updates in Vascular Surgery 2007. Minerva Medica. pp.150-156.
[56] Chisci E, De Donato G, Setacci F, Sirignano P, Galzerano G, Cappelli A, Palasciano G, Setacci C (2009) Standard elective endovascular aortic aneurysm repair (EVAR). In: Setacci C, Gasparini D, Reimers B, Cremonesi A, Rossi P.T, editors. Aortic Surgery New Developments and Perspectives. Minerva Medica. pp.227-147.

[57] Brennan J, Gambardella I (2006) Aortic stent grafts: current availability and applicability. In: Wyatt M.G, Watkinson A.F, editors. Endovascular Therapies. tfm Publishing Ltd. pp.1-11.
[58] Freyrie A, Testi G, Faggioli G, Gargiulio M, Giovanetti F, Serra C, Stella A (2010) Ring-stents supported infrarenal aortic endografts fits well in abdominal aortic aneurysms with tortuous anatomy. J Cardiovasc Surg. 51:467-474.
[59] Ghotbi R, Sotiriou A, Mansur R (2010) New results with 100 Excluder cases. J Cardiovasc Surg. 51:475-480.
[60] Bockler D, Fitridge R, Wolf Y, Hayes P, Silveira P.G, Numan F, Riambau V (2010) Rationale and design of the Endurant Stent Graft Natural Selection Global Postmarket Registry (ENGAGE): interim analysis at 30 days of the first 180 patients enrolled. J Cardiovasc Surg. 51:481-491.
[61] Becquemin J.P, Aksoy M, Marzelle J, Roudot-Thoraval F, Desgranges P, Allaire E, Kobeiter H (2008) Abdominal aortic aneurysm sac behavior following Cook Zenith graft implantation: a five-year follow-up assessment of 212 cases. J Cardiovasc Surg. 49:199-206.
[62] Krajcer Z, Gregoric I (2010) Totally percutaneous aortic aneurysm repair: methods and outcomes using the fully integrated IntuiTrak Endovascular System. J Cardiovasc Surg. 51:493-501.
[63] Moulakakis K.G, Avgerinos E.D, Giannakopoulos T, Papapetrou A, Brountzos E.N, Liapis C.D (2010) Current knowledge on E-vita abdominal endograft. J Cardiovasc Surg. 51:533-538.
[64] Stableford J.A, Maldonado T.S, Berland T, Kim B, Adelman M.A, Pachter H.L, Mussa F (2009) Endograft infection after EVAR. Endovascular Today. 8:35-38.
[65] Franks S.C, Sutton A.J, Bown M.J, Sayers R.D (2007) Systematic review and meta-analysis of 12 years of endovascular abdominal aortic aneurysm repair. Eur J Vasc Endovasc Surg. 33:154-171.
[66] Akkersdijk G.J, Prinssen M, Blankensteijn J.D (2004) The impact of endovascular treatment on in-hospital mortality following non-ruptured AAA repair over a decade: a population based study on 16446 patients. Eur J Vasc Endovasc Surg. 28:41-46.
[67] Gleason T.G (2009) Endoleaks after endovascular aortic stent-grafting: impact, diagnosis and management. Semin Thorac Cardiovasc Surg. 21:363-372.
[68] White G.H, Yu W, May J et al. (1997) Endoleak as a complication of endoluminal grafting of abdominal aortic aneurysms: classification, incidence, diagnosis and management. J Endovasc Surg. 4:152-168.
[69] Ricotta II J, Malgor R.D, Oderich G.S (2009) Traitement endovasculaire des anevrysmes de l'aorte abdominale: 1ere partie. Annales de Chirurgie Vasculaire. 23:864-878.
[70] van Keulen J.W, van Prehn J, Prokop M, Moll F.L, van Herwaarden J.A (2009) Potential value of aneurysm sac volume measurements in addition to diameter measurements after endovascular aneurysm repair. Journal of Endovascular Therapy. 16:506-513.
[71] Wolf Y.G, Tillich M, Lee A, Fogarty T.J, Zarins C.K, Rubin G.D (2002) Changes in aneurysm volume after endovascular repair of abdominal aortic aneurysm. Journal of Vascular Surgery. 36:305-309.

[72] Qu L, Raithel D (2008) Experience with the Endologix Powerlink endograft in endovascular repair of abdominal aortic aneurysms with short and angulated necks. Perspectives in Vascular Surgery and Endovascular Therapy. 20:158-166.

[73] Droc I, Raithel D, Pinte F, Nita D, Deaconu S, Popovici A, Molnar F, Finichi R, Candea B, Goleanu V (2008) Abdominal aortic aneurisms treatment - new devices for endovascular treatment. Romanian Journal of Cardiovascular Surgery. 7:235-242.

[74] Harkin D.W, Dillon M, Blair P.H, Ellis P.K, Kee F (2007) Endovascular ruptured abdominal aortic aneurysm repair (EVRAR): a systematic review. Eur J Vasc Endovasc Surg. 34:673-681.

[75] Richards T, Goode S.D, Hinchliffe R, Altaf N, MacSweeney S, Braithwaite B (2009) The importance of anatomical suitability and fitness for the outcome of endovascular repair of ruptured abdominal aortic aneurysm. Eur J Vasc Endovasc Surg. 38:285-290.

[76] Perrott S, Puckridge P.J, Foreman R.K, Russell D.A, Spark J.I (2010) Anatomical suitability for endovascular AAA repair may affect outcomes following rupture. Eur J Vasc Endovasc Surg. 40:186-190.

[77] Veith F.J, Cayne N (2009) Endovascular repair for ruptured abdominal aortic aneurysms: why the results vary. Vascular Disease Management. 6:165-170.

[78] Amiot S, Haulon S, Becquemin J.P, Magnan P.E, Lermusiaux P, Goueffic Y, Jean-Baptiste E, Cochennec F, Favre J.P (2010) Fenestrated endovascular grafting: the french multicentre experience. Eur J Vasc Endovasc Surg. 39:537-544.

[79] Greenberg R.K, Sternbergh W.C, Makaroun M, Ohki T, Chuter T, Bharadwaj P, Saunders A (2009) Intermediate results of a United States multicenter trial of fenestrated endograft repair for juxtarenal abdominal aortic aneurysms. Journal of Vascular Surgery. 50:730-737.

[80] O'Neill S, Greenberg R.K, Haddad F, Resch T, Sereika J, Katz E (2006) A prospective analysis of fenestrated endovascular grafting: intermediate-term outcome. Eur J Vasc Endovasc Surg. 32:115-123.

[81] Budde R.P.J, Huo F, Cramer M.J.M, Doevendans P.A, Bots M.L, Moll F.L, Prokop M (2010) Simultaneous aortic and coronary assessment in abdominal aortic aneurysm patients by thoraco-abdominal 64-detector-row CT angiography: estimate of the impact on preoperative management: a pilot study. Eur J Vasc Endovasc Surg. 40:196-201.

[82] Jean-Baptiste E, Hassen-Khodja R, Bouillanne P.J, Haudebourg P, Declemy S, Batt M (2007) Endovascular repair of infrarenal abdominal aortic aneurysms in high-risk-surgical patients. Eur J Vasc Endovasc Surg. 34:145-151.

[83] Steinmetz E, Abello N, Kretz B, Gauthier E, Bouchot O, Brenot R (2010) Analysis of outcome after using high-risk criteria selection to surgery versus endovascular repair in the modern era of abdominal aortic aneurysm treatment. Eur J Vasc Endovasc Surg. 39:403-409.

[84] Malkawi A.H, Hinchliffe R.J, Holt P.J, Loftus I.M, Thompson M.M (2010) Percutaneous access for endovascular aneurysm repair: a systematic review. Eur J Vasc Endovasc Surg. 39:676-682.

[85] Raman V.K, Karmarkar P.V, Guttman M.A et al. (2005) Real-time magnetic resonance-guided endovascular repair of experimental abdominal aortic aneurysm in swine. J Am Coll Cardiol. 45:2069-2077.

Section 3

Cerebral Aneurysm

Chapter 10

Simulation of Pulsatile Flow in Cerebral Aneurysms: From Medical Images to Flow and Forces

Julia Mikhal, Cornelis H. Slump and Bernard J. Geurts

Additional information is available at the end of the chapter

http://dx.doi.org/10.5772/47858

1. Introduction

There is a growing medical interest in the prediction of the flow and forces inside cerebral aneurysms [24, 52], with the ultimate goal of supporting medical procedures and decisions by presenting viable scenarios for intervention. The clinical background of intracranial aneurysms and subarachnoid hemorrhages is well introduced in the literature such as [46, 51]. These days, with the development of high-precision medical imaging techniques, the geometry and structure of blood vessels and possible aneurysms that have formed, can be accurately determined. To date, surgeons and radiologists had to make decisions about possible treatment of an aneurysm based on size, shape and location criteria alone. In this chapter we focus on the role of Computational Fluid Dynamics (CFD) for therapeutic options in the treatment of aneurysms. The tremendous potential of CFD in this respect was already anticipated in [29]. The value of numerical simulations for treating aneurysms will likely increase further with better quantitative understanding of hemodynamics in cerebral blood flow.

Ultimately, we aim to support the medical decision process via computational modeling. In particular, CFD allows to add qualitative and quantitative characteristics of the blood flow inside the aneurysm to this complex decision process. We propose to compute the precise patient-specific pulsatile flow in all spatial and temporal details, using a so-called 'Immersed Boundary' (IB) method. This requires a number of steps, from preparing the raw medical imagery to define the complex patient-specific flow domain, to the execution of high-fidelity simulations and their detailed interpretation in terms of flow visualization and the extraction of quantitative measures of relevance to medical practice. We compute the flow inside the aneurysm to predict high and low stress regions, of relevance to the possible growth of an aneurysm. We also visualize vortical structures in the flow indicating the quality of local blood circulation. We show that, as the size of the aneurysm increases, qualitative transitions in the flow behavior can arise, which express themselves as high-frequency variations in the flow and shear stresses. These variations could quantify the level of risk associated with the growing aneurysm. Such computational modeling may lead to a better understanding of the progressive weakening of the vessel wall and its possible rupture after long time.

In this chapter we present a numerical model for the simulation of blood flow inside cerebral aneurysms. A significant amount of work has been done on simulation of flow in the brain and in the cardiovascular system [2, 5, 13, 18, 24, 38, 40]. As a numerical approach, the finite element method is most commonly used to represent geometries of vessels and the flow of blood through them. Often, the data are obtained from rather coarse biomedical imagery. As a result, the highly complex vessel geometry is defined with some uncertainty, and considerable smoothing and interface approximation need to be included to prepare simulations with a body-fitted approach [2, 6, 11]. As an alternative, the IB method was designed primarily for capturing viscous flow in domains of realistic complexity [39]. In particular, we consider a volume penalization method. In this method, fluid is penalized from entering a solid part of a domain of interest by adding a suitable forcing term to the equations governing the fluid flow [21]. This method is also known as 'fictitious domain' method [1] and physically resembles the Darcy penalty method [42] or the Navier-Stokes/Brinkman equations describing viscous flow on the scale of individual pores in porous domains [49]. Here, we consider in particular the limit in which the porous domain becomes impenetrable and flow in complex solid domains can be represented. This method is discussed as one of the IB methods in the recent review chapter by [32], and in the sequel will be referred to as 'volume penalization immersed boundary method', a label that was also adopted in [20].

A primary challenge for any CFD method, whether it is a body-fitted method [16] or an IB method [17, 32, 39], is to capture the flow near solid-fluid interfaces. In this region the highest velocity gradients may occur, leading to correspondingly highest levels of shear stress, but also potentially highest levels of numerical error. In methods employing body-fitted grids, the quality of predictions is directly linked to the degree to which grid-lines can be orthogonal to the solid-fluid interface and to each other. Also, variation in local mesh sizes and shapes of adjacent grid cells is a factor determining numerical error. The generation of a suitable grid is further complicated as the raw data that define the actual aneurysm geometry often require considerable preprocessing steps before any grid can be obtained. These steps include significant smoothing, segmentation and geometric operations eliminating small side vessels that are felt not to be too important for the flow. On the positive side, the main benefit of a body-fitted approach is that discrete variables are situated also at the solid-fluid interface, which makes implementation of no-slip boundary conditions quite straightforward. Hence, in body-fitted approaches the no-slip property can be accurately imposed, but only on a 'pre-processed' smoothed and often somewhat altered geometry [6, 11]. These finite element based approaches can be used to predict the patient's main flow structures of clinical value as suggested by [5, 6, 15, 19].

Capturing flow near complex shaped solid-fluid interfaces is equally challenging in an IB method, as it is in body-fitted approaches. In the IB approach adopted here, the actual geometry of the aneurysm can be extracted directly from the voxel information in the raw medical imagery, without the need for smoothing of the geometry. Grid generation is no issue for IB methods since the geometry of the flow domain is directly immersed in a Cartesian grid. The location of the solid-fluid interface is known only up to the size of a grid cell, and the shape of the interface is approximated using a 'staircase' representation, stemming from the fact that any grid cell is labeled either entirely 'solid' or entirely 'fluid'. Refinements in which a fraction between 0 and 1 of a cell can be fluid-filled [7] are not taken into consideration here. In fact, the medical imagery from which we start has a spatial resolution that is not too high when small-scale details are concerned. This calls for a systematic assessment of the sensitivity of predictions to uncertainties in the flow domain [31] incorporating also the effects due to adaptations of the domain by smoothing and interface reconstruction as is considered in higher-order methods [10]. Without relaxing the staircase approximation, the problem of capturing near-interface properties can only be addressed by increasing the spatial resolution. This gives an insight into the error-reduction by systematic grid-refinement for flow in complex geometries.

We illustrate the process of predicting flow and forces based on incompressible Newtonian fluid to characterize blood properties. Non-Newtonian corrections can be readily included, however, these typically lead only to modest changes in the predictions and will hence be omitted here. Pulsatile flow forcing is obtained from the direct measurement of the time-dependent mean flow velocity in a vessel during a cardiac cycle. Transcranial Doppler (TCD) sonography is a non-invasive technique, which can be used for this purpose, allowing to measure cerebral blood flow velocity near the actual aneurysm [51]. We consider a full range of physiologically relevant conditions. Understanding flow patterns inside an aneurysm may help to describe long-term effects such as the likelihood of the growth [4] or even rupture [44] of the aneurysm, or the accelerated deterioration of the vessel wall due to low shear stress [8]. Regions of high and low shear stress are often visualized as potential markers for aneurysm growth. High shear stress levels were reported near the 'neck' of a saccular aneurysm, and may be relevant during the initiating phase [44]. Low wall shear stress has been reported to have a negative effect on endothelial cells and may be important to local remodeling of an arterial wall and to aneurysm growth [4]. A low wall shear stress may facilitate the growing phase and may trigger the rupture of a cerebral aneurysm by causing degenerative changes in the aneurysm wall. The situation is, however, more complex, as illustrated by the phenomenon of spontaneous stabilization of aneurysms after an initial phase of growth [25]. It is still very much an open issue what the precise relation is between shear stress patterns and general circulation on the one hand, and developing medical risks such as aneurysm rupture, on the other hand. In this complex problem, hemodynamic stimuli are but one of many factors.

Cerebral aneurysms are most often located in or near the Circle of Willis [51] – the central vessel network for the supply of blood to the human brain. Common risk-areas are at 'T' and 'Y'-shaped junctions in the vessels [15]. Treatment of cerebral aneurysms often involves insertion of coils. This coiling procedure represents considerable risk and uncertainty about the long-term stability of coiled aneurysms [45, 47]. Blood vessels and aneurysms are rather complex by their structure and geometrical shapes. The walls of blood vessels contain several layers of different types of biological cells, which provide elasticity to the vessels and play a role in the compliance [40]. The shape of cerebral aneurysms developing in patients can be inferred by using three-dimensional rotational angiography [33]. In this procedure a part of the brain can be scanned, and aneurysms even of a size less than 3 mm can be depicted [3, 48]. This technique allows a reconstruction of three-dimensional arteries and aneurysms and hence an approximate identification of the blood vessels and parts of the soft tissue in the scanned volume. In the IB approach the domain is characterized by a so-called masking function, which takes the value '0' in the fluid (blood) part and '1' in solid (tissue) parts of the domain. The raw angiography data allows for a simple 'staircase approximation' of the solid-fluid interface that defines the vessel and aneurysm shape. Individual voxels in the digital data form the smallest unit of localization of the solid-fluid interface. A computational cell is assigned to be 'solid' or 'fluid' on the basis of the digital imagery. We will adopt the 'staircase' geometry representation in this chapter and do not incorporate any additional smoothing of the geometry or sophisticated reconstruction methods.

For a more complete modeling of the dynamics in the vessel system, flow-structure interaction often plays a role [40]. In that case also parameters and models that characterize, e.g., mechanical properties of arterial tissue, influence of brain tissue and the influence of the cerebrospinal fluid are required. The amplitude of the wall motion in intracranial aneurysms was found to be less than 10% of an artery diameter. Despite the rather modest motion of the vessel, long time effects may accumulate. Even modest movement can affect the vessel walls, which might play a role in possible aneurysm rupture as was hypothesized in [35]. For realistic pulsatile flows some movement of the aneurysm walls was observed during a cardiac cycle [36]. In this chapter we take a first step and restrict to developing the IB approach for rigid geometries. This allows to obtain the main flow characteristics inside relatively large cerebral aneurysms for which the wall movement can be neglected [24].

The organization of this chapter is as follows. In Section 2 we present the computational model, discuss numerical discretization and introduce the IB method for defining complex vessel and aneurysm geometries. We also describe the process of the reconstruction of the geometry from medical imagery. We illustrate steady flow inside a realistic aneurysm geometry in Section 3 and discuss the reliability of numerical predictions. A pulsatile flow and qualitative impression of the flow and forces distribution inside a realistic aneurysm is presented in Section 4. Concluding remarks are in Section 5.

2. Numerical model of blood flow inside human brain

In this section we present the numerical model for simulation of blood flow inside the human brain. We consider blood as an incompressible Newtonian fluid with a constant viscosity. The flow dynamics is governed by the Navier-Stokes equations, which are presented in Subsection 2.1. The numerical method used to solve these equations in 3D is based on skew-symmetric finite-volume discretization and explicit time-stepping using the method as proposed by [50]. This is discussed in Subsection 2.2, in which we also detail the volume penalizing IB method that is adopted to represent the complex vessel structures through which the blood flows. Finally, in Subsection 2.3, we discuss the method used to obtain the precise geometry of realistic blood vessels.

2.1. The Navier-Stokes equations for an incompressible cerebral flow

There are various approaches to model flow of blood in the human brain. A comprehensive overview is given in [40]. In one approach, the blood is approximated as a Newtonian fluid [5]. More refined models, e.g., the Carreau-Yasuda model, include the shear-thinning behavior of blood and allow to capture non-Newtonian rheology [2, 13, 18]. Under physiological flow conditions in sufficiently large arteries non-Newtonian corrections were found to be quite small [6, 13, 18, 38]. The main flow characteristics appeared to be the same as for a Newtonian fluid at somewhat different stress and velocity levels.

We concentrate on the human brain, in particular on arteries of the Circle of Willis. Typical fine-scale structures in the blood are on the order of $10^{-6}m$. A length-scale that characterizes the cross section of a typical cerebral vessel inside the Circle of Willis is on the order of $10^{-3}m$ [19]. This difference in length-scale of three orders of magnitude motivates to approximate blood as an incompressible Newtonian fluid [40].

The Navier-Stokes equations provide a full representation of Newtonian fluid mechanics, expressing conservation of mass and momentum. The total physical domain Ω, consists of a fluid part Ω_f and a solid part Ω_s. The interface between the two will be identified as $\partial\Omega$ at which no-slip conditions apply. The governing equations are given in dimensional form by:

$$\frac{\partial \mathbf{u}^*}{\partial t^*} + \mathbf{u}^* \cdot \nabla^* \mathbf{u}^* = -\nabla^*(\frac{p^*}{\rho^*}) + \nu^* \nabla^{*\,2} \mathbf{u}^* + \frac{\mathbf{f}^*}{\rho^*} \tag{1}$$

$$\nabla^* \cdot \mathbf{u}^* = 0 \tag{2}$$

Here $\mathbf{u}^*$ is the velocity of the fluid, ρ^* its mass density, p^* the pressure and $\mathbf{f}^*$ a forcing term that will play a central role in this chapter as it is used to represent the impenetrability of complex shaped solid vessel walls. We denote variables with a physical dimension by an asterisk and render the formulation dimensionless momentarily. By choosing a reference velocity u_r^* and reference length L_r^* we can express a reference time scale as $t_r^* = L_r^*/u_r^*$. Using as reference density $\rho_r^* = \rho^*$ we will use a reference pressure as $p_r^* = (u_r^*)^2\rho_r^*$. For the forcing term we select a direct volume penalization in which

$$\frac{\mathbf{f}^*}{\rho^*} = -\frac{1}{\varepsilon^*} H \mathbf{u}^* \tag{3}$$

where ε^* is a forcing time scale and H is the masking function: $H(\mathbf{x}) = 1$ if $\mathbf{x} \in \Omega_s$ and $H(\mathbf{x}) = 0$ if $\mathbf{x} \in \Omega_f$. We set the reference forcing time scale $\varepsilon^* = \varepsilon t_r^* \ll t_r^*$, i.e., much smaller than the reference time scale. Here we introduce the dimensionless forcing parameter $\varepsilon \ll 1$.

After choosing all reference parameters we obtain the non-dimensional form of the Navier-Stokes equations:

$$\frac{\partial \mathbf{u}}{\partial t} + \mathbf{u} \cdot \nabla \mathbf{u} = -\nabla p + \frac{1}{Re} \nabla^2 \mathbf{u} - \frac{1}{\varepsilon} H \mathbf{u} \tag{4}$$

$$\nabla \cdot \mathbf{u} = 0 \tag{5}$$

In this chapter we will consider only stationary, i.e., non moving walls. By adding the forcing to the incompressible momentum equations we formally arrive at the Brinkman equation for flow in a porous medium with permeability related to the parameter ε [26]. Note that, with the inclusion of $\mathbf{f}$ as in (3) we arrive at a model for the velocity and pressure fields in the entire domain Ω.

The Reynolds number Re is the only parameter which is required to specify the flow conditions. It quantifies the ratio between the magnitude of the (destabilizing) convective transport and the (stabilizing) viscous processes. It is well known that for relatively low Reynolds numbers flow is laminar and steady [53], which implies a smooth velocity and pressure field. With increasing Reynolds number the flow can develop more detailed vortical structures, e.g., associated with separated flow near abrupt changes in the shape of a vessel. A further increase in Re usually implies that the flow becomes unsteady and the range of vortices becomes much wider [12]. The range of Reynolds numbers arising in the flow in the Circle of Willis, corresponds to laminar, possibly unsteady flow. This will be discussed in more detail momentarily.

2.2. Numerical method for flow simulation using an immersed boundary approach for representing complex geometries

In this subsection we sketch the numerical method used for the simulation of flow through complex shaped domains. First, we describe the direct numerical simulation approach and specify the volume penalization IB method afterwards.

We employ a staggered allocation of the flow variables $(\mathbf{u}, p) = (u, v, w, p)$ as basis for our flow solver [12]. In two dimensions this is sketched in Figure 1, where a primary grid cell with the pressure defined in the center and the Cartesian velocity components at the cell surfaces is presented. The locations at which the velocities and the pressure are stored are referred to as the velocity- and the pressure-points, respectively.

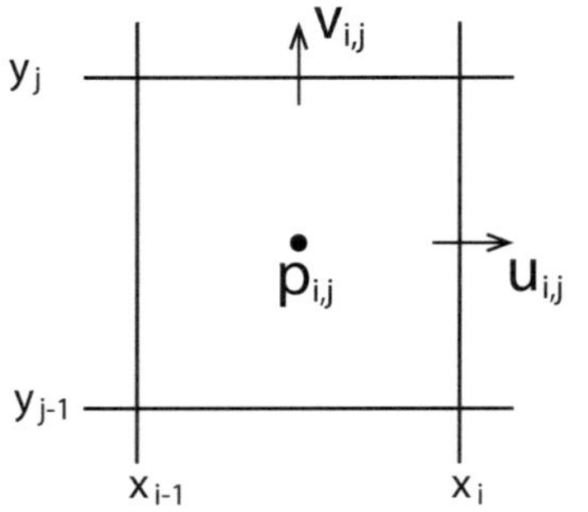

Figure 1. Sketch of a primary grid cell in 2D with staggered allocation of the variables. The pressure p is in the middle of the grid cell, while the velocities (u and v) are defined at the centers of the faces.

The principles of conservation of mass and momentum as expressed in (4) and (5), form the basis for the discrete computational model that is used for the actual simulations. In the Navier-Stokes equations (4) the rate of change of momentum is obtained from the nonlinear convective flux, the linear viscous flux, the gradient of the pressure and the contribution from the forcing term. These contributions to the total flux each have a particular physical character that needs to be represented properly in the discrete formulation. In particular, the convective flux is skew-symmetric, implying that this flux only contributes to the transport of kinetic energy of the solution in physical space; it does not generate nor dissipate this energy. Likewise, the viscous flux contributes only to dissipation of energy, which has to be strictly maintained in a numerical method. We motivate this in some more detail next.

Starting from the original momentum equation without the forcing term

$$\frac{\partial \mathbf{u}}{\partial t} = -(\mathbf{u} \cdot \nabla)\mathbf{u} - \nabla p + \frac{1}{Re} \nabla \cdot \nabla \mathbf{u} \tag{6}$$

we are interested in the kinetic energy, given by

$$E = \frac{1}{2} \int_{\Omega} dV |\mathbf{u}|^2 = \frac{1}{2} \int_{\Omega} dV \mathbf{u} \cdot \mathbf{u} \tag{7}$$

where $\mathbf{u} \cdot \mathbf{u}$ is the vector inner product. Note, that in (7) we effectively integrate only over Ω_f as $\mathbf{u} = \mathbf{0}$ in Ω_s. The evolution of the kinetic energy follows from

$$\frac{dE}{dt} = \int_{\Omega} dV \mathbf{u} \cdot \frac{\partial \mathbf{u}}{\partial t} \tag{8}$$

In order to obtain the integrand in (8) we multiply the Navier-Stokes equation (6) by $\mathbf{u}$. Integrating by parts we can derive the contribution of each of the fluxes in (6). In fact, the convective and pressure terms do not contribute to the evolution of energy, and we find

$$\frac{dE}{dt} = -\frac{1}{Re}\int_{\Omega} dV(\nabla\mathbf{u} : \nabla\mathbf{u}) \leq 0 \tag{9}$$

where $\nabla\mathbf{u} : \nabla\mathbf{u} = \partial_i u_j \partial_i u_j$ in which we sum over repeated indices. This suggests that the energy of any solution decreases in time because of viscous fluxes only.

A more elaborate derivation can be found in [50], which departs from the expressions

$$E = \frac{1}{2}(\mathbf{u},\mathbf{u}) \quad \text{and} \quad \frac{dE}{dt} = \frac{1}{2}\frac{d}{dt}(\mathbf{u},\mathbf{u}) \tag{10}$$

where energy is written in terms of the function inner product $(\mathbf{u},\mathbf{u})$ as defined in (7). This yields the symmetric expression

$$\begin{aligned}\frac{dE}{dt} &= -\frac{1}{2}\Big(((\mathbf{u}\cdot\nabla)\mathbf{u},\mathbf{u}) + (\mathbf{u},(\mathbf{u}\cdot\nabla)\mathbf{u})\Big) - \frac{1}{2}\Big((\nabla p,\mathbf{u}) + (\mathbf{u},\nabla p)\Big)\\ &+ \frac{1}{2Re}\Big((\nabla\cdot\nabla\mathbf{u},\mathbf{u}) + (\mathbf{u},\nabla\cdot\nabla\mathbf{u})\Big)\end{aligned} \tag{11}$$

Since $(\nabla p,\mathbf{u}) = -(p,\nabla\cdot\mathbf{u})$ and the skew-symmetry $((\mathbf{u}\cdot\nabla)\mathbf{v},\mathbf{w}) = -(\mathbf{v},(\mathbf{u}\cdot\nabla)\mathbf{w})$ we obtain again (9), i.e., no contribution from pressure and the convective flux.

In a discrete setting the Navier-Stokes equations in matrix-vector notation are written as

$$\mathbf{\Lambda}\frac{d\mathbf{u}_h}{dt} = -\mathbf{C}\mathbf{u}_h - \mathbf{D}\mathbf{u}_h + \mathbf{M}^T\mathbf{p}_h \tag{12}$$

$$\mathbf{M}\mathbf{u}_h = \mathbf{0} \tag{13}$$

where $\mathbf{u}_h$ is the vector containing the discrete velocity solutions (u_h, v_h, w_h), $\mathbf{p}_h$ is the discrete pressure, $\mathbf{\Lambda}$ is a matrix with the volumes of the grid cells on its diagonal, $\mathbf{C}$ and $\mathbf{D}$ are the coefficient matrices corresponding to the discretization of the convective $((\mathbf{u}\cdot\nabla)\mathbf{u})$ and diffusive $(-\Delta\mathbf{u}/Re)$ operators, respectively. The discretization of the pressure gradient is given by $-\mathbf{M}^T$, while the coefficient matrix $\mathbf{M}$ itself represents the discretization of the divergence operator, integrated over the control volumes [50].

The discrete approximation for the kinetic energy can be given using the midpoint rule, as

$$E_h = \mathbf{u}_h^T\mathbf{\Lambda}\mathbf{u}_h \tag{14}$$

Similar to the continuous case (11) we compute the evolution of the energy in the discrete model as

$$\frac{dE_h}{dt} = -\mathbf{u}_h^T(\mathbf{C}+\mathbf{C}^T)\mathbf{u}_h - \mathbf{u}_h^T(\mathbf{D}+\mathbf{D}^T)\mathbf{u}_h + \mathbf{u}_h^T(\mathbf{M}^T\mathbf{p}_h) + (\mathbf{M}^T\mathbf{p}_h)^T\mathbf{u}_h \tag{15}$$

For a discrete solution we also require the convective conservation of energy, which implies skew-symmetry of the matrix $\mathbf{C}$ of the convective operator: $\mathbf{C}+\mathbf{C}^T = \mathbf{0}$. The two terms related to the numerical pressure gradient can be rewritten as

$$\mathbf{u}_h^T(\mathbf{M}^T\mathbf{p}_h) + (\mathbf{M}^T\mathbf{p}_h)^T\mathbf{u}_h = (\mathbf{M}\mathbf{u}_h)^T\mathbf{p}_h + \mathbf{p}_h\mathbf{M}\mathbf{u}_h = \mathbf{0} \tag{16}$$

where the numerical divergence operator $\mathbf{M}$ satisfies equation (13). Thus, pressure terms also cancel and do not influence the stability of the spatial discretization. By comparison with the expression for the energy evolution (9), the second term in the right-hand side of (15) should provide a strict decrease of the energy:

$$\frac{dE_h}{dt} = -\mathbf{u}_h^T(\mathbf{D} + \mathbf{D}^T)\mathbf{u}_h \leq 0 \tag{17}$$

This implies that the coefficient matrix $\mathbf{D}$ of the diffusion operator is a positive-definite matrix. Thus, discretely we obtain the same properties for the energy decay as in the continuous case.

In this chapter we employ symmetry preserving finite volume discretization and use central differencing of second order accuracy, which maintains explicitly the skew-symmetry in the discrete equations. Since the energy is preserved under the convective operator the skew symmetric discretization allows to obtain a stable solution on any grid. For proper capturing of the solenoidal property (5) of the velocity field we approximate the gradient operator by the transpose of the numerical divergence operator and use a positive definite discretization of the viscous terms, closely following [50]. The contributions of the convective, viscous and pressure gradient fluxes are integrated in time using a generalization of the explicit second order accurate Adams-Bashforth method. Care is taken of accurately representing the skew-symmetry also in the time-integration. Full incorporation would require an implicit time-stepping, which, however, is computationally too demanding. Instead, time-integration starts from a modification of the leapfrog method [43] with linear inter/extrapolations of the required 'off-step' velocities and an implicit treatment of the incompressibility constraint. Optimization for largest stability region of the resulting scheme yields a particular so-called 'one-leg' time-integration method, with a mathematical structure that is akin to the well-known Adams-Bashforth scheme. More details can be found in [50].

For the total computational domain periodic boundary conditions are applied. A special role is played by the forcing term $\mathbf{f}$ in the Navier-Stokes equations (4), which represents the volume penalization accounting for solid objects inside and at the boundaries of the flow domain. The role of the forcing term is to yield an accurate approximation of the no-slip condition at solid boundaries. In conventional computational fluid dynamics such a forcing term is not needed since the flow domain is endowed with a body-fitted grid on which the equations are discretized. The grid-lines in such cases are defined such that they either closely follow the contours of the solid boundaries, or they are (preferably) orthogonal to them. In such a discrete formulation the no-slip boundary condition can be imposed easily. The body-fitted grid is efficient if the fluid domain Ω_f is not too complex and does not contain too many separate objects around which the fluid should flow [22]. For considerably more complex flow domains or in case the location of the solid-fluid interface is not perfectly known, as in case of medical imagery, the body-fitted grid approach is limited by the generation of suitable meshes. These should not only align with the solid boundaries, but also be sufficiently smooth near these boundaries to allow an accurate solution in the boundary layers [27]. In our discrete model the forcing term contributes strongly to the stiffness of the equations. When an explicit time-stepping method would be adopted for the forcing term, as is done for the other dynamic contributions, this would result in extremely small time-steps in view of numerical stability. Therefore, the linear forcing term is integrated in time using the implicit Euler scheme [28].

We use an IB method based on volume penalization [32] to capture flow in complex aneurysm geometries. A key role in our IB method is played by the so-called 'masking function' H, which is a binary function in 3D with values '0' inside the fluid and '1' in the solid parts of the domain. In regions where $H = 0$ the Navier-Stokes system is solved and thus the fluid domain is defined. In the solid regions $H = 1$ and the forcing is dominant if the non-dimensional parameter ε is very small. We take $\varepsilon = 10^{-10}$ in the sequel. As a result, the momentum equation (4) reduces to $\partial_t \mathbf{u} \approx -\mathbf{u}/\varepsilon$ if $|\mathbf{u}| \gg \varepsilon$ in the solid domain. Hence, any nonzero $\mathbf{u}$ is exponentially sent back to $\mathbf{0}$ on a time-scale ε. If $|\mathbf{u}| \leq \varepsilon$ the forcing is not dominant in the solid, but control over $|\mathbf{u}|$ is already obtained, i.e., $|\mathbf{u}|$ takes on negligible values in the solid.

A schematic representation in 2D of the masking function for a complex domain is presented in Figure 2, where dark cells correspond to fluid cells with masking function $H = 0$, while white cells represent the solid part of the computational domain. For realistic 3D cases uncertainties in defining the geometry arise because of the finite spatial resolution of the images of the vessels. We introduced and applied so-called numerical 'bounding' solutions in [31], where next to the basic constructed geometry we consider slightly smaller ('inner') and slightly bigger ('outer') geometries. These bounding geometries differ from the 'basic' geometry by maximally one grid cell in terms of the location of the numerical solid-fluid interface. This implies very tight bounding of the basic geometry especially at high grid resolution. We routinely compute the flow in the basic geometry and in two bounding geometries in order to quantify the associated level of uncertainty. The solution and its main characteristics in the basic geometry appeared to be bounded by the inner and outer solutions.

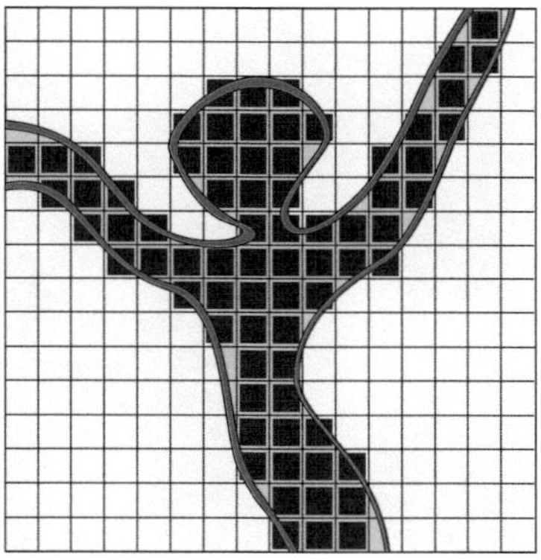

Figure 2. IB method illustrated on a Cartesian grid in 2D for an arbitrary geometry. Dark cells correspond to fluid cells with masking function $H = 0$, while white cells represent solid part of the computational domain, where $H = 1$.

2.3. Masking function of realistic cerebral aneurysm, reconstructed from 3DRA data

In this subsection we describe the process of construction of the masking function from medical imagery. The initial set of data was obtained from three-dimensional rotational angiography (3DRA) applied to the brains of patients suffering from a brain aneurysm. The 3DRA scans were provided by the St. Elizabeth Hospital in Tilburg (The Netherlands). We choose one example to illustrate our numerical method.

Before simulation of flow we need to convert the geometry into the masking function. The 3D volume data was first segmented to obtain a vessel structure suitable for flow simulations. After this step small branch vessels were removed and the main vessel with the aneurysm on it was retained [23]. An illustration of the geometry obtained at this stage is presented in Figure 3(a). On the right hand side downstream of the aneurysm we observe the vessel to split. Currently, our approach only allows for a single inflow and a single outflow. Therefore the next steps of the construction are 'cutting' a part of the vessel and 'connecting' the 'outflow' of the vessel to its 'inflow' by adding an appropriate, smooth connecting vessel. This way we obtain the desired periodic flow model. Adding an artificial connecting vessel can be avoided by allowing actual inflow and outflow boundary conditions. However, for the flow in the direct vicinity of the aneurysm, we expect the influence of the periodicity assumption relatively 'far' from the aneurysm to be negligible and the remaining computational model to be suitable for illustrating the flow in realistic aneurysms. In Figure 3(b) this connecting vessel is represented in black. Several steps in the specification of the masking function can be a source of error in the flow prediction. Special care needs to be taken to limit these errors and to understand the sensitivity of the predictions to details of the connecting vessel, locations of cuts etc. etc. Through systematic numerical simulations these sensitivities can be assessed and the reliability of the predictions quantified.

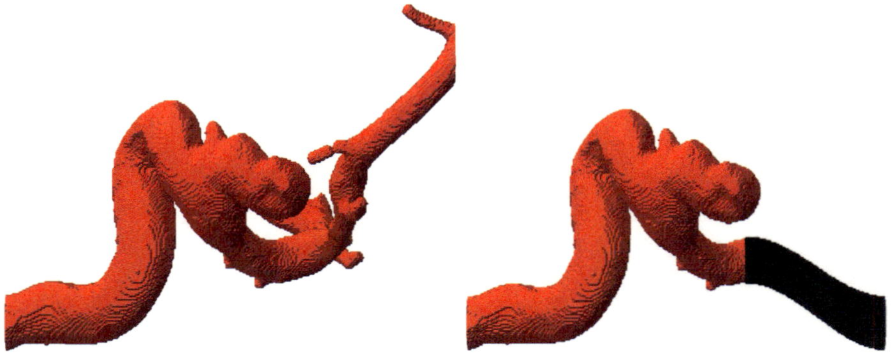

(a) (b)

Figure 3. Three dimensional geometries of realistic aneurysms reconstructed from 3DRA. The segmented data are presented in (a), while in (b) we plot the 'cut'-vessel. The original aneurysm region (red) and the 'connecting' artificial vessel (black) are displayed.

3. Steady flow simulations in realistic cerebral aneurysm

In this section we present numerical results for the flow inside the realistic aneurysm geometry as shown in Figure 3. We simulate steady flow and present the solution (velocity and pressure) and its gradients (in terms of the shear stress) in Subsection 3.1. Subsequently, we consider the reliability of the predictions by presenting the convergence of pressure drop, velocity and shear stress in Subsection 3.2.

3.1. Motivation and exact definition of the reference case

We simulate flow in the geometry as introduced in Figure 3. First, we need to specify the correct scale and corresponding non-dimensional parameters, to define this application in detail. Subsequently, we will visualize the solution in a number of qualitative ways to appreciate the complexity of the flow structures that develop.

In order to specify the computational model we need to choose reference scales for the length and velocity, and specify the kinematic viscosity. These quantities allow to compute the Reynolds number *Re*, which is the only parameter that is required for the dimensionless formulation. From literature one may find a range of values characteristic of these reference scales, which implies some degree of freedom in setting the precise values that are physiologically relevant. In particular, the value of the flow velocity is subject to the largest uncertainty when comparing literature, although also the viscosity displays considerable variation. We motivate our choices next to provide a point of reference.

The raw data of the 3DRA scan of the aneurysm consists of a grid of 256^3 voxels. The voxel width is 0.1213 mm. This implies that the total physical length of the flow domain is 3.10528 cm. As reference length we take a characteristic scale representative of the average radius of the cerebral vessel in this part of the Circle of Willis. We extract $R^* = 1.94\ mm$ from the 3DRA data. This value is quite similar to [11] who adopt 2.5 mm, and also consistent with [19], who suggests a scale of $2.1 \pm 0.4\ mm$. Hence, in the non-dimensional setting we work in a domain of total 'length' of $31.0528/1.94 \approx 16$. The computational domain, enclosing the aneurysm geometry is in fact $16 \times 8 \times 16$ in the non-dimensional formulation. Simulations will be done at grid resolutions $128 \times 64 \times 128$, $64 \times 32 \times 64$ and $32 \times 16 \times 32$. These resolutions define the grid refinements that we use for the convergence analysis.

Next to the length-scale, also the viscosity and the velocity scales need to be set. From literature we infer that the mass density ρ^* is in the range $1025 \leq \rho^* \leq 1125\ kg/m^3$, while the dynamic viscosity of blood is reported to be $3 \cdot 10^{-6} \leq \mu^* \leq 4 \cdot 10^{-6}\ Pa\ s$. Specifically, choosing typical values for the mass density of blood $\rho^* = 1060\ kg/m^3$ and the dynamic viscosity of blood $\mu^* = 3.2 \cdot 10^{-3}\ Pa\ s$ implies a kinematic viscosity $\nu^* = \mu^*/\rho^* = 3.01 \cdot 10^{-6}\ m^2/s$. Finally, the reference flow-rate as proposed by [15] and [34] is $245 \pm 65\ ml/min$, showing an uncertainty of about 25%. This range of values was obtained on the basis of either 3D MR angiograms or TCD measurements. The corresponding range for the velocity scale can be extracted from this as $u^* = Q^*/(\pi(R^*)^2) = 0.345 \pm 0.09\ m/s$. This is consistent with the range $0.34 \pm 0.087\ m/s$ as obtained by [41] on the basis of TCD measurements. Combining these numbers yields a typical Reynolds number range of $175 \lesssim Re \lesssim 300$. For convenience, we adopt $Re = 250$ in the sequel, which, in terms of the chosen reference length-scale and kinematic viscosity, corresponds to a velocity scale of $u_r^* = 0.388\ m/s$, well within the quoted range found in literature. In the sequel we will also consider the dependence of the fluid dynamics in relation to variation in the Reynolds number, particularly when we consider pulsatile flow.

In order to visualize the flow and forces that develop in the aneurysm, a number of options is available. We will start by choosing a more qualitative set of methods, i.e., three-dimensional and two-dimensional views of the velocity and shear stress. Here, we show results obtained at a resolution of $128 \times 64 \times 128$. A quantitative approach, showing the effect of grid refinement will be followed in the next subsection.

Numerically computed velocity streamlines for a steady flow at $Re = 250$ are presented in Figure 4. By properly selecting the initial condition for the streamline at the inflow on the left-hand side of the domain, we can achieve both streamlines that pass through the section with the aneurysm, without actually entering the aneurysm bulb, as well as streamlines that

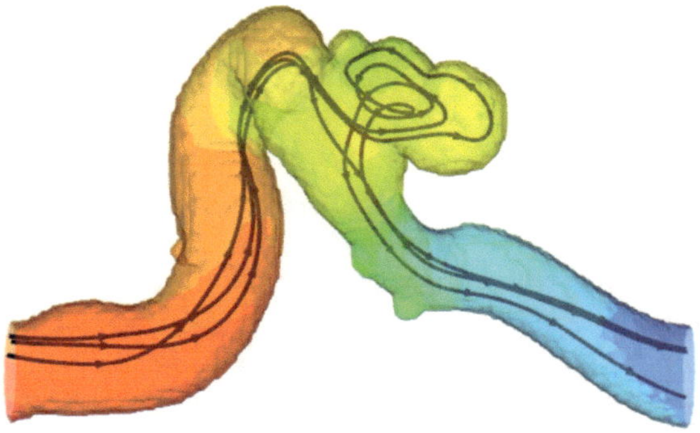

Figure 4. Three characteristic velocity streamlines inside the aneurysm geometry. The geometry is colored with the pressure field which shows a smooth transition from a high pressure (red) to a low pressure (blue) area. Grid resolution is $128 \times 64 \times 128$.

display the rather complex vortical pattern that appears within the aneurysm. The geometry is colored with the value of the local pressure. A smooth transition from a high pressure to a low pressure can be observed, driving the flow inside the geometry.

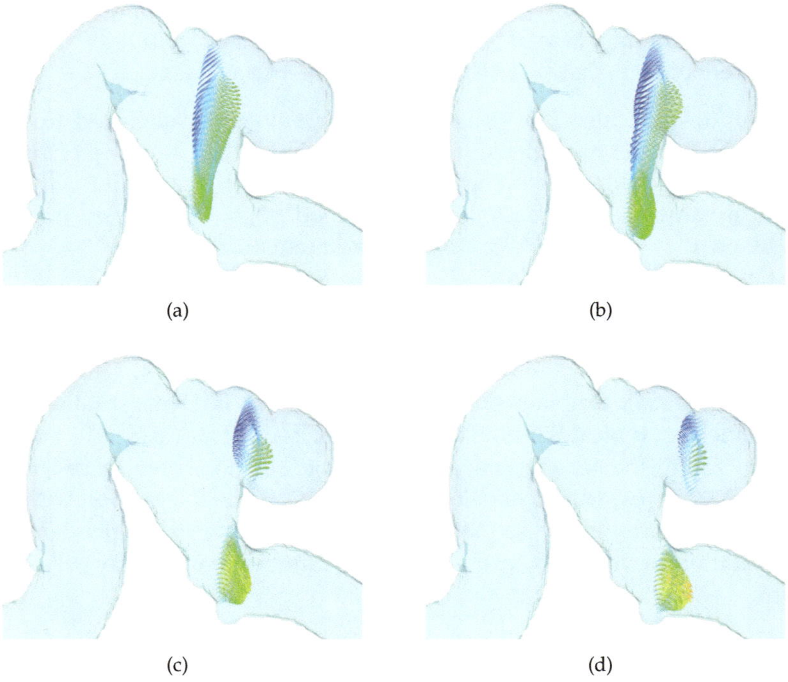

Figure 5. Velocity vector field in a few cross-sections along the aneurysm geometry. The cross-sections are taken at several x locations in yz planes, largely perpendicular to the flow direction. Green and yellow arrows show the middle range of flow velocities. Areas of slightly higher velocity are shown in red, while blue arrows indicate negative velocities related to the recirculating flow that develops. Grid resolution is $128 \times 64 \times 128$.

To get an alternative impression of the velocity field, in Figure 5 we present the velocity vector field in a few cross-sections near the aneurysm bulb. The cross-sections are taken in yz planes, largely perpendicular to the mean flow direction. The flow in more or less cylindrical tube sections of the local vessel system shows similarity to a parabolic profile, reminiscent of Hagen-Poiseuille flow. We notice that the dominant flow still follows what used to be the non-diseased tract (Figure 5(c),(d)). However, also within the aneurysm there is considerable dynamics, showing regions of forward and backward flow, as illustrated in the velocity vectors. In the middle cross-sections (Figure 5(a),(b)) the flow dynamics is nicely illustrated with flow entering (green arrows) as well as exiting (blue arrows) the aneurysm in a complex vortical sweep; the flow partially comes back from the aneurysm after having circulated in it. The flow structure inside the aneurysm also leads to higher residence times of red blood cells, and possibly a reduced quality of circulation. This is correlated with regions of lower levels of wall-shear stress, as the flow-intensity in the aneurysm is rather low. From this general visualization one may already appreciate the frequently expressed observation that regions of low wall-shear stress are a marker of increased likelihood of aneurysm growth, possibly since the endothelial cells lining the vessel walls are (slightly) less well supplied with oxygen and nutrients, leading to their gradual degeneration [8].

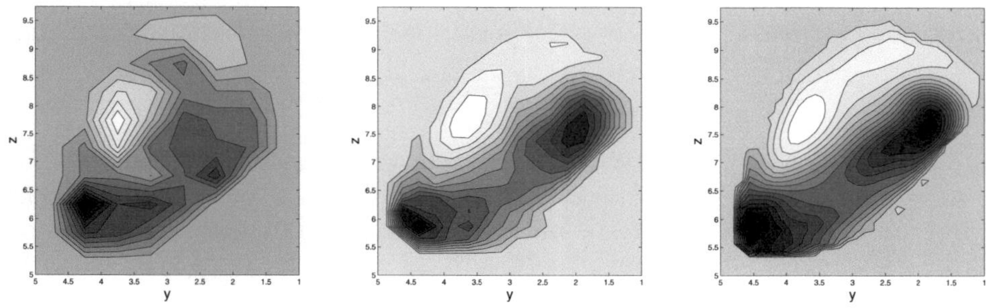

(a) (b) (c)

Figure 6. Contour plot of the streamwise u-velocity in a yz cross-section in the middle of the geometry at $x = 8$. Dark regions correspond to high positive velocities, while the lightest contours are related to regions of negative velocity; we adopt the same color-coding for all figures. The flow structures show a vortex inside the aneurysm. We present the velocity contours in the same plane for different grid resolutions: $32 \times 16 \times 32$ (a), $64 \times 32 \times 64$ (b) and $128 \times 64 \times 128$ (c).

A closer impression of the flow inside the aneurysm can be obtained by considering contour plots of velocity components. In Figure 6 we show a particular contour of the streamwise velocity component at $x = 8$, which is through the actual aneurysm, i.e., a section through the middle in Figure 5(a). We show a cross-section in the yz-plane at a number of spatial resolutions. The grid refinement shows a clear qualitative convergence toward the grid-independent solution. The resolution $32 \times 16 \times 32$ is seen to be insufficient to capture the full complexity of the flow. However, the main features are already captured properly at a resolution of $64 \times 32 \times 64$, while high accuracy results can only be expected by further increase of the resolution. We notice both dark and light colors in this contour plot, corresponding to positive and negative streamwise velocities. These show a region of recirculating flow in the aneurysm, next to the main through-flow represented by the dark region in the lower left corner of each contour plot. We also investigated the dependence of the flow prediction on spatial resolution at other streamwise locations and found similar qualitative convergence. A more precise assessment of the level of convergence is considered momentarily.

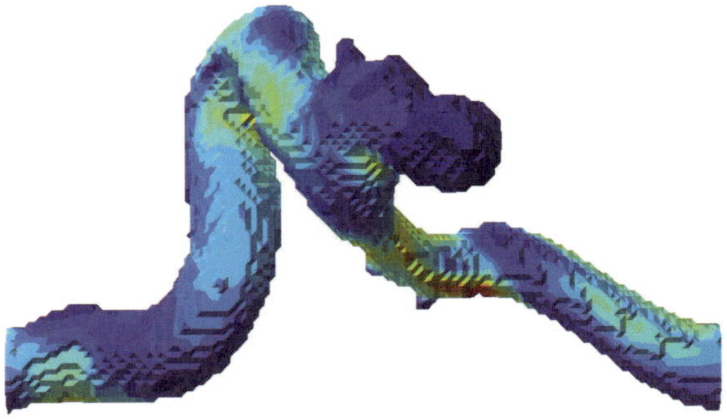

Figure 7. Distribution of the non-dimensional shear stress, computed at $Re = 250$. The grid resolution is $128 \times 64 \times 128$. Red and yellow areas correspond to the locations of high shear stress, while blue areas are related to the low stresses.

Regions of relatively high and relatively low shear stress are considered as important markers for the risk of aneurysm growth. These can be obtained from the simulations as well, by post-processing the velocity field. The shear stress τ is defined in non-dimensional form as

$$\tau = \frac{1}{Re}\sqrt{2S_{ij}S_{ij}} \tag{18}$$

where $S_{ij} = (\partial_i u_j + \partial_j u_i)/2$ denotes the rate of strain tensor. A global impression of the wall shear stress distribution is given in Figure 7. Regions of high shear stress are concentrated near relatively sharp bends in the vessel and near the 'neck' of the aneurysm (red and yellow), where the bulge connects to the previously unaffected vessel. Inside the aneurysm the shear stress is rather low (uniform blue), consistent with the rather low velocities that are observed inside the aneurysm bulge. Such a region of low (wall) shear stress is reported to be connected to aneurysm growth, associated with a slow degeneration of endothelial cells at the vessel walls. Further research in this direction is highly needed to clarify the precise mechanisms and to quantify possible growth-paths of the aneurysm.

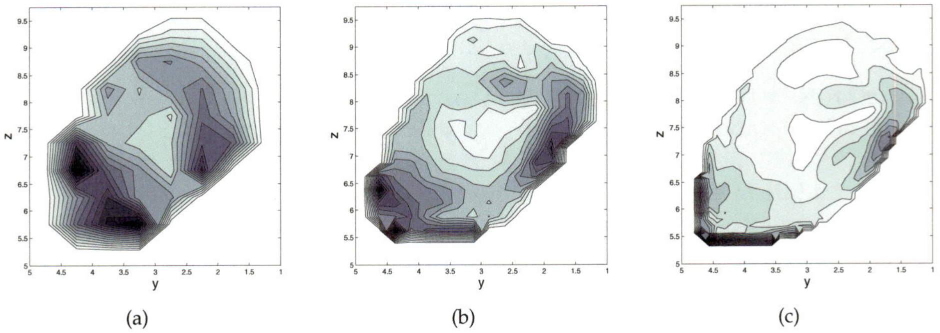

Figure 8. Contour plot of shear stress τ in a yz cross-section in the middle of the geometry $x = 8$. Dark regions correspond to high levels of shear stress, while the lightest contours are related to low shear regions. We present the distribution of stress contours in the same plane for different grid resolutions: $32 \times 16 \times 32$ (a), $64 \times 32 \times 64$ (b) and $128 \times 64 \times 128$ (c).

A more precise impression of the shear stress distribution can be obtained in terms of contour plots. In Figure 8 we show the steady state shear stress distribution in a yz-plane through the middle of the aneurysm at $x = 8$. We observe a qualitative convergence of the shear stress, although the degree of convergence seems to be slightly less compared to the velocity field as shown in Figure 6. For the shear stress we need to approximate the derivative of the velocity, which is more demanding on the spatial resolution, especially close to the aneurysm wall. The aneurysm region shows one focal point of somewhat higher shear stress, while elsewhere the level of the shear stress is seen to be rather low. In addition, quite high shear stress levels are observed in the lower left corner of each contour plot, corresponding to the main flow through what remains of the original vessel structure prior to the development of the aneurysm.

In order to quantify more precisely the level of convergence, in the next section we consider the reliability of the flow simulations by investigating the quality with which the actual local solution is obtained.

3.2. Reliability of IB predictions: a grid refinement study

In this subsection we concentrate on a more quantitative analysis of the reliability of the numerical flow prediction. We consider the convergence of the driving pressure drop as well as profiles of velocity and shear stress at different grid resolutions.

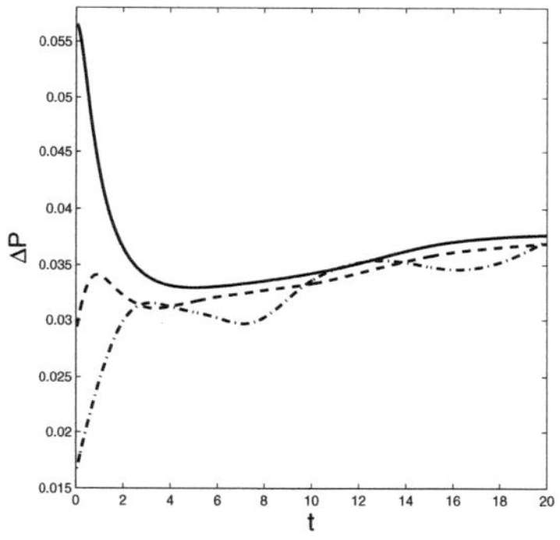

Figure 9. Convergence of the pressure drop across the whole flow domain, computed at different grid resolutions: $32 \times 16 \times 32$ (dash-dot), $64 \times 32 \times 64$ (dash) and $128 \times 64 \times 128$ (solid).

In order to maintain a constant mass flow rate through the aneurysm, a pressure drop ΔP needs to be supplied. In Figure 9 we show the evolution of the forcing pressure drop at different spatial resolutions. The initial solution from which each simulation starts uses $u = 1$ and $v = w = p = 0$. Hence, we deliberately set the streamwise velocity equal to unity everywhere, i.e., also inside the solid part of the domain. This presents a strict test for the robustness of the method, in which the solution in the solid has to adapt and reduce completely to zero within the solid. Moreover, a realistic flow in the fluid part needs to build up. There is considerable difference between the solution at different spatial resolutions in the initial stage due to the strong acceleration of the flow to rectify the non-physical aspects of the initial condition. As the flow settles into the steady state we notice a clear convergence of the pressure drop levels. Since the non-dimensional size of the domain is 16 and the velocity is maximally on the order of 0.7, a typical flow-through time, i.e., the time needed to pass from one side of the domain to the other, can be expected to be in the range of 20 or more. To reach a fully steady state, a simulation covering several flow-through times is needed. In Figure 9 we notice already a fair agreement for ΔP at different spatial resolutions after about one flow-through time.

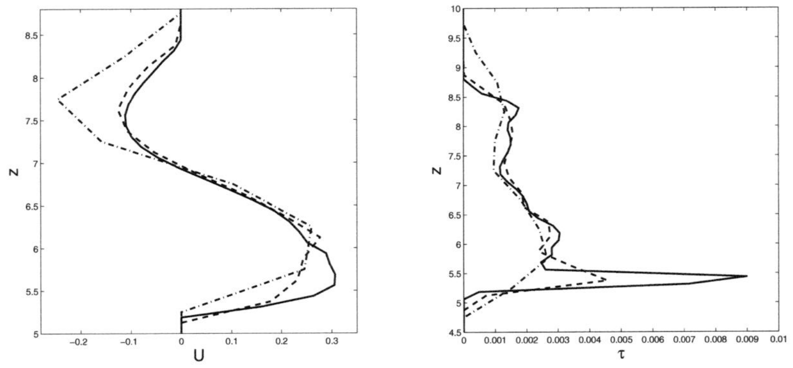

(a) (b)

Figure 10. Streamwise velocity (a) and shear stress (b) profiles as a function of z, in the middle of the domain at $x = 8$ and $y = 4$. The profiles were computed at $t = 20$ using different grid resolutions: $32 \times 16 \times 32$ (dash-dot), $64 \times 32 \times 64$ (dash) and $128 \times 64 \times 128$ (solid).

To further assess the reliability of the solution we turn to profiles of velocity and shear stress in a characteristic region in Figure 10. This provides a quantitative measure for the convergence of the numerical solution. We observe that the coarsest resolution of $32 \times 16 \times 32$ is not capable to capture more than the main flow pattern of recirculating flow. Increasing the resolution shows a much closer correspondence between the different velocity predictions. This is also seen in the profiles for the shear stress. The general agreement is quite close, as long as we do not include the coarsest resolution. Convergence of the sharp stress peak near the lower wall in this particular profile is seen to be most challenging to our IB method. We also investigated convergence by considering profiles in a range of other locations and observed similarly close agreement of the numerical solutions at different spatial resolutions. This establishes that a first quantitatively acceptable solution can be obtained using a grid of $64 \times 32 \times 64$, while higher accuracy requires further refinement.

In the next section we turn our attention to realistic pulsatile flow in the given cerebral aneurysm geometry.

4. Pulsatile flow simulations in realistic cerebral aneurysm

In this section we will focus on pulsatile flow. We first consider the pulsatile velocity pattern and translate this into the volumetric flow rate used in the simulations. Then we will present the dynamics of the shear stress at different, physiologically relevant Reynolds numbers. Next to $Re = 250$ as used up to now, we include $Re = 200$ and $Re = 300$ to probe the variability of predictions when alternative values for the blood viscosity, the vessel sizes and/or velocity scales are taken from literature. We also compute the flow at $Re = 100$ and $Re = 400$, which are expected to be indicative of diseased conditions. A striking transition to very complex time-dependence at higher Re is observed, which may be of interest for medical monitoring.

The velocity of the blood flow in cerebral arteries can be measured by different techniques, e.g., phase-contrast (MR) angiography [15] or TCD sonography as presented in [41]. In the current study the velocity was recorded in the middle cerebral artery by [9] using TCD. In Figure 11(a) we plotted a segment of 10 seconds of the pulsating velocity wave. The mean velocity value, obtained by integrating this signal, is found to be 38.66 cm/s, which is very close to the reference scale selected in Section 3.

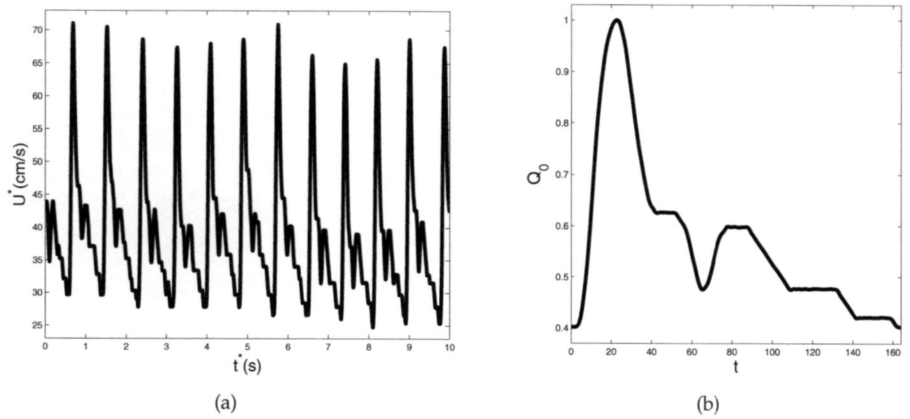

Figure 11. Pulsatile wave measured in the human brain using TCD sonography. The 10 seconds velocity signal measured in the MCA is presented in (a). The unit pulse mass-flow wave was chosen from the original signal and normalized for the computations (b).

The computed pulsatile flow is maintained by using the actually recorded velocity signal as forcing. We choose a typical pulse from Figure 11(a) and repeat it periodically. We need to convert the recorded velocity values into a time-dependent volumetric flow rate, which we specify next. The selected pulse has a maximal velocity $u^*_{max} \approx 67.94\ cm/s$, which corresponds to a peak flow rate of $Q^*_{max} \approx 8.033 \cdot 10^{-6}\ m^3/s$, using the selected radius $R^* = 1.94\ mm$ and assuming a perfectly circular cross section. If we take the reference velocity $u^*_r = 0.388\ m/s$ corresponding to a Reynolds number $Re = 250$, we find similarly as reference flow rate $Q^*_r \approx 4.59 \cdot 10^{-6}\ m^3/s$. For convenience, we split the forcing signal in the non-dimensional formulation into a normalized flow rate pattern Q_0 and an amplitude Q^*_{max}/Q^*_r such that the forcing used in the simulations becomes $Q(t) = (Q^*_{max}/Q^*_r)Q_0(t) \approx 1.75Q_0(t)$. The normalized pulsatile wave Q_0 is illustrated in Figure 11(b). The physical duration of one pulse is $t^* = 0.82\ s$. The reference time-scale can be computed as $t^*_r = R^*/u^*_r = 0.005\ s$. Thus at $Re = 250$ one pulse requires 164 non-dimensional time units.

The procedure to define the pulsatile flow rate can be extended to also address other Reynolds numbers. We take as reference Reynolds number Re and fix the reference length-scale to R^* (since we consider the same geometry) and the kinematic viscosity to ν^*_r (since we still consider the flow of blood). If we wish to simulate at another Reynolds number Re' this implies that the reference velocity scale is changed according to $(u^*)'_r = (Re'/Re)u^*_r$. Correspondingly, the time-scale changes into $(t^*)'_r = (Re/Re')t^*_r$ and hence, the 'new' number of dimensionless time-steps to take in order to complete one cycle of 0.82 s of the pulsatile flow decreases with decreasing Reynolds number. Another consequence of changing the Reynolds number at constant length-scale and kinematic viscosity is that $(Q^*)'_r = (Re'/Re)Q^*_r$, as well as $(Q^*)'_{max} = (Re'/Re)Q^*_{max}$. Hence, the dimensionless forcing does not alter with changing Reynolds number and remains at $Q(t) \approx 1.75Q_0(t)$. The factor 1.75 denotes the 'contrast' in the pulsatile flow rate, i.e., the ratio between the maximal and the average velocity during a cycle - this quantity varies from one person to another and even per heartbeat.

We compute the pulsatile flow in a range of Reynolds numbers $100 \leq Re \leq 400$ while keeping the viscosity of the blood and the size of the vessel constant. In Section 3 we discussed the uncertainty in physical parameters, when consulting literature. This leads to a range of Reynolds number $175 \lesssim Re \lesssim 300$ of physiologically realistic values. Including also unhealthy changes in the blood vessels, e.g., narrowing of the vessel diameter, or the development of an aneurysm and corresponding increase in the size of the vessel, but also changes in the viscosity of blood, or in the velocity of the flow, we propose to also compute the flow at $Re = 100$ and $Re = 400$. This total range of Reynolds numbers gives a complete set of flow conditions relevant to flow in the Circle of Willis. For all simulations we use a spatial resolution of $64 \times 32 \times 64$, which we showed to be the lower limit at which quantitatively reliable results can be obtained for the case considered here.

The translation 'back' from non-dimensional units to physical units requires scaling of the time and of the shear stress values. For the indicated range of Reynolds numbers Re a single pulse of 0.82 s requires $\#_t$ dimensionless time steps with $(Re, \#_t) = (100, 65.6), (200, 131.2), (250, 164), (300, 196.8)$ and $(400, 262.4)$. Moreover, the change in Re corresponds to a change in u_r^*, which affects the scale for the shear stress which is $\rho_r^*(u_r^*)^2$. The final result is a wall shear stress in Pa and time measure in s, which allows a more direct assessment than the fully dimensionless representation.

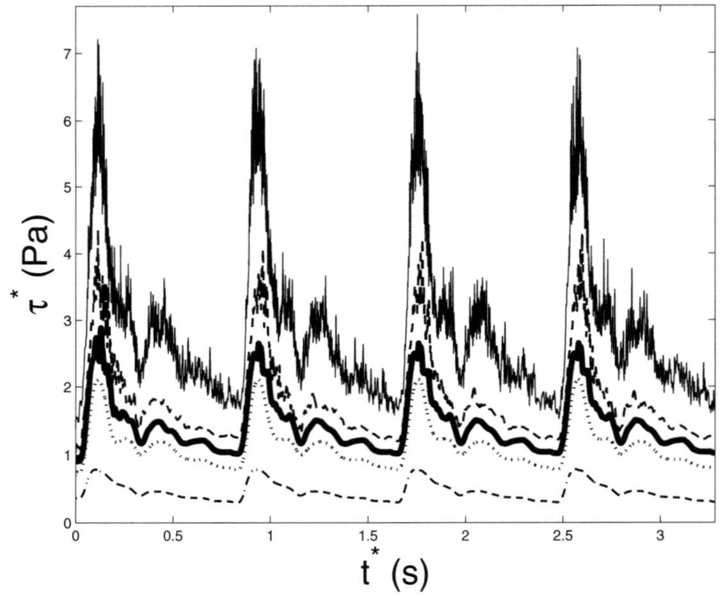

Figure 12. Maximal shear stress for realistic pulsatile flow in the aneurysm geometry. The reference $Re = 250$ is shown (bold, solid). Lower values are shown as $Re = 200$ (dot), $Re = 100$ (dash-dot), while higher value are displayed as $Re = 300$ (dash) and $Re = 400$ (thin, solid). The average stress levels decrease with decreasing Reynolds number.

After these preparations, we show the dynamic response of the maximum shear stress in Figure 12 for 4 full pulse cycles. The initial condition is that of quiescent flow, i.e., $u = v = w = 0$ - we observe that this leads to a short transient, e.g., seen because the response in the first cycle differs slightly from that in later cycles. After this transient we observe for our reference case $Re = 250$ (solid bold line) that the maximum shear stress closely follows the imposed volumetric flow rate profile. The mean value is found to be around 1.4 *Pa* with peak values near 2.9 *Pa*. These values show the same general magnitude as reported in [14, 37].

Increasing or decreasing the Reynolds number has a marked effect on the dynamic response. At the lower Reynolds numbers the response of the shear stress maximum is seen to be smooth, following the imposed pulsatile profile. At the higher Reynolds numbers the natural Navier-Stokes nonlinearity seems to become dominant, which makes the shear stress response lively by the emergence of relatively high frequency components to the solution. In addition, the level of the shear stress rises considerably. Such rapid transition in flow regime within the physiologically relevant *Re*-range may contribute to an increased risk of aneurysm rupture. This transition was also seen in simulations of other realistic aneurysms and even for simplified model aneurysms consisting of curved vessel to which a spherical cavity was added [30].

5. Concluding remarks

We presented computational modeling of cerebral flow based on a volume penalizing IB method, aimed at understanding the flow and forces that emerge in aneurysms that may form on the Circle of Willis. We sketched how medical imagery can serve as point of departure for a sequence of numerical representations and modeling steps, ultimately leading to the full simulation of pulsatile flow in a realistic cerebral aneurysm, which was used as a case study in this chapter.

Taking data from literature we identified physiologically relevant flow conditions and their general uncertainty. Data concerning sizes of vessels, kinematic viscosity of blood and flow speeds in the region of the Circle of Willis during the cardiac cycle, can not be obtained with very high accuracy. This leaves considerable uncertainty as to the precise flow conditions. However, consensus seems to exist that the Reynolds number, which is the crucial parameter for incompressible flow, should be in the range $175 \leq Re \leq 300$ for non-diseased situations. This is a rather wide range, but throughout this range the flow in the blood vessels is pulsatile and laminar, i.e., sharing quite comparable dynamics. The main challenge for computational modeling is not just to predict a certain flow under specified conditions, but to reckon also with the variability in flow conditions due to a variety of possible changes in key parameters. This approach was taken in this chapter.

Settling for $Re = 250$ as characteristic point of reference, we analyzed a particular, realistic cerebral aneurysm in detail. First, the main flow features and the reliability of predictions were considered for steady flow at fixed volumetric flow rate. This is not a realistic flow condition, as in reality interest is with pulsatile flow, but it does allow to investigate the sensitivity of the predicted solution on things such as spatial resolution. We visualized both qualitatively and quantitatively the steady flow in the aneurysm, as well as the shear stress field that emerges. It was shown that the main flow follows a path that is close to what used to be the original vessel before the formation of the aneurysm. Next to this 'main' flow, a complex circulation was shown to develop inside the aneurysm bulge. By considering contour plots and also profiles of velocity and shear stress at different spatial resolutions, the degree of reliability of the numerical simulation was discussed. The current IB method is first order accurate. Developments in which sub-grid forcing is included [42] can be used to increase the formal order of accuracy to two - this appears a relevant extension of the IB approach and will be considered in more detail in the near future, allowing to cut down on the computational cost and/or increase the accuracy of flow predictions.

A complete model was obtained by incorporating realistic pulsatile flow, obtained from direct TCD measurements of the velocity of blood flow in the brain. The recorded velocity in a vessel near the Circle of Willis was used to impose a proper time-dependent volumetric flow rate, representing a cardiac cycle. Repeating a characteristic pulse periodically, leads to a model with which the time-dependent flow and shear stresses can be determined. As regards the flow structures, for pulsatile flow at $Re = 250$ one basically notices the same dominant flow features as in case of steady flow forcing, with the exception that the 'amplitude' of the motion becomes time-dependent. As an example, the recirculating flow in the aneurysm was observed throughout the entire cycle, but with a time-dependent intensity and a slight 'meandering' of the precise vortical structures. We sketched the extension of the pulsatile flow model to other flow conditions, i.e., other Re and other time-scales. If the flow is in the physiologically relevant regime $Re \leq 300$, the response of, e.g., the shear stress, closely follows that of the input flow-rate forcing. At higher Reynolds numbers, indicative of possible diseased states, the flow develops considerable complexity and shows a transition toward much higher frequencies. This goes hand in hand with increased levels of shear stress and may be monitored as a potential indication of increased risk to the patient. By recording the spectrum of these frequencies an easy monitoring concept may become available.

The application of computational support in the monitoring and treatment of cerebral aneurysms is a field of ongoing research. Accessibility of time-dependent flow fields in all relevant detail is a crucial point from which to depart toward developing predictive capability for the associated slow growth of the aneurysm bulge. This requires a new kind of 'flow-structure interaction' in which degradation of endothelial cells due to reduced quality of blood circulation typically triggers a further expansion of the aneurysm bulge, and generally leads to an increase in the risk of rupture. The latter type of 'flow-structure interaction' is subject of ongoing research. In order to achieve a closer connection with medical practice several computational modeling steps still need to be taken, such as the development of higher order accurate methods, multi inflow/outflow configurations, flow-structure interaction in which a full coupling to slow degenerative processes of endothelial cells is made, as well as modeling of mechanical properties of brain tissue to also address aneurysm compliance during the pulsatile cycle. This brief listing shows the various developments that are still needed in order to make the pathway from medical imagery to quantitative decision support both reliable as well as fully automated.

Acknowledgements

The authors gratefully acknowledge many fruitful discussions with Prof. Dr. Hans Kuerten (Eindhoven University of Technology and University of Twente). We are also grateful to Willem Jan van Rooij, MD, PhD and Menno Sluzewski, MD, PhD (St. Elizabeth Hospital, Tilburg, the Netherlands) for providing angiographic data and to Dr. Ir. Dirk-Jan Kroon (Focal, Oldenzaal, the Netherlands) for segmentation of the data. Computations at the Huygens computer at SARA were supported by NCF through the project SH061.

Author details

Julia Mikhal, Cornelis H. Slump and Bernard J. Geurts
Faculty EEMCS, University of Twente, P.O.Box 217, 7500 AE, Enschede, The Netherlands

6. References

[1] Angot, P.; Bruneau, C.H.; Frabrie, P. (1999). A penalization method to take into account obstacles in viscous flows. *Numerical Mathematics*, Vol. 81, pp. 497-520

[2] Bernsdorf, J. & Wang, D. (2009). Non-Newtonian blood flow simulation in cerebral aneurysms. *Computers & Mathematics with Applications*, Vol. 58, pp. 1024-1029

[3] Bescós, J.O.; Slob, M.J.; Slump, C.H.; Sluzewski, M.; van Rooij, W.J. (2005). Volume Measurement of Intracranial Aneurysms from 3D Rotational Angiography: Improvement of Accuracy by Gradient Edge Detection. *AJNR American Journal of Neuroradiology*, Vol. 26, pp. 2569-2572

[4] Boussel, L.; Rayz, V.; McCulloch, C.; Martin, A.; Acevedo-Bolton, G.; Lawton, M.; Higashida, R.; Smith, W.S.; Young, W.L.; Saloner, D. (2008). Aneurysm Growth Occurs at Region of Low Wall Shear Stress: Patient-Specific Correlation of Hemodynamics and Growth in a Longitudinal Study. *Stroke*, Vol. 39, pp. 2997-3002

[5] Cebral, J.R.; Castro, M.A.; Burgess, J.E.; Pergolizzi, R.S.; Sheridan, M.J.; Putman, C.M. (2005). Characterization of Cerebral Aneurysms for Assessing Risk of Rupture By Using Patient-Specific Computational Hemodynamics Models. *AJNR American Journal of Neuroradiology*, Vol. 26, pp. 2550-2559

[6] Cebral, J.R.; Castro, M.A.; Appanaboyina, S.; Putman, C.M.; Millan, D.; Frangi, A.F. (2005b). Efficient Pipeline for Image-Based Patient-Specific Analysis of Cerebral Aneurysms Hemodynamics: Technique and Sensitivity. *IEEE Transactions on Medical Imaging*, Vol. 24, No. 4, pp. 457-467

[7] Cheny, Y.; Botella, O. (2010). The LS-STAG method: A new immersed boundary/level-set method for the computation of incompressible viscous flows in complex moving geometries with good conservation properties. *Journal of Computational Physics*, Vol. 229, No. 4, pp. 1043-1076

[8] Doenitz, C.; Schebesch, K.M.; Zoephel, R.; Brawanski, A. (2010). A mechanism for the rapid development of intracranial aneurysms: a case study. *Neurosurgery*, Vol. 67, No. 5, pp. 1213-1221

[9] Duijvenboden, S., Schaafsma, A., Geurts, B.J. (2011). Usefulness of Schrodingerś operator for assessing new parameters in Transcranial Doppler sonography, University of Twente, Internal Report

[10] Gao, T.; Tseng, Y.H.; Lu, X.Y. (2007). An improved hybrid Cartesian/immersed boundary method for fluid-solid flows. *International Journal for Numerical Methods in Fluids* Vol. 55, No.12, pp. 1189-1211

[11] Gambaruto, A.M.; Janela J.; Moura A.; Sequeira A. (2011). Sensitivity of Hemodynamics in a Patient Specific Cerebral Aneurysm to Vascular Geometry and Blood Rheology. *Mathematical Biosciences and Engineering*, Vol. 8, No. 2, pp. 409-423. doi:10.3934/mbe.2011.8.409

[12] Geurts, B.J. (2003). Elements of Direct and Large-Eddy Simulation. Edwards Publishing, ISBN: 1-930217-07-2

[13] Gijsen, F.J.H.; van de Vosse, F.N.; Janssen, J.D. (1999). The influence of the non-Newtonian properties of blood on the flow in large arteries: steady flow in a carotid bifurcation model. *Journal of Biomechanics*, Vol. 32, pp. 601-608

[14] Goubergrits, L.; Schaller, J.; Kertzscher, U.; van der Bruck, N.; Poethkow, K.; Petz, Ch.; Hege, H.-Ch.; Spuler, A. (2012). Statistical wall shear stress maps of ruptured and unruptured middle cerebral artery aneurysms. *Journal of the Royal Society Interface*, Vol. 9, No. 69, pp. 677-688. doi: 10.1098/rsif.2011.0490

[15] Hendrikse, J.; van Raamt, A.F.; van der Graaf, Y.; Mali, W.P.T.M.; van der Grond, J. (2005). Distribution of Cerebral Blood Flow in the Circle of Willis. *Radiology*, Vol. 235, pp. 184-189. doi: 10.1148/radiol.2351031799

[16] Hirsch, C. (1988). Numerical computation of internal and external flows. Wiley and Sons, ISBN: 0471-917621

[17] Iaccarino, G.; Verzicco, R. (2003). Immersed boundary technique for turbulent flow simulations. *Applied Mechanics Reviews, ASME*, Vol. 56, No. 3, pp. 331-347. doi: 10.1115/1.1563627

[18] Janela, J.; Moura, A.; Sequeira, A. (2010). A 3D non-Newtonian fluid-structure interaction model for blood flow in arteries. *Journal of Computational Applied Mathematics*, Vol. 234, No. 9, pp. 2783-2791. doi: 10.1016/j.cam.2010.01.032

[19] Kamath, S. (1981). Observations on the length and diameter of vessels forming the Circle of willis. *Journal of Anatomy*, Vol. 133, No. 3, pp. 419-423

[20] Keetels, G.H.; DÓrtona, U.; Kramer, W.; Clercx, H.J.H.; Schneider, K.; van Heijst, G.J.F. (2007). Fourier spectral and wavelet solvers for the incompressible Navier-Stokes equations with volume-penalization: Convergence of a dipole-wall collision. *Journal of Computational Physics*, Vol. 227, No. 2, pp. 919-945. doi: 10.1016/j.jcp.2007.07.036

[21] Khadra, K.; Angot, P.; Parneix, S.; Caltagirone, J.P. (2000). Fictitious domain approach for numerical modelling of Navier-Stokes equations. *International Journal for Numerical Methods in Fluids*, Vol. 34, No. 8, pp. 651-684. doi: 10.1002/1097-0363

[22] Kovalev, K. (2005). Unstructured hexahedral non-conformal mesh generation. PhD Thesis, Vrije University of Brussels

[23] Kroon, D.J.; Slump, C.H.; Sluzewski, M.; van Rooij, W.J. (2006). Image based hemodynamics modelling of cerebral aneurysms and the determination of the risk of rupture. *SPIE Medical Imaging 2006: Physiology, Function, and Structure from Medical Images*, Vol. 6143, Manduca, A; Amini, A.A. (Ed.), Proc. of SPIE, 61432B. doi: 10.1117/12.648062

[24] Ku, D.N. (1997). Blood flow in arteries. *Annual Review Fluid Mechanics*, Vol. 29, pp. 399-434

[25] Koffijberg, H.; Buskens, E.; Algra, A.; Wermer, M.J.H.; Rinkel, G.J.E. (2008). Growth rates of intracranial aneurysms: exploring constancy. *Journal of Neurosurgery*, Vol. 109, No. 2, pp. 176-185

[26] Liu, Q.; Vasilyev, O.V. (2007). A Brinkman penalization method for compressible flows in complex geometries. *Journal of Computational Physics*, Vol. 227, No. 2, pp. 946-966. doi: 10.1016/j.jcp.2007.07.037

[27] Löhner, R.; Baum, J.D.; Mestreau, E.L.; Rice, D. (2007). Comparison of body-fitted, embedded and immersed 3-d euler predictions for blast loads on columns. *American Institute of Aeronautics and Astrounatics*, pp. 1-22

[28] Lopez Penha, D.J.; Geurts, B.J.; Stolz, S.; Nordlund, M. (2011). Computing the apparent permeability of an array of staggered square rods using volume-penalization. *Computers & Fluids*, Vol. 51, No. 1, pp. 157-173. doi: 10.1016/j.compfluid.2011.08.011

[29] Metcalfe, R.W. (2003). The Promise of Computational Fluid Dynamics As a Tool for Delineating Therapeutic Options in the Treatment of Aneurysms. *AJNR Editorials*, Vol. 24, pp. 553-554

[30] Mikhal, J. & Geurts, B.J. (2011). Pulsatile flow in model cerebral aneurysms. *Procedia Computer Science*, Vol. 4, pp. 811-820. doi: 10.1016/j.procs.2011.04.086

[31] Mikhal, J. & Geurts, B.J. (2011). Bounding Solutions for Cerebral Aneurysms. *New Archive for Mathematics*, Vol. 5(12), No. 3, pp. 163-168

[32] Mittal, R. & Iaccarino, G. (2005). Immersed Boundary Methods. *Annual Review of Fluid Mechanics*, Vol. 37, pp. 239-261. doi: 10.1146/annurev.fluid.37.061903.175743

[33] Moret, J.; Kemkers, R.; Op de Beek, J.; Koppe, R.; Klotz, E.; Grass, M. (1998). 3D rotational angiography: Clinical value in endovascular treatment. *Medicamundi*, Vol 42, No 3, pp. 8-14

[34] Oktar, S.O.; Yücel, C.; Karaosmanoglu, D.; Akkan, K.; Ozdemir, H.; Tokgoz, N.; Tali, T. (2006). Blood-flow volume quantification in internal carotid and vertebral arteries: comparison of 3 different ultrasound techniques with phase-contrast MR imaging. *AJNR American Journal of Neuroradiology*, Vol. 27, No. 2, pp. 363-369

[35] Oubel, E.; De Craene, M.; Putman, C.M.; Cebral, J.R.; Frangi, A.F. (2007). Analysis of intracranial aneurysm wall motion and its effects on hemodynamic patterns. *SPIE Medical Imaging 2007: Physiology, Function, and Structure from Medical Images*, Vol. 6511, Manduca, A; Hu, X.P. (Ed.), San Diego, CA: SPIE Press, 10–11

[36] Oubel, E.; Cebral, J.R.; De Craene, M.; Blanc, R.; Blasco, J.; Macho J.; Putman, C.M.; Frangi, A.F. (2010). Wall motion estimation in intracranial aneurysms. *Physiological Measurement*, Vol. 31, pp. 1119-1135. doi: 10.1088/0967-3334/31/9/004

[37] Oyre, S.; Ringgaard, S.; Kozerke, S.; Paaske, W.P.; Erlandsen, M.; Boesiger, P.; Pedersen, E.M. (1998). Accurate Noninvasive Quantification of Blood Flow, Cross-Sectional Lumen Vessel Area and Wall Shear Stress by Three-Dimensional Paraboloid Modeling of Magnetic Resonance Imaging Velocity Data. *Journal of the American College of Cardiology*, Vol. 32, No. 1, pp. 128-134

[38] Perktold, K.; Peter, R.; Resch, M. (1989). Pulsatile non-Newtonian blood flow simulation through a bifurcation with an aneurysm. *Biorheology*, Vol. 26, No. 6, pp. 1011-1030

[39] Peskin, C.S. (2002). The immersed boundary method, *Acta Numerica*, pp. 1-39. doi: 10.1017/S0962492902000077

[40] Quarteroni, A. & Formaggia, L. (2004). Mathematical Modelling and Numerical Simulation of the Cardiovascular System. *Handbook of Numerical Analysis*, North-Holland, Amsterdam

[41] Ringelstein. E.B.; Kahlscheuer, B.; Niggemeyer, E.; Otis, S.M. (1990). Transcranial Doppler Sonography: Anatomical landmarks and normal velocity values. *Ultrasound in Medicine & Biology*, Vol. 16, No. 8, pp. 745-761

[42] Sarthou, A.; Vincent, S.; Caltagirone, J.P.; Angot, P. (2008). Eulerian-Lagrangian grid coupling and penalty methods for the simulation of multiphase flows interacting with complex objects. *International Journal for Numerical Methods in Fluids*, Vol. 56, pp. 1093-1099. doi: 10.1002/fld.1661

[43] Saylor, P.E. (1988). Leapfrog variants of iterative methods for linear algebraic equations. *Journal of Computational and Applied Mathematics*, Vol. 24, pp. 169-193

[44] Shojima, M.; Oshima, M.; Takagi, K.; Torii, R.; Hayakawa, M.; Katada, K.; Morita, A.; Kirino, T. (2004). Magnitude and Role of Wall Shear Stress on Cerebral Aneurysm. Computational Fluid Dynamic Study of 20 Middle Cerebral Artery Aneurysms. *Stroke*, Vol. 35, pp. 2500-2505. doi: 10.1161/01.STR.0000144648.89172.0f

[45] Sprengers, M.E.; Schaafsma, J.; van Rooij, W.J.; Sluzewski, M.; Rinkel, G.J.E.; Velthuis, B.K.; van Rijn, J.C.; Majoie, C.B. (2008). Stability of Intracranial Aneurysms Adequately Occluded 6 Months after Coiling: a 3T MR Angiography Multicenter Long-Term Follow-Up Study. *AJNR American Journal of Neuroradiololgy*, Vol. 29, pp. 1768-1774. doi: 10.3174/ajnr.A1181

[46] van Rooij, W.J. (1998). Endovascular Treatment of Cerebral Aneurysms. PhD Thesis, University of Utrecht. ISBN: 90-393-1818-2

[47] van Rooij, W.J.; Sprengers, M.E.; Sluzewski, M.; Beute, G.N. (2007). Intracranial aneurysms that repeatedly reopen over time after coiling: imaging characteristics and treatment outcome. *Neuroradiology*, Vol. 49, pp. 343-349. doi: 10.1007/s00234-006-0200-2

[48] van Rooij, W.J.; Sprengers, M.E.; de Gast, A.N.; Peluso, A.P.P.; Sluzewski, M. (2008). 3D Rotational Angiography: The New Gold Standard in the Detection of Additional Intracranial Aneurysms. *AJNR American Journal of Neuroradiology*, Vol. 29, pp. 976-979. doi: 10.3174/ajnr.A0964

[49] Vasilyev, O.V.; Kevlahan, N.K.R. (2002) Hybrid wavelet collocation-Brinkman penalization method for complex geometry flows. *International Journal for Numerical Methods in Fluids*, Vol. 40, No. 3-4, pp. 531-538. doi: 10.1002/fld.307

[50] Verstappen, R.W.C.P. & Veldman, A.E.P. (2003). Symmetry-Preserving Discretization of Turbulent Flow. *Journal of Computational Physics*, Vol. 187, pp. 343-368

[51] Wanke, I.; Dörfler, A.; Forsting, M. (2008). Intracranial Aneurysms. *Intracranial Vascular Malformations and Aneurysms*. Springer, ISBN: 978-3-540-32919-0

[52] Wiebers, D.O.; Whisnant, J.P.; Forbes, G. et al. (1998). Unruptured intracranial aneurysms – risk of rupture and risks of surgical intervention. International Study of Unruptured Intracranial Aneurysms Investigators. *New England Journal of Medicine*, Vol. 339, No. 24, pp. 1725-1733

[53] Young, D.F.; Munson, B.R.; Okiishi, T.H. (1997). A brief introduction to fluid mechanics. John Wiley & Sons, Inc., ISBN: 0-471-13771-5

Chapter 11

A (Near) Real-Time Simulation Method of Aneurysm Coil Embolization

Yiyi Wei, Stéphane Cotin, Jérémie Dequidt, Christian Duriez,
Jérémie Allard and Erwan Kerrien

Additional information is available at the end of the chapter

http://dx.doi.org/10.5772/48635

1. Introduction

1.1. Aneurysm

An aneurysm is an abnormal widening of a blood vessel. As the vessel widens, it also gets thinner and weaker, with an increasing risk of rupture. Aneurysms are essentially found in the aorta, the popliteal artery, mesenteric artery, and cerebral arteries. Intracranial aneurysms are smaller than other types of aneurysm and mostly saccular. Though most patients do not experience rupture, it can lead to a stroke, brain damage and potential death. The mortality rate after rupture is considerably high: the incidence of sudden death was estimated to be 12.4% and death rate ranged from 32% to 67% after the hemorrhage [16]. Each year, over 12,000 people die in the United States due to rupture of intracranial aneurysms [17].

In order to prevent the rupture, or rerupture, of an aneurysm, several treatments have proved successful: neurosurgical clipping, endovascular coiling and stenting. The aneurysm can be permanently sealed from the normal blood circulation by placing a tiny metal clip across the aneurysm neck. This open surgery requires to perform a craniotomy, which is invasive and associated with risks of complications during or shortly after surgery. In recent years, the development of interventional radiology techniques made it possible for a growing number of patients to be treated with minimally invasive strategies, essentially endovascular coiling. The procedure of coil embolization starts with the insertion of a catheter into the femoral artery, which is then advanced through the arterial system all the way to the location of the intracranial aneurysm. Then the radiologist delivers the filling material (the coils) through a micro-catheter into the aneurysm sac. The presence of coils in the aneurysm reduces blood velocity, and decreases the pressure against the aneurysmal wall, progressively creating a favorable hemodynamic environment for thrombus embolization. Finally, the formation of a blood clot blocks off the aneurysm, thus considerably reducing the risk of rupture. In the case of irregularly-shaped or fusiform aneurysms, or aneurysms with wide necks, stenting of the parent artery can be used in combination with coils. Although endovascular techniques are less invasive than open surgery, they remain complex and risky to perform, requiring an important expertise and careful planning.

1.2. Computer-based medical simulation

Medical simulation provides a solution to the current need for residency training and procedure planning, by allowing trainees to experience realistic scenarios, and by repeatedly practicing without putting patients at risk. With the ongoing advances in biomechanics, algorithmics, computer graphics, software design and parallelism, computer-based medical simulation is playing an increasingly important role in this area, particularly by providing access to a wide variety of clinical scenarios, patient-specific data, and reduced training cost. Even for experienced physicians, medical simulation has the potential to provide planning and preoperative rehearsal for patient-specific cases. In some cases it can also offer some insight into the procedure outcome. Nevertheless, several fundamental problems remain to be solved for a wide and reliable use of computer-based planning systems in a clinical setup, and in particular for coil embolization. Such a planning system is expected to have a high level of realism and good predictive abilities. In particular we are interested in a prediction of the hemodynamics before and after the procedure, an evaluation of the number of coils required to achieve embolization, and an interactive simulation of coil deployment for rehearsal. This involves the following challenges:

- **Geometry modeling**: although 3D imaging of the patient's vasculature is now widely available under various modalities, extracting the actual geometry of the blood vessels is still an issue due to the limitations in spatial resolution and the presence of noises and artifacts. Particularly, accurate and exact geometry extraction of blood vessel is a challenge in the vicinity of intracranial aneurysms due to the small size and complex shape of the surrounding vascular network.
- ***In vivo* data**: for the purpose of realism, patient-specific *in vivo* data is necessary for biomechanical modeling and hemodynamic simulation, such as mechanical parameters of vessel wall, blood flow rate. Acquisition of *in vivo* data is quite challenging, because imaging techniques are not currently capable to provide images with a high resolution either in space or in time.
- **Fast computation**: the planning system targets at assistance for rapid decision making or rehearsal in a virtual environment. As such it requires fast or even real-time computation of blood flow and blood-structure interaction, which cannot always be guaranteed by modern computers with certain limitations in memory and frequency. Therefore, the need still remains to increase computing speed by optimizing algorithms or proposing alternative numerical methods.
- **Coil modeling**: modeling intracranial coils, which are thin platinum wires, remains challenging, because mechanical parameters are not provided by device manufacturers. As coils are designed to conform to the aneurysm wall, it is also important to compute the multiple contacts (or self-contacts) between the coils and the aneurysm.

1.3. Previous work

Generally speaking, there are three main approaches to obtain hemodynamic data. Experimental techniques have been widely used in clinical analysis, but restricted to idealized geometries or surgically created structures in animals. However, a better method is *in vivo* analysis, which can be provided through medical imaging. For example, angiography can provide *in vivo* flow data, but only in 1D; Magnetic Resonance Imaging (MRI) data is 3D, but quite noisy. Finally, the computational approach, which can provide a 3D representation of detailed flow patterns in patient-specific geometry, becomes more and more attractive in this area.

To obtain patient-specific geometry, excellent review papers [21] reported on the vast literature that addressed blood vessel segmentation. The diversity in the methods reflected the variety of contexts in which the question of blood vessel segmentation araised, requiring us to be more specific about our expectancies. First, the vessel surface model should be smooth enough for its use in the simulation. Implicit surface representations, where the surface was defined as the zero-level set of a known function f, were arguably well suited [5]. C1-continuous models (with C0-continuous normal) allowed for much smoother sliding contacts. Unwanted friction might occur with polyhedral surfaces [26] or level-sets such as vesselness criteria [11, 34] defined on a discrete grid. Implicit surfaces also offered an improved collision management over parametric surfaces [10]. Indeed, the implicit function value at a point telled whether this point was inside or outside the surface, detecting a collision in the latter case. Furthermore, the implicit function gradient gave a natural direction for the contact force used to handle this collision. In many cases, segmentation or vessel enhancement aimed at improving vessel visibility. When quantitative assessment was required, most previous works grounded on the same seminal idea as Masutani [22], which tracked the vessel centerline by fitting local vessel models: graphics primitives [43], convolution kernel [33], or cylinder templates [12]. Both the centerline location and radius estimation might be correct, but such models were unable to accurately cope with irregularities on the vessel surface, especially when the vessel section was not circular (or elliptic). Also, they did not correctly handle pathologies such as aneurysms. Various methods were proposed to improve the vessel delineation in cross-sections. Ray-casting methods were of particular interest, as they were able to extract candidate points at the vessel surface. Indeed, they opened the path to using a wealth of techniques developed by the graphics community to fit an implicit surface to a set of scattered surface points. Radial Basis Functions (RBF) had a promising potential, especially in their variational formulation [37] with the capacity to produce compact models. Closer to our work, Schumann [35] used Multi-level Partition of Unity (MPU) implicits to get a locally defined model. However, RBF or MPU implicit gradients gave appropriate contact directions close to the surface but could mislead contact forces elsewhere. We propose in Section 2 a new and efficient algorithm to model local blood vessels with blobby models [28].

Most computational methods for blood flow simulation relied on the science of Computational Fluid Dynamcis (CFD), and approximated blood flow as a continuous incompressible Newtonian fluid, described by the unsteady incompressible Navier-Stokes equations [23]. For instance, Groden et al. constructed a simple geometrical model by only straight cylinders and spheres to approximate an actual aneurysm, and simulated the flow by solving the Navier-Stokes equations [14]. The geometry model they used could not accurately describe the real patient's case, therefore, had little use in surgery planning for a specific patient. In the last ten years, the successful effort in the research of combining image processing and CFD made it possible to compute patient-specific hemodynamic information in this community. Kakalis et al. employed patient-specific data to get more realistic flow patterns [19]. However, both of their methods, as well as most similar studies, relied on the CFD commercial software to simulate the flow, and the computational times (dozens of hours in general) were incompatible with interactive simulation or even clinical practice. In order to reach fast computation, several template-based methods were designed [24] [25]. These methods pre-computed hemodynamics on a set of similar template geometries, and then interpolated on a patient-specific geometry instead of fluid simulation. However, they required to set up a pre-computed database, and were only tested on simple artery structures. But for the brain vessels around intracranial aneurysm, the network and shape are much more complicated, so the high accuracy cannot be expected.

More methods for fast computation were proposed in the field of computer graphics, essentially required the results to be visually convincing, but not physically accurate. The stable fluids approach [39] was a significant milestone, as it brought in fluid advection and the Helmholtz-Hodge decomposition to ensure the mass conservation law. However, this approach relied on discretization of Eulerian space using a regular grid, thus making it inappropriate for complex geometry with irregular boundaries, as it is usually the case in anatomical structures. Recently, the Discrete Exterior Calculus (DEC) method, based on unstructured mesh for incompressible fluid simulation, was proposed in [9]. It presented several benefits in terms of stability and computational efficiency. However, the context, in which this method was applied, did not aimed at the practical use in medical simulation. We further assess the stability, accuracy and computational time of this method, more importantly, improve the method for medical applications in (near) real-time.

Previous work in the area of real-time or near real-time simulation for interventional radiology mainly focused on training, for instance, [29], [15], [1], [7] and [5], which proposed approaches for modeling either catheter deformation or more general catheter navigation in vascular networks. Real-time simulation of coil embolization was investigated more recently. However, additional difficulties need to be faced: the deformation of the coil is more complex, and the coil is self-colliding during embolization while it also has frictional contact with the vessel wall. A FEM model, based on beam element allowed to adequately capture the deformation of the coil [6]. This model was validated, and an inverse problem was solved to capture the correct rest-shape configuration. Moreover, a solution to contact and self-collision was proposed, which was based on the resolution of Signorini's law and Coulomb friction [4]. A Gaussian deformation, close to the Boussinesq approximation model, allowed to take into account the very small deformation of the aneurysm wall. This approach is developed in more details in Section 3. Recently, a deformation model for the coil, based on inextensible elastic rods was proposed [38], in combination with a geometric approach for coil embolization, based on path-planning [27].

1.4. Our contributions

In our work, we aim at real-time simulations of the blood flow and blood-structure interaction during aneurysm coil embolization in the patient-specific geometry. While the existing studies of aneurysm embolization only concerned the impact of the deployed coil(s) on the blood flow, we also present an effective way to compute the reverse effect of the blood flow on the coil during the medical procedure, and provide higher reality for the simulation of placing coils into the aneurysm compared to the case without considering the interactive force from blood flow.

First of all, a smooth and accurate model of the vessel wall around aneurysm is required. We propose to use a blobby model whose parameterization is constrained so that the implicit function varies with the distance to the vessel surface. Thereafter, a stable blob selection and subdivision process are designed. Also, an original energy formulation is given under closed-form, allowing for an efficient minimization.

Secondly, we present a coil model based on the serially-linked beams that can handle large geometric deformations. Our model can also handle various shape memories in order to simulate different types of coils (like helical, bird-cage or 3D coils). This model is computed efficiently by a backward Euler scheme combined with a linear solver that takes into account the particularities of our model.

Thirdly, in order to achieve accurate and near real-time blood flow simulation, we introduce the DEC method into hemodynamic simulation for the first time. Compared to the DEC method initially applied in the field of computer graphics, we improve the numerical stability by using more advanced backtracking schemes, and more importantly by optimizing quality of the mesh used in the computation. Moreover, a detailed analysis of the results and comparison with a reference software are performed to understand the stability and accuracy of the method, as well as the factors affecting these two aspects.

Finally, based on the DEC method, we propose a framework for real-time simulation of the interventional radiology procedure (Figure 1). We reconstruct 3D models of vascular structures, and propose a real-time finite element approach for computing the behavior of flexible medical devices, such as coils, catheters and guide wires. Then we present the methods for computing contacts between virtual medical devices and virtual blood vessels. Furthermore, we model bilateral interactions between blood flow and deformable medical devices for real-time simulation of coil embolization. Our simulated results of blood-coil interaction show that our approach permits to describe the influence between coils and blood flow during coil embolization, and that an optimal trade-off between accuracy and computation time can be obtained.

2. Geometry modeling

In this section, we present our work on vascular modeling using implicit representations. We show how such models can be obtained from actual patient data (3D rotational angiography, 3DRA).

2.1. Local implicit modeling

2.1.1. Implicit formulation as a blobby model

An implicit isosurface generated by a point-set skeleton is expressed as the zero-level set of a function f, a sum of implicit spheres:

$$f(X;p) = T - \sum_{j=1}^{N_b} \alpha_j \phi\left(\frac{|X - C_j|}{\rho_j}\right),$$

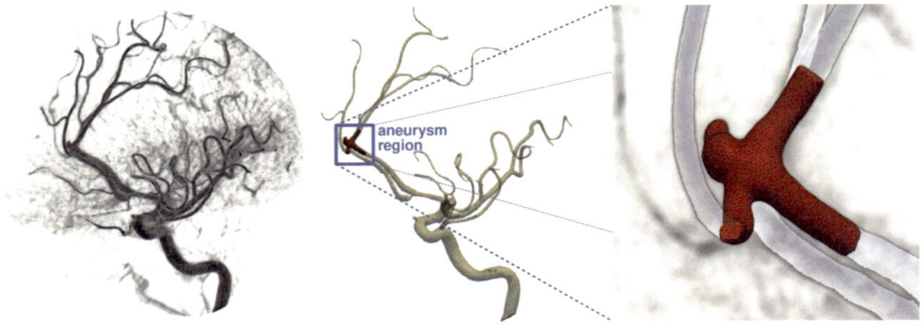

(a) From patient-specific data (left), we reconstruct vessel surface model (middle), and then generate tetrahedral mesh in the region of aneurysm (right).

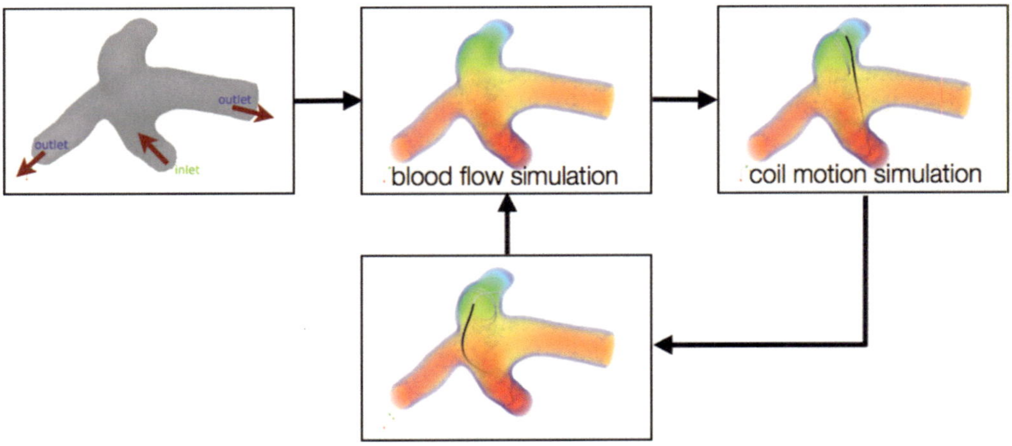

(b) Given the boundary conditions, we simulate the blood flow velocity, from which we compute the interactive force applied on the coil. Until there is a significant increase of coil density, we update the velocity field.

Figure 1. The framework of real-time simulation of coil embolization: (a) mesh generation; (b) simulation of bilateral interaction of blood and medical devices.

where T is the isosurface threshold, $\{\alpha_j\}$ are positive weights, and $\{C_j\}$ is the point set skeleton. Each implicit sphere #j is defined by a symmetric spherical function, centered on C_j, of width ρ_j. The local field function, or kernel, is a function $\phi : \mathbb{R} \rightarrow \mathbb{R}^+$, rapidly decreasing to 0 at infinity. Thus, model locality is ensured: an implicit sub-model can be extracted by merely selecting neighboring blobs. For example, all results presented below are produced using the 'Cauchy' kernel [36]:

$$\phi(x) = (1 + x^2/5)^{-2},$$

where the dividing factor 5 normalizes the kernel such that $\phi''(1) = 0$.

Such objets are called differently depending on the kernel used [36]. Our method is not kernel-dependent, and was successfully used with the computationally less efficient Gaussian kernel. Muraki [28] was the first to use this type of model in the context of object reconstruction. Following this seminal work, we will use the terms *blob* for an implicit sphere, and *blobby models* as a generic name for implicit models.

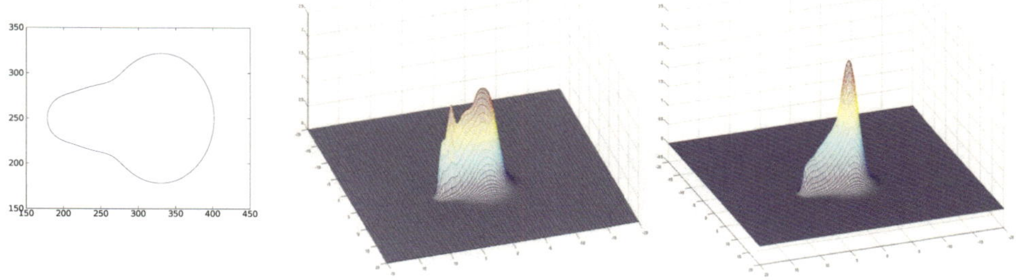

Figure 2. Redundancy in implicit function parameterization: (left): 2D shape to model; middle: implicit modeling using a uniform weight of 1 ($\alpha_j = 1$); right: implicit modeling using weights equal to radii ($\alpha_j = \rho_j$). The implicit function looks more like a distance function in the latter case.

2.1.2. Setting the weights

In the above formulation, there is a redundancy between the weight $\{\alpha_j\}$ and the radii $\{\rho_j\}$. Figure 2 gives an example of a 2D shape (left image) with two different implicit representations ($z = f(x, y)$) only parameterized by the center locations and the radii: for the image in the center, all the weights $\{\alpha_j\}$ were set to 1 ; while on the right we had $\alpha_j = \rho_j, \forall j$. This latter case is particularly interesting when we consider circles of different radii: there is a monotonously increasing relation between the distance function and the implicit function f.

In our particular simulation context, in order to help predict collisions, and have the function give a valid contact force direction, the algebraic value $f(X; p)$ at point X should relate monotonously to the geometric distance of X to the surface.

As a consequence, we set $\alpha_j = \rho_j$. Thereby, as demonstrated in Figure 2, the function gradient gives a valid contact direction anywhere in space (consider the crease in the middle of the shape in the middle image). Meanwhile, redundancy in the parameters of f is also dismissed. This choice for parameterization will also prove useful later to efficiently select the blob to be subdivided.

2.1.3. Energy formulation

Fitting a surface to N points $\{P_i\}_{1 \le i \le N_p}$ can be written as an energy minimization problem [28, 42]. We propose to combine three energy terms:

$$\mathcal{E} = \mathcal{E}_d + \alpha \mathcal{E}_c + \beta \mathcal{E}_a$$

, where $(\alpha, \beta) \in \mathbb{R}^{+2}$, and:

1.
$$\mathcal{E}_d = \frac{1}{N_p} \sum_i f(P_i; p)^2$$

   , which translates the algebraic relation between data points and the zero-level set. It gives a raw expression of the approximation problem.

2.
$$\mathcal{E}_c = \frac{1}{(N_b(N_b - 1))} \sum_{j \neq k} \left(\frac{s\sqrt{\rho_j \rho_k}}{|C_k - C_j|} \right)^{12} - 2 \left(\frac{s\sqrt{\rho_j \rho_k}}{|C_k - C_j|} \right)^{6}$$

, which is Lennard-Jones energy. Each term is minimal (with value -1) for $|C_j - C_k| = s\sqrt{\rho_j \rho_k}$, being repulsive for blobs closer than this distance, and attractive for blobs further away. It imposes some cohesion between neighboring blobs to avoid leakage where data points are missing, while preventing blobs from accumulating within the model.

3.
$$\mathcal{E}_a = \frac{1}{N_p} \sum_i \kappa(P_i)^2$$

$\kappa(P)$ is the mean curvature. It can be computed in a closed form at any point in space from the implicit formulation [13]

$$\kappa(P) = \frac{\nabla f^t H_f \nabla f - |\nabla f|^2 trace(H_f)}{2|\nabla f|^3}$$

, where ∇f is the implicit function gradient and H_f its Hessian matrix, both computed at point P. This energy smoothes the surface according to the minimal area criterion. In particular, the wavy effect that could stem from modeling a tubular shape with implicit spheres, is reduced.

Behind the rather classical form given above for the energy terms, it is important to notice that the whole energy is known under a closed-form expression. As a consequence, closed-form expressions were derived for its gradients with respect to the blobby model parameters $\{\rho_j\}$ and $\{C_j\}$.

2.1.4. Selection-subdivision

The blob subdivision procedure proposed in the seminal work [28] was exhaustive and time consuming. A blob selection mechanism was added in [42], measuring the contribution of each blob to $\mathcal{E}_d$ within a user-defined window, and choosing the main contributor. We experimentally noted that this technique was prone to favor small blobs, thus focusing on details, before dealing with areas roughly approximated by one large blob. This behavior is caused by this selection mechanism using the algebraic distance to the implicit surface. Our criterion relies upon the geometric distance approximation proposed by Taubin [40]:

$$d_T(P, f_0) = \frac{|f(P;p)|}{|\nabla f(P;p)|},$$

where P is a point and f_0 is the 0-level set of implicit function f, parameterized by p. As a consequence, the point P_{i^*} farthest to the surface is such that:

$$i^* = \arg \max_{1 \leq i \leq N_p} d_T(P_i, f_0).$$

The blob $\#j^*$ whose isosurface is the closest to P_{i^*} is selected (according to Taubin's distance d_T). Note that this criterion is valid in large area because we set $\alpha_j = \rho_j$ in the definition of f. The subdivision step then replaces this blob with two new ones. Their width ρ'_{j^*} is chosen such that two blobs, centered on C_{j^*}, of width ρ'_{j^*} would have the same isosurface as one blob centered on C_{j^*}, with width ρ_{j^*} (the formula depends on the kernel). The first new blob is centered on C_{j^*}, while the second is translated by $\rho_{j^*}/10$ towards P_{i^*}.

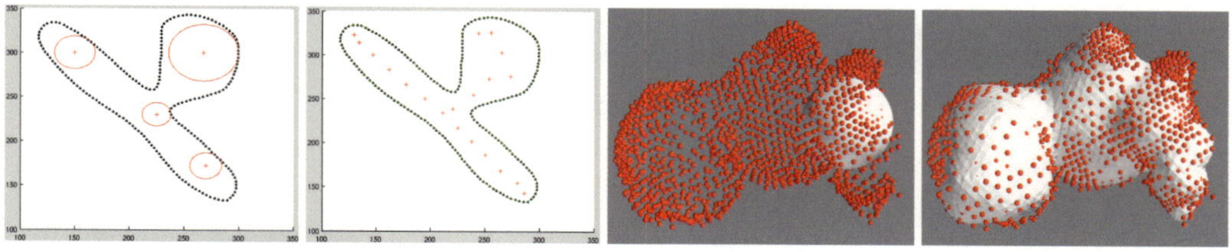

(a) 2D case: initialization with 4 blobs (b) 2D case: final result (c) 3D case: initialization with one blob (d) 3D case: final result

Figure 3. Examples of implicit modeling. In the 2D case (two leftmost images), data points are in black, blob centers are red crosses, and the final implicit curve is in green. In the 3D case (two rightmost images), data points are in red and the implicit surface is in white.

2.1.5. Optimization

Such a gradual subdivision procedure may lead to a dramatic increase in the number of blobs, and hence the size of the optimization problem. The locality of the kernel ϕ allows us to focus the optimization onto the newly created pair of blobs. More exactly, only the new blob that is slightly misplaced is optimized, the other blobs remaining constant. The energy is minimized using Polak-Ribiere conjugate gradient (PR) algorithm, taking advantage of the closed-form expressions of both the energy and its gradients. A single minimization loop consists in one PR minimization over the center (3 variables), followed by one on the width (1 variable). In practice, a maximum of 5 loops proved sufficient.

2.2. Overall modeling algorithm

This fitting procedure proved to be very robust to initialization. Figure 3 gives two examples, one in 2D and the other in 3D, of typical initializations and results obtained.

The 2D case (Figure 3(a) and 3(b)) mimics the neighborhood of an aneurysm. Starting from 4 blobs dispatched on the aneurysm and parent vessel (Figure 3(a)), the final result on Figure 3(b) shows 20 blobs whose centers naturally span the skeletal line of the shape while providing a close fit (green line). The 3D case (Figure 3(c) and 3(d)) is an actual bilobated aneurysm. Starting from one blob located at the entrance of the aneurysm (Figure 3(c)), the procedure ends up on Figure 3(d) with 100 blobs closely fitting all bumps and other details in the shape.

Previous works [44] demonstrated that good candidate points at the vessel surface could be obtained by casting rays from center points inside the vessel, and keeping only the locations of minimal directional gradient (blood vessels are bright onto a darker background in angiographic images). The same strategy was followed, except that rays were thrown in directions regularly spaced on the unit 3D sphere. A user-defined threshold was applied to the gradient amplitude to remove extraneous points detected on small intensity variations that could be captured in large areas, such as the aneurysm sac or when rays were cast along the vessel direction.

As a consequence, modeling the vicinity of an aneurysm takes three steps:

1. Manually place initial blobs inside the aneurysm and related blood vessel. Only an approximate radius is needed for these blobs.
2. Extract data points by casting rays from the blob centers
3. Run the above implicit modeling algorithm

Once we get a smooth surface model, meshing the domain is done using the interleaved optimization algorithm based on Delaunay refinement and Lloyd optimization [41], and implemented using the CGAL library [1]. Each refinement step acts on the size of elements, while each optimization step acts on the shape of elements. Using this method, we can also define a size field to obtain anisotropic and non-uniform mesh. We control the fidelity of the generated mesh to the previously obtained surface model, by specifying the distance tolerance between the two surfaces.

3. Modeling of coil deformations during embolization

In this section, we describe the deformation model that is used to capture the mechanical properties of the coil. Moreover, as the behavior of the coil during embolization strongly depends on the contacts with the vessel wall, we presents a constraint-based collision response.

3.1. Coil model

There are different types of detachable coils but most of them have a core made of platinum, and some are coated with another material or a biologically active agent. All types are made of a soft platinum wire of less than a millimeter diameter and therefore are very soft. The softness of the platinum allows the coil to conform to the arbitrary shape of an aneurysm.

The deformation model of the coil is based on the recent work of Dequidt et. al. [6]. Coil dynamics is modeled using serially linked beam elements:

$$\mathbf{M}\dot{\mathbf{v}} = \mathbf{p} - \mathbb{F}\left(\mathbf{q}, \mathbf{v}, \mathbf{q}_0\right) + \mathbf{Hf}, \tag{1}$$

where $\mathbf{M} \in \mathbb{R}^{(n \times n)}$ gathers the mass and inertia matrices of beams. $\mathbf{q} \in \mathbb{R}^n$ is the vector of generalized coordinates (each node at the extremity of a beam has six degrees of freedom: three of which correspond to the spatial position, and three to the angular position in a global reference frame). The rest position $\mathbf{q}_0$ represents the reference position. Tuning the rest position allows to simulate different families of coil: for instance, helical shape or more complex 3D shape (see Figure 4). $\mathbf{v} \in \mathbb{R}^n$ is the vector of velocity. $\mathbb{F}$ represents internal visco-elastic forces of the beams, and $\mathbf{p}$ gathers external forces. $\mathbf{f}$ is the vector of the contact forces with the aneurysm wall, and $\mathbf{H}$ gathers the contact directions. To integrate this model we use backward Euler scheme with a unique linearization of $\mathbb{F}$ per time step. Moreover the linear solver takes advantage of the nature of our model. All beam elements being serially connected, $\mathbf{F}$ is a tridiagonal matrix with a band size of 12. nd we solve the linear system using the algorithm proposed by Kumar *et al.* [20]. The solution can thus be obtained in $O(n)$ operations instead of $O(n^3)$.

[1] http://www.cgal.org/

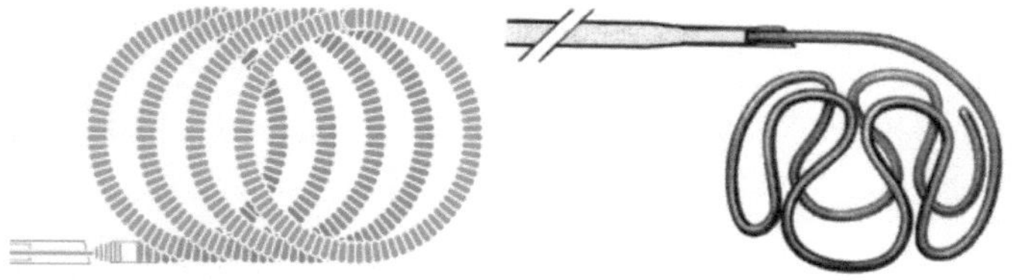

Figure 4. Example of coils used in our simulations: (left) Boston Scientific helical coil GDC 10; (right) 3D GDC built with omega loops [2].

3.2. Simulation of coil deployment

3.2.1. Modeling contacts with aneurysm walls

Simulating coil embolization requires to accurately model contacts that occur between the coil and the aneurysm wall. The contact model must provide the following features: first, account for the stick and slip transitions that take place during the coil deployment, second include a compliant behavior of vessel wall (we choose the one that is close to Boussinesq model [30]) and finally the friction motion of the coil along the aneurysm wall. For modeling contacts with friction, we use two different laws, based on the contact force and on the relative motion between the coil and the aneurysm walls. The contact law is defined along the normal $\mathbf{n}$ and the friction law, along the tangential $(\mathbf{t}, \mathbf{s})$ space of the contact.

The contact model, based on Signorini's law, indicates that there is complementarity between the gaps δ^n and the contact forces f^n along the normal direction, that is,

$$0 \leq \delta^n \perp \mathrm{f}^n \geq 0.$$

With the Coulomb's friction law, the contact force lies within a spacial conical region whose height and direction are given by the normal force, giving two complementarity conditions for stick and slip motion:

$$\begin{array}{ll} [\delta^t \ \ \delta^s] = \mathbf{0} \Rightarrow \|[\mathrm{f}^t \ \ \mathrm{f}^s]\| < \mu \, \|\mathrm{f}^n\| & \text{(stick condition)} \\ [\delta^t \ \ \delta^s] \neq \mathbf{0} \Rightarrow [\mathrm{f}^t \ \ \mathrm{f}^s] = -\mu \, \|\mathrm{f}^n\| \frac{[\delta^t \ \ \delta^s]}{\| [\delta^t \ \ \delta^s] \|} & \text{(slip condition)} \end{array}$$

Where the vector $[\delta^t \ \ \delta^s]$ provides the relative motion in the tangential space and μ represents the friction coefficient.

The obtained complementarity relations could create *singular* events when it changes from one state to another: For instance, when a collision occurs at instant $t^\star$, the velocity $\mathbf{v}(t^\star)$ of the coil, at that point, changes instantaneously. The acceleration could then be ill-defined and we can observe some quick changes in the dynamics. Each friction contact creates three non-holonomic constraints along the normal and tangential directions. Our approach allows for processing simultaneously multiple friction contacts, including self-contacts on the coil.

3.2.2. Simulation steps

The processing of one simulation step begins with solving Equation 1 for all forces except contact forces ($\mathbf{f} = 0$). This *free motion* corresponds essentially to the deformation of the beam elements under gravity and user force input. Once the *free motion* has been computed, collision detection computes the contact points between the coil model and the aneurysm

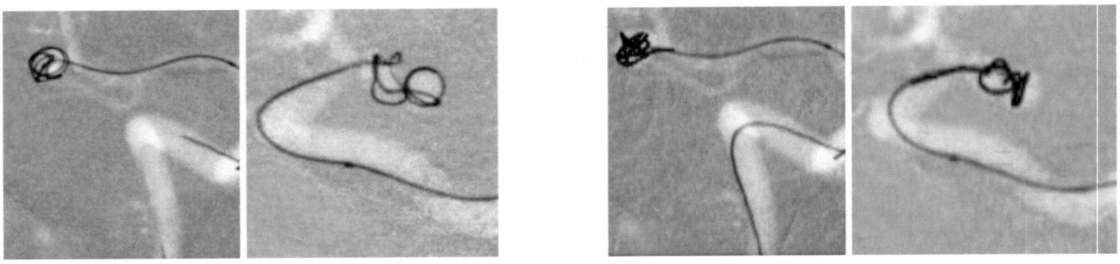

Figure 5. Examples of our simulation results: (left) real coil embolization; (right) our simulated coil embolization with 3D coils.

surface and the points of self-collision. When collisions are detected, the *contact response* is computed. This is a complex aspect that influences greatly the overall behavior of the coil model. To describe the mechanical behavior during contact, the mechanical coupling between the different contact points is modeled. This information is provided by evaluating the compliance matrix in the contact space, called **W**, for both the coil and the aneurysm. Let's consider a contact α on the node i of the coil (with one constraint along the contact normal $\mathbf{n}$ and two along the tangential friction directions $\mathbf{t}, \mathbf{s}$). $\mathbf{H}_\alpha$ is the matrix of the frame $[\mathbf{n}\ \mathbf{t}\ \mathbf{s}]$. The mechanical coupling of this contact with a contact β (with frame $\mathbf{H}_\beta$) on node j can be evaluated with the following 3×3 matrix:

$$\mathbf{W}_{(\alpha,\beta)} = \mathbf{H}_\alpha^T \left(\frac{\mathbf{M}}{h^2} + \frac{d\mathbb{F}}{hd\mathbf{v}} + \frac{d\mathbb{F}}{d\mathbf{q}} \right)^{-1}_{(i,j)} \mathbf{H}_\beta = \mathbf{H}_\alpha^T \mathbf{C}_{(i,j)} \mathbf{H}_\beta,$$

where $\mathbf{C}_{(i,j)}$ is the 3×3 sub-matrix of global compliance matrix **C** (inverse of tangent matrix) at the rows of node i and the columns of node j. For the aneurysm wall, the formulation of the coupling is simpler:

$$\mathbf{W}_{(\alpha,\beta)} = \frac{g(d_{ij})}{e} \mathbf{H}_\alpha^T \mathbf{H}_\beta,$$

where e is an elasticity parameter that is homogeneous to young modulus and $g(d_{ij})$ is a Gaussian function of the distance, defined on the surface, between contact point i and j. The Gaussian function allows a fall-off of the coupling with increasing distance between the contact points. This model is close to the Boussinesq approximation which provides a distribution of the normal contact stress from the elasticity of the surface, around a point of contact [30].

The result of the *contact response* involves finding the friction contact forces that respect Signorini and Coulomb laws. Several works ([18] and [8]) present Gauss-Seidel iterative approaches that solve this problem. The solver needs an evaluation of a global compliance matrix **W**, which is the sum of the compliances of the coil and the aneurysm wall. It also needs the value of the relative displacement of the contacting points during the free motion $\boldsymbol{\delta}^{\text{free}}$. When the contact forces are found, during the last step, called *contact correction* we compute the motion associated to the contact forces.

In this section, we presented an efficient dynamic coil model, *i.e.*, FEM beams based model for the intrinsic mechanical behavior of the coil, combined with a process for computing collision response (with the aneurysm wall) and auto-collision response. However, even if the results are quite encouraging, as illustrated in Figure 5, the mechanical modeling is not fully complete. Indeed, the behavior of the coil is also greatly influenced by the blood flow.

Moreover, we also aim at predicting the influence of the coils on the hemodynamic status near the aneurysm. As a result, it is important to simulate the flow within the aneurysm, and to propose a method for blood-coil coupling.

4. Modeling of blood flow around intracranial aneurysm

The blood is modeled as an incompressible Newtonian fluid of constant density, $\rho = 1.069 \times 10^3 kg/m^3$, and constant viscosity, $\mu = 3.5 \times 10^{-3} kg/(m \cdot s)$. In this work, we only consider the blood flow near intracranial aneurysms with relatively small Reynolds number ranging from 100 to 1,000 [31], which satisfies the laminar assumption. Thus, it is reasonable to describe the behavior of blood flow using the incompressible Navier-Stokes equations. Additionally, the influence of pulsating vessel on the fluid is ignored; hence vessel walls are assumed to be rigid.

We rely on the Discrete Exterior Calculus (DEC) method for numerically solving the equations, as it offers several benefits for our application. First of all, it is based on unstructured tetrahedral mesh, which is more suitable to describe irregular boundary of anatomical geometries than regular grids. From the tetrahedral mesh, referred as primal mesh, the dual mesh is constructed as follows: dual vertices correspond to the circumcenters of primal tetrahedra, dual edges link dual vertices located on neighbor tetrahedra, and dual faces are surfaces of Voronoi cells of primal vertices, which are dual cells as well. More generally, a dual $(n-p)$-cell is associated to a corresponding p-simplex ($p = 0, 1, 2, 3, n = 3$) as depicted in Figure 7.

Secondly, the orthogonality between primal and circumcentric dual is useful to define the physical variables in fluid (Figure 6), such as flux, which is the face integral of velocity orthogonal to the face, and the vorticity (the circulation per unit area at a point), whose direction is orthogonal to the plane of circulation (the line integral of velocity around a closed curve). The discrete version of these physical quantities is not only defined on points, but represented as scalars attached to the primitives of any dimension on primal or dual mesh, *i.e.*, vertex, edge, face or volume. The scalars are integral values of physical quantity over the primitives (except point-wise variable), and the orientation of each primitive represents the local direction of vector variable. For example, velocity is described as flux on each triangle face (2D primal primitive), so it is primal 2-form, and the orientation of the face indicates whether the fluid flows outward or inward. Vorticity is defined as the integral value over the dual face (2D dual primitive), thus it is dual 2-form. According to the Stoke's theorem, this value equals to the circulation along the boundary of dual face. The orientation of the primal edge gives the direction of vorticity.

Thirdly, based on the discretization of space and variables, discrete vector calculus operators, such as curl, divergence, Laplace operators, can be easily expressed by two basic operators, the discrete differentials d and the Hodge stars $\star$. The former, d_p, maps p-forms to $(p+1)$-forms on the primal mesh, represented by signed incidence matrix. The transpose of this matrix operates similarly on the dual mesh. The latter, $\star_p$, maps from primal p-forms to dual $(n-p)$-forms, represented by a diagonal matrix whose element equals to the volume ratio between the corresponding dual and primal elements. And the inverse matrix maps in the opposite (Figure 7).

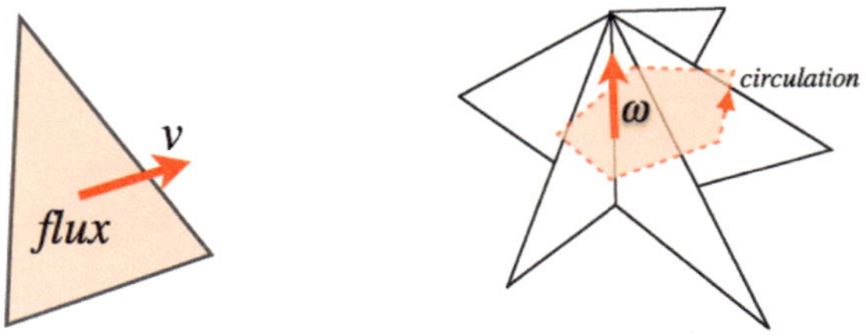

(a) Velocity v and flux $\mathbf{U}$ (b) Vorticity ω and circulation $\mathbf{\Omega}$

Figure 6. Discretization of physical variables in fluid: (a) velocity; (b) vorticity.

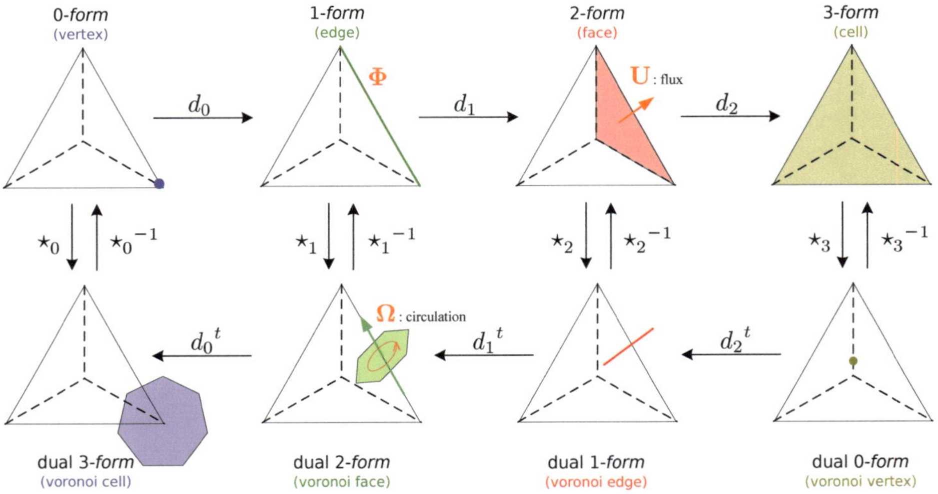

Figure 7. The duality of primal and dual mesh: the first line shows the primal simplex, whose dual elements are below. Physical variables $\mathbf{U}$ and $\mathbf{\Omega}$, defined as discrete forms, can be transferred by two fundamental operators d and $\star$.

Finally, it applies the same idea of Stable Fluids [39], a semi-Lagrangian method, which is much more stable than traditional Eulerian methods, and allows larger time steps and improves the computational efficiency. But instead of dealing with velocity field, the DEC method uses vorticity-based formulations (Equation 2), and preserves the circulation at a discrete level. As a result, to some degree, it overcomes the issue of numerical diffusion, and results in higher accuracy.

$$\begin{aligned} \frac{\partial \boldsymbol{\omega}}{\partial t} &= -\mathscr{L}_{\boldsymbol{v}}\boldsymbol{\omega} + \frac{\mu}{\rho}\Delta\boldsymbol{\omega} \\ \nabla \boldsymbol{v} = 0 \quad & \boldsymbol{\omega} = \nabla \times \boldsymbol{v}, \end{aligned} \tag{2}$$

where $\boldsymbol{\omega}$ is the vorticity, Lie derivative $\mathscr{L}_{\boldsymbol{v}}\boldsymbol{\omega}$ (in this case equal to $\boldsymbol{v} \cdot \nabla\boldsymbol{\omega} - \boldsymbol{\omega} \cdot \nabla\boldsymbol{v}$), is the advection term, and $\frac{\mu}{\rho}\Delta\boldsymbol{\omega}$ is the diffusion term.

Simply speaking, the advection term describes the idea that the local spin is pushed forward along the direction of the velocity, which is consistent with Kelvin's circulation theorem: the circulation around a closed curve moving with the fluid remains constant with time. In this

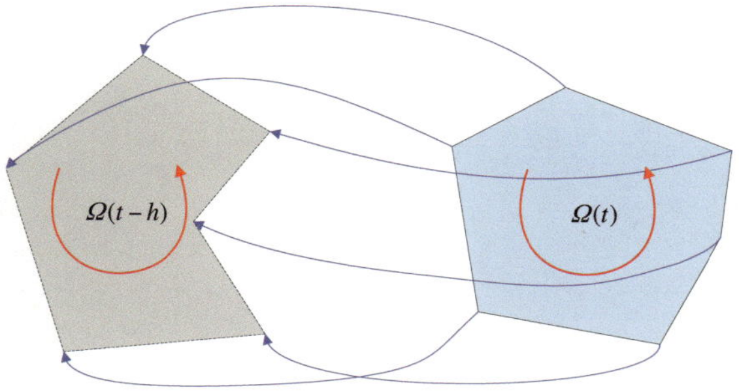

Figure 8. Backtracking. At the current time step $t_n = t$, given the velocity field, each dual vertex (on the right) is backtracked to its position at the previous time step $t_{n-1} = t - h$ (on the left). The circulation around the loop of dual face boundary at time t_n is forced to be equal to the circulation of the backtracked loop at time t_{n-1}, *i.e.*, $\Omega(t) = \Omega(t-h)$.

approach, the discrete vorticity is conserved by extending Kelvin's theorem to the discrete level: the circulation around the loop of each dual face's boundary keeps constant as the loop is advected by fluid flow. So we run a backtracking step (Figure 8) to find out where the current dual face comes from, and accumulate the circulation around the backtracked dual face, and then assign this value to the current one. This step makes the computation circulation-preserving at a discrete level, as well as stable, because the maximum of the new field is never larger than that of the previous field. For the diffusion term, linear solver is used, and an implicit scheme is chosen for the purpose of stability (Equation 3).

$$\omega_{n+1} - \omega_n = \frac{\mu h}{\rho} L \omega_{n+1}, \tag{3}$$

where h is the span of time step, and L is the Laplace operator.

5. Blood-coil interaction

In this section, we illustrate how we simulate the bilateral interaction between coils and blood flow. First, we describe how we compute the impact of the coil onto the blood flow by adding extra terms to the Navier-Stokes equation. Second, we explain how the drag force applied by blood flow onto the coil is computed. Finally, we combine the fluid and structure systems by a loosely-coupled strategy for real-time simulation of coil embolization.

5.1. Porous media model

The typical diameter of coils chosen for intracranial aneurysms ranges from $0.2mm$ to $0.4mm$, which is quite small compared to the aneurysm size (0.02 to 0.11 times of the intracranial aneurysm in diameter). And after inserted into aneurysm, they are randomly distributed, forming the shape of a twisted nest (Figure 9). Considering the relatively small dimension of coils and their random distribution in aneurysm, coils are modeled, from a statistical point of view, as porous media in aneurysm.

We divide the fluid domain $\mathscr{D}$ into 3 sub-domains, a coil-free and a coil-filled sub-domain, as well as a transitory sub-domain between them, which allows the porous parameters to vary

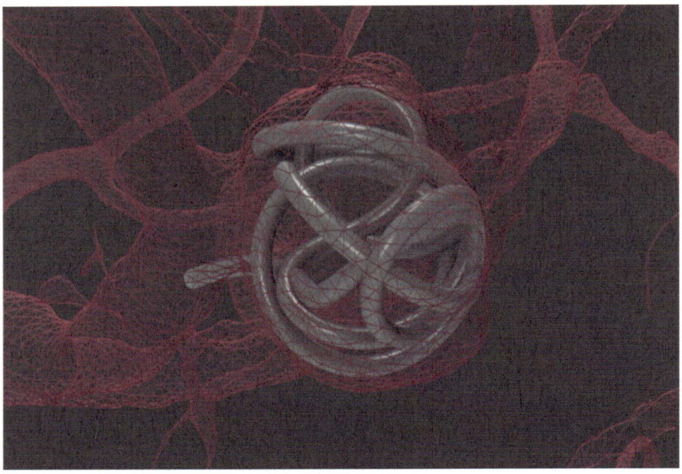

Figure 9. The shape of detachable coils after deployment.

smoothly between the first two sub-domains. However, blood motion in all sub-domains is described uniformly by the Navier-Stokes equations (vorticity-based) of Brinkmann type:

$$\begin{gathered}\frac{\partial \boldsymbol{\omega}}{\partial t} + \mathscr{L}_{\boldsymbol{v}}\boldsymbol{\omega} = \frac{\mu}{\rho}\Delta\boldsymbol{\omega} - \frac{\mu\varphi}{\rho k}\boldsymbol{\omega} - \frac{\varphi^2 C_D}{\sqrt{k}}\nabla \times \boldsymbol{b}, \\ \nabla(\varphi \boldsymbol{v}) = 0 \quad \boldsymbol{\omega} = \nabla \times \boldsymbol{v} \quad \boldsymbol{b} = \boldsymbol{v}\,|\boldsymbol{v}|\,,\end{gathered} \tag{4}$$

where three more parameters are used to describe the properties of porous media: porosity φ, permeability k and drag factor C_D. Porosity φ describes the volume ratio of pores to the total coil-filled sub-domain, $\varphi = 1 - V_{coil}/V_{sac}$, where V_{coil} is the accumulated volume of all coils, and V_{sac} is the volume of the aneurysm sac. The permeability k measures the fluid conductivity through porous media, $k = \varphi^3 / cS^2$, where c is the Kozeny coefficient related to the micro-shape of the porous media (for coils, the value of cylinders is chosen, $c = 2$), and S is the ratio of the surface area of all coils to the volume of porous region V_{sac}. The drag factor C_D can be derived from the local Reynolds number. Note that when $\varphi \to 1$ and $k \to \infty$, these porous terms disappear, therefore, Equation 4 is identical to Equation 2, within the coil-free region. The computation of the extended porous terms takes little extra computational time (less than 1% of computing the other terms) when using the DEC method.

5.2. Drag force

In the existing simulations of aneurysm embolization, the interactive force between blood and coil was only studied for the blood from a global view, while the local reacting force on coils during the deployment process was ignored. In fact, the last term of Equation 4 is a description of the interactive force, but treated as an averaged quantity. When computing the reaction on the coil, we apply its local version, which is the drag force of flow over cylinder, since the coil is considered to consist of serially linked cylinder segments:

$$\boldsymbol{F_D} = \frac{1}{2} C_D \rho \boldsymbol{v}_\perp \,|\boldsymbol{v}_\perp|\, A|l,$$

where $\boldsymbol{v}_\perp$ is the velocity orthogonal to the coil, A is the cross-sectional area of the coil, l is the length of one short cylinder segment, and $\boldsymbol{F_D}$ is the drag force applied on this segment. The velocity parallel to the coil is neglected, since it only produces shear force on the coil, which is insignificant compared to the drag force, and has little impact on the movement of the coil in the blood. Hence, the reacting force on the coil only depends on local fluid velocity.

5.3. Fluid-structure coupling

For integrating the two models (coil and blood flow) in one single frame, we design a loosely-coupled strategy with the assumption that the simulation is performed over a series of identical cardiac cycles. Given the periodically time-varying boundary conditions at the inlet and outlet vessels around aneurysm, we solve the Navier-Stokes equations of Brinkmann type with a constant coil packing density by the DEC approach, and obtain the velocity at each tetrahedron center of the mesh at each time step. Then these velocity values are used to interpolate the velocity at the positions of coil segments and apply appropriate drag forces on the coil. The coil can provide real-time feedback inside the aneurysm at any time step during embolization. In this stage, we assume that a small segment of inserted coil does not change the blood flow. Until there is a significant increase of the coil density, the velocity of blood flow is recomputed at the new level of coil packing density. In this stage, we only care about the coil density, but not the coil shape. So the blood velocity field can be pre-computed and stored for real-time simulation of coil deployment. Although we use pre-computation of blood velocity, this process can be done in several minutes to simulate one cardiac cycle at five levels of coil density in our simulation. This is still essential for interactive planning.

The main benefit of the loosely-coupled approach is the relatively independency between the two systems, which allows different time resolution in two systems, independent real-time strategies, as well as pre-computation of the blood flow over one cardiac cycle. For the purpose of real-time refresh rate, we consider using relatively coarse mesh to reduce the size of the linear systems to be solved, and using large time steps to lessen the iterations necessary to simulate one second. As in other applications where real-time computation is sought, the objective is then to reach the best trade-off between accuracy and computational time.

6. Simulations and results

6.1. Blood flow simulation

We have performed comparative tests against FLUENT software [2] both in 2D and 3D space. In this case, we mostly aim at validating numerical accuracy of the DEC method rather than the ability to precisely describe the actual blood flow features near aneurysm, due to the present difficulties in *in vivo* analysis of velocity, particularly in the small cerebral vessels. Each group of the comparison between DEC and FLUENT consists of blood flow simulation on several identical meshes with the same geometry but different resolution.

The first group of simulations using a 2D aneurysm model (generated from the profile of a patient-specific geometry) is performed on three meshes composed of 210177, 19753 and 2160 triangles respectively. The contours of velocity magnitude and streamlines computed by DEC and FLUENT are shown in Figure 10. The unit of velocity displayed in all the figures is mm/s

[2] FLUENT is a commercial product of ANSYS (http://ansys.com), widely used in industries.

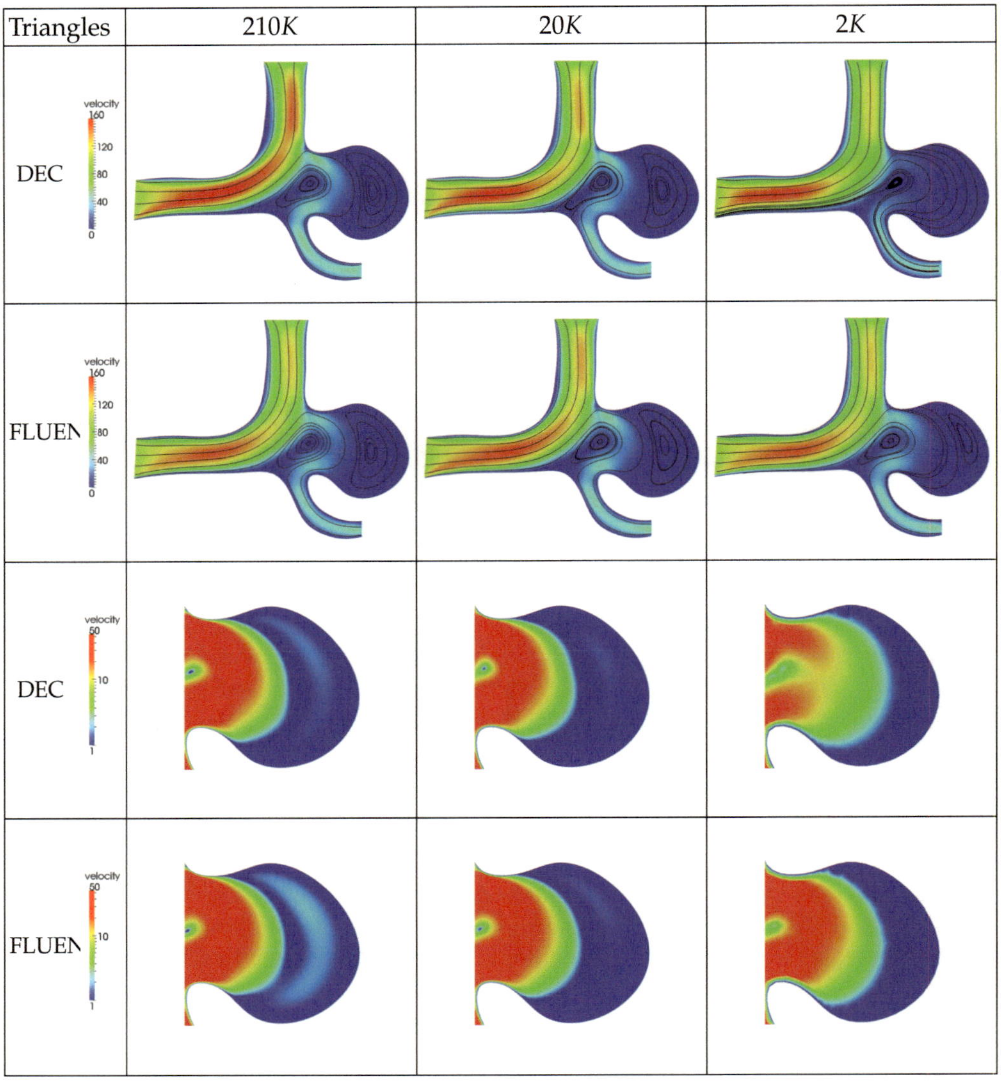

Figure 10. Comparison of velocity field on 2D aneurysm model. The contours of velocity magnitude and streamlines in the whole region (the first two rows) and in the sac (the last two rows) are computed by DEC and FLUENT on the identical meshes of three different resolution.

by default. Besides, we plot the profiles of the velocity magnitude over two lines across the inlet and the aneurysm respectively in Figure 11. When the mesh resolution decreases by 10 times, the contours and profiles are almost the same, and show the similarity between the two methods. In addition, the streamlines show a strong agreement for flow patterns and vortex structures in terms of the positions of the vortex centers. Only when we reduce the mesh resolution by 100 times, the result computed by DEC loses some detail information inside the sac; less fluid flows into the sac, and the vortex inside the sac is missing. But the main features of the velocity field still remain the same, such as the flow pattern (characterized by the streamlines) and the variation of the velocity field in space (characterized by the profiles).

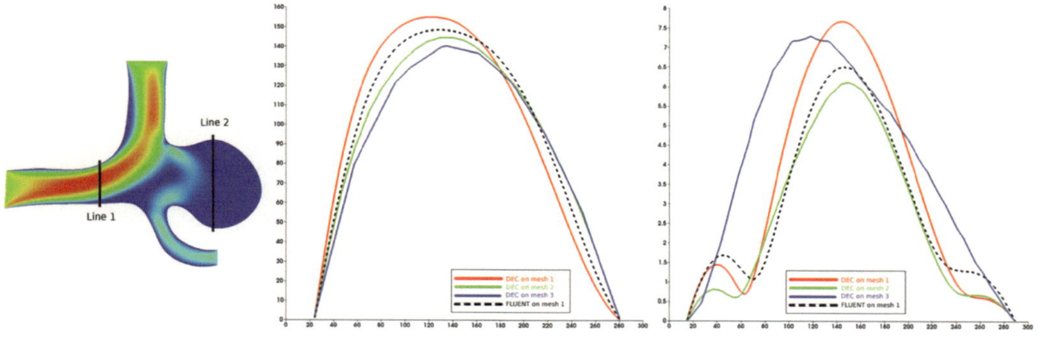

(a) Two lines (b) Profile over line 1 (c) Profile over line 2

Figure 11. Comparison of velocity profiles over two lines across the inlet and aneurysm

The second group of simulations is performed similarly on two meshes of a 3D patient-specific aneurysm with a wide neck. In Figure 12, the streamlines show the similar movement of blood. In both cases there is a low-speed region surrounded by high-speed flows observed on slice 1, which represents a local vortex in this region. There are two obvious vortices in the FLUENT result, reflected both by the low-speed regions observed on slice 2 and the swirls of streamlines, but in the DEC result on the coarser mesh, the smaller vortex is not that obvious. These results show that the DEC method can capture large-scale flow structures, while small-scale differences exist between the two approaches. Considering both accuracy and computational efficiency, we choose the lower-resolution mesh of 34029 tetrahedra for the simulation of coil embolization, and the computational time of simulating $1s$ real time is $44s$ on an Intel i7 $3.33GHz$ processor.

6.2. Real-time simulation of coil embolization

We predict the embolization outcome for an intracranial aneurysm with a small sac of volume $132.1mm^3$ (usually the sac volume of an intracranial aneurysm varies from 100 to $1000mm^3$) and a wide neck of dimension $7.0mm$. From the clinical experience, the final coil packing density is around 25%, *i.e.*, the porosity φ is around 75%. In Figure 13, we show the blood flow without coils, with 10% and 25% volume filled with coils. The velocity magnitude contours are compared on two sections, crossing the neck and the sac respectively. From the comparison on the neck section, we can see that every incremental increase in coil packing density is accompanied by a decrease in cross-neck flow rate. Additionally on the sac section, after inserting the first coil, the velocity magnitude over the whole sac region has been reduced, which creates a favorable hemodynamic environment for the deployment of the following coils.

Then we show the inverse influence of the blood flow on the coil deployment. Figure 14 displays the simulated process of placing the first coil into the small aneurysm. After the catheter is advanced in the vascular network to reach the position of the aneurysm, the coil is delivered through the catheter and inserted into the aneurysm. The contact among the catheter, the coil and the vessel wall, as well as the interaction of the blood flow are all included in this simulation. The pre-computation of blood velocity covering one cardiac cycle at 5 levels of coil density is accomplished in less than 5 minutes, and then using the pre-computed velocity field, the simulation of coil deployment is performed in real time.

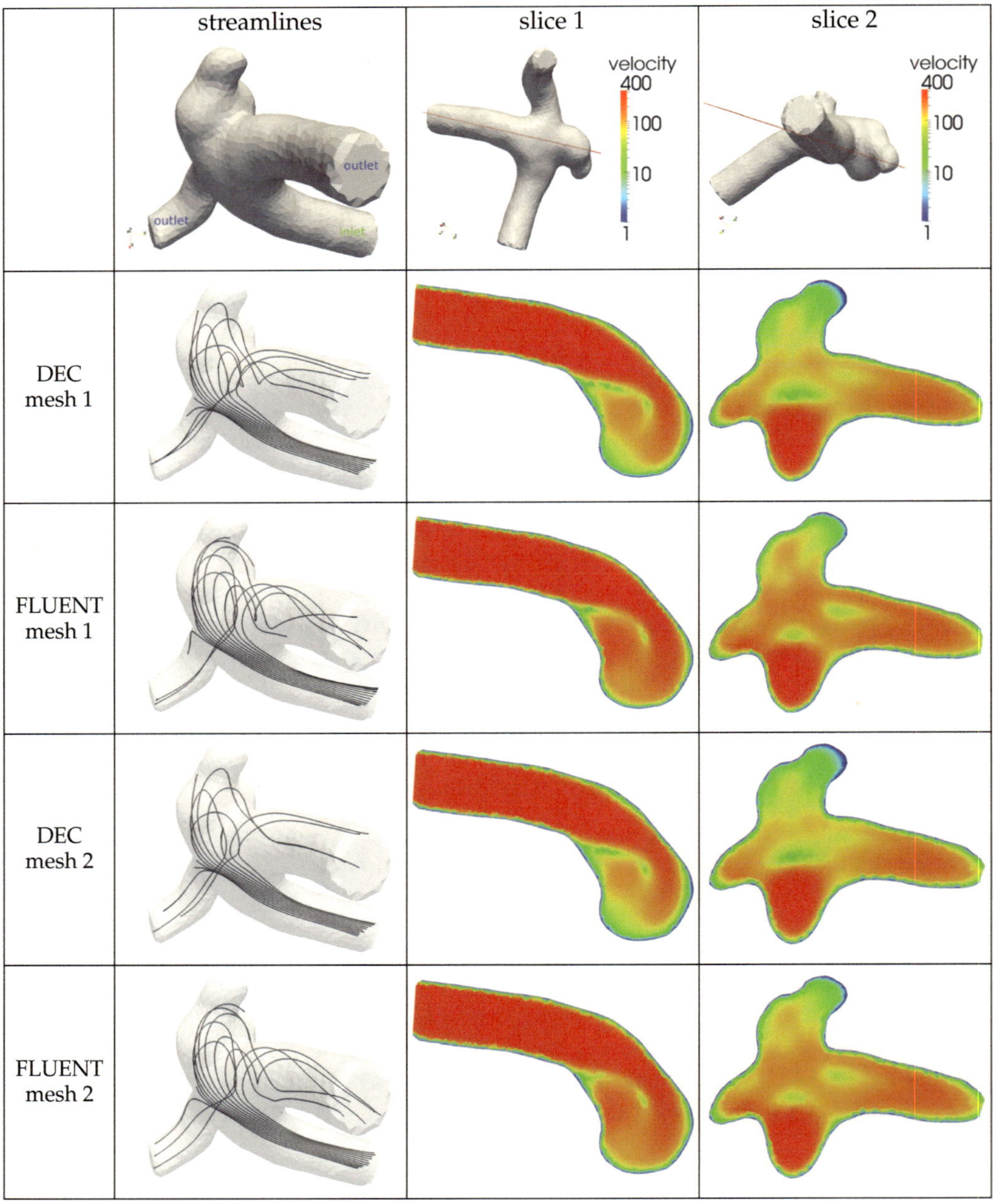

Figure 12. Comparison of velocity field on the 3D patient-specific aneurysm model. The first row displays the geometry of the model and the position of two slices chosen for comparing velocity magnitude contours. In the following rows, streamlines and contours of velocity magnitude are computed by DEC and FLUENT on the identical meshes, which are mesh 1 of 55711 tetrahedra and mesh 2 of 34029 tetrahedra.

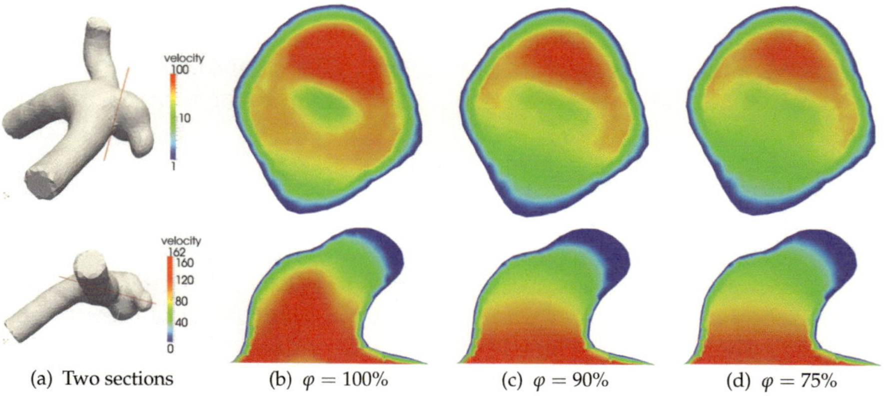

Figure 13. Coil embolization of a small aneurysm. The velocity magnitude on two sections (a) before the embolization (b), after the first coil deployed (c), and after the final coil deployed (d).

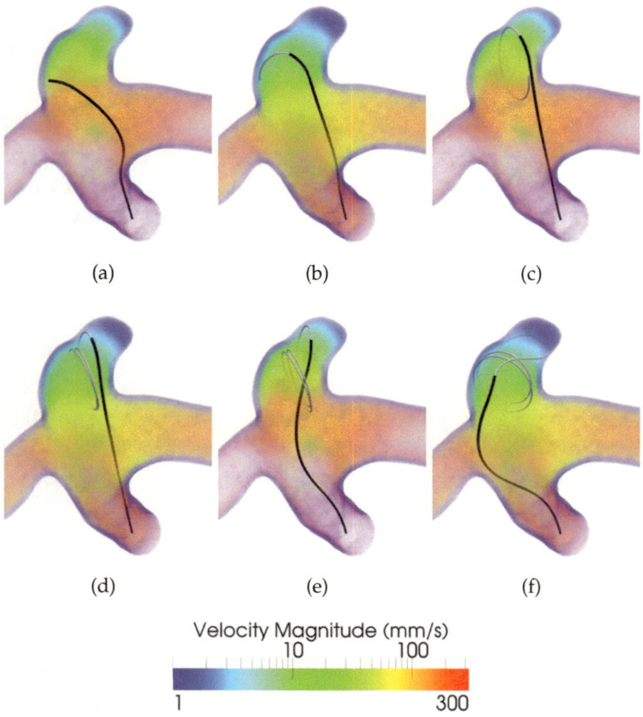

Figure 14. Simulation of coil embolization: (a) The catheter (black) reaches at the aneurysm neck through vessels. (b)-(f) The first coil (silver) is delivered by the catheter and inserted into the aneurysm. The colorful volume displays the periodically varying velocity field.

7. Conclusion and perspectives

7.1. Conclusion

We proposed an approach to accurate and real-time simulation of coil deployment, as well as prediction of coil embolization outcome in a patient-specific environment for clinical planning and rehearsal.

- The geometry of the aneurysm and its parent vessel has been reconstructed as an implicit surface. The proposed blobby model is particularly adapted to simulation; it enables to model complex shapes, as smooth surfaces, with a relatively small number of primitives. Our model improves upon previous works in two ways. First the constrained parameterization closely relates the implicit function to the distance field to the surface, and stabilizes the blob selection and subdivision process. Second, reconstruction is expressed as an energy minimization problem. The closed-form expression given for the energy enables to leverage efficient minimization algorithms with derivatives for faster and more accurate results.
- We have achieved real-time simulation of flexible medical devices, such as the catheter or coil by using a model based on beams that can handle various rest shapes and large geometric deformations. Special care is taken to make this model computationally robust and efficient by using dedicated linear solver and time-integration scheme. Our contributions also include an accurate contact model to handle the collisions between the coil and the vascular surface. This allows computation times of about 2 ms for a coil composed of 100 beam elements.
- While most previous work on hemodynamic simulation aimed at accurate results and required dozens of hours computational time, we have achieved fast simulation of blood flow using the DEC method, which is initially developed in the field of computer graphics. However, a much deeper analysis and improvement has been made for medical application.
- Bilateral interaction between coil and blood flow has been first studied in our work for planning two key steps of the procedure. Firstly, prediction of hemodynamic status after deployment is performed by modeling the inserted coils as porous media. Secondly, the reciprocal force, *i.e.*, the impact of the flow onto the coil, is modeled as drag force and applied on the coil during deployment for interactive choice and placement of the first coil. The results show that our approach permit real-time simulation of the interaction between coils and blood flow during coil embolization.

7.2. Perspectives

Regarding future work, first of all, we are further improving the computational efficiency, since real-time simulation has not been achieved when performed on a mesh consisting of over 8,000 elements. We still want to more deeply investigate various computational strategies to obtain real-time computation by using more advanced numerical schemes, such as parallel implementation on GPU of the backtracking step, optimization of linear solvers by the preconditioning technique coupled with a GPU-based conjugate gradient implementation [3]. Additionally, more advanced techniques to generate a multi-resolution mesh, such as adaptive refinement [32], could also be a solution, as it maximizes the result accuracy while minimizing the computational effort.

Of course, we acknowledge that further validation is required, both on the DEC method and on other elements of the simulation. However, comparison between simulated results and *in vivo* data remains difficult due to the limitations of current medical imaging techniques. We are starting to investigate the use of fluoroscopic imaging to assess the simulation of medical devices used in interventional radiology procedures. Regarding the specific validation of the flow computation, a possible direction is MR imaging which, under some modalities, can measure flow patterns. Although quite noisy, such data could provide interesting insights and help validate our results.

Before put to wide clinical utilization, our method should be further improved. The boundary conditions obtained from patient-specific real data will improve the realism of the simulated results. To obtain such real data, we can benefit from the imaging techniques or the state-of-the-art medical instruments, such as the ultra-miniature pressure catheter, which is a so small sensor on the catheter that it does not significantly change the blood flow. Furthermore, standards of assessment and metrics of evaluation should be set up to offer doctor the information on the minimal number of coils required to achieve embolization in long term, and to evaluate the doctor's performance on the procedure.

Finally, when using stent-assisted coiling, the stent acts as scaffolding, and prevents the coils from falling out. Our work could be easily extended to simulate the outcome by taking the collision contact between coils and the stent into account.

Acknowledgments

The authors are grateful to Prof. Anxionnat who provided them with the 2D and 3D angiographic patient data used in this paper. Prof. Anxionnat is with the therapeutic and interventional neuroradiology department of the University Hospital of Nancy, France.

Author details

Yiyi Wei, Stéphane Cotin, Jérémie Dequidt, Christian Duriez, Jérémie Allard
Shacra Team, INRIA, France

Erwan Kerrien
Magrit Team, INRIA, France

8. References

[1] Alderliesten, T. [2004]. *Simulation of Minimally-Invasive Vascular Interventions for Training Purposes*, PhD dissertation, Utrecht University.

[2] Cloft, H. J., Joseph, G. J., Tong, F. C., Goldstein, J. H. & Dion, J. E. [1999]. Use of three-dimensional guglielmi detachable coils in the treatment of wide-necked cerebral aneurysms, *American Journal of Neuroradiology* .

[3] Courtecuisse, H., Allard, J., Duriez, C. & Cotin, S. [2011]. Preconditioner-based contact response and application to cataract surgery, *Medical Image Computing and Computer-Assisted Intervention–MICCAI 2011* pp. 315–322.

[4] Dequidt, J., Duriez, C., Cotin, S. & Kerrien, E. [2009]. Towards interactive planning of coil embolization in brain aneurysms, *Proceedings of the 12th International Conference on Medical Image Computing and Computer-Assisted Intervention: Part I*, MICCAI '09, Springer-Verlag, Berlin, Heidelberg, pp. 377–385.

[5] Dequidt, J., Lenoir, J. & Cotin, S. [2007]. Interactive contacts resolution using smooth surface representation, *Proc. Medical Image Computing and Computer-Assisted Interventions (MICCAI)*, pp. 850–857.

[6] Dequidt, J., Marchal, M., Duriez, C., Kerien, E. & Cotin, S. [2008]. Interactive simulation of embolization coils: Modeling and experimental validation, *Medical Image Computing and Computer-Assisted Intervention–MICCAI 2008* pp. 695–702.

[7] Duriez, C., Cotin, S., Lenoir, J. & Neumann, P. F. [2006]. New approaches to catheter navigation for interventional radiology simulation, *Computer Aided Surgery* 11: 300–308.

[8] Duriez, C., Dubois, F., Kheddar, A. & Andriot, C. [2006]. Realistic haptic rendering of interacting deformable objects in virtual environments, *IEEE Transactions on Visualization and Computer Graphics* 12(1): 36–47.

[9] Elcott, S., Tong, Y., Kanso, E., Schröder, P. & Desbrun, M. [2007]. Stable, circulation-preserving, simplicial fluids, *ACM Transactions on Graphics (TOG)* 26(1): 4.

[10] Frangi, A., Niessen, W., Hoogeveen, R., van Walsum, T. & Viergever, M. [1999]. Model-based quantitation of 3-D magnetic resonance angiographic images, *IEEE Trans. Med. Imaging* 18(10): 946–956.

[11] Frangi, A., Niessen, W., Vincken, K. & Viergever, M. [1998]. Multiscale vessel enhancement filtering, *Medical Image Computing and Computer-Assisted Intervention – MICCAI 1998*, number 1496 in *LNCS*, pp. 130–137.

[12] Friman, O., Hindennach, M., Kühnel, C. & Peitgen, H.-O. [2010]. Multiple hypothesis template tracking of small 3D vessel structures, *Medical Image Analysis* 14(2): 160 – 171.

[13] Goldman, R. [2005]. Curvature formulas for implicit curves and surfaces, *Computer Aided Geometric Design* 22: 632–658.

[14] Groden, C., Laudan, J., Gatchell, S. & Zeumer, H. [2001]. Three-dimensional pulsatile flow simulation before and after endovascular coil embolization of a terminal cerebral aneurysm, *Journal of Cerebral Blood Flow & Metabolism* 21(12): 1464–1471.

[15] Hoefer, U., Langen, T., Nziki, J., Zeitler, F., Hesser, J., Mueller, U., Voelker, W. & Maenner, R. [2002]. Cathi - catheter instruction system, *Computer Assisted Radiology and Surgery (CARS)*, Paris, France, pp. 101 – 06.

[16] Hop, J., Rinkel, G., Algra, A. & van Gijn, J. [1997]. Case-fatality rates and functional outcome after subarachnoid hemorrhage: a systematic review, *Stroke* 28(3): 660–664.

[17] Huang, J. & van Gelder, J. [2002]. The probability of sudden death from rupture of intracranial aneurysms: a meta-analysis, *Neurosurgery* 51(5): 1101.

[18] Jourdan, F., Alart, P. & Jean, M. [1998]. A gauss-seidel like algorithm to solve frictional contact problems, *Comp. Meth. in Appl. Mech. and Engin.* pp. 33–47.

[19] Kakalis, N., Mitsos, A., Byrne, J. & Ventikos, Y. [2008]. The haemodynamics of endovascular aneurysm treatment: a computational modelling approach for estimating the influence of multiple coil deployment, *Medical Imaging, IEEE Transactions on* 27(6): 814–824.

[20] Kumar, S. & Petho, A. [1993]. An algorithm for the numerical inversion of a tridiagonal matrix, *Communications in Numerical Methods in Engineering* 9(4): 353–359.

[21] Lesage, D., Angelini, E., Bloch, I. & Funka-Lea, G. [2009]. A review of 3D vessel lumen segmentation techniques: Models, features and extraction schemes, *Medical Image Analysis* 13(6): 819–845.
[22] Masutani, Y., Masamune, K. & Dohi, T. [1996]. Region-growing based feature extraction algorithm for tree-like objects, *Visualization in Biomedical Computing*, Vol. 1131 of *LNCS*, Springer, pp. 159–171.
[23] Mazumdar, J. [1992]. *Biofluid mechanics*, World Scientific Pub Co Inc.
[24] McGregor, R., Szczerba, D., Muralidhar, K. & Székely, G. [2009]. A fast alternative to computational fluid dynamics for high quality imaging of blood flow, *Medical Image Computing and Computer-Assisted Intervention–MICCAI 2009* pp. 124–131.
[25] McLeod, K., Caiazzo, A., Fernández, M., Mansi, T., Vignon-Clementel, I., Sermesant, M., Pennec, X., Boudjemline, Y. & Gerbeau, J. [2010]. Atlas-based reduced models of blood flows for fast patient-specific simulations, *Statistical Atlases and Computational Models of the Heart* pp. 95–104.
[26] Montagnat, J. [1999]. *Deformable Modelling for 3D and 4D Medical Image Segmentation*, PhD thesis, Nice – Sophia Antipolis University, Nice, France.
[27] Morales, H., Larrabide, I., Kim, M., Villa-Uriol, M., Macho, J., Blasco, J., Roman, L. & Frangi, A. [2011]. Virtual coiling of intracranial aneurysms based on dynamic path planning, *Medical Image Computing and Computer-Assisted Intervention–MICCAI 2011* pp. 355–362.
[28] Muraki, S. [1991]. Volumetric shape description of range data using Blobby Model, *SIGGRAPH Comput. Graph.* 25: 227–235.
[29] Nowinski, W. & Chui, C. [2001]. Simulation of interventional neuroradiology procedures, *MIAR*, pp. 87 – 94.
[30] Pauly, M., Pai, D. & Leonidas, G. [2004]. Quasi-rigid objects in contact, *Proceedings of ACM SIGGRAPH Symposium on Computer Animation*, pp. 109–119.
[31] Penney, D. [2002]. Hemodynamics.
[32] Prakash, S. & Ethier, C. [2001]. Requirements for mesh resolution in 3d computational hemodynamics, *Journal of biomechanical engineering* 123: 134.
[33] Preim, B. & Oeltze, S. [2008]. 3d visualization of vasculature: An overview, *Visualization in Medicine and Life Sciences*, Mathematics and Visualization, Springer, pp. 39–59.
[34] Sato, Y., Nakajima, S., Atsumi, H., Koller, T., Gerig, G., Yoshida, S. & Kikinis, R. [1998]. 3D multi-scale line filter for segmentation and visualization of curvilinear structures in medical images, *Medical Image Analysis* 2: 143–168.
[35] Schumann, C., Neugebauer, M., Bade, R., Preim, B. & Peitgen, H.-O. [2008]. Implicit vessel surface reconstruction for visualization and CFD simulation, *Int. J. of Computer Assisted Radiology and Surgery* 2(5): 275–286.
[36] Sherstyuk, A. [1999]. Kernel functions in convolution surfaces: A comparative analysis, *The Visual Computer* 15(4): 171–182.
[37] Slabaugh, G., Dinh, Q. & G., U. [2007]. A variational approach to the evolution of radial basis functions for image segmentation, *Conference on Computer Vision and Pattern Recognition*, pp. 1–8.
[38] Spillmann, J. & Harders, M. [2009]. Inextensible elastic rods with torsional friction based on lagrange multipliers, *Computer Animation and Virtual Worlds* 21(6): 561–572.

[39] Stam, J. [1999]. Stable fluids, *Proceedings of the 26th annual conference on Computer graphics and interactive techniques*, ACM Press/Addison-Wesley Publishing Co., pp. 121–128.

[40] Taubin, G. [1991]. Estimation of planar curves, surfaces, and nonplanar space curves defined by implicit equations with applications to edge and range image segmentation, *IEEE Trans. on PAMI* 13: 1115–1138.

[41] Tournois, J., Wormser, C., Alliez, P. & Desbrun, M. [2009]. Interleaving delaunay refinement and optimization for practical isotropic tetrahedron mesh generation, *ACM Transactions on Graphics (TOG)* 28(3): 1–9.

[42] Tsingos, N., Bittar, E. & Cani, M.-P. [1995]. Implicit surfaces for semi-automatic medical organ reconstruction, *Computer Graphics Internat. (CGI'95)*, pp. 3–15.

[43] Tyrrell, J., di Tomaso, E., Fuja, D., Tong, R., Kozak, K., Jain, R. & Roysam, B. [2007]. Robust 3-D modeling of vasculature imagery using superellipsoids, *IEEE Trans. Med. Imag.* 26(2): 223–237.

[44] Wink, O., Niessen, W. & Viergever, M. [2000]. Fast delineation and visualization of vessels in 3-D angiographic images, *IEEE Trans. Med. Imag.* 19(4): 337–346.

Chapter 12

Endovascular Treatment of Internal Carotid and Vertebral Artery Aneurysms Using Covered Stents

Ivan Vulev and Andrej Klepanec

Additional information is available at the end of the chapter

http://dx.doi.org/10.5772/48733

1. Introduction

1.1. Epidemiology

Internal carotid artery (ICA) and vertebral artery (VA) aneurysms are most frequent aneurysmatic lesions. Especially intracranial aneurysms are pathologic focal dilatations of the cerebrovasculature that are prone to rupture. These vascular abnormalities are classified by presumed pathogenesis. Saccular, berry, or congenital aneurysms constitute 90% of all cerebral aneurysms and are located at the major branch points of large arteries. Dolichoectatic, fusiform, or arteriosclerotic aneurysms account for 7% of all cerebral aneurysms. Infectious or mycotic aneurysms are situated peripherally and comprise 0.5% of all cerebral aneurysms. Other peripheral lesions include neoplastic aneurysms, rare sequelae of embolized tumor fragments, and traumatic aneurysms. Saccular intracranial aneurysms are situated in the anterior circulation in 85-95% of cases, whereas dolichoectatic aneurysms predominantly the vertebrobasilar system. Multiple saccular aneurysms are noted in 20-30% of patients with cerebral aneurysms. Aneurysmal rupture can result most often in subarachnoid hemorrhage, but may also present as intraparenchymal, intraventricular, or subdural hemorrhage. Giant saccular aneurysms, defined as greater than 25 mm in diameter, may cause SAH, but these lesions more frequently produce mass effect and may result in distal thromboembolism.

On the other hand, extracranial internal carotid and vertebral artery aneurysms usually may present with cerebral embolism, transient ischemic attack, cerebrovascular insufficiency, continued enlargement with compression syndrome, vessel occlusion or hemorrhage. Aneurysms may be also often asymptomatic until the time of rupture. In the past, most of these aneurysms were treated surgically. Surgery, however, is often difficult because of the location and the damaged arterial wall and may result in sacrifice of the internal carotid or vertebral artery. Vertebral artery (VA) aneurysms constitute 0.5 to 3% of intracranial aneurysms and 20% of posterior circulation aneurysms [1]. The causes of aneurysms are multiple and may occur following trauma, mycotic infection, as a result of atherosclerosis, tumor invasion or radiation necrosis or iatrogenic. Among these, dysplastic lesions appeared to be the main cause of extracranial internal carotid artery aneurysms, associated or not with spontaneous dissection. VA aneurysms include VA-PICA (posterior inferior cerebellar artery) aneurysms, vertebro-basilar junction aneurysms, distal PICA aneurysms and those aneurysms located along the distal VA. Dissecting aneurysms of the intradural vertebral arteries often present with subarachnoid haemorrhage. A second episode of bleeding (rebleeding) is common and deadly. Rebleeding rates were estimated at 71% of cases with subsequent re-rupture of the aneurysms in 57% [2]. Ruptured posterior circulation aneurysms are technically difficult to expose and clip and their management and surgical outcomes are poorer as compared to anterior circulation aneurysms [3]. They often need expertise with various skull base approaches to improve the exposure, to minimize brain retraction and to achieve better outcome. Certain subset of posterior circulation aneurysms are considered at even higher risk for surgery due to their location and the size, prompting recourse to other modalities of therapy.

1.2. Diagnostic imaging

Early diagnosis and evaluation of anatomical characteristics of the internal carotid and vertebral artery aneurysms are essential in terms of surgical or endovascular treatment planning.

Ultrasound imaging is initially useful in the diagnostic process for cases with suspicion for extracranial internal carotid artery aneurysm palpable pulsatile mass at neck region. It serves for determination of the size and extension of the aneurysm. Although ultrasound is a valuable diagnostic tool for definition of anechoic structure and pulsation of the aneurysm, it may become insufficient in defining thrombosed aneurysm, relation of the aneurysm with its neighboring structures. Duplex ultrasound scanning is the most simple investigation in the detection of vertebral and extracranial internal carotid artery aneurysms, but this may fail if the lesion is located high, especially if the patient has a short neck or when the examination is focused on stenosis diagnostic and if the size of the aneurysm is small.

In diagnosing and characterizing the aneurysms, DSA is still the gold standard imaging method. But, since DSA is an invasive method, persistant neurological complications can develop and that´s why nowadays it is mostly used just for endovascular treatment. DSA most often provides the diagnosis of the lesion, specifies the localization, and detects any associated lesion, stenosis, or wall irregularities inducing a carotid dysplasia. The disadvantage of DSA is showing only the patent lumen and the risk of complications associated with invasive catheterization. Therefore, recently noninvasive or minimally invasive methods, such as CT angiography and MR angiography are more popular to detect and demonstrate the aneurysms.

Contrast enhanced CT scanning with three-dimensional reconstructions allows analysis of the aneurysm and assesses the possible existence of a false lumen channel, representing the existence of a previous dysplastic or traumatic dissection. Analysis of the slices at the osseous window allows the assessment of the distance between the upper limit of the aneurysm and the temporal bone. Currently, contrast enhanced CT scanning with reconstruction is the most sophisticated examination available and gives the most information. CT angiography (CTA) has advantages such as easy and rapid applicability, being a minimally invasive method, having no manifest complication besides contrast medium allergy, capability of rotating the images 360° [4]. The most important advantage of CT angiography is its capability of evaluating images on preferred planes and angles on the screen. Therefore, superimposed vessel images in DSA making it hard to evaluate are easily evaluated with CT angiography. Moreover, capability of rotating the CT angiographic images on preferred planes and angles helps the surgeon or interventional radiologist in orientation to approach the aneurysm and in the treatment planning (Figure 1). Contrary, CT angiography has some limitations. Differentiation of small aneurysms from neighboring bones is not possible each time and CT angiography is not capable of showing the collateral circulation as seen in DSA [5]. Both arteries and veins are visible in CT angiography and sometimes it is not easy to differentiate either of them. CT angiography has also limitations in the postoperative management of aneuryms, especially in patients receiving coil embolisation because of coil artefacts.

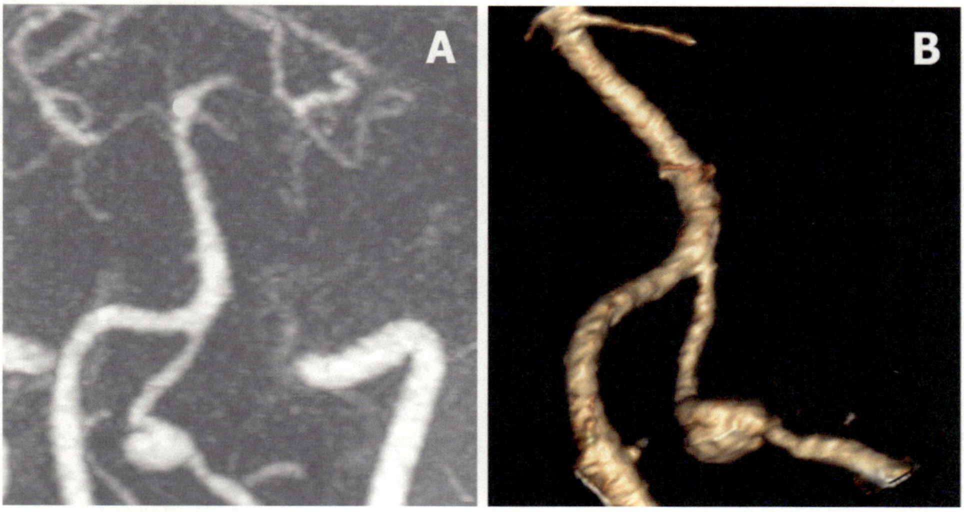

Figure 1. Maximum intensity projection (A) and virtual rendering technique (B) reconstructions of aneurysm of left intradural part of vertebral artery.

Magnetic resonance angiography (MRA) is a non-invasive method that can visualize vascular structures without a need for contrast medium injection or radiation. MRA can manifest the thrombosed portions of aneurysms, residual lumina and flow characteristics. MRA is particularly useful in suspicion of carotid artery dissection due to its characteristic of detecting the old blood in dissected area. MRA and CT angiography mainly replaced the conventional angiography. Promiment factors that emphasize superiority of MRA to arteriography are that it excludes the risk of stroke associated with angiography and also possible access site complications and it gives information about the surrounding tissues. MRA also provides reconstruction and rotation of images of intracranial circulation and evaluation of collateral circulation better than angiography.

1.3. Endovascular treatment

The current treatment options include surgical treatment and endovascular treatment, but these are not without significant problems [6]. For instance, a randomised, multicentre trial compared the safety and efficacy of endovascular coiling with standard neurosurgical clipping for intracranial aneurysms found that the outcome in terms of survival free of disability at 1 year is significantly better with endovascular coiling [7]. In addition, neurosurgery is associated with significantly longer length of stay and significantly higher total hospital charges [8]. Surgical treatment of extracranial internal carotid artery aneurysms located near skull base is technically challenging with high morbidity and mortality rates. In addition, surgical approach often requires an extended cervicotomy, mandibular subluxation, resection of the styloid process, and sometimes a transection of the external auditory canal with resection of the mastoid and vaginal process of the styloid bone to expose the first vertical intrapetrous segment of the ICA and risk of cranial nerve injury. Over the past decades, with advances in technologies, endovascular therapy is becoming the first-line treatment in the treatment of internal carotid and vertebral artery aneurysms and offers a minimally invasive alternative to open surgery.

Endovascular treatment options includes covered stent placement, flow diverting device (FDD) placement, parent vessel sacrifice with detachable balloons and coils, coil embolisation of the aneurysm with or without a stent placement. Endovascular techniques are usually performed via a femoral access route with placement of either covered stent, FDD or stent extending from the normal artery site to the distal vessel beyond the aneurysm. Despite the trend toward endovascular treatment the rate of recurrence and complications can be high.

This article describes current possibilities in endovascular treatment of vertebral and internal carotid artery aneurysms, with special focus on covered stents with our experience and description of used techniques in the treatment of internal carotid and vertebral artery aneurysms.

2. Body

2.1. CASE 1

A 52-year-old female with a pulsatile palpable mass in the left retromandibular space was referred to our hospital. Computed tomography angiography revealed a giant false aneurysm of the left cervical segment of the internal carotid artery (ICA) that was probably due to arterial injury caused by an elongated Styloid process. CTA revealed significant elongation and tortuosity of the left and right proximal ICA and a large supra-ophthalmic aneurysm of the right ICA (Figure 2).

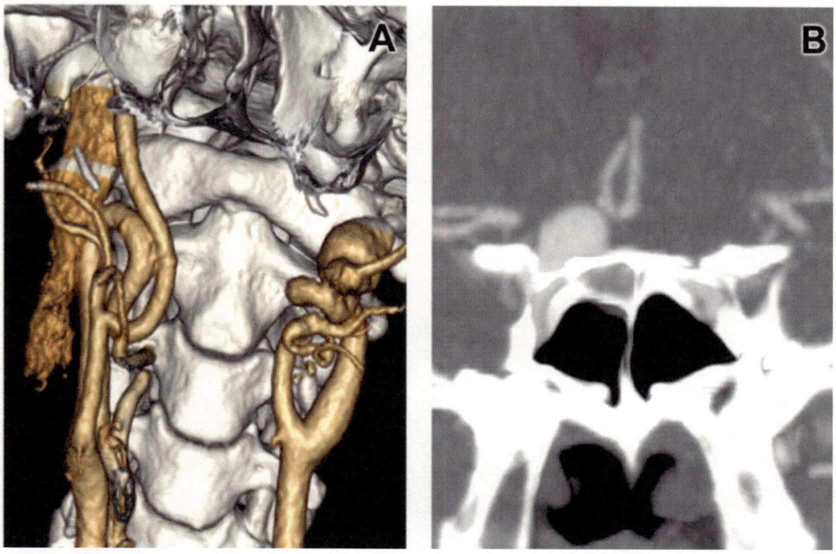

Figure 2. CTA finding of a styloid process causing a false aneurysm of the left ICA, elongation of both proximal parts of the ICA and a large aneurysm of the supra-ophthalmic part of the right ICA (A, B).

A four-step, multidisciplinary therapeutic plan combining surgical and endovascular modalities was selected: (i) resection and straightening of proximal tortuosity of the right ICA; (ii) endovascular coiling of intracranial aneurysms (Figure 3); (iii) resection and straightening of the proximal left ICA; and (iv) endovascular treatment of the false aneurysms in the left retromandibular space using covered stent.

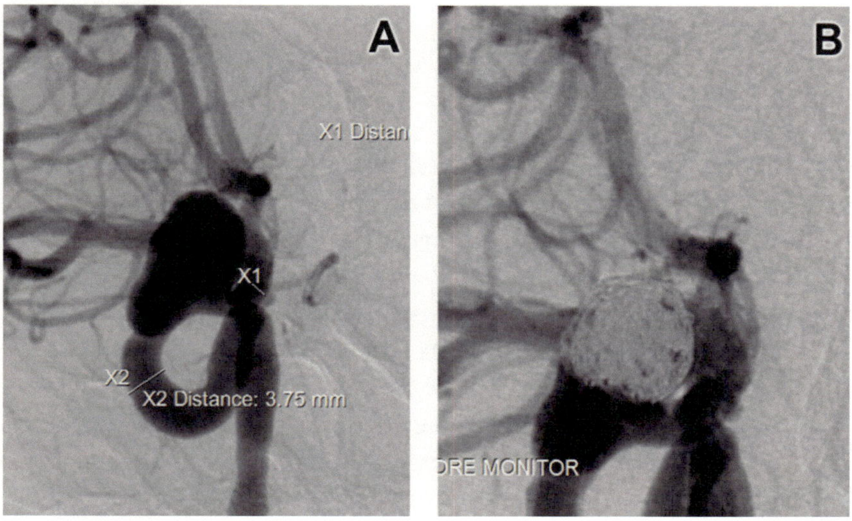

Figure 3. DSA before coiling of the aneurysm of the supra-ophthalmic part of the right ICA (A) and after endovascular treatment (B).

Before implantation of the pericardium civered stent (PCS), the patient was given 100 mg aspirin and 300 mg clopidogrel. Right femoral access was used and digital subtraction angiography (DSA) of the left carotid artery confirmed the findings of the CTA (Figure 4A, 4B). A 6-F guiding catheter (Guider Softip™ XF, Boston Scientific Corp., Fremont, CA, USA) was advanced in the distal part of the common carotid artery (CCA). A 0.014 guidewire (Synchro, Boston Scientific Corp., Fremont, CA, USA) was then passed distal to the neck of the aneurysm. The length of the aneurysm neck necessitated two PCS, and resulted in complete exclusion of the aneurysm demonstrated on post-procedure angiography (Figure 4C).

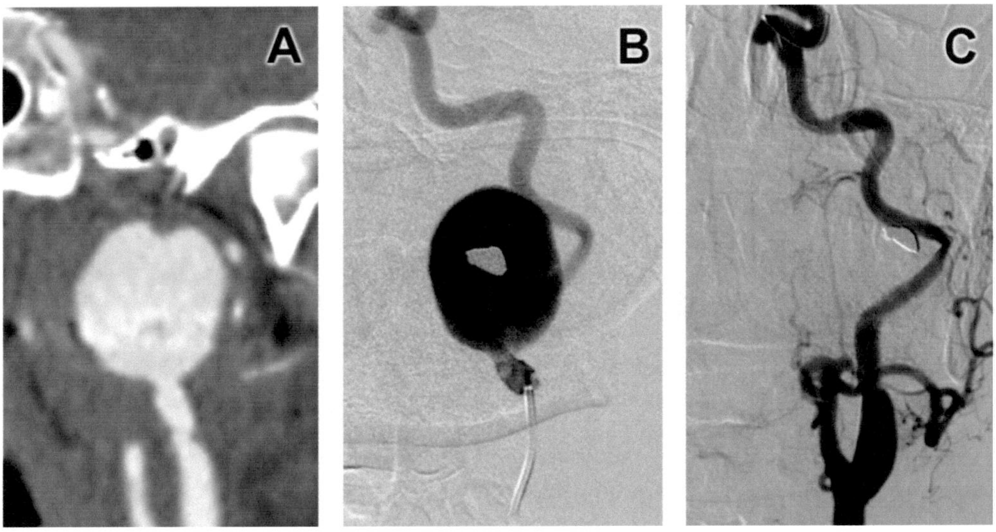

Figure 4. CTA (A) and DSA (B) of a giant false aneurysm of the cervical segment of the left ICA and post-procedure angiography after placement of a covered stent (C).

2.2. CASE 2

A 44-year-old female was referred to our hospital after suffering a subarachnoid hemorrhage. Coiling of a small aneurysm of the communicating segment of the left ICA had been done. A giant (20 × 18 mm), large-neck aneurysm was discovered on CTA at the intradural fourth segment of the left vertebral artery (VA) proximal to the posterior inferior cerebellar artery (PICA). Endovascular treatment was considered to be first-line treatment for this VA aneurysm. The patient received 100 mg aspirin and 75 mg clopidogrel for 3 days before the procedure. Right femoral access was used and a 6-F guiding catheter (Neuron, Penumbra Inc, San Leandro, California, USA) advanced to the V3 segment of the left VA. DSA showed a giant, large-neck aneurysm of the V4 segment of the VA (Figure 5A). After passage of a 0.014 guidewire (Synchro, Boston Scientific Corp., Fremont, CA, USA) distal to the aneurysm neck, a 4 × 27 mm PCS was deployed and inflated to 12 atm. The aneurysm was completely excluded and this was demonstrated at control angiography (Figure 5B). Follow-up CTA at 3 months demonstrated complete exclusion and shrinkage of the aneurysm to 18 × 16 mm (Figure 6).

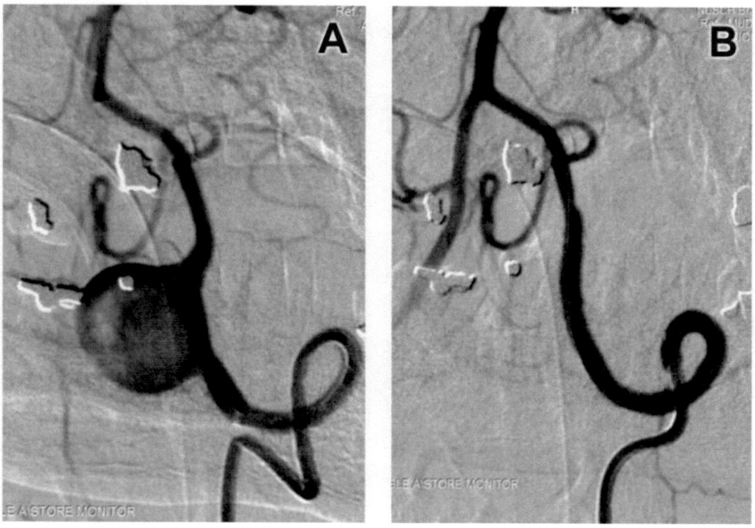

Figure 5. Preoperative DSA of a giant aneurysm of the V4 segment of the left VA (A) and DSA after placement of a covered stent with no filling of the aneurysm (B).

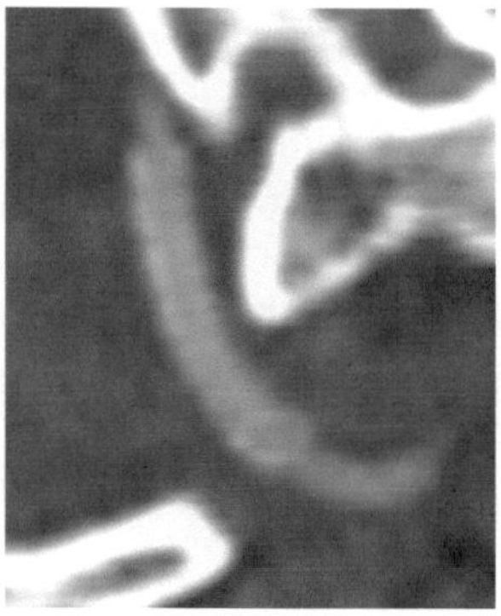

Figure 6. Three-month follow-up CTA showing aneurysm exclusion, a patent covered stent with no intimal hyperplasia, and aneurysm shrinkage.

2.3. CASE 3

An 85-year-old female was admitted to our hospital for endovascular therapy of a symptomatic large-neck aneurysm of the cervical segment of the ICA subsequent to a stroke in the left middle cerebral artery (MCA). The patient was pre-medicated with 100 mg aspirin and 75 mg clopidogrel for 3 days before the procedure. Endovascular treatment was undertaken after gaining access via the femoral artery and placement of a 6-F guiding sheath (Guider Softip™ XF, Boston Scientific Corp., Fremont, CA, USA) in the CCA. DSA confirmed the CTA findings of an aneurysm of the cervical segment of the ICA (Figure 7A, 7B). A 0.014 guidewire (Synchro, Boston Scientific Corp., Fremont, CA, USA) was passed distal to the aneurysm and a PCS (4 × 27 mm) advanced over the wire and placed in the optimal position. The balloon was slowly inflated to 10 atm and the PCS successfully deployed. Control DSA confirmed complete exclusion of the aneurysm with preservation of ICA patency (Figure 7C).

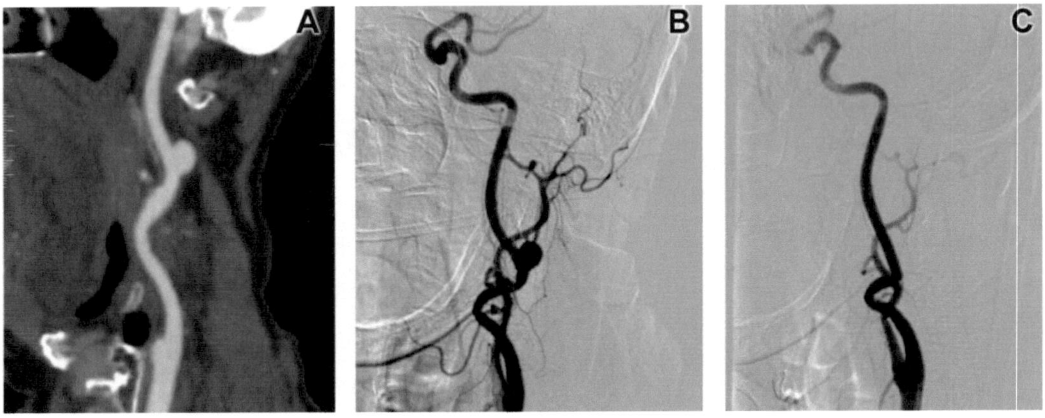

Figure 7. CTA (A) and DSA (B) before endovascular treatment of an aneurysm of the left cervical segment of the ICA and final angiogram after implantation of a covered stent (C).

2.4. CASE 4

An 55-year-old male was admitted to our centre for endovascular treatment of a symptomatic dissecting aneurysm of the cervical segment of the ICA subsequent to a stroke. The patient was pre-medicated with 100 mg aspirin and 75 mg clopidogrel for 3 days before the endovascular procedure. Endovascular treatment was performed after gaining access via the right femoral artery and placement of a 6-F guiding sheath (Guider Softip™ XF, Boston Scientific Corp., Fremont, CA, USA) in the CCA. DSA confirmed the CTA findings of an aneurysm of the cervical segment of the ICA (Figure 8A). A 0.014 guidewire (Synchro, Boston Scientific Corp., Fremont, CA, USA) was passed distal to the aneurysm and a 5x26mm Jostent Graftmaster (Abbott Vascular, Abbott Park, Ill, USA) advanced over the wire and successfully deployed after balloon inflation. Control DSA confirmed exclusion of the aneurysm with patent ICA (Figure 8B).

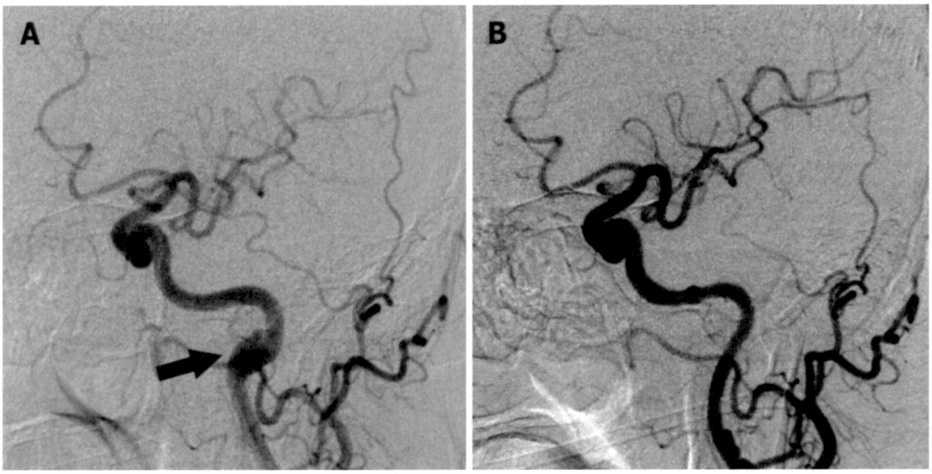

Figure 8. DSA before (A) endovascular treatment of an aneurysm of the left cervical segment of the ICA and angiogram after endovascular treatment with implantation of a covered stent (B).

2.5. CASE 5

A 44-year-old female was referred to our hospital for treatment of an asymptomatic fusiform aneurysm at the intradural fourth segment of the right vertebral artery. Endovascular treatment was considered to be first-line treatment for this VA aneurysm. The patient received 100 mg aspirin and 75 mg clopidogrel for 3 days before the procedure. Left femoral access was used and a 6-F guiding catheter (Neuron, Penumbra Inc, San Leandro, California, USA) advanced to the V3 segment of the right VA. DSA confirmed fusiform aneurysm of the V4 segment of the VA (Figure 9A). After passage of a 0.014 guidewire (Synchro, Boston Scientific Corp., Fremont, CA, USA) distal to the aneurysm neck, a flow diverting device Silk ((Balt, Montmorency, France) was deployed. The aneurysm was excluded and this was demonstrated at control angiography with no filling of the aneurysm (Figure 9B).

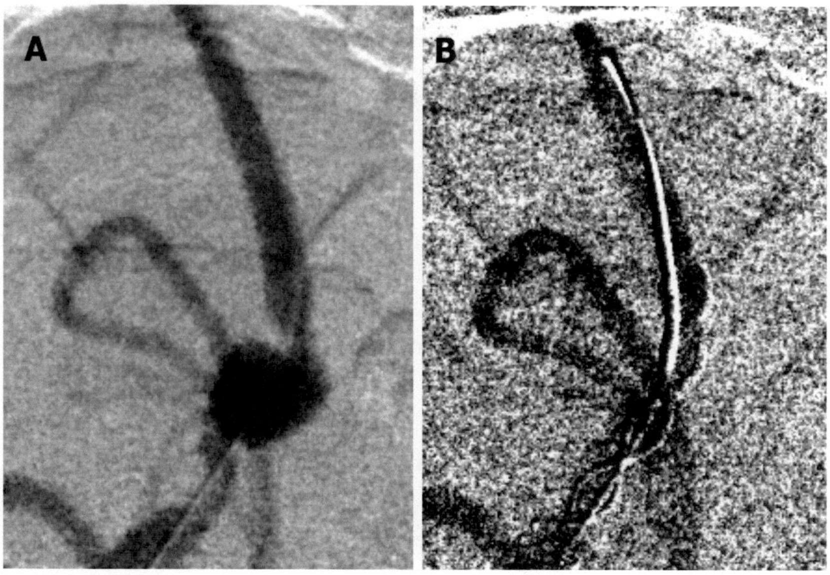

Figure 9. DSA before (A) endovascular therapy of an aneurysm of the intradural segment of right vertebral artery and angiogram after implantation of flow diverting device (B).

3. Discussion

Different endovascular techniques have been used in the treatment of vertebral and internal carotid artery aneurysms. These include covered stent placement, flow diverting device (FDD) placement, parent vessel occlusion with detachable balloons or coils, coil embolisation of the aneurysm with or without a stent placement.

3.1. Covered stents

In the past decade, covered stent placement has been proved to be effective for managing arteriovenous fistulas, aneurysms, and aortic dissections. Covered stents consist of a synthetic material that either covers or is attached to a metallic stent to create a graft endoprosthesis. There are two different types of stent-deployment system - balloon-expandable or self-expanding. Balloon-expandable system represent Jostent Graftmaster (Abbott Laboratories, Abbott Park, Ill) and iCast (Atrium Medical, Hudson, NH), self-expanding covered stents are Fluency stent (Bard Peripheral Vascular, Tempe, Ariz), GORE VIABAHN (W.L. Gore & Assoc, Newark, Del), Wallgraft (Boston Scientific, MA) and Willis covered stent (MicroPort, Shanghai, China). Compared with aneurysm coil embolization, a covered stent has the following advantages: (1) a relatively simple and rapid performance; (2) a low risk of procedural-related rupture or rebleeding; (3) no coil herniation, delayed migration, and coil loop protrusion; (4) disappearance or reduction of mass effects in large or giant aneurysms; and (e) no aneurysm recanalization and recurrence.

The Jostent graft is a composite stent with an ultrathin layer of expandable PTFE sandwiched between two stainless steel stents. It is balloon-expandable, covered-tube stent with radial strength. Jostent has been used for aneurysms up to the ophthalmic artery or up to the vertebrobasilar junction [9,10]. The Graftmaster has also been used for carotido-cavernous fistulas and dissections [11]. Bergeron et al. recently published a series of six patients with EICA in which stent-grafts were used. They had no adverse event perioperatively and the long follow-up revealed patency of all grafts without sign of in-stent stenosis [12]. Chan et al. also reported two cases of successful endovascular treatment of distal internal carotid aneurysms using Jostent, with both patients remaining symptom-free at 1 year and no signs of graft restenosis [13]. Th disadvantage of Jostent is, that it might cause intimal damage at the stent edges as a result of irritation from vessel motion or anatomic distortion and also requires a relatively straight delivery path and is not well suited for use in very tortuous vessels.

The Willis covered stent is specifically designed for use in the intracranial vasculature and consists of 3 parts: a bare stent, an expandable polytetrafluoroethylene (ePTFE) membrane, and a balloon catheter. The bare stent was constructed from a strand of cobalt chromium super alloy wire, which was 0.06mm in diameter. The ePTFE membrane, which was in a tubular configuration with a thickness of 30 to 50μm is glued along the length of the stent struts with use of organic agglomerate. To facilitate the membrane gluing along the stent, the diameter of tubular membrane is generally 0.05mm, which is wider than that of the inflated stent. To prevent the balloon from scaling the inner wall of the stent on withdrawal, the balloon is made into 5 valvae, instead of the commonly used 3 valvae. The whole body of the stent is radiopaque under fluoroscopy to facilitate precise placement of the stent. The stent can be manufactured in any diameter from 3 to 5mm and in any length from 7 to 15 mm . The stent is mounted on a deflated balloon catheter with an outside diameter of 3.8F. Li at. al. performed successfull endovascular treatment of pseudoaneurysms of cranial internal carotid artery in 8 patients without procedural-related complications, and all of the stents were easily navigated to the targeted lesions. Complete resolution of the pseudoaneurysm was observed in 6 patients immediately after the procedure, and a minimal endoleak into the aneurysm persisted in 2 patients. No morbidity or mortality and no technical adverse event occurred. A follow-up angiogram confirmed complete reconstruction of the internal carotid artery, with no recurrent aneurysmal filling and no occurrence of stenosis in the area of the stent [14]. The efficacy of the Willis covered stent in the treatment of traumatic pseudoaneurysms of the internal carotid artery was evaluated in 13 patients with 14 delayed pseudoaneurysms with succesfull covered stent placement in all 14 pseudoaneurysms. The initial angiographic results showed complete exclusion in 9 patients with 10 aneurysms and incomplete exclusion in 4 patients. The angiographic mean follow-up 15 months findings exhibited a complete exclusion in 12 patients with 13 aneurysms and an incomplete exclusion in 1 patient and maintained patency of the ICA in all patients with no procedure-related complications or deaths occurred during follow-up [15]. In another study, the navigation and deployment of the Willis covered stents were successful in 97.6% (41 of 42) of the patients with most of the aneurysms located at the C5 through C7 segment. Although some complications occurred, the 93.5% (29 of 31 aneurysms) final complete occlusion rate with no recanalization during follow-up addressed the effectiveness of the Willis covered stent for managing DICA aneurysms. In addition, endoleak occurred in 21.9% (7 of 32) of the patients owing to the tortuous segment of C5 through C7, but it could not been eliminated by means of postprocedural dilation and additional stent implantation [16].

The Wallgraft consists of a PET (Dacron; E.I. duPont de Nemours and Co., Wilmington, DE) covered self-expanding cobalt super alloy stent. Wallgraft was utilized in 4 cases of inernal carotid artery trauma or disease leading to contained rupture or pseudoaneurysm formation. During a mean 16-month follow-up (range 6–24), duplex ultrasound and CT scanning found no evidence of restenosis, occlusion, or persistent perfusion of the pseudoaneurysm, which was noted to decrease in all cases [17]. Wallgraft was also used in the treatment of tandem aneurysms of the extracranial internal carotid artery near the skull base with successfully exclusion with deployment of a single Wallgraft across both lesions with no complications encountered. At 2-year follow-up, the patient is doing well, without any sign of aneurysm reperfusion [18]. The Wallgraft has several disadvantages. First, PET is immunogenic which animal studies suggest, increases the rate of vessel thrombosis [19]. Second, the Wallgraft delivery system requires a 9-French arterial sheath in the carotid and vertebral arteries, which may increase the risk of pseudoaneurysms or groin hematomas at the femoral puncture site. Finally, the PET covering is initially porous until a clot forms to seal the fabric.

Viabahn endograft is a PTFE covered nitinol stent with extreme flexibility and conformability to vessel configuration. Covered stents have also shown better closure and shorter procedure time in clinical investigations [20]. Current published evidence of the use of covered stent is limited to stents covered with polytetrafluoroethylene (PTFE) [21]. Synthetic materials are used in biological settings with limited success. Studies have shown that polyester covered stent graft with 50% re-stenosis and e-PTFE covered stent with 24% re-stenosis in a sheep iliac model [22]. It has also been shown that PTFE retards endothelization and that Dacron is prone to infection, due to adherence to and survival of bacteria on its rough surface [23]. Baldi et al. in their three cases had no periprocedural complications and all three PTFE Viabahn endografts were patent at 9 month follow-up without evidence of intimal hyperplasia [24].

A novel CE marked coronary stent covered with pericardium (Aneugraft: ITGI Medical limited, Or Akiva, Israel) is available, which so far shows promising clinical results. The pericardium covered stent (PCS) is a percutaneous implantable device consisting of a 316L stainless steel stent covered by a 100μ thick equine pericardium cylinder which makes this device flexible and trackable. It is available in diameters of 2.5mm, 3.0mm, 3.5mm, and 4.0mm, and lengths of 13, 18, 23 and 27mm. The stent is mounted on a balloon catheter. Gluteraldehyde treated pericardium has been widely used for many years due to its desirable features such as low immunogenicity and durability [25-27]. It has been shown that there is significantly less inflammatory cytokine, significantly less antibody response and inflammatory response compared to un-crosslinked decellularized pericardium [28]. It is now recognized that mammalian extracellular matrix represents an excellent scaffold material suitable for many therapeutic applications [29]. In Neurosurgery, serous sheets are used as dural substitute. An investigation involving 200 patients undergoing a surgical procedure with the application of horse pericardium as a dural prosthesis found that they are free from antigenic effects and do not produce any toxic catabolites [30]. The pericardium proved to be resistant to surgical suture, impermeable to cerebrospinal fluid, transparent and does not cause any clinical evidence or radiological artifacts. Pericardium has also shown decreased intraoperative suture line bleeding compared to Dacron [31]. The PCS has shown to be safe and effective in 2 registries [32], and there is also published evidence attesting to this in other indications [33-36].

There are several disadvantages regarding the use of covered stents in the cranial and extracranial vasculature. First, more clinical trials are required to determine the long-term outcomes. Second, the covered stents may not be flexible and conformable enough to navigate entirely through the extremely tortuous ICA and to fully conform to the configuration of the tortuous targeted arteries. Third, the possibility of a closure of the side branches stemming from the covered segment of the artery might occur after the stent placement. Therefore, balloon occlusion tests and angiography examinations from multiple projections should be routinely performed to avoid coverage of the side branches. In addition, in-stent restenosis might occur in patients who are not following the regular anticoagulation medication regimen after stent placement.

3.2. FDD

Flow diversion is a new approach to the endovascular treatment of intracranial aneurysms which uses a high density mesh stent to induce sac thrombosis. These devices have been designed for the treatment of complex shaped and large size aneurysms. Flow diversion aims to cure aneurysms by endovascular reconstruction of the parent vessel, without even performing endosaccular embolisation. The primary intent of a flow diversion device (as opposed to a stent) is to optimally alter the flow exchange between the parent artery and the aneurysm so as to promote complete thrombosis of the sac as rapidly as possible while eliciting minimal neointimal hyperplasia. The principal goal of the flow divertor is placement in the parent artery in order to reconstruct the vessel wall [37]. The concept of flow diversion appears promising in challenging lesions, including fusiform and/or giant aneurysms. However, this stent presents major limitations: (a) the aneurysm occlusion process is unpredictable; (b) an associated complication rate much higher than those previously reported with conventional treatments (coiling, balloon- or stent-assisted coiling, parent artery occlusion, clipping); and (c) a high rate of significant parent artery stenosis.

In contrast to an ideal stent, an ideal flow diversion device has low porosity and high pore density values optimized to promote intraaneurysmal thrombosis while maintaining patency of the parent vessel and side branches. Moreover, lower radial forces are required of this device as compared to a stent, which facilitates the optimization of other device characteristics such as longitudinal flexibility, trackability, and conformability. Recognition of the potential for aneurysm treatment by flow diversion is evidenced by the recent development of these devices by various groups.The major complications with flow divertors have been found to be perforator artery stroke, aneurysm re-rupture, and in-stent stenosis and thrombosis [38,39].

The Pipeline stent (EV3, Irvine, Calif) is the first released flow-diverter stent and it has been evaluated in some series [40,41]. These authors showed that the Pipeline stent represents a safe, durable, and curative treatment of selected wide-necked, large, and giant aneurysms. The Pipeline stent has been used for the treatment of two male patients transferred after acute SAH and dissecting aneurysm on the V4 segment of the dominant vertebral artery with 3 Pipeline stents deployed in each vertebral artery. One dissecting aneurysm was excluded immediately after 3 stents and one patient had complete exclusion demonstrated at the 48 hour control. No morbidity directly related to the procedure was observed and no recanalization and no re-bleeding occurred during the 3 months follow-up [42]. In the recent publication, Yeung et al. demonstrated favourable long-term clinical and angiographic outcomes of FDD use and the ability to maintain parent artery and side branch patency for the endovascular treatment of unruptured dissecting intracranial vertebral aneurysms. In their series, total of 4 aneurysms were successfully obliterated by using flow-diverting devices alone, two devices were deployed in a telescoping fashion in each of 2 aneurysms, whereas only 1 device was inserted in each of the other 2 aneurysms with no periprocedural complications. No patient showed any angiographic evidence of recurrence, in-stent thrombosis, or side-branch occlusion in angiographic reassessment at a mean of 22 months after treatment (range 18-24 months) [43].

The other available flow-diverter device is the Silk stent (Balt, Montmorency, France) and little information is available concerning its use [44-46]. By the use of telescopic catheters, the Silk stent may be placed in most patients. Silk opening and wall apposition frequently require pushing back the delivery catheter. This is particularly mandatory within curved vessel such as the ICA siphon. Because of its low radial force, the Silk stent must be placed with great caution if the vessel shows a stenotic portion because vessel occlusion may occur. Moreover, careful size and length selection is mandatory because stent shortening and migration may happen. For all these reasons, Silk stent placement is more difficult than nonflow-diverter self-expandable stent.

3.3. Parent vessel occlusion

One of the treatment options available for patients with internal carotid or vertebral artery aneurysms is parent vessel occlusion, either surgical or endovascular. The goal of parent vessel occlusion for the treatment of fusiform aneurysms is intra-aneurysmal thrombosis and involution of the aneurysm. Endovascular occlusion can be achieved with detachable balloons or coils or with a combination of the two. Studies reporting patient outcomes after parent vessel occlusion for treatment of fusiform aneurysms of the vertebrobasilar circulation have been limited. A few series have reported the results of parent vessel occlusion in the posterior circulation, although not exclusively for intracranial fusiform aneurysms. In one study the long-term outcomes for 21 patients with unclippable posterior circulation aneurysms treated with either unilateral or bilateral parent vessel occlusion of the vertebral artery, with a mean follow-up of 2 years (range, 6 months to 6 years) were examined [47]. Six of the patients had fusiform aneurysms, and the remaining 5 had aneurysms that were of saccular morphology. All occlusions in this series were performed by using latex balloons. Thirteen (61.9%) of 21 patients achieved good outcomes, including angiographic cure and clinical improvement. Twenty-eight and six-tenths percent of the patients had partial thrombosis of their aneurysm. One death and one treatment failure occurred.

Occlusion of the internal carotid artery may lead to severe cerebrovascular events and therefore a balloon occlusion test should be performed in advance; if a temporary occlusion test is successful, trapping or parent artery occlusion is an option. However, it has been shown that 5–22% of patients passing the balloon occlusion test develop ischemic complications, including cerebral infarct, while some reports have revealed cerebral aneurysm formation after permanent carotid occlusion [48,49]. The placement of detachable balloons in the ICA above and below the false aneurysm can completely eliminate blood flow. Disadvantages with this endovascular approach include the possibility of embolic cerebrovascular accidents. If the patient cannot tolerate the occlusion test, an extracranial-to-intracranial bypass should be contemplated.

3.4. Coil embolisation and stent placement

Another treatment option in the management of aneurysms represents stent placement with or without coil embolisation and coil embolisation without stent placement. Findings of experimental studies have shown that a metallic stent, bridging the aneurysmal neck, may alter the flow pattern within the aneurysm, promoting thrombus formation and aneurysmal occlusion [50,51]. Although immediate aneurysmal occlusion can be seen after single stent placement for treatment of extracranial pseudoaneurysms, in some cases, 3–6 months or longer may pass before occlusion occurs. To achieve faster complete aneurysmal occlusion, the combination of stents and detachable coils has been suggested for extracranial, as well as intracranial aneurysms [2,52,53] and the combination is currently considered an alternative to single stent placement or other techniques such as the remodeling technique or parent vessel occlusion. Lanzino et al [52] reported 10 cases managed with stent-supported coil embolization; they achieved aneurysmal occlusion of more than 90% in eight patients. In four of these patients, treated with stent placement only, no evidence of intraaneurysmal thrombosis was found either immediately or during follow-up studies performed 48 hours (two patients), 4 days (one patient), and 3 months (one patient) after treatment. Phatouros et al [2] reported a series of seven patients with fusiform aneurysms, wide-neck aneurysms, or pseudoaneurysms who underwent stent-supported coil embolization; technical success was achieved in six. In one patient, a coil became entangled with the stent, resulting in partial coil delivery into the parent artery with no neurologic sequelae.

However, certain limitations, may be encountered when stents are used in conjunction with coils. In some cases, a microcatheter can be navigated through the stent interstices only with difficulty. Packing of the aneurysm sac can be inaccurate because of the density of platinum detachable coils. Multiple projections with big amount of used contrast medium may become necessary, particularly with fusiform aneurysms, and in some cases, complete packing of the aneurysm cannot be achieved. Coil loops may become entangled with the stent struts and unravel during attempts to retrieve them, leading to the risk of moving the stent or leaving coils within the parent artery. A report by Phatouros et al [2] shows the successful use of stent-supported coil embolization in the treatment of fusiform and wide neck aneurysms. The stent mesh allows for attenuated packing of the aneurysm with less concern for herniation of coils into the parent artery. Phatouros et al reported technical success in six of the seven patients treated, with 0% 30-day periprocedural morbidity and mortality. After a mean follow-up of 14.5 months, all the patients treated with stent-supported coil embolization were at their neurologic baseline or had improved. The authors acknowledged the current limitations of this therapy, including the concern for occluding small but important perforators with the struts of the stent. Kurata et al. published their findings in a series of 24 ruptured dissecting vertebral artery aneurysms. Endosaccular embolisation was performed within 4 days of onset of symptoms with no experienced complications with coil embolisation. Radiologic investigation showed complete occlusion of the dissection and patency of the unaffected artery at a mean follow-up of 9 months [54].

The use of double stent placement for complete exclusion of wide-neck aneurysms has been reported in only a single case to date [55], however double stent placement may be a relatively simple technique to more effectively change intraaneurysmal flow and achieve subsequent thrombosis. The influence of stent porosity on changing the local hemodynamics between the aneurysm and the parent vessel was shown in the experimental study [56].

4. Conclusion

In conclusion, endovascular treatment of vertebral and carotid artery aneurysms with covered stents is very promising, safe and feasible treatment option. So called flow diverting devices despite their "slow mode" of action, but according to their special features (as is high flexibility and very low profile), seems to be very effective tool in endovascular treatment of carotid and vertebral artery aneurysms. On the other hand, covered stents with for example a novel pericardium covered stent, allow complete occlusion of the aneurysm, fistula or dissection in one action. This approach in the treatment of aneurysms seems to be very promising. Therapeutic decision making in the treatment of vertebral and carotid artery aneurysms must balance endovascular or surgical morbidity and mortality rates with the risk of hemorrhage and other considerations on an individual basis. Evolving technologies move towards increased covered stents flexibility with pushing down their profiles. This evolution followed with future studies of these advanced endovascular approaches will probably increase the role of covered stents in the field of endovascular treatment of vertebral and carotid artery aneurysms in the future. More detailed clinical studies will need to be conducted to confirm the overall performance and long-term effect of covered stents in the treatment of internal carotid and vertebral artery aneurysms.

Author details

Ivan Vulev and Andrej Klepanec
Department of Diagnostic and Interventional Radiology,
National Institute of Cardiovascular Diseases Bratislava, Slovakia

5. References

[1] Vega C, Kwoon JV, Lavine SD. Intracranial aneurysms: current evidence and clinical practice. American Family Physician 2002;66(4): 601-608.

[2] Phatouros CC, Sasaki TY, Higashida RT, Malek AM, Meyers PM, Dowd CF, Halbach VV. Stent-supported coil embolization: the treatment of fusiform and wide-neck aneurysms and pseudoaneurysms. Neurosurgery 2000;47: 107-115.

[3] Nichols DA, Brown RD, Thielen KR, Meyer FB, Atkinson JL, Piepgras DG. Endovascular treatment of ruptured posterior circulation aneurysms using electrolytically detachable coils. Journal of Neurosurgery 1997;87: 374-380.

[4] Matsumoto M, Sato M, Nakano M, Endo Y, Watanabe Y, Sasaki T, Suzuki K, Kodama N. Three-dimensional computerized tomography angiography-guided surgery of acutely ruptured cerebral aneurysms. Journal of Neurosurgery 2001;94: 718-727.

[5] Villablanca JP, Martin N, Jahan R, Gobin YP, Frazee, Duckwiler G, Bentson J, Hardart M, Coiteiro D, Sayre J, Vinuela F. Volume rendered helical computerized tomography angiography in the detection and characterisation of intracranial aneurysms. Journal of Neurosurgery 2000;93: 254-264.

[6] Rinkel GJ. Natural history, epidemiology and screening of unruptured intracranial aneurysms. Journal of Neuroradiology 2008;35(2): 99-103.

[7] Molyneux A, Kerr R, Stratton I, Sandercock P, Clarke M, Shrimpton J, Holman R; International Subarachnoid Aneurysm Trial (ISAT) Collaborative Group. International Subarachnoid Aneurysm Trial (ISAT) of neurosurgical clipping versus endovascular coiling in 2143 patients with ruptured intracranial aneurysms: a randomised trial. Lancet 2002;60: 1267-1274.

[8] Hoh BL, Chi YY, Lawson MF, Mocco J, Barker FG 2nd. Length of stay and total hospital charges of clipping versus coiling for ruptured and unruptured adult cerebral

aneurysms in the Nationwide Inpatient Sample database 2002 to 2006. Stroke 2010;41(2): 337-342.
[9] Saatci I, Cekirge SH, Ozturk MH, Arat A, Ergungor F, Sekerci Z, Senveli E, Er U, Turkoglu S, Ozcan OE, Ozgen T. Treatment of Internal Carotid Artery Aneurysms with a Covered Stent: Experience in 24 Patients with Mid-Term Follow-up Results. American Journal of Neuroradiology 2004;25: 1742-1749.
[10] Greenberg E, Katz, JM, Janardhan, V, Riina, H, Gobin, YP. Treatment of a giant vertebrobasilar artery aneurysm using stent grafts. Journal of Neurosurgery 2007;107: 165-168.
[11] Gomez F, Escobar W, Gomez AM, Gomez JF, Anaya CA. Treatment of Carotid Cavernous Fistulas Using Covered Stents: Midterm Results in Seven Patients. American Journal of Neuroradiogy 2007;28: 1762-1768.
[12] Bergeron P, Khanoyan P, Meunier J-P, Graziani JN, Gay J. Long term results of endovascular exclusion of extracranial internal carotid artery aneuryms and dissecting aneurysm. Journal of Interventional Cardiology 2004;17: 245–252.
[13] Chan AW, Yadav JS, Krieger D, Abou-Chebl A. Endovascular repair of carotid artery aneurysm with Jostent covered stent: Initial experience and one year result. Cathteterization and Cardiovascular Interventions 2004;63: 15–20.
[14] Li MH, Li YD, Gao BL, Fang C, Luo QY, Cheng YS, Xie ZY, Wang YL, Zhao JG, Li Y, Wang W, Zhang BL, Li M. A new covered stent designed for intracranial vasculature: application in the management of pseudoaneurysms of the cranial internal carotid artery. American Journal of Neuroradiology 2007;28(8): 1579-1585.
[15] Wang, W, Li MH, Li YD, Gu BX, Wang J, Zhang PL, Li M. Treatment of Traumatic Internal Carotid Artery Pseudoaneurysms With the Willis Covered Stent: A Prospective Study. Journal of Trauma-Injury Infection and Critical Care 2011;70(4): 816-822.
[16] Li MH, Li YD, Tan HQ, Luo QY, Cheng YS. Treatment of Distal Internal Carotid Artery Aneurysm with the Willis Covered Stent: A Prospective Pilot Study. Radiology 2009;253: 470-477.
[17] Kubaska SM 3rd, Greenberg RK, Clair D, Barber G, Srivastava SD, Green RM, Waldman DL, Ouriel K. Internal Carotid Artery Pseudoaneurysms: Treatment With the Wallgraft Endoprosthesis. Journal of Endovascular Therapy 2003;10(2): 182-189.
[18] Fischer B, Palkovic S, Wassmann H. Endovascular Management of Tandem Extracranial Internal Carotid Artery Aneurysms With a Covered Stent. Journal of Endovascular Therapy 2004;11: 739–741.
[19] Hussain FM, Kopchok G, Heilbron M, Daskalakis T, Donayre C, White RA. Wallgraft endoprosthesis: Initial canine evaluation. The American Surgeon 1998;64: 1002–1006.
[20] Li MH, Leng B, Li YD, Tan HQ, Wang W, Song DL, Tian YL. Comparative study of covered stent with coil embolization in the treatment of cranial internal carotid artery aneurysm: a nonrandomized prospective trial. European Radiology 2010;20(11): 2732-2739.
[21] Tan HQ, Li MH, Zhang PL, Li YD, Wang JB, Zhu YQ, Wang W. Reconstructive endovascular treatment of intracranial aneurysms with the Willis covered stent:

medium-term clinical and angiographic follow-up. Journal of Neurosurgery 2011;114(4): 1014-1020.

[22] Cejna M, Virmani R, Jones R. Biocompatibility and Performance of the Wallstent and Several Covered Stents in a Sheep Iliac Artery Model. Journal of Vascular and Interventional Radiology 2001;12: 351–358.

[23] Shintani H. Modification of Medical Device Surface to attain Anti-Infection Trends. Biomaterials, Artificial Cells, and Artificial Organs 2004;18(1): 1-8.

[24] Baldi S, Rostagno RD, Zander T, Llorens R, Schonholz C, Maynar M. Endovascular Treatment of Extracranial Internal Carotid Aneurysms Using Endografts. Cardiovascular and Interventional Radiology 2008;31: 401–403.

[25] Butany J, Luk A, Leong SW, Leong MM, Singh G, Thangaroopan M, Williams W. A Carpentier-Edwards porcine-valved dacron conduit: at twenty-five years. International Journal of Cardiology 2007;117(1): 13-16.

[26] Jamieson WR, Burr LH, Munro AI, Miyagishima RT. Carpentier-Edwards standard porcine bioprosthesis: a 21-year experience. Annals of Thoracic Surgery 1996;66(6 Suppl): S40-3.

[27] Cribier A, Eltchaninoff, Tron C. Early experience with percutaneous transcatheter implantation of heart valve prosthesis for the treatment of end-stage inoperable patients with calcific aortic stenosis. Journal of the American College of Cardiology. 2004;43: 698-703.

[28] Umashankar PR, Arun T, Kumari TV. Short duration gluteraldehyde cross linking of decellularized bovine pericardium improves biological response. Journal of Biomedical Materials Research Part A 2011;97(3): 311-320.

[29] Badylak SF, Freytes DO, Gilbert TW. Extracellular matrix as a biological scaffold material: Structure and function. Acta Biomaterialia 2009;5(1): 1-13.

[30] Montinaro A, Gianfreda CD, Proto P. Equine pericardium for dural grafts: clinical results in 200 patients. Journal of Neurosurgical Sciences 2007;51(1): 17-19.

[31] Marien BJ, Raffetto JD, Seidman CS, LaMorte WW, Menzoian JO. Bovine pericardium vs dacron for patch angioplasty after carotid endarterectomy: a prospective randomized study. Archives of Surgery 2002;137(7): 785-788.

[32] Colombo A, Almagor Y, Gaspar J, Vonderwalde C. The pericardium covered stent (PCS). EuroIntervention 2009;5(3): 394-399.

[33] Summaria F, Romagnoli E, Preziosi P. Percutaneous antegrade transarterial treatment of iatrogenic radial arteriovenous fistula. Journal of Cardiovascular Medicine (Hagerstown) 2012;13(1): 50-2.

[34] Adlam D, Hutchings D, Channon KM. Optical coherence tomography-guided stenting of a large coronary aneurysm: images at implantation and at 6 months. J. Invasive Cardiol. 2011;23(4): 168-169.

[35] Siregar S, Hoseyni Guyomi S, van Herwerden LA. Covered stents in giant coronary artery aneurysm. European Heart Journal 2010;31(22): 2823.

[36] Ferlini M, Russo F, Marinoni B, Repetto A, Canosi U, Ferrario M, Visconti LO, Bramucci E. Percutaneous coronary aneurysm obliteration using a novel pericardium-covered stent. Journal of the American College of Cardiology 2010;14;56(25): 2139.

[37] Wong GK, Kwan MC, Ng RY, Yu SC, Poon WS. Flow diverters for treatment of intracranial aneurysms: Current status and ongoing clinical trials. Journal of Clinical Neuroscience 2011; 18(6):737-740.

[38] Walcott BP, Pisapia JM, Nahed BV, Kahle KT, Ogilvy CS. Early experience with flow diverting endoluminal stents for the treatment of intracranial aneurysms. Journal of Clinical Neuroscience 2011;18(7): 891-894.

[39] Byrne JV, Beltechi R, Yarnold JA, Birks J, Kamran M. Early experience in the treatment of intra-cranial aneurysms by endovascular flow diversion: a multicentre prospective study. PLoS One 2010;5(9): e12492.

[40] Fiorella D, Woo HH, Albuquerque FC, Nelson PK. Definitive reconstruction of circumferential, fusiform intracranial aneurysms with the pipeline embolization device. Neurosurgery 2008;62: 1115–1120.

[41] Lylyk P, Miranda C, Ceratto R, Ferrario A, Scrivano E, Luna HR, Berez AL, Tran Q, Nelson PK, Fiorella D. Curative endovascular reconstruction of cerebral aneurysms with the pipeline embolization device: the Buenos Aires experience. Neurosurgery 2009;64: 632–642.

[42] Narata AP, Yilmaz H, Schaller K, Lovblad KO, Pereira VM. Flow Diverter Stent for Ruptured Intracranial Dissecting Aneurysm of Vertebral Artery. Neurosurgery 2011;70(4): 982-989.

[43] Yeung TW, Lai V, Lau HY, Poon WL, Tan CB, Wong YC. Long-term outcome of endovascular reconstruction with the Pipeline embolization device in the management of unruptured dissecting aneurysms of the intracranial vertebral artery. Journal of Neurosurgery 2012;116(4):882-887.

[44] Appelboom G, Kadri K, Hassan F, Leclerc X. Infectious aneurysm of the cavernous carotid artery in a child treated with a new-generation of flow-diverting stent graft: case report. Neurosurgery 2010;66: 623–624.

[45] Turowski B, Macht S, Kulcsár Z, Hänggi D, Stummer W. Early fatal hemorrhage after endovascular cerebral aneurysm treatment with a flow diverter (SILK-Stent): do we need to rethink our concepts? Neuroradiology. 2011;53(1): 37-41.

[46] Lubicz B, Collignon L, Raphaeli G, Pruvo JP, Bruneau M, De Witte O, Leclerc X. Flow-Diverter Stent for the Endovascular Treatment of Intracranial Aneurysms A Prospective Study in 29 Patients With 34 Aneurysms. Stroke 2010;41: 2247-2253.

[47] Aymard A, Gobin YP, Hodes J, Bien S, Rüfenacht D, Reizine D, George B, Merland JJ. Endovascular occlusion of vertebral arteries in the treatment of unclippable vertebrobasilar aneurysms. Journal of Neurosurgery 1991;74: 393–398.

[48] Eckert B, Thie A, Carvajal M, Groden C, Zeumer H. Predicting hemodynamic ischemia by transcranial Doppler monitoring during therapeutic balloon occlusion of the internal carotid artery. American Journal of Neuroradiology 1998;19: 577–582.

[49] Larson JJ, Tew JM Jr, Tomsick TA, van Loveren HR. Treatment of aneurysms of the internal carotid artery by intravascular balloon occlusion: Long-term follow-up of 58 patients. Neurosurgery 1995;36: 26–30.

[50] Geremia G, Haklin M, Brennecke L. Embolization of experimentally created aneurysms with intravascular stent devices. American Journal of Neuroradiology 1994;15: 1223-1231.

[51] Wakhloo AK, Schellhammer F, de Vries J, Haberstroh J, Schumacher M. Self-expanding and balloon-expandable stents in the treatment of carotid aneurysms: an experimental study in a canine model. American Journal of Neuroradiology 1994;15: 493-502.

[52] Lanzino G, Wakhloo AK, Fessler RD, Hartney ML, Guterman LR, Hopkins LN. Efficacy and current limitations of intravascular stents for intracranial internal carotid, vertebral, and basilar artery aneurysms. Journal of Neurosurgery 1999;91: 538-546.

[53] Lylyk P, Ceratto R, Hurvitz D, Basso A. Treatment of a vertebral dissecting aneurysm with stents and coils: technical case report. Neurosurgery 1998;43: 385-388.

[54] Kurata A, Ohmomo T, Miyasaka Y, Fujii K, Kan S, Kitahara T. Coil embolisation for the treatment of ruptured dissecting vertebral aneurysms. American Journal of Neuroradiology 2001;22: 11-18.

[55] Benndorf G, Lehmann T, Schneider G, Wellnhofer E. Double stenting: technique to accelerate occlusion of a dissecting carotid artery aneurysm. Neuroradiology 1999;41: (suppl) 77.

[56] Lieber BB, Stancampiano AP, Wakhloo AK. Alteration of hemodynamics in aneurysm models by stenting: influence of stent porosity. Annals of Biomedical Engineering 1997;25: 460-469.

Chapter 13

Complications and Adverse Events Associated with Stent-Assisted Coiling of Wide-Neck Intracranial Aneurysms

Xu Gao and Guobiao Liang

Additional information is available at the end of the chapter

http://dx.doi.org/10.5772/50571

1. Introduction

Endovascular treatment of intracranial aneurysm has been increasingly performed worldwide. The recent publication of a multiple center randomized trial showing improved safety and clinical outcome of patients treated with endovascular methods as compared with open clipping is encouraging to endovascular neurosurgeons and accelerates this trend. [1] Stent-assisted coil embolization, which is earliest reported by Higashida in 1997 [2] and now widely accepted, has expanded the treatment possibilities. It allows for adequate coil placement, prevents coil protrusion into the parent vessel, and also helps prevent aneurysm recanalization. In the last decade, the development of intracranial stents has increased the options for the treatment of wide-necked aneurysms. Successful experiences of the stent-assisted coiling have been reported by many teams in endovascular neurosurgery centers throughout the world. However, most of the reported complications involved a limited number of patients and varied among reports.[3,4] There has been no systematic report of a relatively larger number of patients treated at a single institution, to provide an overview of these complications. The purposes of this article are to systematically document and analyze the periprocedural and follow-up complications of stent-assisted coiling of cerebral aneurysms at our institution and to tentatively answer the following question: is the incidence of complications with stent-assisted coiling acceptable, compared with the benefits?

2. Patients and methods

2.1. Patient population

Between Jul 2003 and Dec 2009, 232 consecutive patients with 239 wide-neck aneurysms underwent stent-assisted coil embolization at our institution. Therapeutic alternatives were discussed between neurosurgical and neurointerventional teams. Informed consent from the patients and institutional review board approval was obtained. The medical records, radiographic studies and endovascular procedure reports were reviewed. Patient and aneurysm characteristics are summarized in table 1.

No. of patients	232
Age (y)	
Mean	55.1
Range	18-81
Gender	
Female	142
Male	90
Ruptured aneurysms (%)	129 (54.0)
Hunt and Hess grade	
I	39
II	46
III	34
IV	7
V	3
Unruptured aneurysms (%)	110 (46.0)
Headache	35
Previous SAH	29
Incidental	22
CN paisy	13
TIA	11
Aneurysm location (%)	
Anterior Circulation	195 (81.6)
PcomA	49
AcomA	12
Paraclinoid ICA	41
Cavernous ICA	20
Ophthalmic	37
ICA bifurcation	14
AchoA	17
A1 segment of ACA	5
Posterior Circulation	44 (18.4)
BA	18
VA	12
VB junction	9
PICA	5
Aneurysm size (%)	
Small	164(68.6)
Large	43(18.0)
Giant	32(13.4)
Neck size (mm)	
Mean	5.9
Range	2-24

Note: SAH, subarachnoid hemorrhage; TIA, transient ischemic attack; PcomA, posterior communicating artery; AcomA, anterior communicating artery; Acho: anterior choroidal artery; ICA, internal carotid artery; ACA , anterior cerebral artery; BA, basilar artery; VA, vertebral artery; VB, vertebrobasilar; PICA, posterior inferior cerebellar artery, small, <10 mm; large, >10-25 mm; giant, >25 mm.

Table 1. Patient and aneurysm characteristics

2.2. Treatment procedures

All procedures were performed under general anesthesia. Patients having unruptured aneurysms were premedicated with antiplatelet therapy consisting of aspirin 300 mg and clopidogrel 75 mg for 3 days before the procedure. Patients with SAH were loaded with aspirin 300 mg and clopidogrel 225 mg via nasogastric tube after general anesthesia. All patients received systemic heparinization to raise the activated clotting time (ACT) at about 300 seconds and continuous intravenous infusion of Nimodipine, 2mg/hour to prevent vasospasm during the procedure. In patients with ruptured aneurysms, heparinization started before puncture, and in patients who presented with acute SAH, heparinization started after aneurysm catheterization. A full three- or four-vessel cerebral angiogram was performed to permit a complete evaluation of the aneurysm, measure the aneurysm neck, width, and height, and measure the parent artery proximal and distal to the aneurysm. A 6F or 8F sheath was introduced in the right femoral artery following a standard Seldinger puncture. A 6F or 8F Envoy guiding catheter (Johnson & Johnson) was then guided into either the cervical internal carotid or vertebral artery, depending on the location of the aneurysm. The microcatheters were Prowler series (Johnson & Johnson), Excelsior SL-10, or Excelsior 1018 (Boston Scientific/Target Therapeutics). In all cases, embolization was completed by packing the aneurysm sac with a variety of commercially available coils. After the procedure, the patient was moved to the neurosurgery intensive care unit for monitoring and received low-molecular weight heparin calcium 4000IU/12h for the next 48 hours. Clopidogrel 75 mg each day was orally taken for an additional 30 days, and aspirin 100 mg for 6 months.

2.3. Stenting strategies

Stent deployment was successful in 237 of 239 aneurysms, and failed in two aneurysms. Strategies used regarding the sequence of stenting and coiling in 237 treated aneurysms were the following:

1. Stents were delivered before coiling in 205 of 237 aneurysms (86.5%).

a. Stenting before coiling in the same session in 191 aneurysms (80.6%). In 67 of 191 aneurysms, the sequential technique was used, by which the microcatheter was introduced into the sac through the struts of the stent. In 93 of 191 aneurysms, the jailing technique was used, by which the coiling catheter was "jailed" between the vessel wall and the stent. Other 31 of 191 aneurysms were treated using the semi-deployment technique. It consisted of the delivery microcatheter into the aneurysm sac and navigating a self-expandable stent into the parent vessel, and subsequently partially deploying (approximate 50%-60% of its opening) the stent, which covered the distal part of the aneurysm to narrow the neck and leaves room to modify the coil delivery microcatheter position during embolization. After a homogeneous coil framing or complete embolization is achieved, the stent was fully deployed. If necessary, coiling could be continued using traditional jailing technique to obtain circulatory exclusion of the lesion. A illustrated case of the whole semi-deployment technique is shown in Figure 1.

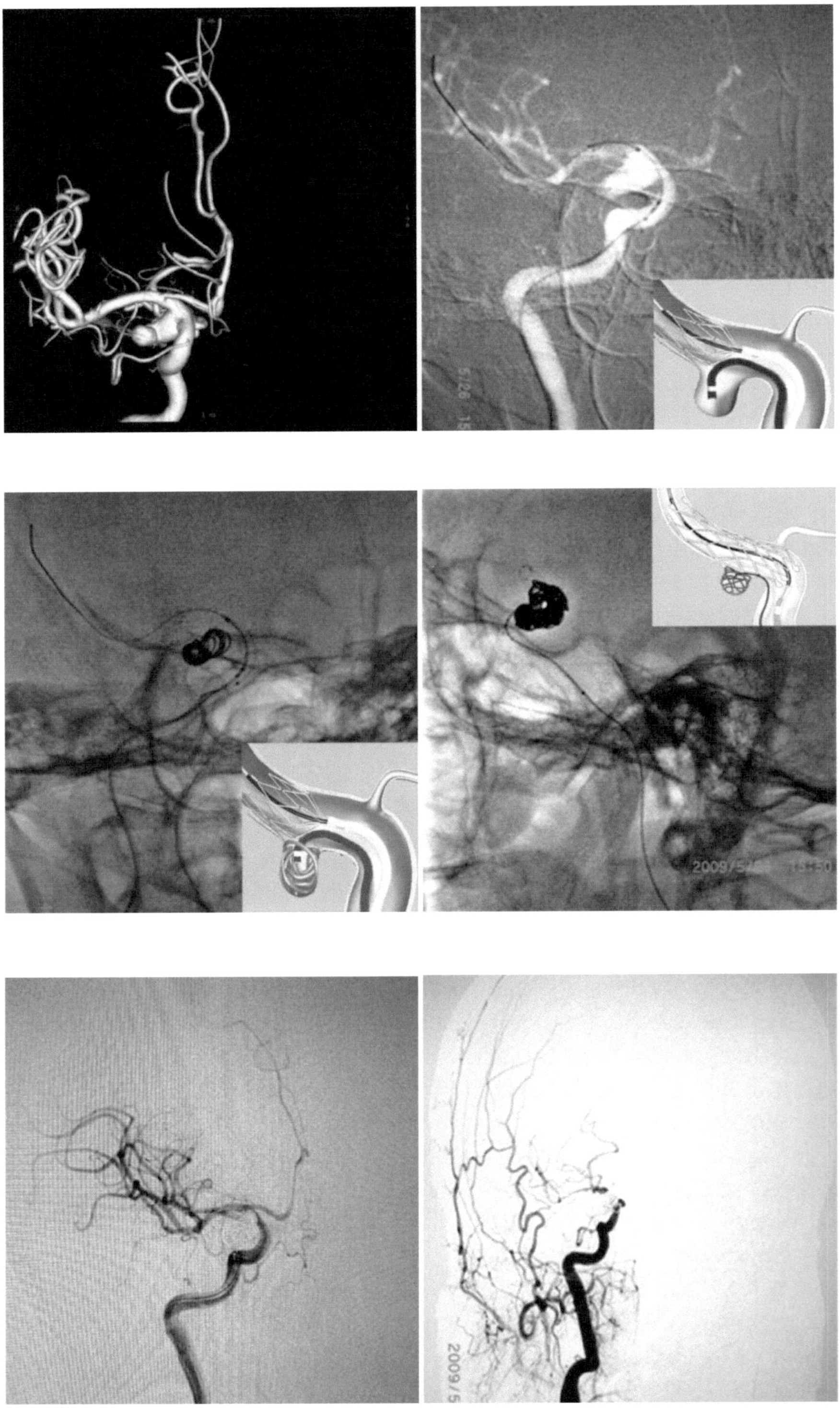

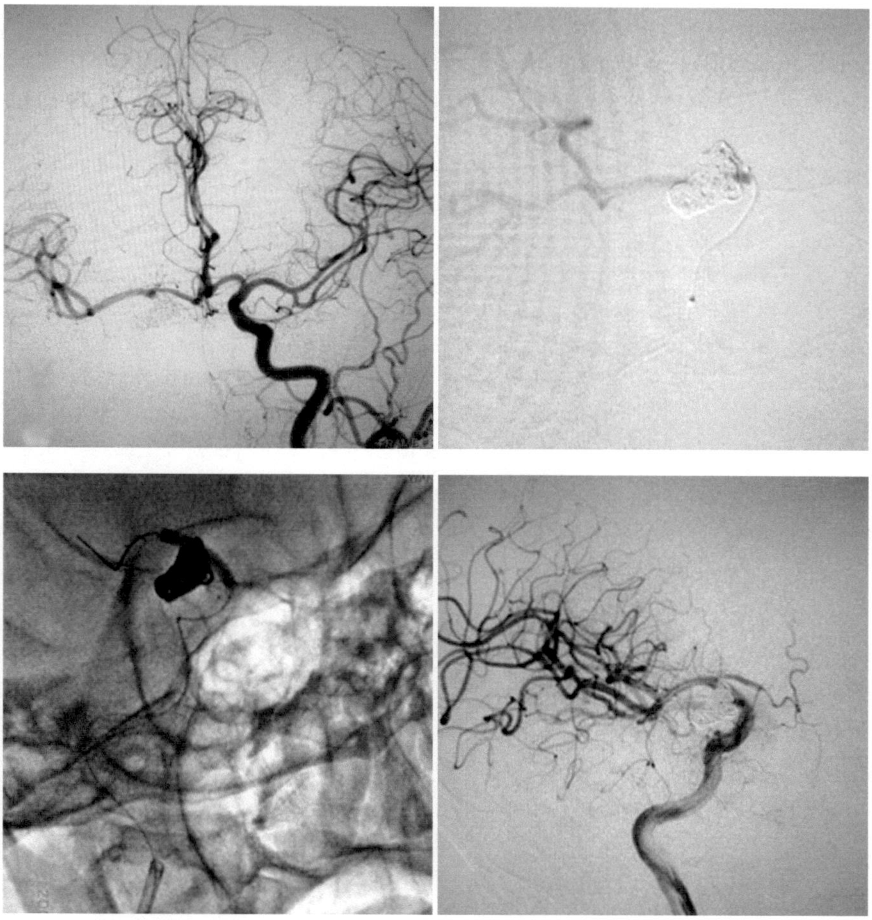

Figure 1. Three dimensional reconstruction (A) of the right ICA in anteroposterior view demonstrated a posterior communicating artery aneurysm. The Neuroform stent delivery system was brought up over the exchange microguidewire to cross the aneurysm neck. The stent was partly deployed to narrow the aneurysm neck after aneurysm catheterization (B). Homogeneous coil framing was achieved without coil prolapse by the limitation of the partially-deployed stent. (C). After several coils were placed, the stent was fully deployed and coiling continued using traditional jailing technique (D). Postprocedure angiogram (E) revealed complete occlusion. 13 months follow-up right common carotd artery angiogram (F) revealed high-grade stenosis within the stented segments of right ICA. Collateralisation was seen over the anterior communicating artery from the left side (G). Superselective angiogram (H) demonstrated that right ICA was not completely occluded. Then, balloon angioplasty of the right ICA was performed (I). Postangioplasty control angiography demonstrated substantial improvement in the caliber, but flow to right cerebral anterior artery was still delayed (J).

b. Stenting before coiling in a second session in 14 aneurysms (5.9%). The main reason for using this option was the difficulties of accessing the aneurysm for coiling after initial stent placement, especially when the parent artery was tortuous, or the aneurysm was small. The coiling procedure was usually performed from 1 to 2 months after the stenting procedure.

2. Stents were delivered after coiling in 31 of 237 aneurysms (13.1%).
   a. Stenting after coiling with balloon remodeling technique in 24 aneurysms. The choice of this option was to decrease the risk of thromboembolism complications in some partially thrombosed aneurysms.
   b. Bail-out stenting in 7 aneurysms. In these cases, the deployment of the stent was not planned in advance. Trapping of an extruded coil or coil mass by means of stent placement could prevent parent vessel closure and obviate the need for coil removal.
3. Stent was delivered alone in one aneurysm (0.4%). A 38-year-old woman with a basilar aneurysm was planned to treat with sequential technique. Because trans-stent aneurysm catheterization was difficult and caused stent movement, coil embolization was postponed to a second session. Fortunately, intraaneurysmal spontaneous thrombosis was noted by angiography 3 months later, and coiling was no more an option for her. Complete occlusion was observed at 1-year follow-up angiography (Figure 2).

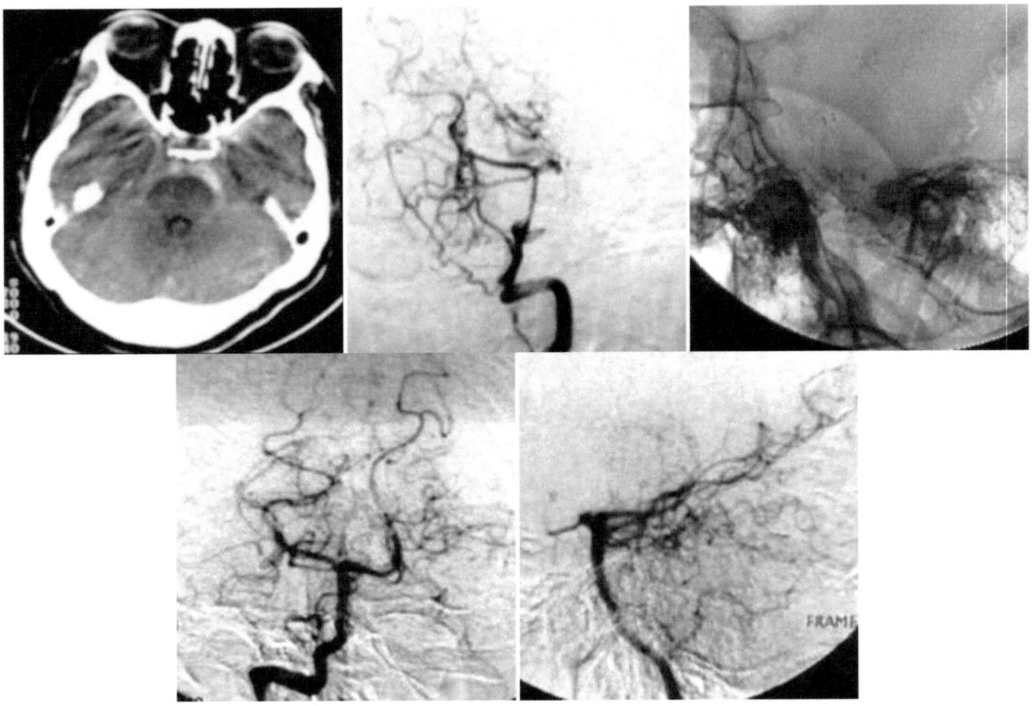

Figure 2. Angiography demonstrated a basilar trunk aneurysm in a 38-year-old woman with SAH (A B). A Neuroform stent (4.5 × 20 mm) was deployed across the aneurysm neck, and coil embolization was postponed to a second session due to difficulty in trans-stent aneurysm catheterization (C). One-year follow-up angiography demonstrated complete occlusion (D E).

2.4. Data collection

All patients underwent CT scanning within 6 hours after the procedure. During the hospital stays, physicians performed neurological examinations of the patients once each day. After discharge, clinical follow-up data were collected by clinic visitation, follow-up angiography, or telephone interview. Clinical outcome was graded according to modified Rankin score (mRS), as follows: excellent (mRS 0-1), good (mRS 2), poor (mRS 3-4) and death (mRS 5). For each patient, 6 months, 1 year, 3 year and 5 year follow-up angiogram were recommended. The pre-embolization, post-embolization and follow-up (if possible) angiograms were reviewed and compared by 2 senior endovascular neurosurgeons not involved in the procedure for initial and follow-up occlusion grade, which was classified as class 1: complete occlusion (no contrast filling the aneurysmal sac); class 2: neck remnant (residual contrast filling the aneurysmal neck); class 3: residual flow (residual contrast filling the aneurysmal body). [5] Recanalization was defined as more than 10 % increase in contrast filling of the aneurysm; less than 10 % increased filling was defined as unchanged. [6]

Angiographic results and clinical outcome were evaluated. Cases with complications were analyzed, including radiological findings, clinical presentations, management experience and clinical sequelae.

2.5. Statistical analysis

SPSS 11.0 software (SPSS, Inc, Chicago, IL) was used for statistical analysis. A chi-square test was used to compare the incidences of intraprocedural rupture and thromboembolic complications between ruptured unruptured aneurysms and to compare the incidences of complete occlusion rate between different stenting strategies.

3. Results

3.1. Angiographic results

Immediate angiographic results of the 236 aneurysms treated with stent-assited coiling are summarized in Table 2.

		class 1	class 2	class 3
Overall	236	162	45	29
Small	162	128	21	13
Large	41	22	11	8
Giant	33	12	13	8
Ruptured	128	82	26	18
Unruptured	108	80	19	11
Overall (%)	236	162(68.6)	45(19.1)	29(12.3)

Table 2. Immediate angiographic occlusion classification

Aneurysm occlusion rate was analyzed in relation to different stenting techniques, bail-out stenting cases excluded. Stenting before coiling was performed in 205 aneurysms and angiographic results showed class 1 occlusion in 142 (69.3%) aneurysms, class 2 in 39

(19.0%) aneurysms, and class 3 in 24 (11.7%) aneurysms. Stenting after balloon-assisted coiling was performed in 24 aneurysms and angiographic results showed class 1 occlusion in 19 (79.2%) aneurysms, class 2 in 3 (12.5%) aneurysms, and class 3 in 2 (8.3%) aneurysms. On comparative analysis of stenting before coiling versus stenting after balloon-assisted coiling, the complete occlusion rate did not show statistical difference (P=0.315, X^2 test).

3.2. Procedure-related complications

Of the total of 239 procedures for 232 patients, 34 procedural complications occurred, of which 26 were in the anterior circulation and 8 in the posterior circulation. Table 3 summarizes the procedural complications. Procedure-related morbidity and mortality were 4.2% and 1.3%, respectively.

Complication	No sequela	Morbidity	Mortality	Total	Incidence(%)
Thomboembolism	8	4	1	13	5.4
Intraprocedural rupture	3	3	2	8	3.3
Coil protrusion	5	0	0	5	2.1
New mass effect	1	2	0	3	1.3
Vessel injury	2	1	0	3	1.3
Stent dislodgement	2	0	0	2	0.8
Total	21	10	3	34	14.2

Note: Results include patients with more than one complication.

Table 3. Procedure-related complications in aneurysms

3.2.1. Thomboembolism

Thirteen periprocedual thromboembolic events occurred; 9 were in ruptured aneurysms and 4 in unruptured ones. Nine thromboembolic complications were evident during the procedure, and four were clinically and angiographically noted after the procedure. Complete or partial recanalization was achieved in 9 cases by local or systemic administration of abciximab or urokinase and mechanical disruption of clot with microwire immediately. On last follow-up, eight patients completely recovered, two patients developed residual mild neurological deficit and independent daily activity, and two patients developed hemiplegia and became dependent. A 68-year-old woman with ruptured PcomA aneurysm (Hunt-Hess grade I) developed right hemiparesis six hours after the procedure. A thrombus in the distal stent segment of right ICA was confirmed by angiography and the left cerebral hemisphere infarction was noted by MRI. She developed severe brain herniation eventually, and decompressive craniotomy failed to save her life.

3.2.2. Intraprocedural rupture

Intraprocedural aneurysmal rupture occurred in eight aneurysms due to coil extrusion (n=2), microcatheter protrusion (n=5), or inflation of the balloon (n=1): three in the PcomA, two in the ophthalmic artery, one in the AComA, one in the AchoA, and one in the basilar tip. All eight ruptures occurred during embolization of acutely ruptured small aneurysms, four of which occurred when coiling microcatheter accessed the aneurysm through the struts of the stent. All intraprocedural ruptures were managed with a protamine injection for heparin reversal and further coil embolization. External ventricular drainage (EVD) surgery was preformed in four cases with postprocedural Fisher grades of III or IV. Five of these ruptures resulted in adverse outcome (3 neurological sequelae, 2 death).

3.2.3. Coil protrusion

Coil protrusion occurred in five procedures, in four of which the last several loops of a small coil (diameter 2 mm) in part protruded through the interstice after detachment, and in one of which the coil was unraveled when a second stent-assisted coiling was performed on a 71-year-old female with bilateral PComA aneurysms. During positioning of the third coil (3 mm × 6 cm), the microcatheter was repelled from the aneurysm from the aneurysm into the parent vessel, and it was noted that the trailing end of the coil was unraveled, with several loops in the parent vessel, which affected the blood flow. After attempts to pull back the coil or to replace the coil failed, a balloon catheter was introduced into the guiding catheter, and the trailing end of the coil was caged in the guiding catheter by inflation of the balloon. Then the coil was stretched into the aorta. Fortunately, none of these patients had sequela.

3.2.4. New mass effect

Cranial nerve III palsy occurred in three large PComA aneurysms, which thought to be the result of the compressive effect of a coiled aneurysm. Only one patient recovered under steroid therapy.

3.2.5. Vessel injury

Vessel injury occurred in three procedures. Two cases of small vessel dissections developed during balloon manipulations. Each involved the carotid siphon. Both dissections spontaneous healed on angiographic follow-up, with no clinical consequence. One case of intracranial hematoma was noted in a 67-year-old woman with a ruptured right PcomA aneurysm (Hunt-Hess grade II). She developed conscious disturbance about one hour after treatment. Intracranial CT showed 30 ml hematoma in the right ipsilateral fissure, most probably due to MCA injury with the microguidewire used for stent introducement. Surgical evacuation was performed and she discharged with mild hemiparesis.

3.2.6. Stent dislodgement

Stent dislodgement during treatment occurred in two procedures: one caused by aneurysm catheterization through the stent struts and the other caused by retrieving the coiling catheter jailed between the stent and vessel wall. In the former case, the stent still covered the aneurysm neck and embolization was completed successfully. In the latter case, the coil mass partially herniated to the parent artery, which blocked the blood flow, during treatment for a left paraclinoid ICA aneurysm. Fortunately, we did not pull back the exchange microwire over which the stent delivery system was brought up. Another Neuroform stent (4.5 × 30 mm) was advanced through that exchange microwire and successfully deployed across the aneurysm neck. The herniated coil mass was pushed back against the vessel wall, and complete flow recanalization was achieved, with no clinical consequence (Figure 3).

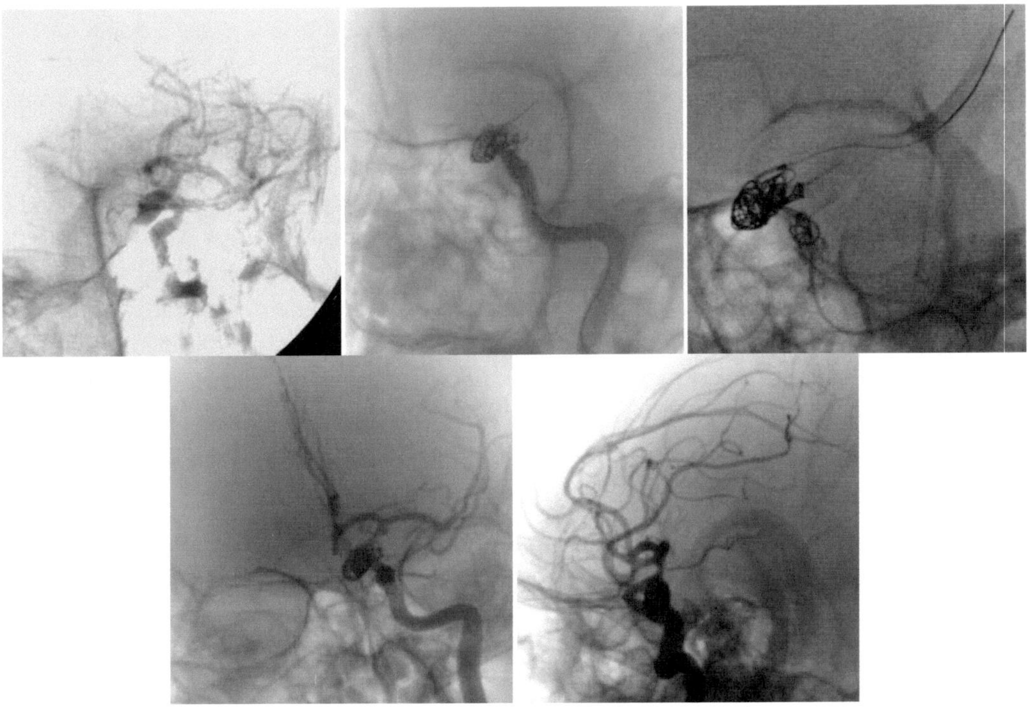

Figure 3. Angiography showed a left paraclinoid ICA aneurysm in a 62-year-female (A). Retrieving the coiling catheter jailed between the stent and vessel wall caused Enterprise stent dislodgement and the coil mass partially herniated to the parent artery, which blocked the blood flow (B). A Neuroform stent (4.5 × 30 mm) was advanced through the exchange microwire and successfully deployed across the aneurysm neck to push back the coil mass against the vessel wall (C). Frontal and lateral angiogram (D E) showed complete flow recanalization of the parent artery and class2 occlusion of the aneurysm.

3.3. Nonprocedural complications attributable to SAH

3.3.1. Vasospasm

Though all 129 patients with SAH were managed with systemic administration of Nimodipine and/or lumbar drainage of cerebrospinal fluid, twenty-four (18.6%) had systematic vasospasm, resulting in five cases of parent artery occlusion during the procedure. one aneurysm was located at AComA, Two at PcomA, and two at basilar tip. They were managed with local administration of Nimodipine 3mg and narceine 30mg immediately. Three patients resolved well after administration and had no deficit. In a 58-year-old woman with ruptured basilar tip aneurysm (Hunt-Hess grade Ⅲ), after a successful stent deployment vasospasm was noted in the basilar trunk. After immediate management, angiogram showed vasospasm completely resolved. However, she did not recover from the transient ischemia. Fellow-up MR showed infarct in the pons. Eventually, she discharged to a skilled nursing facility, not cognitively able to participate in her care. In a 70-year-old man with ruptured left paraclinoid ICA aneurysm (Hunt-Hess grade Ⅲ), vasospasm was noted in the left supraclinoid ICA during post-procedure angiography. After immediate management, angiogram showed vasospasm completely resolved. However, decreased level of consciousness occurred 24 hours later after the treatment. CT scan showed left cerebral hemisphere infarction. Cerebral angiography revealed diffuse severe bilateral anterior and posterior circulation vasospasm. An emergent decompressive craniotomy was performed. This patient had a long recovery with right hemiplegia and expressive aphasia, and then discharged to a skilled nursing facility.

3.3.2. *Hydrocephalus*

Of the 129 patients with SAH, nine (6.9%) had shunt-dependent hydrocephalus. All these nine patents received EVD only. One poor-grade patient died of the initial effect of SAH, and other patients recovered gradually. no patients developed chronic hydrocephalus at clinical follow-up.

3.4. Clinical outcome

Three patients died of procedure-related complications, and eight patients with acute SAH (high Hunt-Hess grade) died because of the severity of their initial hemorrhage during hospitalization. All other 221 patients were clinically evaluated. Clinical follow-up was obtained from < 1 month to 81 months with a mean of 57.7 months. The mRS score was excellent in 167 patients, good in 38 patients, and poor in 11 patients at last follow-up. Five died of other diseases. No rehemorrhage of treated aneurysm occurred.

3.5. Follow-up complications

3.5.1. *Aneurysm recanalization*

Follow-up angiography was obtained using DSA or MRA in 155 patients with 159 treated aneurysms. Angiographic follow-up was obtained from 3 to 62 months, with a mean of 39.2 months. 131 of the 155 patients (84.5 %) had >1 year follow-up. The main reasons that patients were lost to follow-up were the patients' refusal to return, economical problem and travel distance. In these 159 angiographic followed aneurysms, the follow-up angiograms of 23 aneurysms (14.5 % of the follow-up angiograms) demonstrated recanalization (Table 4). Of note, 8/22 (36.4 %) class 2 and class 3 aneurysms converted to class 1 on last follow-up. Seventeen of these aneurysms underwent successful re-embolization. The other six patients' angiogram showed an increasing remnant neck on the first follow-up examination, but the subsequent follow-up angiogram showed a stable appearance. Therefore, re-embolization was not a treatment option for them. No symptomatic procedural complications were seen in the retreatment.

Aneurysm size	Recanalized
Small	9/102
Large	6/31
Giant	8/26
Overall	23/159(14.5)
Immediate aneurysm result	**Recanalized (%)**
Class 1	9 /108
Class 2	9/32
Class 3	5 /19
Overall	23/159 (14.5)

Table 4. Recanalization rates

3.5.2. Chronic effect on parent artery

In-stent stenosis was confirmed in two patients by follow-up angiography. In a 45-year-old man, after stent-assisted coiling of a VB aneurysm, delayed in-stent stenosis was seen at 3-month follow-up but had resolved spontaneously at 12-month follow-up. Fortunately, he patient had no symptom. In a 65-year-old man, a 4.5 mm x15 mm Neuroform stent was deployed in the paraclinoid and communicating segments of right ICA to treat a PcomA aneurysm. High-grade stenosis within the stented segments of right ICA was present 13 months after the procedure. He suffered from a mild left hemiparesis. In view of the severity of the stenosis and symptoms while on aspirin, balloon angioplasty of the right ICA was performed. Postangioplasty control angiography demonstrated substantial improvement in the caliber and the patient recovered fully (Figure 1).

One patient developed ophthalmic artery occlusion 6 months after the procedure in whom the ophthalmic artery origin was bridged with the stent. Fortunately no clinical problem occurred because of the reconstruction of the ophthalmic artery via external carotid artery collaterals.

A case of Déjérine syndrome occurred in a 52-year-old woman with a VB junction aneurysm treated by stent-assisted coiling eight month after the procedure. She suffered from vertigo, bilateral deep sensory disturbance and right mild hemiparasis. Diffusion-weighted MRI demonstrated increased signal in the medial medulla. The mechanism was suggested that unusually aggressive neointimal response to the stent resulted in occlusion of a small penetrating artery from the stented segment of the vertebral artery, though direct evidence was not found by angiography. (Figure 4)

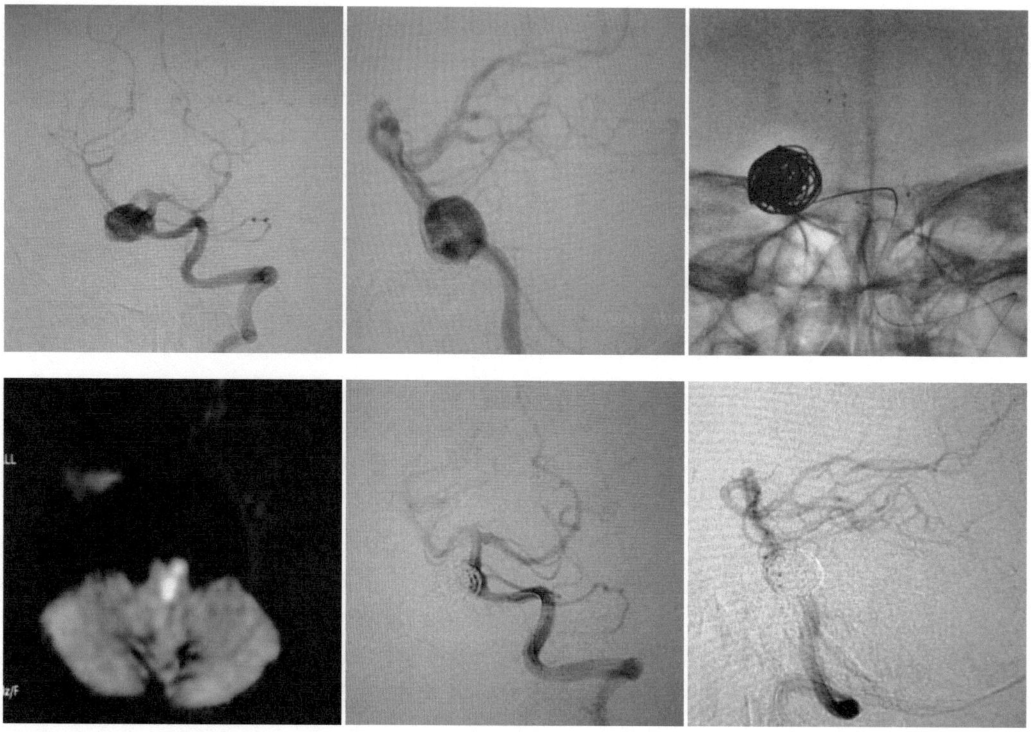

Figure 4. Frontal and lateral angiogram (A B) showed VB junction aneurysm in a 52-year-old woman. Complete occlusion was achieved by stent-assisted coiling (Neuroform 4.5mm x30mm) (C). Diffusion-weighted MRI demonstrated increased signal in the medial medulla eight month after the procedure (D). Fowllow-up angiogram demonstrated that the stented segment of the parent artery appeared intact, with no evidence of dissection or in-stent stenosis (E F).

3.5.3. Hemorrhagic events

No rehemorrhage of treated aneurysm occurred. One 73-year-old male died of contralateral putaminal hemorrhage 7 months after discharge. Though he had a history of hypertension for nearly 20 years, posttreatment antiplatelet might be a precipitating factor.

3.6. Incidences of thromboembolism and intraprocedural rupture in ruptured vs unruptured aneurysms

All 8 intraprocedual ruptures, and 9 of 13 thromboembolic events were in the SAH group. The incidence of intraprocedural rupture and thromboembolism were 6.2% and 6.9%, respectively, in the ruptured group and 0% and 3.6%, respectively, in the unruptured group. There was a statistically significant difference in the incidence of intraprocedural rupture between two groups (P =0.008). The incidence comparison for thromboembolism between these groups, however, gave a P value of 0.256.

4. Discussion

Endovascular and surgical treatment of wide-neck and fusiform intracranial aneurysms has remained technically challenging. Stent-assisted aneurysm embolization is a new tool in the treatment of intracranial aneurysms and maybe particularly useful in the case of wide-necked or dissecting aneurysm. The earliest clinical report of stent-assisted coiling of an intracranial ruptured cerebral aneurysm is by Higashida et al, in 1997[2]. From then on, with improvements in microstent technology, more reports from various centers describing the experimental and clinical use of different stents for embolization assistance has reported good results in the literature.[7-13] Up till now, several literatures have demonstrated the technical feasibility, efficacy of treating complicated intracranial aneurysms. [14-17] The stent can provide a permanent scaffold across the aneurysm neck, which may prevent coil prolapse into the parent artery and allow for safer packing of the aneurysm with a denser coil mesh. In addition, the stent may help prevent recanalization by hemodynamic changes and stent endothelialization. [17]However, as a new device, there is limited knowledge about the complications and the long-term effects of the stent on the cerebrovasculature.

We have found that the overall procedure-related complication, morbidity and mortality were 14.2 %, 4.2 % and 1.3 %, respectively, and that a cumulative excellent or good clinical outcome rate is 88.3 %, which reflect better outcome than open surgical series. Most of our complication cases were treated during the first half of our experience period.

4.1. Ischemic events

Ischemic event is a significant problem in periprocedural period. Usually, thromboembolism is the main cause of ischemic event. [18] Park observed nine thromboembolic events among 27 complications during coiling of 118 ruptured aneurysms.[19] The acute or subacute thrombogenicity of endovascular stents also represents an important limitation with respect to the treatment of aneurysms and appears to be the main drawback of stent-assisted coil embolization. [20-24] According to these literatures, incidence of thromboembolic event ranged from 4.2 to 17.1%. In our series, we observed a relatively low rate of thromboembolic events (5.4%), with 1.6% morbidity and 0.4% mortality. Our findings suggest stent-assisted coiling does not increase the risk of thromboemblism with proper management, which is similar to those of some reports. [18]This low rate of thromboembolic events has been achieved with enough heparinisation, dual pre- and postoperative antiplatelet therapy, shorten duration of endovascular manipulation, and sufficient prevention from injection of embolus into circulation. Additionally, the use of bioactive coils (e.g. Matrix coil) in conjunction with the stent should be avoided. Partially thrombosed aneurysms can be coiled using the balloon remodeling technique, and then the stent is delivered across the aneurysm neck at the end of the procedure. Once thromboembolism is noted, local intra-artery administration of abciximab or urokinase and mechanical disruption of clot with microwire are necessary. Sometimes mechanical dilation with balloon angioplasty can be performed.

Delayed in-stent stenosis is likely a rare event. Biondi et al [16] reported one (2.4%) asymptomatic stenosis of the parent artery at the proximal end of the stent, which was observed on follow-up angiography and successfully treated by angioplasty. Fiorella et al [25] reported a 5.8% rate (9 of 156 patients) of delayed moderate to severe (>50%) in-stent stenosis after 2 to 9 months, of which two patients needed retreatments to control ischemic symptoms. In our series, in-stent stenosis was confirmed in two patients, one of whom underwent angioplasty. The Wingspan study[26], reported a rate of in-stent stenosis of 29.7% and an additionally 4.8% of in-stent thrombosis after an average of 5.9 months on the treatment for symptomatic intracranial atheromatous disease. Endothelian disruption and denudation of the vascular wall during stenting in the absence of functional endothelium in an atheromatous vessel resulting in neointimal tissue formation may play an important role. This action is mediated by proliferation and activation of regional smooth muscle cells. It is unclear whether similar reaction is also responsible for delayed in-stent stenosis after the stent placement, which has much lower radial force, as an aneurysm neck bridging device covering the normal vessel wall. Additional follow-up will be critical to delineate the incidence of this phenomenon.

Delayed ischemic neurological deficit associated with vasospasm is a major cause of morbidity and mortality in patients with SAH. Symptomatic vasospasm is reported in 22–40% of patients with SAH, resulting in 34% morbidity and 30% mortality rates. [27-31] Murayama et al [32] reported a 23% incidence of symptomatic vasospasm after endovascular coil occlusion of acutely ruptured; this rate compares favorably with that found in conventional surgical series. Gruber et al[33], however, noted an increased incidence of vasospasm-related infarctions in patients treated endovascularly (37.7% vs. 21.6% with surgery). However, when patients with Fisher grade 4 and Hunt and Hess grade V lesions were excluded, the difference between the treatment groups was no longer significant. Other authors [19,34,35] have not found an increased risk of vasospasm with endovascular therapy as well. They concluded that the type of treatment was not associated with an increased risk of cerebral vasospasm. Rabinstein et al [36] studied 415 consecutive patients with aneurysmal SAH. Symptomatic vasospasm occurred in 39% treated with surgical clip placement and 30% treated with endovascular coil occlusion. In a univariate analysis, the incidence of vasospasm did not differ between the groups. In our study, the incidence of symptomatic vasospasm among 129 patients with SAH was 18.6%. It seems that the stent-assisted coiling does not increase the risk of symptomatic vasospasm, compared with open clipping and other endovascular techniques.

4.2. Stenting techniques

Different stategies regarding the timing of stent deployment in relation to coiling are practiced. In majority of reports, stenting was performed before coiling in the same session, including the sequential technique and the jailing technique.[9, 20-22] The strategy of stenting after balloon-assisted coiling is less frequently reported. [21, 16] In our series, several main options were practiced and the strategy of stenting before coiling was predominantly used.

On comparative analysis of stenting before coiling versus stenting after balloon-assisted coiling, the complete occlusion rate did not show significant difference ($P>0.05$, X^2 test). However, balloon remodeling technique have some drawbacks according to our experience (maybe bias). Coil mass herniation is sometimes a limitation of balloon-assisted coiling once the balloon is deflated or removed. Repeated inflation and deflation of the balloon may cause intimal damage[37], which has occurred in our series. Furthermore, balloon inflation, which results in complete blood flow arrest in the parent artery, can increases the risk of thromboembolic events[38, 39], although this is still controversial. In our series, a novel stent-assisted coiling technique, the semi-deployment technique, was used in 31 aneurysms. Compared to the conventional techniques, this technique has several advantages. First, it increases maneuverability of the coiling catheter, allowing more controlled coil positioning. Second, the coil basket can be optimized and there is less likelihood for coil migration when the aneurysm neck is narrowed by the partially deployed stent. Last, it decreases the risk of the stent herniating into the aneurysm in treatment of large or giant aneurysm. Nevertheless, further experience is necessary to determine complication rate and suitable selection of patients to different strategies.

4.3. Dual antiplatelet regimen

There are controversial reports about benefit of the dual antiplatelet therapy. [40, 41] The optimal regimen has not yet been defined. It is intuitive that the aneurysms are fragile and parent vessels are less healthy in patients in the acute phase of SAH. A meta-analysis of published reports, from retrospective data has also suggested the risk of intraprocedure rupture is significantly higher in patients with ruptured aneurysms. Our data suggest that the incidence of intraprocedual rupture is significantly higher in patients with ruptured aneurysm ($P<0.01$), and the incidence of thromboembolism between those with and without ruptured aneurysms is not statistically significant. This finding may advocate for a more cautious preprocedural antiplatelet treatment for patients with ruptured aneurysms. Katsaridis V has reported a very low thromboembolic complication rate (1.8%) in the Neuroform2 stent-assisted embolization of 54 aneurysms without antiplatelet pretreatment.[40] In our practice, it is after general anesthesia that dual antiplatelet treatment (aspirin 300 mg and clopidogrel 225 mg via nasogastric tube) initiates for accurately ruptured aneurysms.

Because of a prolonged posttreatment antiplatelet regimen, if there is any evidence that the patient will need EVD surgery due to SAH, this should be done before interventional therapy. On the basis of our experience, this might not only prevent fatal increase of intracranial pressure, but might also reduce subsequent bleeding complications if the patient is on a strong anticoagulation and antiplatelet regimen. However, in our series, a total of seven patients underwent additional emergent surgical treatment after interventional therapy. Five patients received EVD and two patients underwent decompressive craniotomy. Protamine chloride and minirin were used to reverse the anticoagulation and antiplatelet drugs before surgery. Fortunately, there were no surgical complications or special difficulties due to abnormal intraoperative bleeding during the operation. Taking into account relatively more ischemic events, a more aggressive anticoagulation and antiplatelet therapy should be used after the procedure.

In our opinion, the risk of periprocedual antiplatelet therapy should be weighed against the potential benefit and that antiplatelet and anticoagulation therapy should be tailored according to the results of ongoing researches.

4.4. Aneurysm recanalization

The goal of aneurysm treatment should be permanent exclusion of the aneurysm from the circulatory system to prevent rupture or rerupture. Aneurysm recanalization must be acknowledged as a failure to achieve this goal. However, not a single one of treated aneurysms experienced rehemorrhage during the follow-up time, in our series, despite incomplete occlusion and recanalization. Lylyk et al reported that follow-up was obtained in 63% of their patients and stressed that there were no cases of repeated hemorrhage.[21] Biondi et al [16] also reported that no aneurysm bled after stent-assisted coiling during the follow-up period, though complete or subtotal aneurysm occlusion was not always obtained. Based on these results, we therefore conclude that the risk of rupture after occlusion of aneurysms may be substantially reduced. Aneurysm follow-up angiography and reembolization, if necessary, still should be done, though. Fiorella et al [22] reported initial (3-6 mo) angiographic follow-up in 58% of aneurysms treated with Stent-assisted coiling showing progressive thrombosis in 52% of patients, recanalization in 23%, and no change in 25%. In the series of Biondi et al [16], recanalization was observed in 13% of wide-neck aneurysms treated with stent-assisted coiling. We observed 23 cases (14.5%) of aneurysm recanalization on follow-up angiograms, which was acceptable compared with most publications. In our experience, the recanalization rate of none-stented wide-neck aneurysms is high. Murayama et al reported that the overall recanalization rate of coiling without stenting was 20.9%.[6] A stent placed across the aneurysm neck may prevent recanalization because of the hemodynamic changes and stent endothelialization. The stent is used not only to assist in coil delivery, but also to prevent recanalization. In our series 60.9% (14/23) of the recanalized aneurysms were not initially completely occluded (class2 or class3) and no recanalization occurred in small aneurysms which was completely occluded. Therefore, sequential follow-up angiograms are mandatory, especially for those aneurysms showing incomplete occlusion. In our series, no adverse events were shown on follow-up angiograms or occurred during retreatment with detachable coils. Recently, Renowden et al [42] and Henkes et al [43] reported complication rates of 2% to 3% in their large series of retreatment of previously embolized aneurysms. Follow-up procedures can be done safely, and the risk from retreatment with detachable coils does not negate the advantages of initial use of coil embolization. During initial treatment discussions, patients should aware that wide-neck aneurysms, especially large and giant ones, may require multiple treatment and will certainly require a significant course of long-term follow-up.

5. Conclusion

Our study indicates that stent-assisted coil embolization of intracranial aneurysm is a safe technique with low morbidity and mortality rates. Our results are consistent with those reported in the literature (Table 5). The main cause of morbidity and mortality is thromboembolism (38.2% of all procedure-related complications are thromboembolic in our study). In our hand, this technique does not increase the risk of symptomatic vasospasm, compared with open clipping and other endovascular techniques. The recanalization rate is relatively low. The delayed in-stent stenosis seems a rare complication, compared to stent deployment in atherosclerotic lesions. Nevertheless, additional, large series with long-term follow-up are necessary to determine the durability of these promising results.

Series (ref no)	No of patients (aneurysms)	Rate
Fiorella et al. 2004 (15)	19 (22)	10.5% thromboembolism rate (10.5% thromboembolic morbidity)
dos Santos et al. 2005(17)	18 (17)	23.5% technical complication rate (5.8% morbidity)
Lee et al. 2005(23)	22 (23)	9.1% procedure-related complication rate
Akpek et al. 2005(20)	32 (35)	25% adverse event rate, 9.3% morbidity, 3.1% mortality
Lylyk et al. 2005(21)	50 (50)	8.6% morbidity, 2.1% mortality
Katsaridis et al. 2006(38)	44 (54)	4% stent-related complication rate
Biondi et al. 2007(16)	42 (46)	4.3% procedural morbidity, 2.2% procedural mortality
Yahia et al. 2008 (3)	67(67)	7.4% procedure-related complication rate
Mordasini et al. 2008 ([4]4)	18(18)	22.2% thromboembolism rate(no morbidity and mortality)
Wajnberg et al. 2009 (24)	24 (24)	4.2% procedure-related thromboembolism rate
Seadt J et al. 2009 (45)	42(42)	2.4% procedural morbidity

Table 5. Published complication rates for Neuroform stent-assisted coiling of intracranial aneurysms

Author details

Xu Gao and Guobiao Liang

Department of Neurosurgery, the General Hospital of Shenyang Military Command, Shenyang, P. R. China

6. References

[1] Wolstenholme J, Rivero-Arias O, Gray A, et al: Treatment pathways, resource use, and costs of endovascular coiling versus surgical clipping after aSAH. *Stroke* 39:111-119, 2008.

[2] Higashida RT, Smith W, Gress D, et al: Intravascular stent and endovascular coil placement for a ruptured fusiform aneurysm of the basilar artery. Case report and review of the literature. *J Neurosurg* 87: 944-949, 1997.

[3] Yahia AM, Gordon V, Whapham J, Malek A, Steel J, Fessler RD: Complications of Neuroform stent in endovascular treatment of intracranial aneurysms. *Neurocrit Care* 8:19-30, 2008.

[4] Yahia AM, Latorre J, Gordon V, Whapham J, Malek A, Fessler RD: Thromboembolic events associated with Neuroform stent in endovascular treatment of intracranial aneurysms. *J Neuroimaging* 20:113-117, 2010.

[5] Roy D, Milot G, Raymond J: Endovascular treatment of unruptured aneurysms. *Stroke* 32:1998-2004, 2001.

[6] Murayama Y, Nien YL, Duckwiler G, et al: Guglielmi detachable coil embolization of cerebral aneurysms: 11 years' experience. *J Neurosurg* 98:959-966 ,2003.

[7] Mericle RA, Lanzino G, Wakhloo AK, Guterman LR, Hopkins LN. Stenting and secondary coiling of intracranial internal carotid artery aneurysm: technical case report. *Neurosurgery* 43:1229-1234, 1998.

[8] Sekhon LH, Morgan MK, Sorby W, Grinnell V: Combined endovascular stent implantation and endosaccular coil placement for the treatment of a wide-necked vertebral artery aneurysm: technical case report. *Neurosurgery* 43:380-383, 1998.

[9] Lownie SP, Pelz DM, Fox AJ: Endovascular therapy of a large vertebral artery aneurysm using stent and coils. *Can J Neurol Sci*27:162-165, 2000.

[10] Barras CD, Myers KA. Nitinol: its use in vascular surgery and other applications. *Eur J Vasc Endovasc Surg* 19:564-569, 2000.

[11] Mocco J, Snyder KV, Albuquerque FC, et al: Treatment of intracranial aneurysms with the Enterprise stent: a multicenter registry. *J Neurosurg* 110:35-39, 2009.

[12] Lv X, Li Y, Jiang C, Yang X, Wu Z: Potential advantages and limitations of the Leo stent in endovascular treatment of complex cerebral aneurysms. *Eur J Radiol* 2010; [Epub ahead of print].

[13] Lubicz B, Collignon L, Raphaeli G, Bandeira A, Bruneau M, De Witte O: Solitaire stent for endovascular treatment of intracranial aneurysms: immediate and mid-term results in 15 patients with 17 aneurysms. *J Neuroradiol*37:83-88, 2010.

[14] Liang G, Gao X, Li Z, Wei X, Xue H: Neuroform stent-assisted coiling of intracranial aneurysms: a 5 year single-center experience and follow-up. *Neurol Res* 32: 721-727, 2010.

[15] Fiorella D, Albuquerque FC, Han P, McDougall CG: Preliminary experience using the Neuroform stent for the treatment of cerebral aneurysms. *Neurosurgery* 54:6-16, 2004.

[16] Biondi A, Janardhan V, Katz JM, Salvaggio K, Riina HA, Gobin YP: Neuroform stent-assisted coil embolization of wide-neck intracranial aneurysms: strategies in stent deployment and midterm follow-up. *Neurosurgery* 61:460-468, 2007.

[17] dos Santos Souza MP, Agid R, Willinsky RA, et al: Microstent-assisted coiling for wide-necked intracranial aneurysms. *Can J Neurol Sci* 32:71-81, 2005.

[18] Ross IB, Dhillon GS: Complications of endovascular treatment of cerebral aneurysms. *Surg Neuro l*64:12-18, 2005.

[19] Park HK, Horowitz M, Jungreis C, et al: Periprocedural morbidity and mortality associated with endovascular treatment of intracranial aneurysms. *AJNR Am J Neuroradiol* 26:506-514, 2005.

[20] Akpek S, Arat A, Morsi H, Klucznick RP, Strother CM, Mawad ME: Self-expandable stent-assisted coiling of wide-necked intracranial aneurysms: A single-center experience. *AJNR Am J Neuroradiol* 26:1223–1231, 2005.

[21] Lylyk P, Ferrario A, Pasbón B, Miranda C, Doroszuk G: Buenos Aires experience with the Neuroform self-expanding stent for the treatment of intracranial aneurysms. *J Neurosurg* 102:235–241, 2005.

[22] Fiorella D, Albuquerque FC, Deshmukh VR, McDougall CG: Usefulness of the Neuroform stent for the treatment of cerebral aneurysms: Results at initial (3–6-mo) follow-up. *Neurosurgery* 56:1191–1201, 2005.

[23] Lee YJ, Kim DJ, Suh SH, Lee SK, Kim J, Kim DI: Stent-assisted coil embolization of intracranial wide-necked aneurysms. *Neuroradiology* 47:680-689, 2005.

[24] Wajnberg E, de Souza JM, Marchiori E, Gasparetto EL: Single-center experience with the Neuroform stent for endovascular treatment of wide-necked intracranial aneurysms. *Surg Neurol* 72:612-9, 2009

[25] Fiorella D, Albuquerque FC, Woo H, Rasmussen PA, Masaryk TJ, McDougall CG: Neuroform in-stent stenosis: incidence, natural history, and treatment strategies. *Neurosurgery* 59:34–42, 2006.

[26] Levy EI, Turk AS, Albuquerque FC, et al: Wingspan in-stent restenosis and thrombosis: incidence, clinical presentation, and management. *Neurosurgery* 61:644–50, 2007.

[27] Kassell NF, Torner JC, Haley EC, Jane JA, Adams HP, Kongable G: The International Cooperative Study on the Timing of Aneurysm Surgery, I: overall management results. *J Neurosurg* 73:18–36, 1990.

[28] Adams HP Jr, Kassell NF, Torner JC, Haley EC Jr: Predicting cerebral ischemia after aneurysmal subarachnoid hemorrhage: Influences of clinical condition, CT results, and antifibrinolytic therapy—a report of the Cooperative Aneurysm Study. *Neurology* 37:1586–1591, 1987.

[29] Dorsch NWC, King MT: A review of cerebral vasospasm in aneurismal subarachnoid hemorrhage, I: incidence and effects. *J Clin Neurosci* 1:19–26, 1994.

[30] Ljunggren B, Brandt L, Sundbarg G, Saveland H, Cronqvist S, Stridbeck H: Early management of aneurysmal subarachnoid hemorrhage. *Neurosurgery* 11:412–418, 1982.

[31] Taneda M: Effect of early operation for ruptured aneurysms on prevention of delayed ischemic symptoms. *J Neurosurg* 57: 622–628, 1982.

[32] Murayama Y, Malisch T, Guglielmi G, et al: Incidence of cerebral vasospasm after endovascular treatment of acutely ruptured aneurysms: report on 69 cases. *J Neurosurg* 87:830–835, 1997.

[33] Gruber A, Ungersbo¨ck K, Reinprecht A, et al: Evaluation of cerebral vasospasm after early surgical and endovascular treatment of ruptured intracranial aneurysms. *Neurosurgery*42:258–268, 1998.

[34] Charpentier C, Audibert G, Guillemin Civit T, et al: Multivariate analysis of predictors of cerebral vasospasm occurrence after aneurysmal subarachnoid hemorrhage. *Stroke* 30:1402–1408, 1999.

[35] Yalamanchili K, Rosenwasser RH, Thomas JE, Liebman K, McMorrow C, Gannon P: Frequency of cerebral vasospasm in patients treated with endovascular occlusion of intracranial aneurysms. *AJNR Am J Neuroradiol* 19:553–558,1998.

[36] Rabinstein AA, Pichelmann MA, Friedman JA, et al: Symptomatic vasospasm and outcomes following aneurysmal subarachnoid hemorrhage: A comparison between surgical repair and endovascular coil occlusion. *J Neurosurg* 98:319–325, 2003.

[37] Mu SQ, Yang XJ, Li YX, Zhang YP, Lü M, Wu ZX: Endovascular treatment of wide-necked intracranial aneurysms using of "remodeling technique" with the HyperForm balloon. *Chinese Medical Journal* 121:725-729, 2008.

[38] Sluzewski M, van Rooij WJ, Beute GN, Nijssen PC: Balloon-assisted coil embolization of intracranial aneurysms: Incidence, complications, and angiography results. *J Neurosurg* 105:396–399, 2006.

[39] Soeda A, Sakai N, Sakai H, et al: Thromboembolic events associated with Guglielmi detachable coil embolization of asymptomatic cerebral aneurysms: Evaluation of 66 consecutive cases with use of diffusion-weighted MR imaging. *AJNR Am J Neuroradiol* 24:127–132, 2003.

[40] Albiero R, Hall P, Itoh A, et al: Result of a consecutive series of patients receiving only antiplatelet therapy after optimized stent implantation. comparison of aspirin alone versus combined ticlopidine and aspirin therapy. *Circulation* 95:1145-1156, 1997.

[41] Katsaridis V, Papagiannaki C, Violaris C: Embolization of acutely ruptured and unruptured wide-necked cerebral aneurysms using the neuroform2 stent without pretreatment with antiplatelets: a single center experience. *AJNR Am J Neuroradiol* 27:1123-1128, 2006.

[42] Renowden SA, Koumellis P, Benes V, Mukonoweshuro W, Molyneux AJ, McConachie NS: Retreament of previously embolized cerebral aneurysms: the risk of further embolization does not negate the advantage of the initil embolization. *AJNR Am J Neuroradiol* 29: 1401-1404, 2008.

[43] Henkes H, Fischer S, Liebig T, et al: Repeated endovascular coil occlusion in 350 of 2759 intracranial aneurysms: safety and effectiveness aspects. *Neurosurgery* 62:1532-1537, 2008.

[44] Mordasini P, Walser A, Gralla J, et al: Stent placement in the endovascular treatment of intracranial aneurysms. *Swiss Med Wkly* 138:646-54, 2008.

[45] Sedat J, Chau Y, Mondot L, Vargas J, Szapiro J, Lonjon M: Endovascular occlusion of intracranial wide-necked aneurysms with stenting (Neuroform) and coiling: mid-term and long-term results. *Neuroradiology* 51:401-409, 2009.

Chapter 14

Stent-Assisted Techniques for Intracranial Aneurysms

Igor Lima Maldonado and Alain Bonafé

Additional information is available at the end of the chapter

http://dx.doi.org/10.5772/51295

1. Introduction

The aim of this chapter is to present the current state of stent-assisted techniques for the treatment of intracranial aneurysms. Most of the information that is presented here is based on recent international literature, as well as the personal experience of the authors. It is illustrated with diagrams of key procedures. Since it is a technical chapter, the subject will be discussed from an operative point of view, and the topics will be presented in the order in which they would probably be approached by the operator: *background, indication, patient evaluation and preparation, equipment, operative technique, results, complications and post-operative management*.

2. History

In the early years of endovascular techniques, the main method for the treatment of wide-neck aneurysms was surgical. Attempts at embolization presented significant risks of coil herniation, migration, parent artery occlusion and poor mid-term morphological results with high recurrence rates. A great effort has been made by engineers and manufacturers to develop coils that present a better arrangement inside the aneurysm sac and fulfil two important conditions: a good apposition with the aneurysm wall, and a stable three-dimensional conformation, so that loops do not herniate through the aneurysm neck.

The first issue was approached by the development of coils with a geometry intended to fill the aneurysm sac, even if it is irregular. A good apposition with all regions of the cavity may improve the aneurysm embolization ratio and increase the stability of the coil mass, preventing migration. The second issue was approached through the development of coils with a memory of their three-dimensional shape, so that they may be used to create a relatively predictable cage that would keep the subsequent coils inside. As one may imagine, the above properties are relatively antagonistic. A coil that penetrates irregular spaces and has a good position to the aneurysm wall is also a coil that may herniate through a large aneurysm neck. In this context of technical difficulty, balloon and stent-assisted techniques have been used to provide protection for the parent artery as well as to treat coil mass herniation.

Intracranial stents also serve as scaffolding for neo-endothelization, providing additional reduction of the flow into the aneurysm. Consequently, their use improves intrasaccular thrombosis and decreases the risk of recanalization.

Even if these concepts seem attractive, manufacturers were rapidly confronted with technical difficulties, such as the narrowness and fragility of the intracranial vasculature, the need to navigate tortuous vessels, and the obligation to provide materials that were thin enough so that a microcatheter could be placed simultaneously in the vasculature.

The first case of intracranial stenting for treating a brain aneurysm was reported by Higashida et al. in 1997 (Higashida et al., 2005). In that occasion, the authors used a balloon-expandable cardiac stent in combination with Guglielmi detachable coils to treat a fusiform aneurysm of the vertebrobasilar junction. At that time, other authors had already attempted the placement of stent and coils in a fusiform aneurysm in an experimental context in pigs. Soon after, different groups reported a number of strategies using a combination of balloon-mounted stents and coils. In 2000, the use of stents for managing coil migration during the treatment of wide neck aneurysms was reported (Fessler et al., 2000, Lavine et al., 2000) and the case series became progressively larger.

The first stent specifically designed for the intracranial area to obtain Food and Drug Administration (FDA) approval was the Neuroform™ (Boston Scientific Corporation, Natick, USA). The device was approved for 'humanitarian device exemption' in 2002. This means that its use was complicit to the additional approval of an Institutional Review Board and was supposed to be limited to use on no more than 4000 individuals per year in the United States of America (USA).

Outside the USA, especially in Europe and in the context of clinical research, other stents became rapidly available. That was the case with the Leo™ (Balt, Montmorency, France), the first self-expanding closed cell design stent released in Europe in 2003, and then the Enterprise™ (Cordis Neurovascular I., Miami Lakes, USA), which was approved by the FDA in the US in 2007.

Flow diverters are the last technical advances bringing the concept of 'reverse remodeling' for intracranial aneurysm treatment. Silk™ (Balt, Montmorency, France) and Pipeline™ (Chestnut Medical Technologies Incorporation, Menlo Park, CA, USA) are in this category. These devices are intended to exclude the aneurysm sac from the parent artery by creating significant flow disruption, so that blood significantly stagnates inside the aneurysm sac and thromboses.

3. Indications

For treatment of intracranial aneurysms, stents are used mainly in two different situations: wide neck aneurysm and unfavourable anatomy. Wide neck aneurysm has been defined as a saccular aneurysm in the diameter of the neck larger than 4 mm, in which the dome–to-neck ratio is less than 2, or in which the ASPECT ration is superior to 1.6. These circumstances are associated with an increased risk of coil migration and compromising of parent artery patency during non-assisted endovascular coiling. Both situations are not uncommon with large and giant sacciform aneurysms. Circumstances for unfavourable anatomy are MCA trifurcation, neck-to-parent artery diameter <1 and fusiform aneurysms.

The indication stent-assisted endovascular treatment of cerebral aneurysms goes beyond vascular morphology. In the last few years, issues regarding patient selection have received progressively more attention, with the aim of reducing perioperative complications. A candidate for such a procedure must understand the risks and benefits, and be capable of following medical recommendations, especially the use of double antiplatelet therapy. As a consequence, any social and psychiatric conditions in which the compliance of the use of such medications and follow-up are significantly compromised should be considered as relative contra-indications.

Caution should be taken with individuals who may need surgery or a ventricular drainage shortly after the aneurysm treatment - situations that are more frequent with ruptured aneurysms. As the use of antiplatelet medication is mandatory, significant controversy exists on the placement of intracranial stents in the acute phase of intracranial haemorrhage. If subtotal embolization of the aneurysm sac may be performed with coils only, a valuable strategy is to complete treatment in a different session. In such a case, stenting would be performed far from the subarachnoid haemorrhage. Other relative contra-indications are exaggerated; vessel tortuosity, significant atherosclerotic disease and coagulation disorders.

4. Pre and per-operative evaluation

The decision to deploy an intracranial stent is taken after considering the feasibility of performing the treatment without it (e.g. aneurysm coiling to be safely treatable using balloon remodeling techniques), or the possibility of not completing the treatment due to technical difficulties such as poor navigability. The diameter and length of each device is chosen according to the diameter of the native vessel and the extension of the pathological segment.

Important issues for treatment planning are: exact aneurysm anatomical location, parent artery morphology and presence of side branches and perforators. These factors are studied on CT, MRI or DSA images before the operative procedure. The size and shape of the aneurysm, as well as the diameter of the neck, are recorded. The diameter of the parent artery is then measured, as well as the segment of the artery that will be covered by the stent. The operator will then be able to choose the adequate diameter and length of the device to use so that adequate covering of the neck can be assured.

The tortuosity of the parent artery and the technique for coiling (e.g. jailing, semi-jailing, 'X' and Y' stents, etc.) also influences the type of stent used (open cell versus closed cell, self-expandable versus balloon-mounted, etc). It is particularly important to detect potential irregularities due to other vascular pathologies such as atherosclerosis or fibromuscular dysplasia. Part of the assessment of feasibility of the stent-assisted treatment is the study of branches presenting with sharp angle of bifurcation or incorporation of its origin into the neck of the aneurysm. Such vessels may be very difficult to catheterize. If it needs to be stented, this may result in a longer and more laborious procedure. If the progression of a microguidewire and a microcatheter inside a recurrent branch is impossible after numerous attempts, other treatment modalities (e.g. surgical) must be considered. As a consequence, the patient must be properly informed before the endovascular procedure that his or her treatment presents elements of technical complexity, and that endovascular treatment may not be feasible.

5. Pre-operative preparation

A baseline neurological examination is performed and neurological scores are attributed when applicable (e.g. modified Rankin and NIHSS score), which are useful for follow-up , especially for patients who have a past history of neurological disease.

Antiplatelet agents are highly recommended in the preparation patients undergoing intracranial stenting. Insufficient platelet inhibition (PI) has been associated with an augmented risk of thrombus formation and embolic complications. As a consequence, patients receive either a loading-dose or a period of antiplatelet therapy. A loading-dose of 300 or 600 mg of clopidogrel is then administered the day before the endovascular treatment. Alternatively a dose of 75mg PO QD for five or more days has also been proposed for some authors. This is supported by both literature to date and previous experience in the cardiology field.

Since double antiaggregation is recommended, administration of acethyl-salicic acid (ASA) is also performed perioperatively. Some authors have suggested the use of preparations of 325mg or more for three or more days before the procedure, concomitant with clopidogrel. Other teams have preferred to administer a single intravenous bolus of 250-500 mg of injectable ASA at the moment of the endovascular procedure. This presents the advantage of avoiding the use of double antiaggregation in the pre-operative period, in which the aneurysm is not yet secured. However, injectable preparations are not available in all countries worldwide.

Whilst ASA resistance seems relatively uncommon, clopidogrel resistance seems to be frequent. The prevalence of low-response to this drug varies from 28% to 66% in literature. Little data is available specifically for patients undergoing stent-assisted treatment of intracranial aneurysms, but thromboembolic adverse events do seem highly concentrated in the low responder group. Some authors have consequently recommended a level of at least 40% of platelet inhibition.

Individual response to clopidogrel may be evaluated using different techniques. Recently, point-of-care assays have been commercially available, allowing practitioners to perform prompt measurements pre-operatively. The level of PI is now routinely assessed before intracranial stenting in a number of centers. In selected cases, the doses of antiplatelet agents might be adapted in order to achieve the desired levels. Another advantage of these point-of-care assays is the fact that they may be performed per-operatively, so that the operator is informed of the percentage of antiaggregation at the moment of stent deployment.

Such an approach requires systematic blood sampling, subsequent drug administration and financial investment. At present, no prospective study assessed the potential benefits in achieving a level of anti-aggregation over 40% in patients undergoing intracranial procedures. The same applies for the assessment of the risk of hemorrhagic adverse events that may be related to the combination of intravenous heparin and double antiaggregation.

We have witnessed a proliferation of portable devices and this technology is increasingly being used, and particularly in the cardiology field. Different assays are now commercially available: VerifyNow (Accumetrics, San Diego,USA), PlateletWorks (Helena Lab.; Beaumont,USA), IMPACT-R (with and without ADP stimulation, DiaMed AG, Cressier sur Morat,Switzerland), DADE PFA collagen/ADP test (Siemens Healthcare Diagnostics Products, Marburg,Germany) and others. Even so, there is some evidence that only measurements using light transmittance aggregometry (VerifyNow and PlateletWorks) are significantly correlated to the occurrence of ischemic adverse events in interventional cardiology as suggested by the POPULAR study in 2010 (Breet et al., 2010). Other studies, such as the BOCLA (Neubauer et al., 2011), showed that the concept of clopidogrel resistance may be relative, and that more than half of poor responders may have a good response by increasing (two-fold) the dose.

In the field of interventional neuroradiology, studies specifically focused on the importance of antiaggregation are rare. Four case series were published in 2008 (Lee et al., 2008, Muller-Schunk et al., 2008, Pandya et al., 2008, Prabhakaran et al., 2008). Only two have studied the incidence of thromboembolism using techniques and different cut-offs. We recently performed a study on 271 procedures in which the VerifyNow assay was used and observed a significant association between thromboembolism and poor antiagregation. The ability to predict the risk of a thromboembolic event occuring does exist, but it is moderate given the multifactorial nature of these events. In our experience, body weight should be considered as an important factor to observe. After a homogenous, single loading dose of 300mg of clopidogrel, the prevalence of low-response (<40% of PI) is significantly lower in patients weighing less than 60 kilograms (43% versus 29%). If a stent has to be deployed urgently and the patient has not been prepared with antiplatelet agents, the risk of thromboembolic events may be significant, since post-operative aspirin and clopidogrel will take time to act. Some authors have suggested the use of a loading dose just after the procedure. Others have preferred to use a GPIIb/IIIa inhibitor . A bolus of 0.025 mg/Kg of intravenous abciximab may be administered and followed by infusion at 10 mcg/min per 12 hours. Evidently, this strategy should be used with caution and not as routine in view of the well-known hemorrhagic side effects of intravenous GPIIb-IIIa inhibitors.

6. Equipment

6.1. Leo™

Leo™ (Balt, Montmorency, France) was the first closed-cell stent to be released in the market. A second generation was released thereafter as Leo+™. This is a self-expandable device made of nitinol (nickeltitanium) wires with a braided design. Its main features are good visibility and the availability of long devices (up to 75 mm). According to the manufacturer, the following product characteristics should be noted:

- Available in four nominal diameters: 2.5, 3.5, 4.5 and 5.5 mm, for vessels from 2.0 to 6.5 mm;
- Available in nine lengths: 12, 18, 25, 30, 35, 40, 50, 60, 75 mm;
- Braided design of nitinol wires;
- Self-expandable;
- Good wall apposition;
- Very good visibility;
- Significant shortening after deployment;
- Retrievable up to its 90% deployment;
- Equipped with a double helix radio-opaque, easily visible strands;
- Equipped with delivery microguidewire with a radio-opaque distal tip;
- Compatible and recommended to be delivered with a Vasco+ microcatheter;
- Recommended to be used in a triaxial system with a distal access system 6F Fargo-Fargomax.

6.2. Neuroform™

The first version of the Neuroform stent was approved in 2002 for the treatment of wide-neck, intracranial aneurysms. It was designed for vessels with diameters from 2 to 4.5 mm. It was the first self-expandable device specifically designed for assisting the treatment of brain aneurysms with coils. Made of nitinol, the Neuroform stent has an open-cell design. In its first version, a low radial force resulted in a number of cases of inadequate support for the coil mass within the aneurysm and technical problems such as stent migration. The Neuroform2 stent was launched in 2003 and the Neuroform3 in 2005. According to the manufacturer, the following product characteristics should be noted:

- Available in a range of sizes from 10 to 30 mm in length;
- Available in a range of diameters from 2.5 to 4.5 mm;
- Open cell geometry;
- Minimal shortening after deployment;
- Self-expandable;
- Flexibility and conformable in tortuous distal anatomy;
- Capable of apposition in tapered vessels;
- Interstices of 2–2.5 F (<1mm), allowing the positioning of a microcatheter through the stent;

- Proximal and distal stent markers
- Thin mesh;
- Minimal radial force;
- Not retrievable.
- Equipped with 131cm delivery microcatheter (3F proximal, 2.8F distal)
- Compatible and more appropriate for use with 0.014" Transend 300 Floppy microguidewire
- Equipped with a 150cm (2F) stabilizer (pusher) catheter with a marker band at the distal tip that indicates the proximity of the stabilizer catheter to the proximal end of the stent.

In 2010, the fourth version of the Neuroform stent was released: Neuroform EZ™. This newest version eliminated the need for an exchange maneuver using a 3m microguidewire. It may be delivered using a standard 3F microcatheter. As a consequence, the following features should be noted:

- Equipped with a Neuro Renegade™ Hi-Flo™ Microcatheter for deployment (total usable length 150cm, flexible tip length 10 cm)
- Equipped with a 185cm stainless stent delivery wire with a radio-opaque 19mm 45º pre-shaped distal tip and two radio-opaque positioning bumpers, one proximal, the other distal to the stent.

6.3. Enterprise™

The Cordis Enterprise Vascular Reconstruction Device and Delivery System consists of a self-expanding closed-cell stent and a delivery system. Its design is that of tubular mesh made of nitinol. The delivery system is composed of a delivery wire that acts also as a pusher. A major characteristic of this device is its easy placement, with good wall apposition and excellent support of the coil mass. A partially deployed device can be recaptured once and redeployed. A disadvantage of the delivery system is the absence of a very long microguidewire distal to the parent artery. In the context of very tortuous vessels, this may be a factor of instability during deployment. According to the manufacturer, the following product characteristics should be noted:

- Available in one diameter, 4.5 mm and can be used in vessels from 2.5 to 4 mm;
- Available in four lengths: 14, 22, 28, and 37 mm;
- Closed-cell geometry;
- Self-expandable;
- Good wall apposition;
- May present significant shortening after deployment, from 1.1 to 4.7mm, depending on the length of the stent and the diameter of the parent vessel;
- Proximal and distal stent markers;
- Equipped with a delivery wire with three radio-opaque segments (distal, at the tip of the wire; intermediate, long radio-opaque segment for stent positioning; and proximal marker, just before the proximal stent markers)

- Retrievable once, if the proximal end of the stent-positioning marker the (intermediate marker on the delivery wire) is not beyond the distal microcatheter markerband.
- Compatible and recommended with a 0.021 Prowler Select Plus Infusion Catheter, positioned at least 12 mm beyond aneurysm neck before stent delivery.

6.4. Solitaire AB™

The Solitaire AB (aneurysm bridging) Neurovascular remodeling Device (ev3 Cooperate, Plymouth, USA) is the first fully deployable and retrievable device for assisting intracranial aneurysm embolization with coils. It is a nitinol self-expanding stent that can be delivered and deployed by a single operator. The stent works with an open longitudinal split and is fixed to its pusher. There is no guidewire beyond the distal markers. It can be detached electrolytically using a dedicated detachment system. According to the manufacturer, the following product characteristics should be noted:

- Available in two diameters, 4mm for vessels from 3 to 4mm, and 6 mm for vessels from 5 to 6mm. Since recently, a new 3mm version is also available.
- Available in three lengths: 15 (only with 4mm diameter), 20 (both 4 and 6 mm diameter) and 30mm (only with 6 mm diameter);
- Closed-cell geometry;
- Self-expandable;
- Presence of a longitudinal split with overlapping of the stent cells, depending on the diameter of the parent vessel;
- Good wall apposition;
- High cell deformation resistance;
- Presents significant shortening after deployment, depending on the length of the stent and the diameter of the parent vessel;
- One Proximal and three distal stent markers;
- Equipped with a delivery wire, with a detachment zone just before the proximal marker;
- Can be retrieved and repositioned before detachment, even when fully deployed;
- Compatible and recommended with a Rebar 18-27 Microcatheter (*but also compatible with a 0.021 Prowler Select Plus Infusion Catheter).

6.5. Pharos™

The Pharos stent (Micrus, San Jose, USA) was launched in 2006 in Europe for the treatment of ischemic disease. The Pharos Vitesse stent is the second generation of this balloon-expandable stent for both intracranial ischemic stenosis and wide-neck aneurysm treatment. It is a rapid exchange balloon-delivered device, which enables the operator to deliver and deploy the stent in one step. Made of cobalt chromium, the stent is opened by the radial force of the balloon. There is no self-expansion of the device. According to the manufacturer, the following product characteristics should be noted:

- Available in eight diameters: 2, 2,5, 2,75, 3, 3,5, 4, 4,5 and 5 mm, for vessels from 2 to 5 mm;
- Available in six lengths: 8, 10, 13, 15, 18 and 20 mm;
- Double helix geometry with thin struts (60 micra);
- Not self-expandable;
- Good wall apposition;
- High radial force
- Good visibility;
- Compatible with a 0.014" microguidewire
- Very low shortening after deployment (<1%);
- Proximal and distal stent markers;

6.6. LVIS™

The Low-profile Visualized Intraluminal Support (MicroVention Incorporation, Tustin, USA) is a very recent generation of devices intended for use with embolic coils, now available in Europe. It is a hybrid closed-cell stent in nitinol with flared ends and a double helix of tantalum strands to assist full-length visualization. It presents a high metal-to-surface coverage intended to help promote neo-endothelization. However, the sliding design of its cells ensures the feasibility of crossing the struts with a microcatheter. According to the manufacturer, the following product characteristics should be noted:

- Available in three nominal diameters, 2,5, 3.5, and 4.0 mm, respectively for vessels from 2 to 3 mm, 2.5 to 3.5 mm and 3.5 to 4.5 mm;
- Available in six lengths, 17 and 25 mm for the 2.5 mm diameter, 15, 25 and 41 mm for the 3.0 mm diameter, 35 and 49 mm for the 4.0 diameter stent;
- Hybrid, compliant closed-cell geometry with thin struts;
- Self-expandable;
- Good wall apposition;
- Flared ends;
- Good visibility;
- High metal-to-surface coverage;
- Significant shortening after deployment;
- Retrievable up to 80% deployment;
- Proximal and distal stent markers, as well as double helix radio-opaque tantalum strands;
- Equipped with delivery microguidewire with a radio-opaque distal tip;
- Compatible with a 0.021 Headway microcatheter.

6.7. Flow diverters

These are braided, tubular stents with very small struts that are intended to provide significant flow disruption along the aneurysm neck, but allow preservation of both large branches and small perforators. Such devices may reduce shear stress on the aneurysm wall and promote intra-aneurysmal blood stagnation and thrombosis (Pierot, 2011). Besides their effects on flow, these devices also provide significant scaffolding for neo-endothelization across the aneurysm neck. They are high-cost devices and their main characteristic is the very high metal-to-artery coverage in comparison to conventional stents. Two devices are currently available, as follows.

6.7.1. Silk™

The Silk and its more recent version Silk Plus (Balt, Montmorency, France) are self expanding stents made of braided nitinol strands, with the following technical characteristics.

- Available in eight nominal diameters: 2.0, 2.5, 3.0, 3.5, 4.0, 4.5, 5.0 and 5.5 mm, for vessels from 1.5 to 5.75 mm;
- Available in six nominal lengths, 15, 20, 25, 30, 35 and 40 mm;
- Also available in tapered version (Tapered Silk+) in three combinations of diameters: 4.0 mm proximal and 3.0 mm distal (30mm long), 4.5 mm proximal and 3.0 distal (25 mm long), 4.5 proximal and 3.5 distal (30 mm long);
- Dense mesh geometry with very high metal-to-surface coverage;
- High radial force (Silk Plus has 15% more radial force than Silk) thanks to a different strut configuration;
- Good wall apposition;
- Good visibility;
- Slight flared ends
- Double helix radio-opaque markers through the entire body of the stent, combined with extra Platinum small wires in the Silk Plus version, that allow visualization of the borders of the stent;
- Equipped with delivery pusher/microguidewire with a radio-opaque distal tip;
- Compatible and recommended with a Vasco+ microcatheter for delivery and a triaxial system with a long introducer and a distal access system 6F Fargo-Fargomax;
- Compatible with concentric Leo+ stents for lumen reconstruction before deployment of Silk or Silk Plus, if needed in fusiform aneurysms.

6.7.2. PED – Pipeline Embolisation Device™

The Pipeline Embolisation Device (ev3-MTI, Irvine, USA) is a newer, self-expanding, flexible device, composed of 25% platinum tungsten and 75% cobalt chromium in interwoven strands. According to the manufacturer, the following product characteristics should be noted:

- Available in eleven nominal diameters: 2.0, 2.75, 3.0, 3.25, 3.5, 3.75, 4.0, 4.25, 4.5, 4.75 and 5.0;
- Available in nine nominal lengths, 10, 12, 14 , 16, 18, 20, 25, 30 and 35 mm;

- Dense mesh geometry with braided construction and very high metal-to-surface coverage, which can be customized according to the push that is imposed to the microcatheter (increased push narrows stent cells);
- High radial force and flexibility, resistant to kinking;
- Good wall apposition;
- Uniform visibility through entire device;
- Ability to telescope multiple devices, one inside another to create longer constructs;
- Equipped with delivery pusher/microguidewire with a radio-opaque distal tip and a 'capture coil' that keeps the device in contact to the guidewire until significant length is deployed;
- Compatible and recommended with a 2.8F/3.2F Marksman™ microcatheter for delivery and deployment.

6.8. Other

It is worth noting that a number of stents that were not specifically designed for use with intracranial aneurysms have non-rarely been used as adjunctive devices. This situation was much more frequent in the early times of stent-assisted aneurysm embolization, when a lesser variety of devices were available. That is the case with the Jostent GraftMaster Stent Graft (Abbott Vascular, Redwood City, Calif), a balloon-mounted system consisting of two stainless steel flexible devices with an expandable layer of polytetrafluoroethylene between them. It was developed for use within the coronary circulation, particularly for cases of leakage or vessel perforation. However, cases of repair of internal carotid artery, middle cerebral artery and vertebral artery aneurysms were regularly reported with this system (Chan et al., 2004, Mehta et al., 2003, Pero et al., 2006, Saatci et al., 2004, Wang et al., 2009). During the advancement of neurointerventional tools for wide-neck aneurysms, several stents initially designed for the cervical carotid or coronary circulation were also used as adjunctive devices, such as Wallstent™ (Boston Scientific, Natick, USA), Multilink™ (Abbott Vascular, Redwood City, Calif), and others (Lavine & Meyers, 2007, Morizane et al., 2000, Wanke & Forsting, 2008).

7. Operative technique

7.1. Coiling and stenting: 'finishing stent' and 'rescue stent'

An intracranial stent may be used at the end of an aneurysm embolization when coils have been used, which is particularly useful in cases in which the aneurysm neck was not fully respected by the coil mass, or to insure protection of the parent artery against coil migration. In addition, when a stent is deployed after an aneurysm coil, significant scaffolding for neo-endothelisation is provided and an increase in pack density may be observed. This technique may be particularly useful for small aneurysms, in which the introduction of a microcatheter and repetitive manipulations may be dangerous. The coil is deployed first and then a preloaded stent is released, pushing the coil loop into the sac. This method has been also been known as a 'stent-jack' technique.

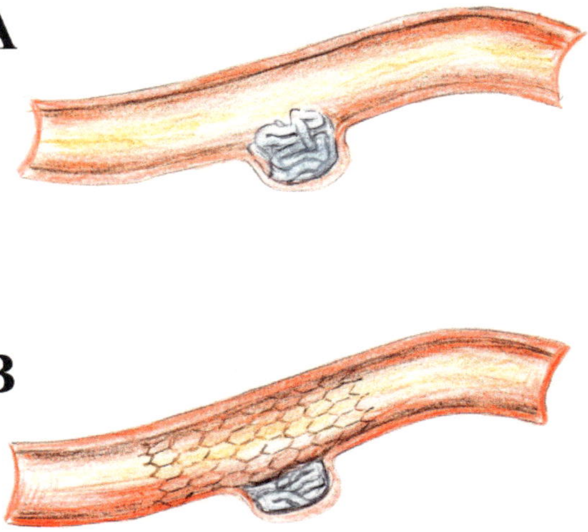

Figure 1. 'Finishing stent'. *A*, The coil mass protrudes slightly in the lumen of the parent vessel. *B*, The coils are pushed back into the aneurysm sack with a 'finishing stent'.

When non-assisted coiling is performed, coil migration or herniation of the coil mass may be observed, even if the neck is not very wide. This may also be observed during balloon-assisted embolization. If a large amount of material is present in the lumen of the parent artery, its patency may be threatened, or the patient may be exposed to a risk of embolic phenomena. In such a situation, a valuable technique can be the deployment of what is called a 'rescue stent', which pushes the herniated coils against the vessel wall or back inside the aneurysm sac.

7.2. Stenting and coiling: crossing a deployed stent with a microcatheter

When stent-assisted coiling is performed, the microcatheter tip may be placed inside the aneurysm the through the stent struts. The choice between this method and placement of the microcatheter before stenting depends on the operator's experience, the vascular morphology and aneurysm size. Placement of a microcatheter into the aneurysm is evidently more difficult after stenting, especially if a closed-cell device was used. In this last case, a thinner microcatheter may be necessary. Some practitioners prefer using a Neuroform stent in such situations, for the same reason. Furthermore, with a Neuroform stent, it is easier to regain access to the aneurysm sac in cases of microcatheter kickback into the parent vessel.

If the operator experiences difficulty in penetrating the aneurysm sac, especially when the angle of penetration is not favorable, caution should be taken in order to avoid abrupt release of energy accumulated in the system, which may have disastrous consequences, especially with small or ruptured cerebral aneurysms.

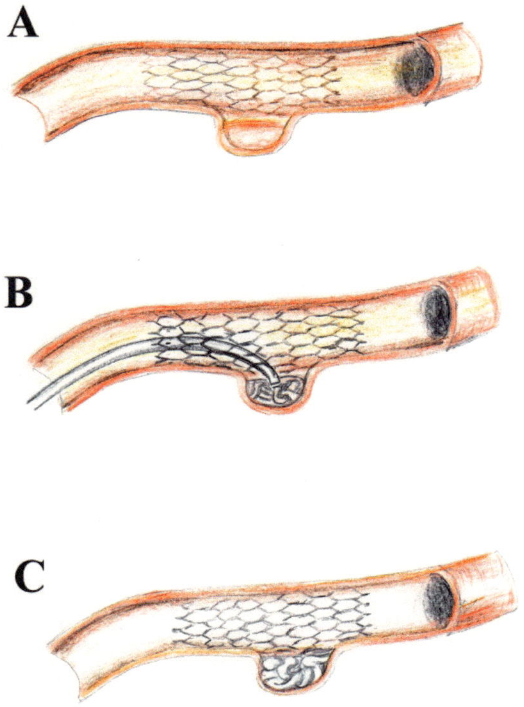

Figure 2. Crossing a deployed stent with a microcatheter. *A,* A stent is deployed, bridging the aneurysm neck. *B,* A microcatheter is introduced into the aneurysm sac through the stent struts allowing treatment with coils. *C,* Final result, after removal of the microcatheter.

7.3. 'Jailing' technique

The technique of placement of the microcatheter tip inside the aneurysm before deployment of the stent has the advantages of being technically easier and being less susceptible to microcatheter kickback phenomena. However, when significant kickback occurs, it may be problematic to regain access to the aneurysm sac. Some authors argue that the previous deployment of coil loops before stent placement may be useful. The previously deployed coil may be used as a guidewire and allow reintroduction of the microcatheter in case of early kickback (Kim et al., 2011).

7.4. 'Semi-jailing' technique

In this technique, a stent is partially deployed in front of the aneurysm neck to act as a remodeling device. For this, the operator chooses a retrievable device such as Solitaire AB or Enterprise (retrievable if the proximal end intermediate marker of the delivery wire is not beyond the distal microcatheter markerband). This technique presents several advantages: the possibility to regain access to the aneurysm sac in case of kickback by a slight repositioning of the stent; the absence of blood flow arrest as observed with balloon-remodeling techniques; the possibility to chose to either retrieve or definitely deploy the stent after coiling; and the possibility of not using double antiplatelet treatment if the stent is retrieved at the end of the procedure.

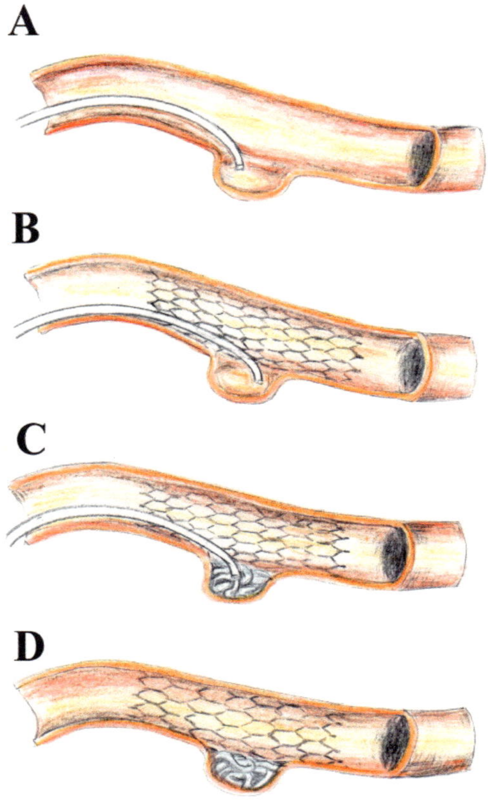

Figure 3. The 'jailing technique'. ***A***, A microcatheter is positioned inside the aneurysm. ***B***, The stent is deployed. ***C***, The aneurysm is treated with coils. ***D***, Final result.

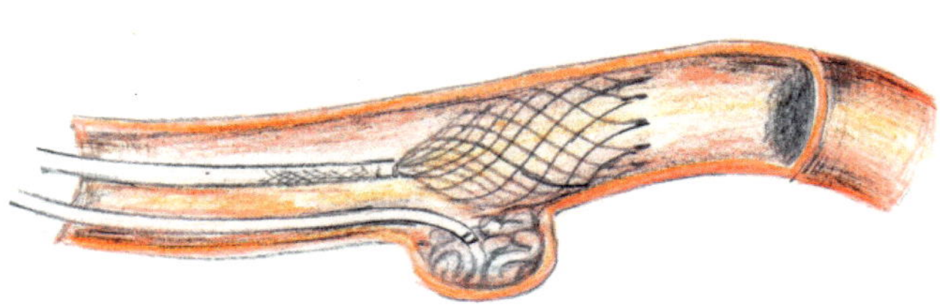

Figure 4. The 'semi-jailing' technique with a partially deployed stent.

7.5. 'Y' and 'X' stenting

If one stent is not able to adequately protect the parent artery or a bifurcation branch, a possible solution is the deployment of two devices in a 'Y' configuration. A first stent is deployed in one of the branches, preferably an open-cell device. A microcatheter is then navigated into the other branch and a second stent is released. Another possibility is to place both stents in a parallel configuration, without crossing the first one. For confluent vessels such as in the anterior communicating territory, crossing stents are also possible, what has been called an 'X' configuration (Kim et al., 2011).

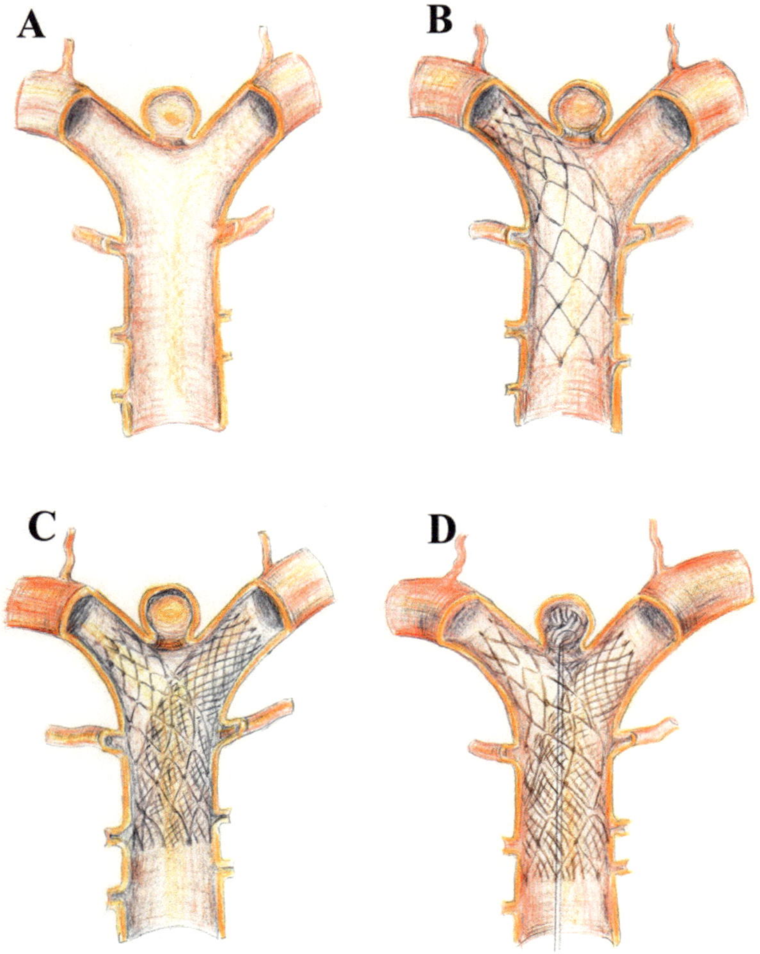

Figure 5. The 'Y' Stent Technique. *A*, A basilar tip aneurysm. *B*, An open-cell stent is deployed into the basilar artery and right posterior cerebral artery, but is not sufficient to provide adequate protection against coil herniation or migration. *C*. A second (closed-cell) stent is placed in the basilar artery (concentric to the first stent) and left posterior cerebral artery. *D*. A microcatheter is positioned inside the aneurysm sac, which is treated with coils.

7.6. Temporary stenting (Solitaire AB™)

Similar to the 'semi-jailing' technique, temporary stenting consists of using a stent as a remodeling device, with full retrieval of the device at the end of the procedure. Up to date, only stents from the Solitaire group may be retrieved after full deployment. It is worth noting that with this kind of stent (but not exclusive to this brand) the use of a dynamic push in the delivery wire increases notoriously the apposition to the vascular walls, an effect that is important to remember when using this device as a remodeling tool.

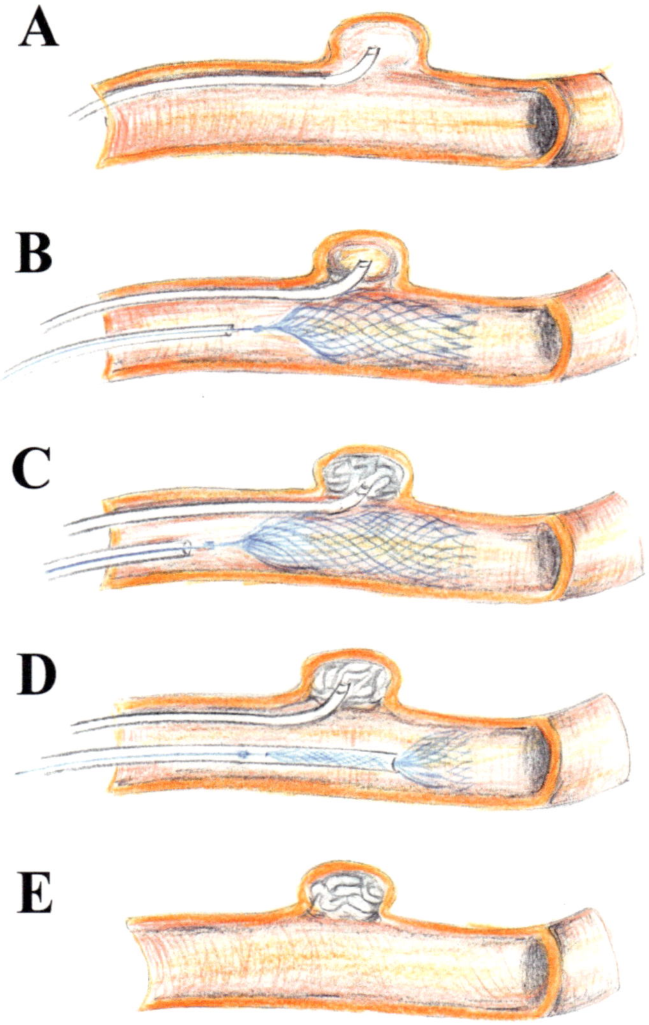

Figure 6. Temporary stenting with a Solitaire AB device. *A,* The microcatheter is positioned inside the aneurysm. *B,* The microcatheter is 'jailed' in the aneurysm by the Solitaire AB stent, which is completely deployed but not detached. *C,* The aneurysm is treated with coils. *D,* The Solitaire AB device is retrieved. *E,* Final result, no stent is left in the parent vessel.

7.7. Flow diversion

Even though a large part of the deployment steps are common for the majority of intracranial stents, the technique for flow diverters differs in some details that make the method more challenging. The operator must work within a technique of pushing the delivery microguidewire forward, of pulling the microcatheter back, and pushing the entire system so that the stent opening and apposition are optimal. In addition, the phenomenon of shortening after deployment must be taken into consideration for the adequate selection of the stent length.

For the Pipeline Embolization Device, adequate pushing on the microcatheter is also important to release the distal extremity of the device from the capture coil that keeps it attached to the delivery microguidewire. In addition, forward pushing may increase mesh density, and accounts for the customization that is possible with this type of device. With an adequate push at the right site, one may deploy a PED with an increased metal-to-artery coverage at the aneurysm neck.

A

B

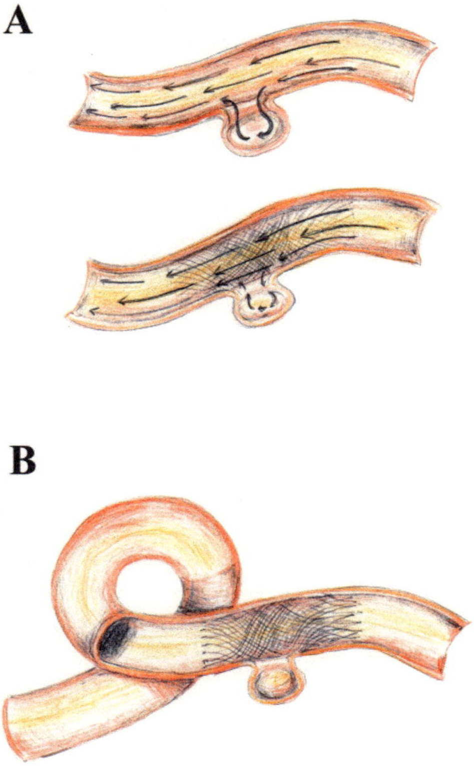

Figure 7. Treatment of a cerebral aneurysm using flow diversion with a Pipeline Embolization Device. *A*, Aspect of blood flow before and after placement of the device. *B*, Final result with thrombosis of the aneurysm. Note the higher density of the mesh near the aneurysm neck, which can be obtained with proper deployment technique.

8. Results

The morphological results on immediate and late post-operative angiograms are categorized according to the revised Raymond classification into 1 of the following groups: complete occlusion, neck remnant, and residual aneurysm. Follow-up examinations with Digital Substraction Angriography or Magnetic Resonance Angiograms are then scheduled at minimum intervals of 6, 18 and 36 months. In cases of early recanalization, a DSA would be preferred in order to properly assess the need for retreatment.

The rates of complete occlusion differ significantly from the results observed on the immediate postoperative angiogram after stent-assisted coiling. In a recent study on the Neuroform Stent in our institution, we observed that the percentage of complete occlusion tends to stabilize after six months. However, progressive thrombosis and subsequent increase of the degree of aneurysm occlusion between the immediate postoperative and six-month angiograms are observed in roughly 50% of the aneurysms treated with stent-assisted techniques (Maldonado et al., 2010). Of 76 aneurysms studied, 31.6% were completely occluded in the initial embolization, 63.8 at six months and 64.7% at 18 months. However, in three years of follow-up, six aneurysms with an initial complete occlusion and five with a neck remnant recanalized. The analysis by type of coil did not demonstrate any association between complete occlusion and coil type.

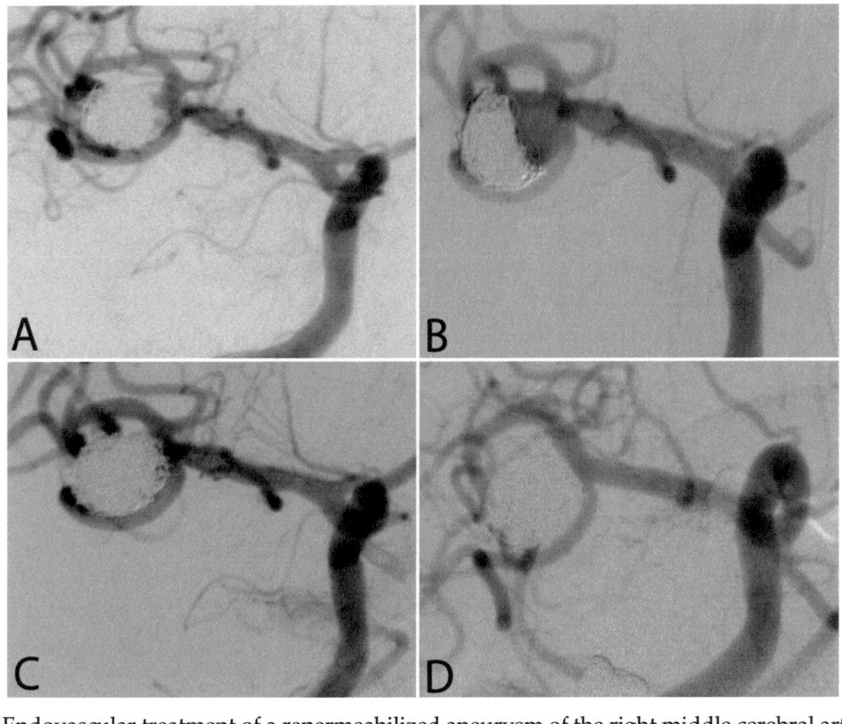

Figure 8. Endovascular treatment of a repermeabilized aneurysm of the right middle cerebral artery using the Neuroform Stent System. ***A***, after initial embolization; ***B***, repermeabilization seven months later; ***C***, after re-treatment using a Neuroform stent and a 'jailing' technique; ***D***, angiographic control 14 months after retreatment, showing adequate reconstruction and re-endothelization of the bifurcation zone.

Stents may contribute to the progression of thrombosis, independent to the size of the aneurysm and type of coils used. Fiorella et al (Fiorella et al., 2005) reported an improvement of anatomic results with progressive thrombosis in 52% of cases of patients treated with the Neuroform stent. Lubicz et al (Lubicz et al., 2009) observed progressive thrombosis in 53% of aneurysms coiled with MicroPlex bare coils or GDCs using the Leo stent.

The overall complete occlusion rate obtained with stent-assisted coiling seems superior to results obtained with coils alone or other adjunctive devices in cases of large or complex aneurysms. Sedat et al (Sedat et al., 2009) documented 9.5% of aneurysmal regrowth at a mean follow-up of 42 months.

9. Complications

Recent case series report incidences of adverse events ranging from 8.4 to 18.9%. Risk factors for complications are age, presence of significant atherosclerotic disease, subarachnoid hemorrhage, small aneurysm and large/giant aneurysm. The most common of those adverse events in the peri-operative phase are navigation problems, stent misplacement, stent migration, vessel dissection or perforation, and thromboembolic events.

Delayed stroke due to intrastent thrombosis or intrastent stenosis are less frequent but may be observed, especially in patients with irregular use of antiplatelets. In a recent study published by the authors on 76 aneurysms treated with a Neuroform Stent-assisted technique, a five-month delayed symptomatic stroke and three clinically silent in-stent stenosis were observed.

There is currently significant concern about the risk of delayed rupture after flow-diversion treatment. The exact mechanism of this adverse event is not completely understood. There are two main hypotheses for this phenomenon. First, the mural thrombus may act as a source of inflammatory substances such as proteases leading to chemical degradation and weakening of the aneurysm wall. Second, flow diversion may induce changes in intra-aneurysmal flow pattern with a consequent increase in stress to areas that were not previously exposed. In a series of recent international cases of rupture after flow diversion, the following risk factors seemed to be important (Kulcsar et al., 2010):

- Large or giant aneurysm;
- Symptomatic aneurysm;
- Saccular aneurysm with AR>1.6;
- Morphologic characteristics predisposing to an inertia-driven inflow.

10. Post-operative management

During the procedure, patients are anticoagulated with a bolus of standard heparin (70–100 IU/kg) followed by an intravenous drip through an automated syringe (40–60 IU/kg/h) to maintain an activated clotting time of 250 seconds, which may be continued for 12-24 hours. At the end of the procedure, they receive an IV dose of 250–500 mg of ASA unless they are already using oral Aspirine. A daily dose of clopidogrel (75 mg) and ASA (75 mg) is then administered for two or three months. After that period, only one of those antiplatelet agents is continued, for a period of time that has varied in literature from three months to indefinitely.

Author details

Igor Lima Maldonado
Universidade Federal da Bahia, Brazil

Alain Bonafé
Université Montpellier 1, France

11. Acknowledgement

We would like to express our thanks to Mr José Alberto Maldonado Via for his assistance with the illustrations.

12. References

Breet N. J., van Werkum J. W., Bouman H. J., Kelder J. C., Ruven H. J., Bal E. T., Deneer V. H., Harmsze A. M., van der Heyden J. A., Rensing B. J., Suttorp M. J., Hackeng C. M.& ten Berg J. M. (2010). Comparison of platelet function tests in predicting clinical outcome in patients undergoing coronary stent implantation. *JAMA*, Vol. 303, No. 8, pp. 754-62.

Chan A. W., Yadav J. S., Krieger D.& Abou-Chebl A. (2004). Endovascular repair of carotid artery aneurysm with Jostent covered stent: initial experience and one-year result. *Catheter Cardiovasc Interv*, Vol. 63, No. 1, pp. 15-20.

Fessler R., Ringer A., Qureshi A., Guterman L.& Hopkins L. (2000). Intracranial stent placement to trap an extruded coil during endovascular aneurysm treatment: Technical note. *Neurosurgery*, Vol. 46, No., pp. 248-251.

Fiorella D., Albuquerque F. C., Deshmukh V. R.& McDougall C. G. (2005). Usefulness of the Neuroform stent for the treatment of cerebral aneurysms: results at initial (3-6-mo) follow-up. *Neurosurgery*, Vol. 56, No. 6, pp. 1191-201; discussion 1201-2.

Higashida R., Halbach V., Dowd C., Juravsky L.& Meagher S. (2005). Initial clinical experience with a new self-expanding nitinol stent for the treatment of intracranial cerebral aneurysms: The Cordis Enterprise stent. *American Journal of Neuroradiology*, Vol. 26, No., pp. 1751-1756.

Kim B. M., Kim D. J.& Kim D. I. (2011). Stent application for the treatment of cerebral aneurysms. *Neurointervention*, Vol. 6, No. 2, pp. 53-70.

Kulcsar Z., Houdart E., Bonafe A., Parker G., Millar J., Goddard A. J., Renowden S., Gal G., Turowski B., Mitchell K., Gray F., Rodriguez M., van den Berg R., Gruber A., Desal H., Wanke I.& Rufenacht D. A. (2010). Intra-Aneurysmal Thrombosis as a Possible Cause of Delayed Aneurysm Rupture after Flow-Diversion Treatment. *AJNR Am J Neuroradiol*, Vol., No., pp.

Lavine S., Larsen D., Giannotta S.& Teitelbaum G. (2000). Parent vessel Guglielmi detachable coil herniation during wide-necked aneurysm embolization: Treatment with intracranial stent placement: Two technical case reports. *Neurosurgery*, Vol. 46, No., pp. 1013-1017.

Lavine S. D.& Meyers P. M. (2007). Application of new techniques and technologies: stenting for cerebral aneurysm. *Clin Neurosurg*, Vol. 54, No., pp. 64-9.

Lee D. H., Arat A., Morsi H., Shaltoni H., Harris J. R.& Mawad M. E. (2008). Dual antiplatelet therapy monitoring for neurointerventional procedures using a point-of-care platelet function test: a single-center experience. *AJNR Am J Neuroradiol*, Vol. 29, No. 7, pp. 1389-94.

Lubicz B., Bandeira A., Bruneau M., Dewindt A., Balériaux D.& De Witte O. (2009). Stenting is improving and stabilizing anatomical results of coiled intracranial aneurysms. *Neuroradiology*, Vol. 51, No., pp. 419-25.

Maldonado I. L., Machi P., Costalat V., Mura T.& Bonafé A. (2010). Neuroform Stent - Assisted Coiling of Unruptured Intracranial Aneurysms: Short- and Midterm Results from a Single-Center Experience with 68 Patients. *American Journal of Neuroradiology*, Vol. 32, No., pp. 131-136.

Mehta B., Burke T., Kole M., Bydon A., Seyfried D.& Malik G. (2003). Stent-within-a-stent technique for the treatment of dissecting vertebral artery aneurysms. *AJNR Am J Neuroradiol*, Vol. 24, No. 9, pp. 1814-8.

Morizane A., Sakai N., Nagata I., Nakahara I., Sakai H.& Kikuchi H. (2000). [Combined endovascular stent implantation and coil embolization for the treatment of a vertebro-basilar fusiform aneurysm: technical case report]. *No Shinkei Geka*, Vol. 28, No. 9, pp. 811-6.

Muller-Schunk S., Linn J., Peters N., Spannagl M., Deisenberg M., Bruckmann H.& Mayer T. E. (2008). Monitoring of clopidogrel-related platelet inhibition: correlation of nonresponse with clinical outcome in supra-aortic stenting. *AJNR Am J Neuroradiol*, Vol. 29, No. 4, pp. 786-91.

Neubauer H., Kaiser A. F., Endres H. G., Kruger J. C., Engelhardt A., Lask S., Pepinghege F., Kusber A.& Mugge A. (2011). Tailored antiplatelet therapy can overcome clopidogrel and aspirin resistance--the BOchum CLopidogrel and Aspirin Plan (BOCLA-Plan) to improve antiplatelet therapy. *BMC Med*, Vol. 9, No., pp. 3.

Pandya D. J., Fitzsimmons B. F., Wolfe T. J., Hussain S. I., Lynch J. R., Ortega-Gutierrez S.& Zaidat O. O. (2008). Measurement of antiplatelet inhibition during neurointerventional procedures: the effect of antithrombotic duration and loading dose. *J Neuroimaging*, Vol. 20, No. 1, pp. 64-9.

Pero G., Denegri F., Valvassori L., Boccardi E.& Scialfa G. (2006). Treatment of a middle cerebral artery giant aneurysm using a covered stent. Case report. *J Neurosurg*, Vol. 104, No. 6, pp. 965-8.

Pierot L. (2011). Flow diverter stents in the treatment of intracranial aneurysms: Where are we? *J Neuroradiol*, Vol. 38, No. 1, pp. 40-6.

Prabhakaran S., Wells K. R., Lee V. H., Flaherty C. A.& Lopes D. K. (2008). Prevalence and risk factors for aspirin and clopidogrel resistance in cerebrovascular stenting. *AJNR Am J Neuroradiol*, Vol. 29, No. 2, pp. 281-5.

Saatci I., Cekirge H. S., Ozturk M. H., Arat A., Ergungor F., Sekerci Z., Senveli E., Er U., Turkoglu S., Ozcan O. E.& Ozgen T. (2004). Treatment of internal carotid artery aneurysms with a covered stent: experience in 24 patients with mid-term follow-up results. *AJNR Am J Neuroradiol*, Vol. 25, No. 10, pp. 1742-9.

Sedat J., Chau Y., Mondot L., Vargas J., Szapiro J.& Lonjon M. (2009). Endovascular occlusion of intracranial wide-necked aneurysms with stenting (Neuroform) and coiling: mid-term and long-term results. *Neuroradiology*, Vol. 51, No. 6, pp. 401-9.

Wang C., Xie X., You C., Zhang C., Cheng M., He M., Sun H.& Mao B. (2009). Placement of covered stents for the treatment of direct carotid cavernous fistulas. *AJNR Am J Neuroradiol*, Vol. 30, No. 7, pp. 1342-6.

Wanke I.& Forsting M. (2008). Stents for intracranial wide-necked aneurysms: more than mechanical protection. *Neuroradiology*, Vol. 50, No. 12, pp. 991-8.

Chapter 15

Retroperitoneal Haemorrhage as a Dangerous Complication of Endovascular Cerebral Aneurysmal Coiling

Yasuo Murai and Akira Teramoto

Additional information is available at the end of the chapter

http://dx.doi.org/10.5772/46036

1. Introduction

Retroperitoneal haemorrhage has been reported as a complication of interventional surgery in less than 3% of all interventional procedures (Ellis et al. 2006, Farouque et al. 2005, Haviv et al. 1996, Kent et al. 1994, Lubavin et al. 2004, Murai et al. 2010, Nasser et al. 1995, Popma et al. 1993, Tiroch et al. 2008, Trimarchi et al. 2010, Witz et al. 1999). Technical advances in neuroendovascular therapy including aneurysm coiling (Bejjani et al.1998, Murai et al. 2005, Umeoka et al. 2010) or embolization of tumor feeders (Murai et al. 2011) have led to an overall improvement in short- and long-term outcomes of aneurysmal subarachnoid haemorrhage. However, iatrogenic complications such as haematoma or vascular dissections may still occur(Sakai et al. 2001). Although most cases of retroperitoneal haematoma are associated with blunt trauma or rupture of a diseased abdominal artery, interventional surgical accidents are another aetiology (Haviv et al. 1996, Kent et al. 1994, Lodge et al. 1973, Sreeram et al. 1993, Tomlinson et al. 2000). Retroperitoneal haematoma is a relatively rare but serious complication of femoral artery catheterization Bejjani et al. 1998, Haviv et al. 1996, Illescas et al. 1986, Kalinowski et al et al. 1998, Kent et al. 1994, Lin et al. 2001, Lodge et al. 1963, Lubavin et al. 2994, Mak et al. 1993, Quint et al. 1993, Raphael et al, 2001, Sreeram et al. 1993, Swayne et al. 1994, Trerotola et al. 1990, Wasay et al. 2001). Tiroch et al. reported a mortality rate of 12% for retroperitoneal haemorrhage patients compared with 1.3% for non-Retroperitoneal haemorrhage patients(Tiroch et al 2008). Ellis et al. reported 17 patients (10.4%) with retroperitoneal haemorrhage who expired during hospitalization (Ellis et al. 2006). Interventional radiologists and cardiologists have identified the predisposing factors, typical presentation and clinical course of this iatrogenic complication (Haviv et al. 1996, Kalinowski et al. 1998, Kent et al. 1994, Lubavin et al. 2004, Quint et al. 1993, Wita et al. 1999). However, only a small number of cases of retroperitoneal haemorrhage have been reported following interventional neurovascular therapy because of the low incidence of this complication (Lubicz et al. 2011, Murai et al. 2010). Post-angiographic retroperitoneal haemorrhage is often difficult to diagnose (Illescas et al. 1986, Sharp et al. 1984, Swayne et al. 1994, Trerotola et al. 1990, Witz et al. 1999) and can masquerade as other abdominal diseases. Symptoms are nonspecific (Kent et al. 1994, Kim et al. 2010, Murai et al. 2010, Paul et al. 2010, Raymond et al. 2001) and include abdominal, back and lower extremity pain, with abdominal distension being the most common sign. We report here a case of retroperitoneal haemorrhage following endovascular coiling of a ruptured anterior communicating artery aneurysm, with emphasis on the difficulty in diagnosing retroperitoneal haemorrhage in patients with disturbed consciousness.

2. Representative case presentation

Computed tomography performed at the time of admission on a male patient who complained of headaches revealed a slight subarachnoid haemorrhage (figure 1). His WFNS (the World Federation of Neurosurgical Societies) grade (Teasdale et al. 1988) was I.

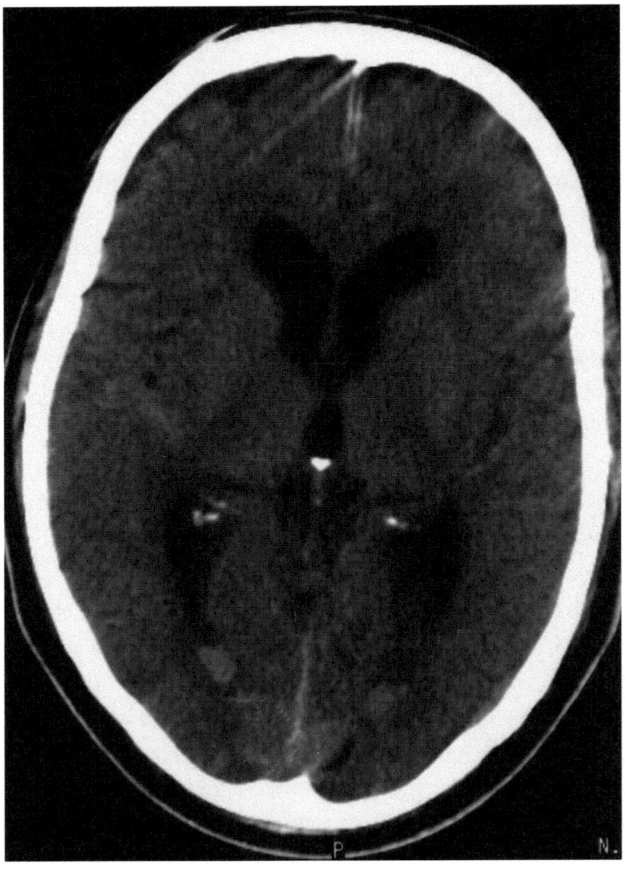

Figure 1. Initial brain computed tomography. Brain computed tomography revealed subarachnoid hemorrhage in the sylvian fissure and lateral ventrile hematoma.

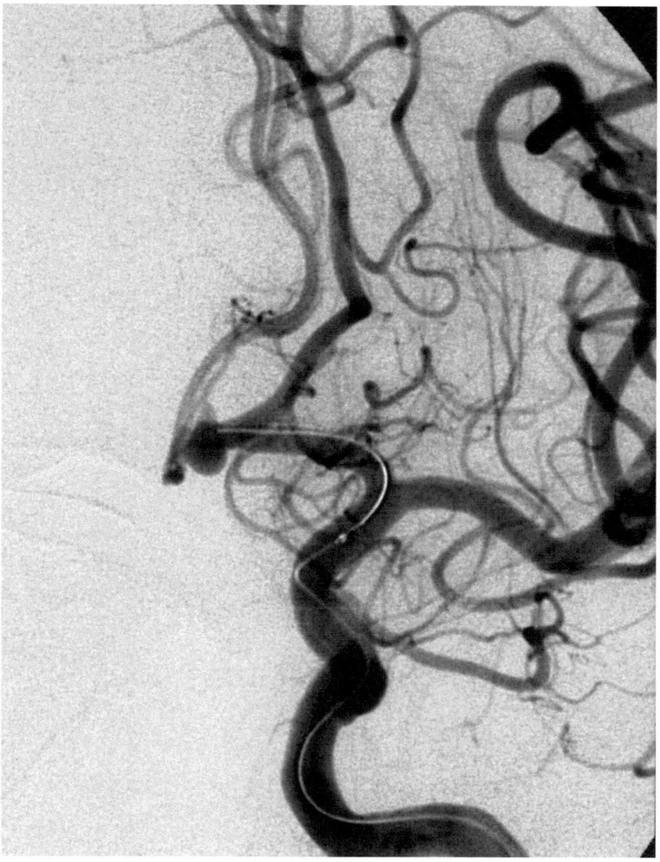

Figure 2. Left carotid angiography. Oblique view of left carotid angiogram indicated anterior communicating artery aneurysm.

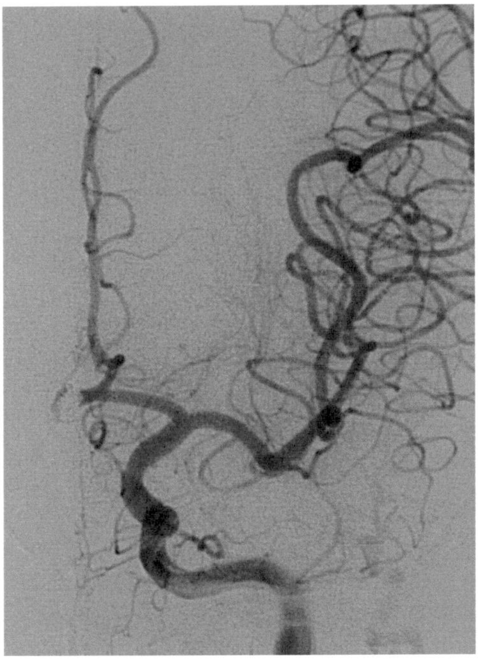

(a)

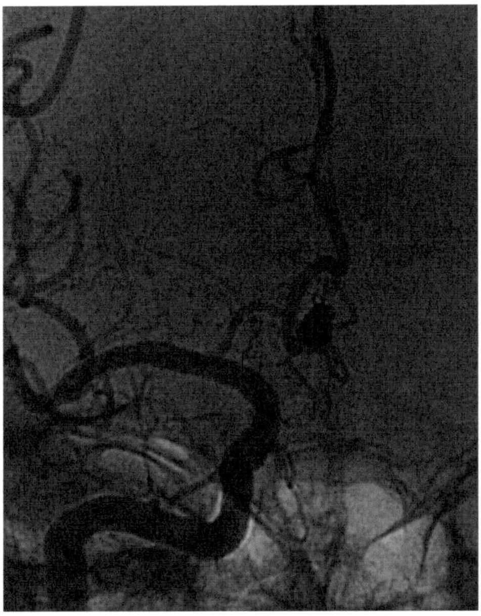

(b)

Figure 3. a) Left carotid angiogram after the coiling. Anterior posterior view of left carotid angiogram indicated coiled anterior communicating artery aneurysm and no perfusion of right distal anterior cerebral artery. b) Right carotid angiogram after the coiling. Anterior posterior view of right carotid angiogram indicated coiled anterior communicating artery aneurysm and perfusion of right distal anterior cerebral artery.

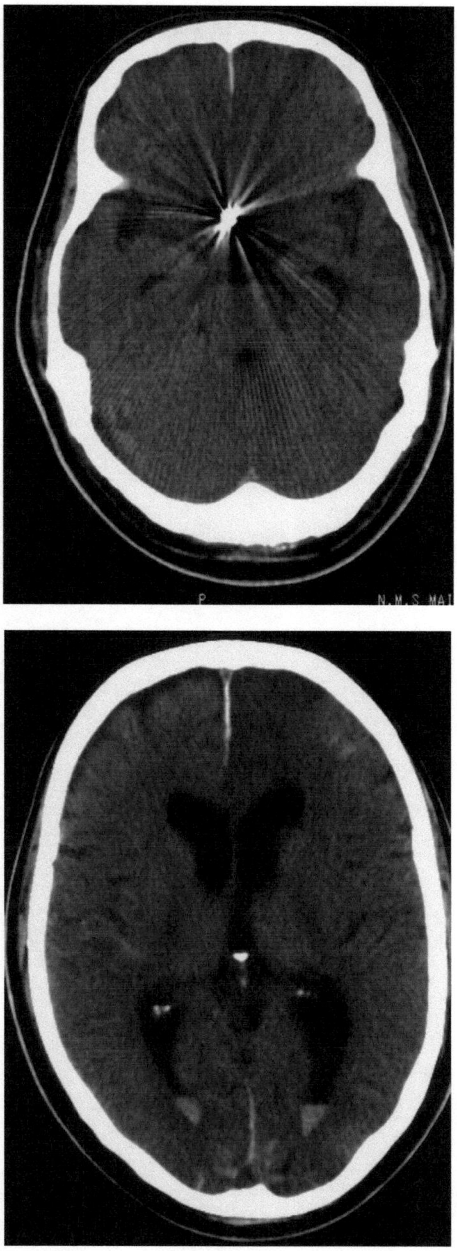

Figure 4. Brain computed tomograpic study 20 hours after interventional aneurysmal coiling of anterior communicating artery aneurysm. A low density area is seen on the left anterior cerebral artery territory.

Left internal carotid digital subtraction angiography via right femoral artery access revealed an aneurysm of the anterior cerebral artery. Endovascular aneurysm coiling was performed (figure 2) the following day via right femoral artery access. A 6 French sheath was inserted and the left internal carotid artery was catheterized with the patient under general anaesthesia. Three complex coils were delivered within the lumen of the aneurysm (figure

3.a, 3.b). The patient received a bolus of 5000 units of heparin immediately following the procedure, and thereafter, heparin was infused at a rate of 10000 units per day.

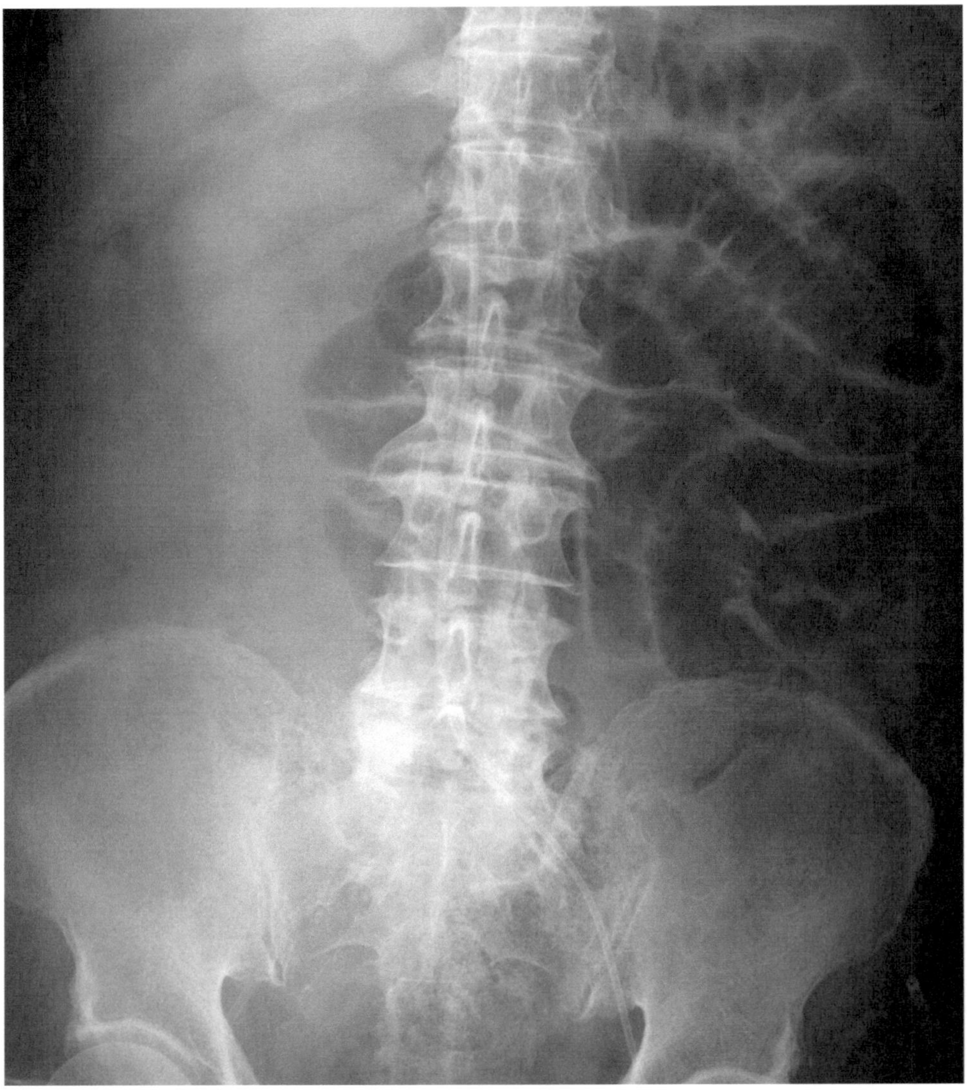

Figure 5. Abdominal X-ray. Abdominal X-ray showing a huge retroperitoneal mass on the right side.

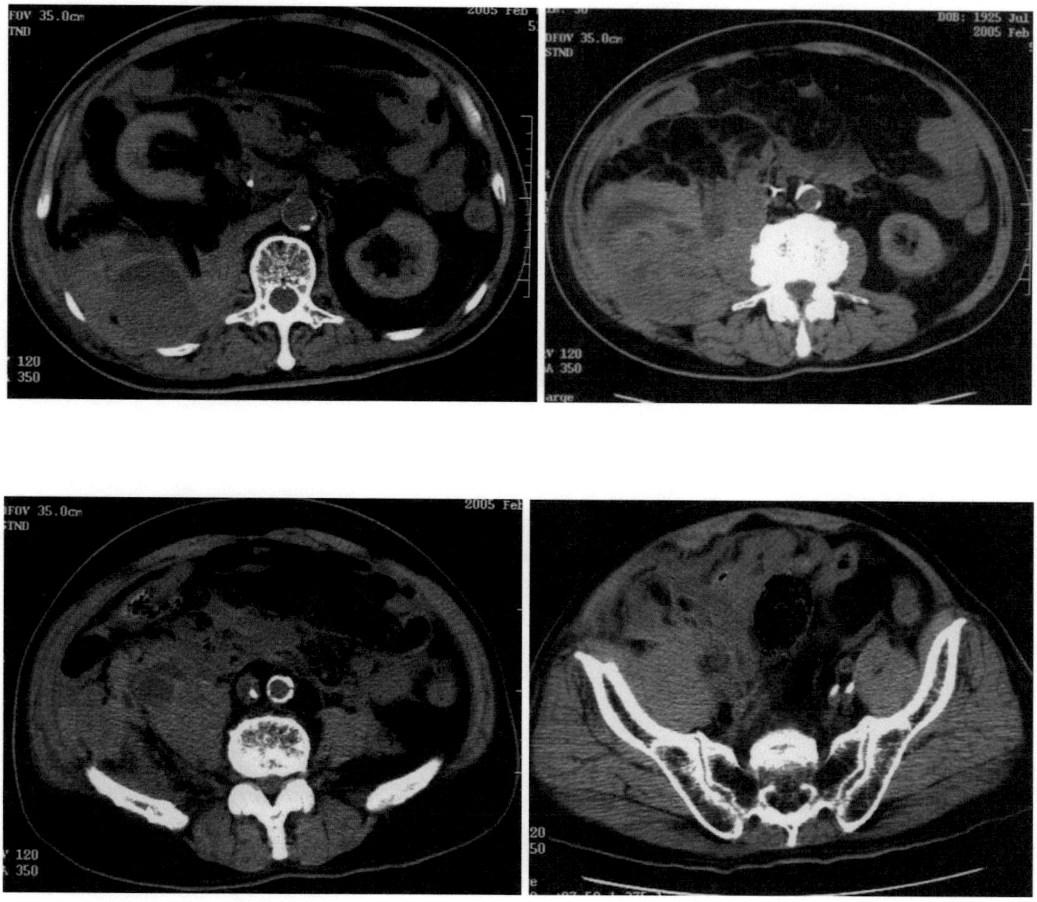

Figure 6. Axial images of abdominal computed tomography.

Abdominal computed tomography 26 hrs after endovascular coiling of an anterior communicating artery aneurysm. A huge retroperitoneal haematoma in the posterior abdominal wall is visible on the right side.

The patient failed to regain consciousness, and brain CT 20 (Fig. 4) hrs after coiling revealed iatrogenic cerebral infarction in the area of distribution of the left anterior cerebral artery. The patient began to become increasingly hypotensive 25 hrs after coiling. He was pale on physical examination and had marked abdominal distension. Abdominal/pelvic roentgenograms (Fig. 5) and CT (Fig. 6) revealed a large retroperitoneal mass on the right side. Abdominal angiography (Fig. 7) was conducted via right femoral artery access.

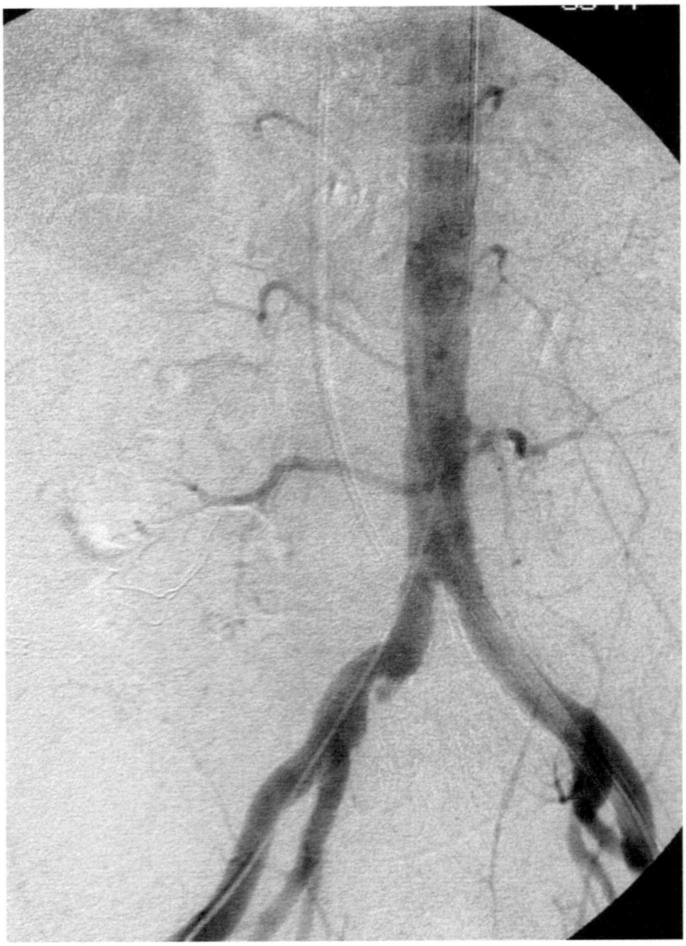

Figure 7. Pervic angiogram. Anterior posterior view of pelvic angiogram indicated no extravasation, abnourmal arterial injury, or actie bleeding focus.

Author(S)/year	Number of cases	Retroperitoneal hematoma	Rate of complications
AbuRahma/2006	101	1	1%
Ellis / 2006	28378	76	0.26%
Farouque/2003	3508	26	0.74%
Sreeram/1993	7334	11	0.15%
Popma/1993	1413	6	0.5%
Kent/1994	9585	45	0.47%

Table 1. Comparison of incidence of retroperitoneal hematoma in large series.

We did not identify the source of the haemorrhage. The puncture site for endovascular coiling was under the inguinal ligament. The haematocrit continued to fall, and the patient remained hypotensive even with multiple blood transfusions. An emergency laparotomy was performed, but the patient died of multiple organ failure five days after surgery.

3.1. Incidence of retroperitoneal haemorrhage

The low incidence of this complication has made it difficult to study in large numbers of patients. Retroperitoneal haemorrhage complicating percutaneous coronary intervention has been reported to occur in ~0.8% of all procedures (Ellis et al. 2006, Tiroch et al. 2008, Farouque et al. 2005). Ellis et al. reported 163 cases (0.57%) of retroperitoneal haemorrhage out of 28378 percutaneous coronary interventions and confirmed that female gender, body weight and location of sheath placement were risk factors of retroperitoneal haemorrhage (Ellis et al. 2006). Tiroch et al. also reported that the risk factors of RH following percutaneous coronary intervention are chronic renal insufficiency and high arterial puncture, with an incidence rate of 0.49% (17 of 3482 cases)(Tiroch et al. 2008).

3.2. Risk factor of retroperitoneal haemorrhage

Farouque et al. reported that the risk factors of retroperitoneal haemorrhage following percutaneous coronary intervention are female gender, higher femoral artery puncture and low body surface area (Farouque et al. 2005). The incidence of retroperitoneal haemorrhage in their study was 0.74% (26 of 3508 cases). In these studies (Cil et al. 2007, Ellis et al. 2006, Tiroch et al. 2008, Farouque et al. 2005), antithrombotic therapy and vascular closure devices after percutaneous coronary intervention were considered for all cases(Table). Kent et al. reviewed 9585 femoral artery catheterizations and reported 45 cases (0.5%) of retroperitoneal haemorrhage (Kent et al. 1994). These authors also reported the incidence of retroperitoneal haemorrhage after coronary artery stent placement with anticoagulation as less than 2% (Kent et al. 1994). Bejjani et al. reported one case of retroperitoneal haemorrhage after angioplasty where anticoagulant therapy was administered for cerebral vasospasm following subarachnoid haemorrhage (Bejjani et al. 1998). Quint et al. reported the role of femoral vessel catheterization and altered haemostasis in the development of extraperitoneal haematomas (Quint et al. 1993). On the basis of these reports, anticoagulant or thrombolytic therapy should be considered a risk factor of post-catheterization retroperitoneal haemorrhage (Cura et al. 2000, Park et al. 2011, Lodge et al. 1973, Luvian et al. 2004, Sharp et al. 1984, Tomlinson et al. 2000, Wasay et al. 2001, Witz et al. 1999).

3.3. Puncture site and retroperitoneal haemorrhage

Quint et al. studied 44 cases of retroperitoneal haemorrhage with catheterization and altered haemostasis and suggested that these haematomas usually arise from a vessel that is distant to the puncture site (Quint et al. 1993). When the haematoma is not adjacent to the punctured vessels, a haemorrhagic diathesis is the most likely aetiology of the haemorrhage. Sreeram et al. also found that post-catheterization antcoagulation and high arterial puncture were significant risk factors (Sreeram et al/ 1993). It has been suggested that some cases of retroperitoneal hematomas after angiography may be unrelated to femoral artery puncture and are more likely due to altered hemostasis. With computed tomographic findings, Quint et al. suggested (Quint et al. 1993) that 25% of retroperitoneal hematomas were remote from the site of femoral artery puncture, with the majority of these being on the contralateral side to the puncture site. Farouque et al. reported (Farouque et al. 2005) that all instances of retroperitoneal haemorrhage were ipsilateral to the femoral puncture site and contiguous with the presumed site of vessel puncture in the inguinal region. Farouque et al. (Farouque et al. 2005) also suggested that their observations imply that femoral artery puncture was an integral element to the formation of retroperitoneal haemorrhage in all cases.

3.4. Diagnosis and Symptoms of retroperitoneal haemorrhage

The diagnosis of retroperitoneal haemorrhage is difficult because its symptoms mimic other conditions (Akata et al. 1998, Cho et al. 2011, Haviv et al. 1996, Illescas et al. 1986, Kent et al. 1994, Murai et al. 2010). Signs and symptoms are nonspecific and include anaemia in 100%, back pain in 23%, groin pain in 46% and lower abdominal pain in 42% of patients according to Farouque's report (Farouque et al. 2005). Sharp et al. documented six cases of haematomas following femoral vein cannulation for haemodialysis (Sharp et al. 1984). In all cases, the diagnosis was made based on symptoms and abdominal radiography. Haviv et al. reported a case of acute right lower quadrant abdominal pain which was misdiagnosed as acute appendicitis on the basis of abdominal CT (Haviv et al. 1996). Neurological signs, such as lower extremity pain, can result from compression of the femoral nerves. Cho et al reported (Cho et al, 2011) that retroperitonal hemorrhage can present a diagnostic dilemma because it can present with a variety of symptoms, which, in order of frequency, include abdominal pain, hip and thigh pain, hypotension, anemia, and back pain. These vague symptoms can cause delay of diagnosis and treatment; consequently, it can lead to severe morbidity or mortality (Cho et al, 2011). Kim et al. suggested that anesthesiologists should be aware of the occurrence of retroperitoneal hemorrhage as a consequence of interventional procedures such as femoral arterial puncture. When On clinical suspicion, immediate imaging should be performed to determine the site and extent of the hematoma; fluid and blood product resuscitation is also essential(Kim et al. 2010).

Tiroch et al. also reported on the severity of retroperitoneal haemorrhage (Tiroch et al. 2008). In their study, patients with retroperitoneal haemorrhage had a mortality rate of 12% compared with 1.3% for non-retroperitoneal haemorrhage patients (Tiroch et al. 2008). Ellis et al. reported 17 patients (10.4%) of retroperitoneal haemorrhage who expired during hospitalization (Ellis et al. 2006). Even when patients cannot complain of pain, a definitive diagnosis can still be made by CT (Illescas et al. 1986, Kent et al. 1994). A disturbance in the level of consciousness is not uncommon in patients with subarachnoid haemorrhage, acute phase middle cerebral artery embolism, cerebral vasospasms after subarachnoid haemorrhage or ruptured arteriovenous malformations. Anticoagulant or thrombolytic therapy is commonly administered after interventional procedures have been completed. Such patients are at increased risk of developing retroperitoneal haematomas.

In our case, we continued to monitor the patient's vital signs, conduct physical examinations and record neurological findings during the perioperative period; however, we could not find evidence of a retroperitoneal haematoma(Murai et al. 2010). Unfortunately, disturbance of consciousness due to post-operative cerebral infarction and general anaesthesia makes it more difficult to find indications of a retroperitoneal haematoma perioperatively. Situations involving disturbance of consciousness, as in this case, are not rare for patients who undergo coiling for a ruptured aneurysm. When the level of consciousness is depressed, physical examination, serial haematocrits and close monitoring of systemic blood pressure should be routinely performed (Murai et al. 2010).

4. Conclusion

Retroperitoneal haematoma following interventional radiology for neurological diseases is relatively rare and can be difficult to diagnose, especially if consciousness is disturbed. This case demonstrates the importance of performing routine physical examinations, sequentially measuring the haematocrit and closely monitoring systemic blood pressure following interventional radiological procedures in patients with altered mental status.

Author details

Yasuo Murai and Akira Teramoto
Department of Neurosurgery, Nippon Medical School, Tokyo, Japan

5. References

AbuRahma AF, Hayes JD, Deel JT, Abu-Halimah S, Mullins BB, Habib JH, Welch CA, AbuRahma Z (2006). Complications of diagnostic carotid/cerebral arteriography when performed by a vascular surgeon. Vasc Endovascular Surg. 40:189-95.

AbuRahma AF, Elmore M, Deel J, Mullins B, Hayes J (2007). Complications of diagnostic arteriography performed by a vascular surgeon in a recent series of 558 patients. Vascular. 15:92-7.

Akata T, Nakayama T, Kandabashi T, Kodama K, Takahashi S (1998). Massive retroperitoneal hemorrhage associated with femoral vein cannulation. J Clin Anesth. 10:321-326.

Bejjani GK, Bank WO, Olan WJ, Sekhar LN (1998). The efficacy and safety of angioplasty for cerebral vasospasm after subarachnoid hemorrhage. Neurosurgery. 42:979-986.

Cho YD, Lee JY, Seo JH, Kang HS, Han MH (2011). Spontaneous peritoneal and retroperitoneal hemorrhage, rare serious complication following carotid angioplasty with stent. J Neurol Sci. 306:160-163.

Cil BE, Türkbey B, Canyiğit M, Geyik S, Yavuz K (2007). An unusual complication of carotid stenting: spontaneous rectus sheath hematoma and its endovascular management. Diagn Interv Radiol.13:46-48.

Cura FA, Kapadia SR, L'Allier PL, Schneider JP, Kreindel MS, Silver MJ, Yadav JS, Simpfendorfer CC, Raymond RR, Tuzcu EM, Franco I, Whitlow PL, Topol EJ, Ellis SG (2000). Safety of femoral closure devices after percutaneous coronary interventions in the era of glycoprotein IIb/IIIa platelet blockade. Am J Cardiol. 86:780-782.

Ellis SG, Bhatt D, Kapadia S, Lee D, Yen M, Whitlow PL (2006). Correlates and outcomes of retroperitoneal hemorrhage complicating percutaneous coronary intervention. Catheter Cardiovasc Interv. 67:541-545.

Farouque HM, Tremmel JA, Raissi Shabari F, Aggarwal M, Fearon WF, Ng MK, Rezaee M, Yeung AC, Lee DP (200). Risk factors for the development of retroperitoneal hematoma after percutaneous coronary intervention in the era of glycoprotein IIb/IIIa inhibitors and vascular closure devices. J Am Coll Cardiol. 45:363-368.

Haviv YS, Nahir M, Pikarski A, Shiloni E, Safadi R (1996). A late retroperitoneal hematoma mimicking acute appendicitis--an unusual complication of coronary angioplasty. Eur J Med Res 1:591-592.

Illescas FF, Baker ME, McCann R, Cohan RH, Silverman PM, Dunnick NR (1986). CT evaluation of retroperitoneal hemorrhage associated with femoral arteriography. AJR Am J Roentgenol. 146:1289-1292.

Kalinowski EA, Trerotola SO (1998). Postcatheterization retroperitoneal hematoma due to spontaneous lumbar arterial hemorrhage. Cardiovasc Intervent Radiol 21:337-339.

Kent KC, Moscucci M, Mansour KA, DiMattia S, Gallagher S, Kuntz R (1994) Retroperitoneal hematoma after cardiac catheterization: prevalence, risk factors, and optimal management. J Vasc Surg. 20:905-910.

Kim HY, Kim MH, Jung SH, Ryu J, Jeon YT, Na HS, Hwang JY (2010). Retroperitoneal hematoma after coil embolization of cerebral aneurysm -A case report-. Korean J Anesthesiol. 59 Suppl:S187-90.

Lin PH, Dodson TF, Bush RL, Weiss VJ, Conklin BS, Chen C (2001). Surgical intervention for complications caused by femoral artery catheterization in pediatric patients. J Vasc Surg. 34:1071-1078.

Lodge JP, Hall R (1973). Retroperitoneal haemorrhage: a dangerous complication of common femoral arterial puncture. Eur J Vasc Surg. 7:355-357.

Lubavin BV (2004). Retroperitoneal hematoma as a complication of coronary angiography and stenting. Am J Emerg Med. 22:236-238.

Lubicz B, Collignon L, Raphaeli G, De Witte O(2011). Pipeline flow-diverter stent for endovascular treatment of intracranial aneurysms: preliminary experience in 20 patients with 27 aneurysms. World Neurosurg. 76:114-119.

Mak GY, Daly B, Chan W, Tse KK, Chung HK, Woo KS (1993). Percutaneous treatment of post catheterization massive retroperitoneal hemorrhage. Cathet Cardiovasc Diagn. 29:40-43.

Murai Y, Adachi K, Yoshida Y, Takei M, Teramoto A (2010) Retroperitoneal hematoma as a serious complication of endovascular aneurysmal coiling. J Korean Neurosurg Soc. 48:88-90.

Murai Y, Kominami S, Yoshida Y, Mizunari T, Adachi K, Koketsu K, Kobayashi S, Teramoto A (2011) Preoperative liquid embolization of cerebeller hemangioblastomas using N-butyl cyanoacrylate. Neuroradiology. 2012, in print

Murai Y, Kominami S, Kobayashi S, Mizunari T, Teramoto A(2005). The long-term effects of transluminal balloon angioplasty for vasospasms after subarachnoid hemorrhage: analyses of cerebral blood flow and reactivity. Surg Neurol.64:122-127.

Nasser TK, Mohler ER 3rd, Wilensky RL, Hathaway DR (1995). Peripheral vascular complications following coronary interventional procedures. Clin Cardiol 18:609–614

Park SH, Lee SW, Jeon U, Jeon MH, Lee SJ, Shin WY, Jin DK (2011). Transcatheter arterial embolization as treatment for a life-threatening retroperitoneal hemorrhage complicating heparin therapy. Korean J Intern Med. 26:352-5.

Paul AR, Colby GP, Radvany MG, Huang J, Tamargo RJ, Coon AL (2010). Femoral access in 100 consecutive subarachnoid hemorrhage patients: the "craniotomy" of endovascular neurosurgery. BMC Res Notes. 3:285.

Popma JJ, Satler LF, Pichard AD, Kent KM, Campbell A, Chuang YC, Clark C, Merritt AJ, Bucher TA, Leon MB (1993). Vascular complications after balloon and new device angioplasty. Circulation 88:1569 –78.

Quint LE, Holland D, Korobkin M, Cascade PN (1993). Role of femoral vessel catheterization and altered hemostasis in the development of extraperitoneal hematomas: CT study in 44 patients. AJR Am J Roentgenol. 160:855-858.

Raymond J, Guilbert F, Roy D(2001). Neck-bridge device for endovascular treatment of wide-neck bifurcation aneurysms: initial experience. Radiology. 221:318-326.

Raphael M, Hartnell G (2001). Femoral artery catheterization and retroperitoneal haematoma formation. Clin Radiol. 56:933-934.

Sakai N, Murai Y, Suzuki N, Kominami S, Mizunari T, Kobayashi S, Teramoto A, Kamiyama H(2001). A case of iatrogenic carotid artery dissection treated with radial artery graft. No Shinkei Geka. 29:837-41.

Sharp KW, Spees EK, Selby LR, Zachary JB, Ernst CB (1984). Diagnosis and management of retroperitoneal hematomas after femoral vein cannulation for hemodialysis. Surgery. 95:90-95.

Sreeram S, Lumsden AB, Miller JS, Salam AA, Dodson TF, Smith RB (1993). Retroperitoneal hematoma following femoral arterial catheterization: a serious and often fatal complication. Am Surg. 59:94-98.

Swayne LC, Peterson DP, Pohl C (1994). Scintigraphic localization of the bleeding site of a large retroperitoneal hematoma following renal angioplasty. Clin Nucl Med. 19:490-492.

Teasdale GM, Drake CG, Hunt W, Kassell N, Sano K, Pertuiset B, De Villiers JC (1988). A universal subarachnoid hemorrhage scale: report of a committee of the World Federation of Neurosurgical Societies. J Neurol Neurosurg Psychiatry. 51:1457.

Tiroch KA, Arora N, Matheny ME, Liu C, Lee TC, Resnic FS (2008). Risk predictors of retroperitoneal hemorrhage following percutaneous coronary intervention. Am J Cardiol. 102:1473-1476.Tomlinson MA, Anjum A, Loosemore T (2000). Retroperitoneal haematoma. Eur J Vasc Endovasc Surg. 19:558-559.

Trerotola SO, Kuhlman JE, Fishman EK (1990). Bleeding complications of femoral catheterization: CT evaluation. Radiology. 74:37-40.

Trimarchi S, Smith DE, Share D, Jani SM, O'Donnell M, McNamara R, Riba A, Kline-Rogers E, Gurm HS, Moscucci M; BMC2 Registry (2010). Retroperitoneal hematoma after percutaneous coronary intervention: prevalence, risk factors, management, outcomes, and predictors of mortality: a report from the BMC2 (Blue Cross Blue Shield of Michigan Cardiovascular Consortium) registry. JACC Cardiovasc Interv. 3:845-850.

Umeoka K, Kominami S, Mizunari T, Murai Y, Kobayashi S, Teramoto A (2011). Cerebral artery restenosis following transluminal balloon angioplasty for vasospasm after subarachnoid hemorrhage. Surg Neurol Int :2:43.

Wasay M, Bakshi R, Kojan S, Bobustuc G, Dubey N, Unwin DH (2001). Nonrandomized comparison of local urokinase thrombolysis versus systemic heparin anticoagulation for superior sagittal sinus thrombosis. Stroke. 32:2310-2317.

Witz M, Cohen Y, Lehmann JM (1999) Retroperitoneal haematoma - a serious vascular complication of cardiac catheterisation. Eur J Vasc Endovasc Surg. 18:364-365.

Chapter 16

Intracranial and Extracranial Infectious Pseudoaneurysms

Václav Procházka, Michaela Vávrová,
Tomáš Jonszta, Daniel Czerný,
Jan Krajča and Tomáš Hrbáč

Additional information is available at the end of the chapter

http://dx.doi.org/10.5772/47405

1. Introduction

Intracranial mycotic pseudoaneurysms are rare and generally lethal. The infectious pseudoaneurysms occur more frequently in the anterior circulation and may be multiple. Haemorrhage is rare but is associated with poor neurological outcome. The outcome in children is comparable, or slightly better, than in adults. Mortality reaches up to 80% in some studies. Cerebral mycotic or infectious aneurysms are a complication of infectious diseases (Cloud et al.,2003). Recently, infectious aneurysms occur more frequently in patients with a history of drug abuse (cocaine, heroine, pervitine, etc.), or in patients with Human Immunodeficiency Syndrome (HIV).

Presenting symptoms are typically headache, focal neurological deficit and/or haemorrhage. Headache is the most common presenting complaint in infectious and dissecting aneurysms.

Treatment of mycotic aneurysms is often difficult; they are managed conservatively with a prolonged course of antibiotics. In case of haemorrhage, surgical or endovascular treatment is used. Although surgery has been a traditional treatment of ruptured infectious pseudoaneurysms, it is associated with a higher rate of mortality (up to 80%). Endovascular treatment seems to be more safe. Parent artery occlusion (PAO) with coil embolisation or droplet of glue has become an attractive alternative treatment due to its low rate of morbidity and mortality. Vasospasm associated with haemorrhage is usually well tolerated in young patients.

2. Selective cases

2.1. Case No. 1

A 17-year-old girl, with the history of desoxyephedrine abuse for the last 2 years, was admitted into the hospital due to severe attack of headache, accompanied with a left-sided hemiparesis. The girl was anorectic, with vaginal discharge. Initial CT/CTA scan showed a large right hemisphere intracerebral haematoma (Fig. 1). The presence of pseudoaneurysm was suspected and confirmed by angiography, located in the right M3-MCA segment (Fig. 2). All vessels in the surrounding area were narrowed, with vessel wall irregularities. Due to the rebleeding risk and marked clinical deterioration at the time of the emergency angiography, parent artery occlusion of M3 MCA segmental branch was performed (Fig. 3).

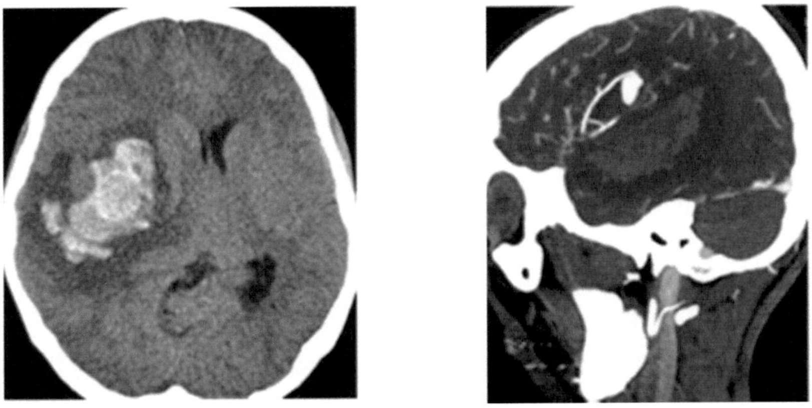

A B

A, CT scan: large intracerebral haematoma in the right hemisphere with midline shift.
B, CTA sagital view: large depo of contrast media in area of M3 segment of right MCA.

Figure 1. Initial CT/CTA scan

Immediately after the embolisation procedure, neurosurgeon evacuated the residual intracerebral haematoma and a decompressive craniectomy was completed (Fig. 4). The blood analysis confirmed latent infectious stage with a high white blood cell count of 17,9 x 10^9/l, CRP 146mg/l and a higher level of fibrinogen 5,252 g/l, with no subsequent shift in coagulation. HIV test was negative.

In addition to the endovascular procedure, intravenous administration of an antibiotic therapy (Claforan, Lek, SLO) was implemented. After a two-month period, the girl was doing quite well, Rankin scale-1, with small residual left-side hemiparesis and completely self-sufficient. All blood tests were normalized. Second control cerebral angiography confirmed a total occlusion of the pseudoaneurysm (Fig.5). At one-year follow-up, digital subtraction angiography was unremarkable, without pseudoaneurysm perfusion and vessel wall inflammation. Surrounding vessels were regular. The girl was back at school and doing well.

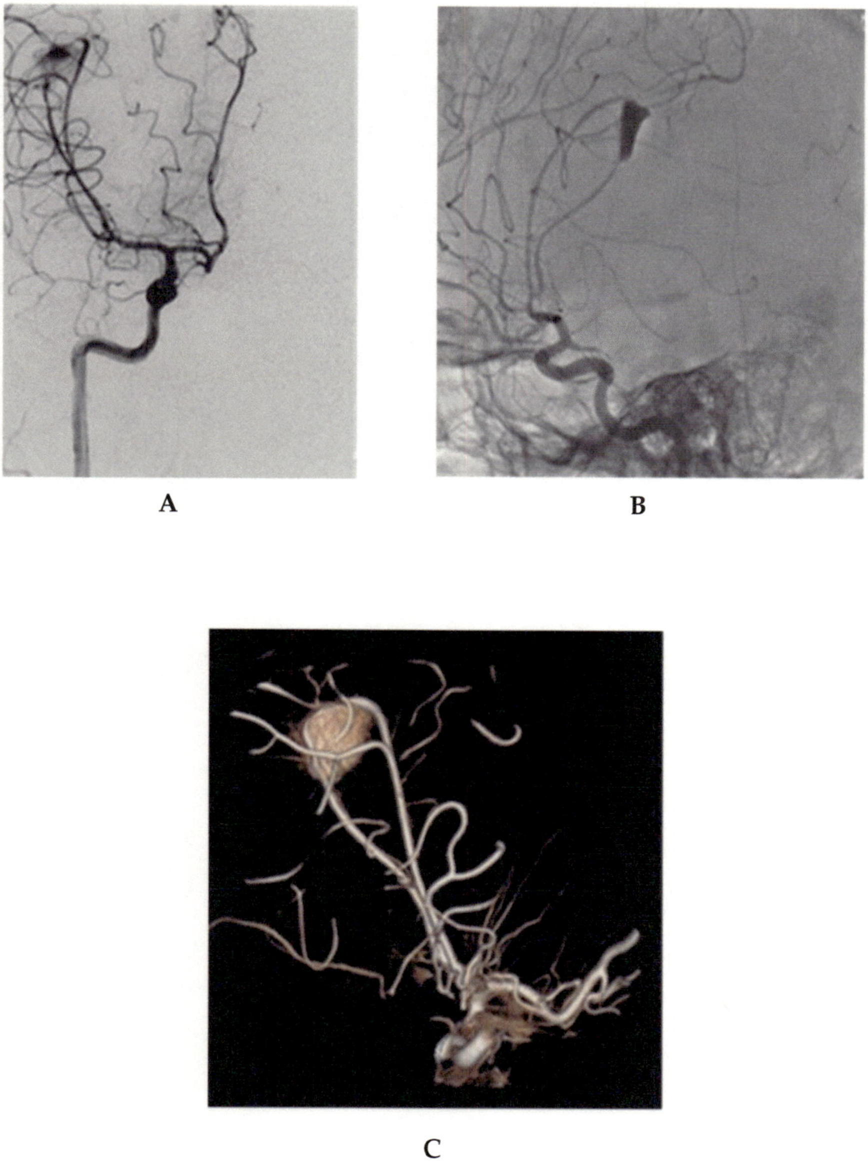

A, Angiography frontal view: M2-3 segment of MCA artery; we see a large pseudoaneurysm, the supplying vessel has irregular shape.
B, Lateral view angiogram with large pseudoaneurysm in the M2-3 segment of the right MCA artery.
C, 3D-XRA reconstruction of the right MCA artery pseudoaneurysm

Figure 2. Digital subtraction angiography with 3D-XRA reconstruction

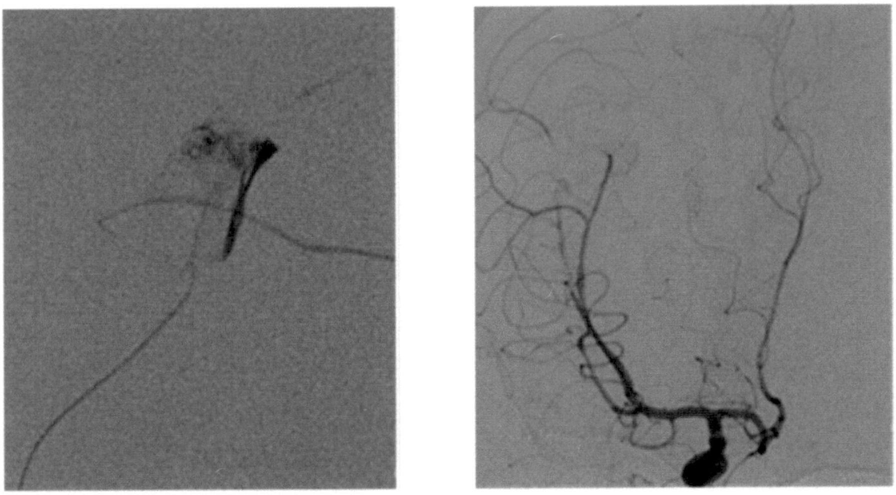

A B

A, Microcatheter in the parent artery. Control angiography confirmed the correct position of microcatheter just below the aneurysm.
B, Frontal view angiogram confirming pseudoaneurysm occlusion.

Figure 3. Embolisation procedure

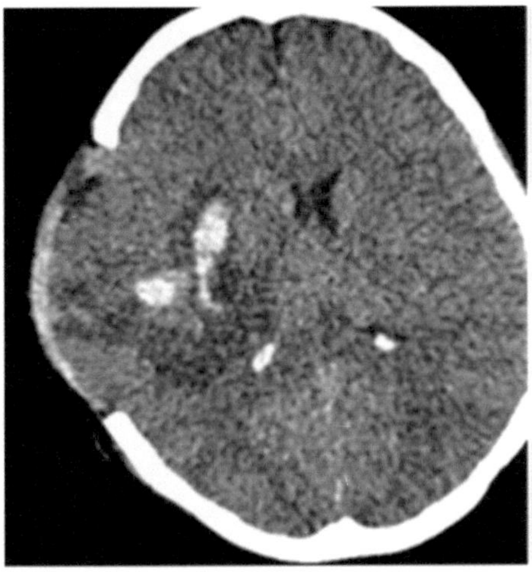

Figure 4. CT scan after neurosurgical removal of large intracerebral haematoma and decompressive craniectomy.

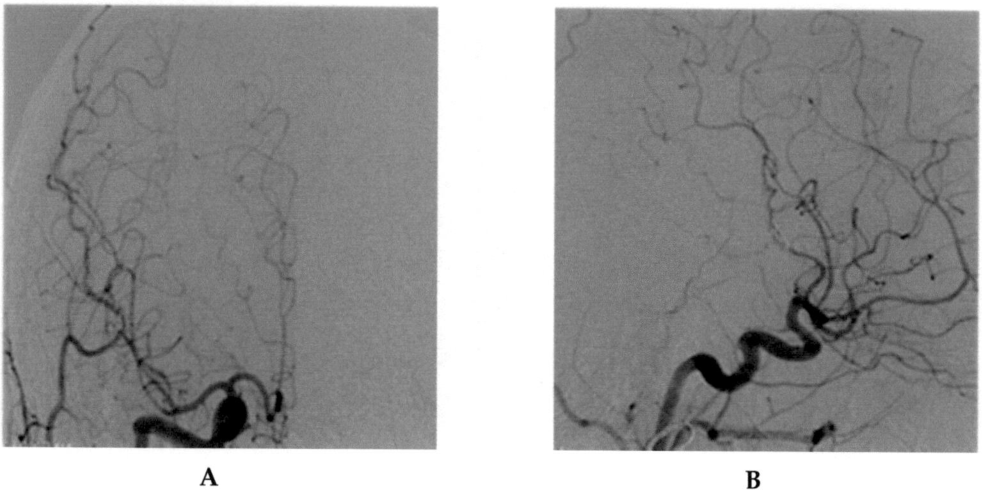

A, One-year follow-up angiography in the AP and lateral view B, shoving no contrast filling of the pseudoaneurysm, normal shape of the vessels in the region of right MCA artery.

Figure 5. Follow-up angiogram

2.2. Case No. 2

A 12-year-old boy, with the history of premature delivery due to the placenta release, (30th week of gestation, having 1300g of body weight and 38cm of height at birth), spent 8 weeks in the incubator on ventilation support and phototherapy due to severe icterus. At 10 months of age, he was admitted into the hospital because of severe pneumonia and was put on assisted ventilation. He also suffered from severe focal seizures, headache, anxiety and impaired locomotion. However, due to the headache deterioration, MRI examination was performed and showed a small area of bleeding in the left opercular insular segment (Fig. 6) suggesting a presence of pseudoaneurysm in the left MCA branch. Peripheral blood counts and CRP levels were in physiological range. Subsequent angiography revealed a mycotic pseudoaneurysm in the left MCA opercular segment (Fig.7) with a straightened supplying artery, while the surrounding vessels were narrowed. Due to the high risk of pseudoaneurysm rupture, the endovascular PAO was directly performed, using coil embolisation. Immediately after the embolization, a weak bradylalia developed due to the Brockas´ area MCA supplying territory perfusion, but the condition rapidly disappeared (Fig.8). Seizure attacks following embolisation stopped, and one-month follow-up MRI confirmed pseudoaneurysm thrombosis (Fig.9).

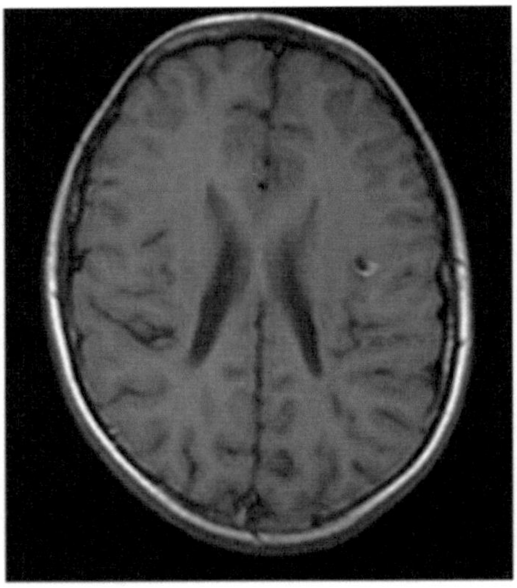

A

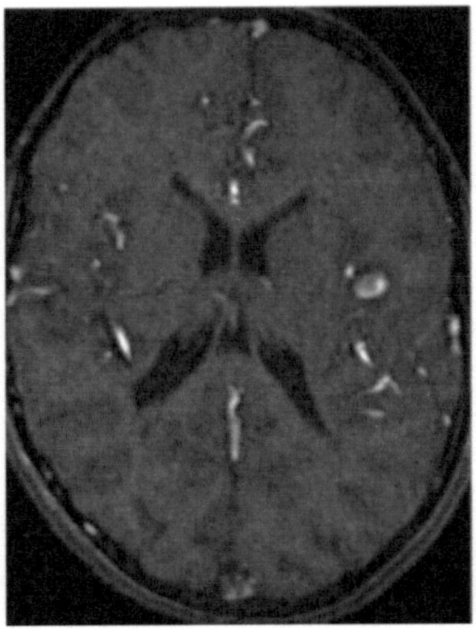

B

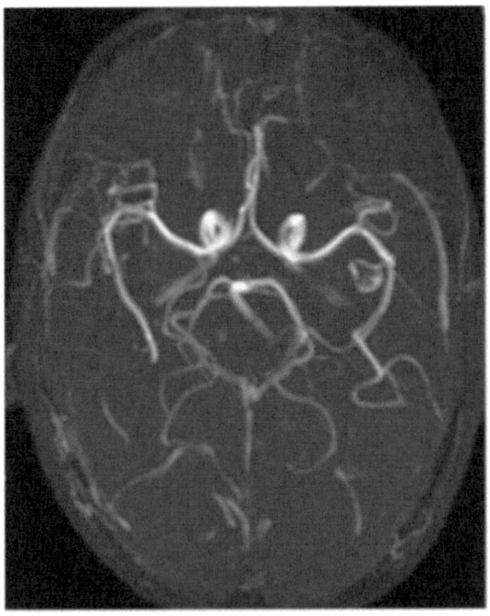

C

A,B MRI + MRA: Pd T2, MRA axial plane confirmed little area of haemorrhage in the left opercular area, deposits of methemoglobine
C, Based on MRA scan, suspicion of pseudoaneurysm in the region of M2,3 segment of the left MCA was confirmed.

Figure 6. MRI/MRA diagnostic scan for seizure and headache.

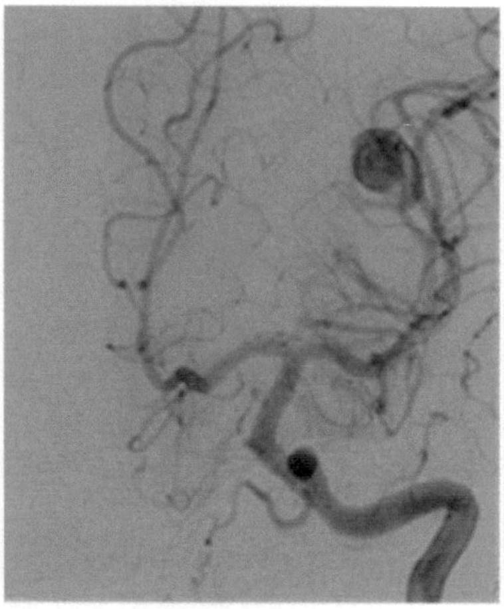

A

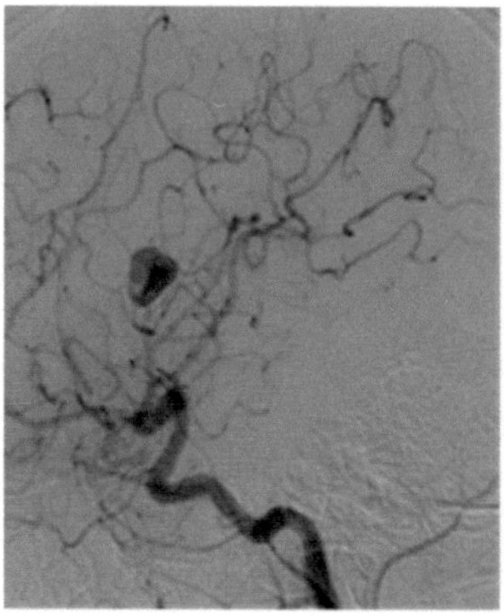

B

A,B, Large pseudoaneurysm in the area of the left MCA artery M3 segment in AP and lateral view, normal size and shape of surrounding vessels.

Figure 7. Digital subtraction angiography of the left intracranial circulation

Six-month follow-up MRA showing no contrast filling of the pseudoaneurysm, and regular shape of the surrounding vessels.

3. Extracranial infectious aneurysms

Pseudoaneurysm of the cervical portion of the internal carotid artery (ICA) is rare but potentially lethal complication of the deep neck infection. Liston was the first to describe pseudoaneurysm in this area in 1843 (Liston,1843). In 1933, Salinger and Pearlman (Salinger & Pearlman, 1933) published a set of 228 pseudoaneurysm cases. This has been the largest group of patients ever reported. Since the introduction of antibiotic treatment, less than 40 pseudoaneurysm cases have been described. In spite of significant advances in the treatment of ICA pseudoaneurysm, this condition is associated with a poor prognosis.

In addition to the systemic antibiotics treatment, surgical management may include ligation of the aneurysm with or without preserving the adjacent vessel wall and an end-to-end anastomosis of the carotid artery. An acceptable alternative treatment to surgery is a stentgraft or bare stent implantation with/without coil embolisation.

4. Selective cases

4.1. Case No. 3

A 56- year-old male, who suffered for one month from sore throat, dysphagia, and left neck stiffness. Parapharyngeal phlegmona was detected on both ultrasound and CT scan, explorative surgery was performed and the patient was put on antibiotics treatment. Ten days later, the patient returned with a painful bulge on his neck. A parapharyngeal abscess was confirmed on CT scan, with subsequent surgical drainage. The infectious agent cultured from the specimen was Staphylococcus species. Five days later, a small fistula in the lower pole of the surgical scar evolved. Prompt follow- up CT scan revealed pseudoaneurysm at the level of the left carotid bifurcation, 18 mm in size (Fig. 10).

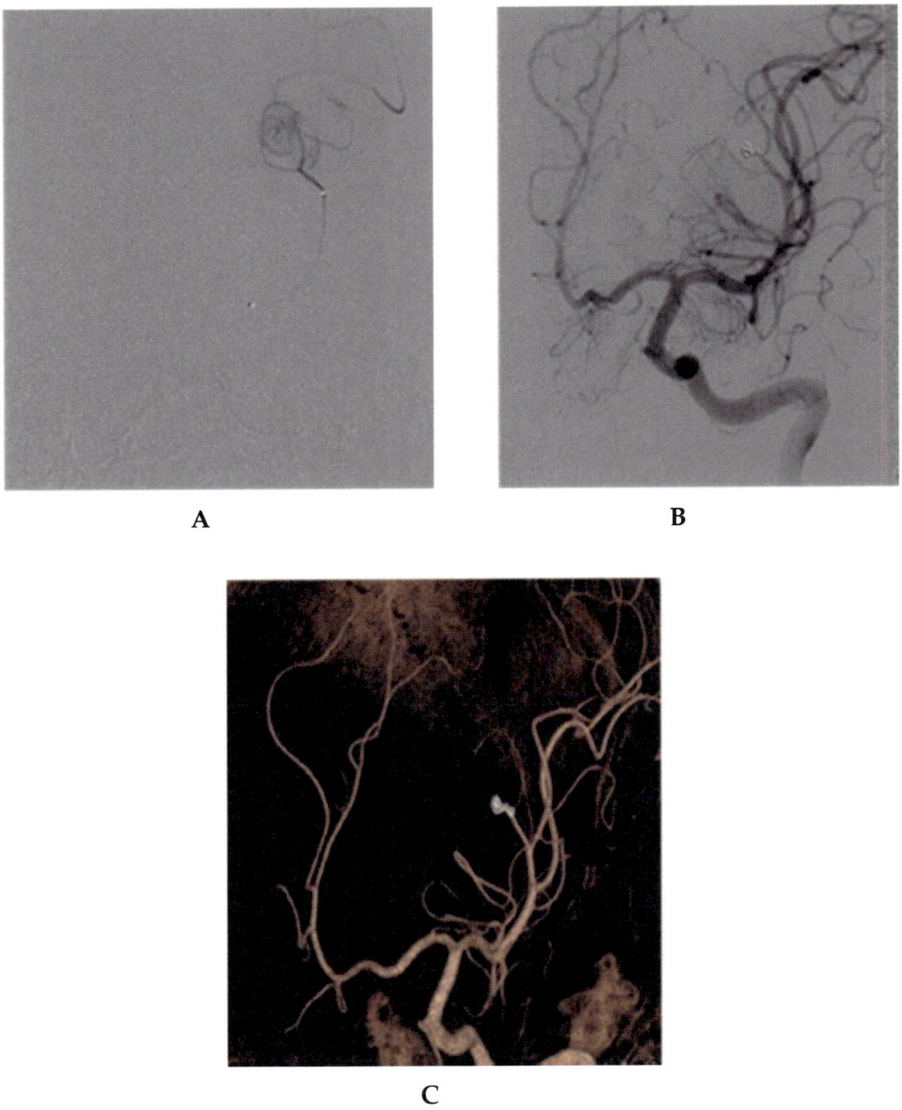

A, Selective angiogram before pseudoaneurysm embolisation. Microcatheter is positioned just below the pseudoaneurysm.
B, Follow-up angiography after embolisation AP view, pseudoaneurysm exclusion.
C, 3D-XRA reconstruction after embolisation.

Figure 8. Parent artery occlusion embolisation procedure

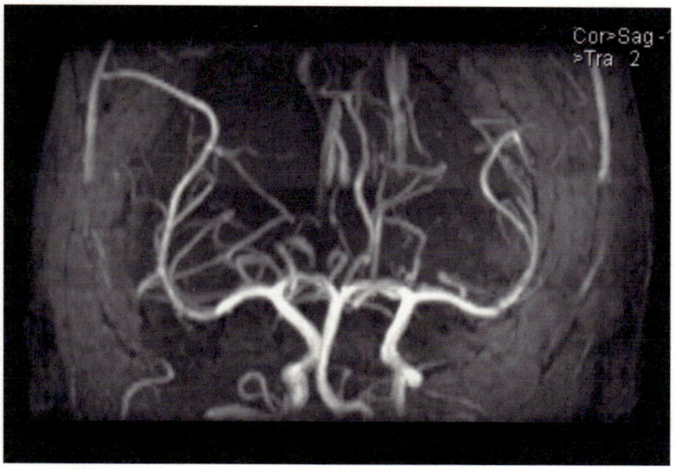

Figure 9. Follow-up MRA

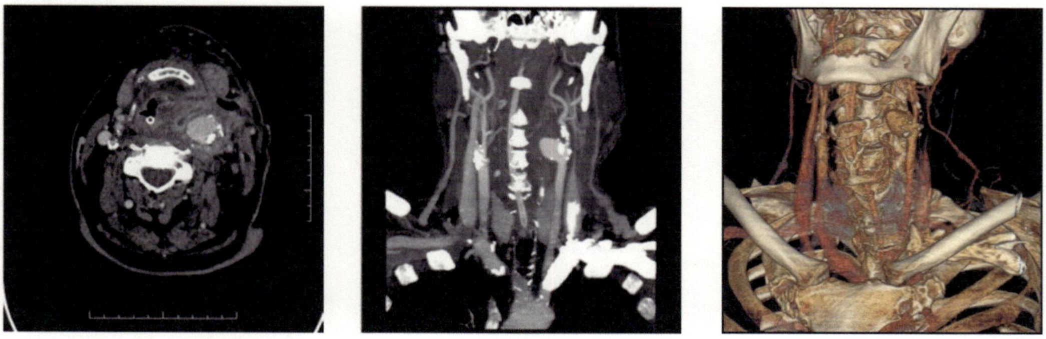

A B C

A, Contrast enhanced CT scan in axial view showing large retropharyngeal inflammation with pseudoaneurysm in the bifurcation of the left common carotid artery.
B, CT scan in MIP projection with large pseudoaneurysm filling
C, CT scan in VRT reconstruction with pseudoaneurysm

Figure 10. Initial CT scan confirming inflammation and pseudoaneurysm

The vascular surgeon and interventional radiologist were consulted and endovascular approach was agreed upon, as the best treatment option at that particular case. The pathological finding was verified with 3D angiography and two interpolated Wallstents 8/29 (Boston Scientific, USA) were implanted into CCA-ICA region (Fig.11,12). Immediate contrast agent stagnation in the pseudoaneurysm sac was observed. The patient was put on Dalteparine, with the dose of 5000 units per day, which was later followed with dual antiplatelet regime. Dual combination of antibiotics was used (cefotaxime and metronidazole) for prolonged treatment.

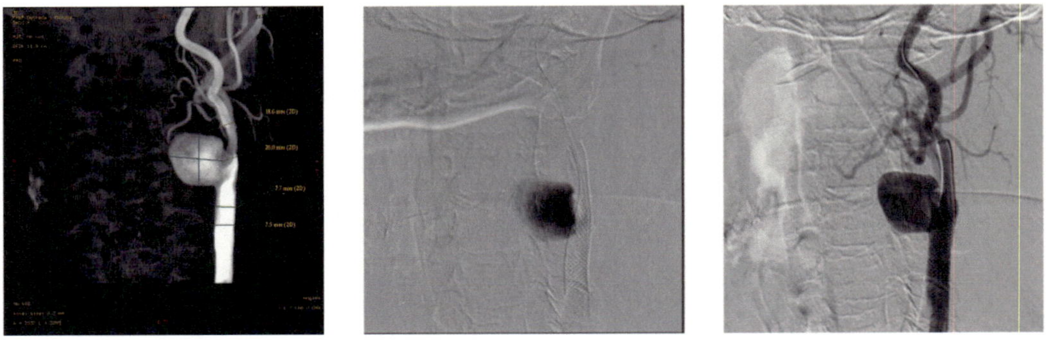

A B C

A, 3D-XRA reconstruction with MIP projection of the left CCA bifurcation pseudoaneurysm.
B, Contrast stagnation in pseudoaneurysm after stenting procedure.
C, Two interpolated Wallstents implanted in ICA-CCA

Figure 11. Stenting procedure

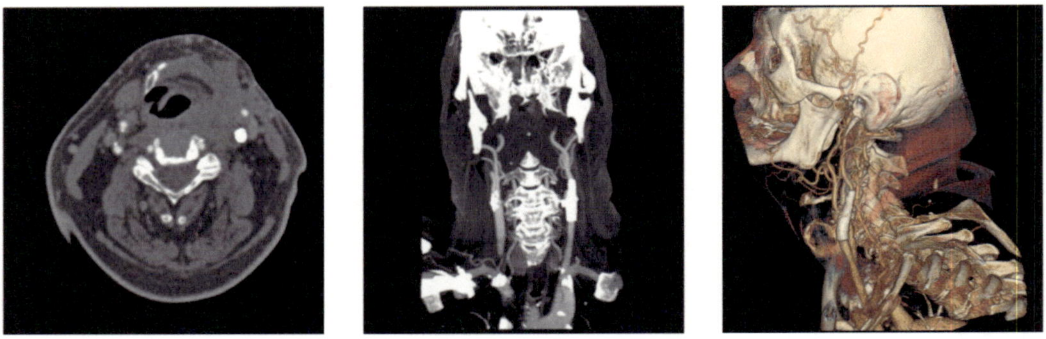

A B C

A, Follow-up CT scan after Wallstent implantation in axial view.
B, CT scan in MIP projection after stent implantation-exclusion of pseudoaneurysm.
C, CT scan in VRT lateral view with normal perfusion in carotid bifurcation.

Figure 12. Follow-up CT scan after stenting procedure with aneurysm exclusion.

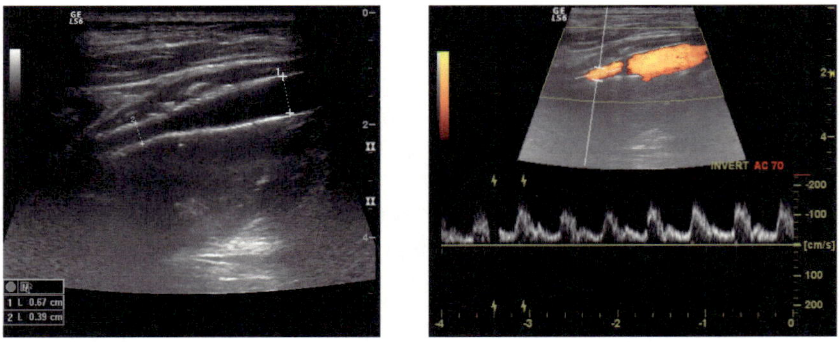

A B

A,B Normal Wallstent perfusion with pseudoaneurysm thrombosis

Figure 13. Ultrasound duplex Doppler follow-up.

The local finding on the vessels was followed with intense ultrasound exams and over the time period of one month, the lesion healed completely with normal carotid vessels patency (Fig. 13).

4.2. Case No. 4

A 17-year-old male with a 5-day history of sore throat, difficult swallowing, pain in the left ear, fever and trismus was examined with CT scan (Fig.14). Inflammation of the left tonsil spreading into the left retrotonsillar and carotid space was confirmed. Laboratory values showed C-reactive protein (CPR) of 175 mg/l and white blood cell count (WBC) of 13,5 x 109/l. Due to worsening of clinical symptoms and continuing fever, an acute tonsillectomy was indicated and tonsillar culture confirmed Neisseria species and Streptoccocus viridans. The patient was discharged on oral Augmentin (Amoxicillinum trihydras and Acidum clavulanicum, Smith Kline Beecham Pharmaceuticals, Worthing, Great Britain) five days later. Laboratory results showed CRP 49 mg/l and WBC 5,8 x 109/l.

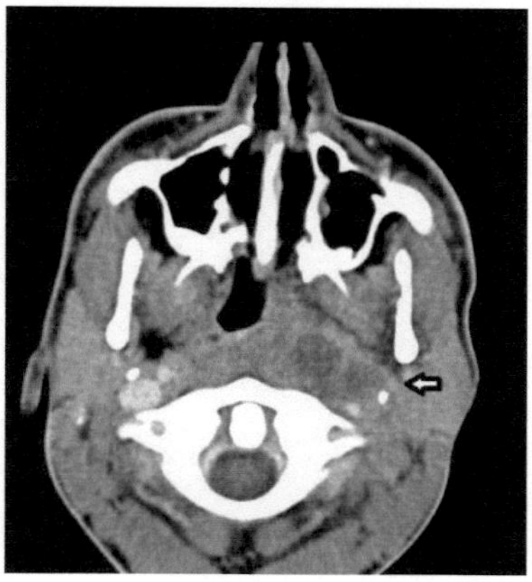

Figure 14. Axial CT scan confirmed an enlarged left tonsil, with an inhomogeneous saturation after i.v. contrast administration. Defiguration of swallowed air-ways and small abscess signs in tonsillar and retrotonsillar space were observed.

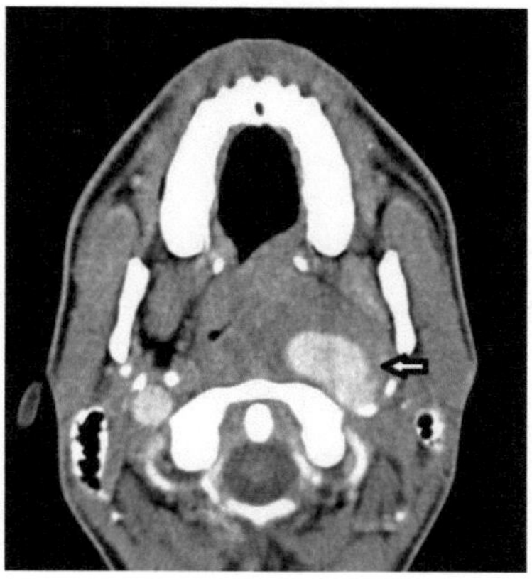

Figure 15. The CT scan shows a large area of pseudoaneurysm in the left retrotonsillar space with a high density.

The patient was readmitted one month later, with a severe pain in the left side of his throat and progressive headache. CT scan was performed with administration of 80 ml of a non-ionic contrast media at a 3.5 ml/s flow rate. A large left ICA pseudoaneurysm was revealed as 18x33 mm dense area in the left retrotonsillar space, extending into the left temporomandibular joint (Fig.15). A vascular surgeon was consulted. However, due to inaccessibility of the skull base pseudoaneurysm, the endovascular treatment was selected as a more feasible approach.

Pseudoaneurysm of the left ICA was visualised (Fig. 16A) and carotid bare Wallstent 7 x 40 mm (Boston Scientific, USA) was promptly implanted into the left ICA. A second angiogram 5 minutes later showed a reduction of the pseudoaneurysm perfusion (Fig 16B). The treatment with Plavix 75 mg and ASA100mg / once a day was continued four weeks. Amoxicillin (Amoxicilinum natricum, Lek Pharmaceuticals, Slovakia) and Klimicin (Klindamycin, Lek Pharmaceuticals, Slovakia) were administered for four weeks. The follow up angiogram in four weeks showed an excellent ICA patency and no pseudoaneurysm filling (Fig 16C). CRP was 17 mg/l, WBC was normal. Patient was discharged doing well.

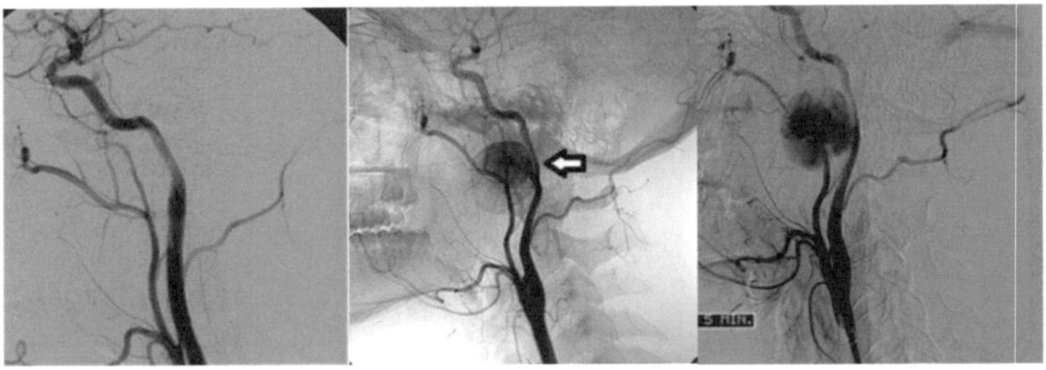

A B C

A, Angiogram of the left common carotid artery confirmed a large pseudoaneurysm at the level of the scull base.
B, The Wallstent immediately after the implantation in the left internal carotid artery.
C, Follow-up angiography after one month confirmed a healed left ICA (C).

Figure 16. Procedure and follow-up angiogram

5. Discussion

Church was the first one to describe an infectious aneurysm in a 13-year-old boy with mitral valve endocarditis in 1869. It has been estimated that infectious aneurysms develop in 3-15% of patients with infectious endocarditis. Intracranial aneurysms are rare in children, accounting for merely 0.5-4.6% of all aneurysms. Several characteristics distinguish them from aneurysms in adults: male predominance; higher incidence of unusual location, such as peripheral or posterior circulation, and a greater count of large or giant aneurysms. These unique features can be attributed to the higher incidence of traumatic, infectious, developmental, and congenital lesions. Subarachnoid haemorrhage is not the exclusive mode of presentation. Neuro-compressive signs and symptoms are frequently observed (Kanaan et al.,1995).

Infectious intracranial pseudoaneurysms develop mostly from the circulating infectious material. The source of this material is obviously located in cardiac valves. Infectious emboli lodges in small distal cerebral arteries and occludes distal arterial flow. Consequently, intense inflammation in the media and adventitia destroys the integrity of the arterial wall and weakens it. The resulting aneurysms are mostly fusiform, eccentric or typical pseudoaneurysms (Chun et al.,2001;Molinari et al.,1973).

Management of the therapy requires multimodality approach. Basically, there exist three possible options. The first one is a medical management of an unruptured infectious pseudoaneurysm with a long course of intravenous antibiotic therapy. This period is usually 6 weeks but may be longer, depending on the impairment of the host immunity. Endovascular therapy is the first line option for patients with ruptured aneurysms. It is a safer, elegant method which decreases the risk of aneurysm rerupture and makes the possible subsequent surgical treatment more safe. In case of multiple aneurysms, there is a benefit of treating more lesions at the same time. Surgical management is the first option for patients in unstable condition, with large intraparenchymal hematoma and increased ICP. The most common location for surgically treated aneurysms is the MCA territory (Lasjaunias et al.,2005;Lasjaunias & Ter Brugge,1997;Rodesch et al.,1987).

Patients with a history of drug abuse desoxyephedrine (Pervitine), cocaine, heroin etc. are frequently affected with brain haemorrhage. These drugs are stimulating. Drugs potentiates dopamine production, which leads to euphoria and high energy, it also suppresses starvation. This drug leads to sympathetic hyperactivity-induced transient hypertension (Gavin,1991;Grinspoon & Bakalar,1981;Lichtenfeld et al.,1984). Hypertension is a predisposing factor for the development and rupture of vulnerable vessels or infectious pseudoaneurysms, which occur more often in drug addicted persons.

Desoxyephedrine, cocaine and its metabolites have been proved as potent cerebral vasoconstrictors (Madden & Powers,1990). In animal models and in human volunteers it was demonstrated that even at a low dose, desoxyephedrine and cocaine can induce cerebrovascular dysfunction and cumulative residual effect in which repeated desoxyephedrine exposure produces delayed and/or prolonged formation and growth of an aneurysm, together with narrowing of vessels. In vivo duration of desoxyephedrine and cocaine-induced vasospasm is unclear (Jain,1963;Nanda et al.,2000). Patients with drug-related aneurysms reportedly have a higher mortality rate than a group of patients with no history of drug abuse.

Pseudoaneurysm of the ICA at the extracranial segment is a rare complication of deep neck area infections, penetrating trauma, tumour invasion and/or radiotherapy. Compared to a true aneurysm, the pseudoaneurysms has no complete native arterial wall. It is composed of extravasated blood that leaked from the area of vessel erosion and is surrounded by inflammatory and fibrous tissues. Pseudoaneurysms of ICA are more frequent in paediatric population. Children are more susceptible to arteritis (Cohen & Rad.,2004). Infection can reach the wall of the carotid artery following a peritonsillar abscesses or pharyngitis. Another pathway for infection may be septicaemia and invasion of the vasa vasorum.

Other possible causes of pseudoaneurysms are penetrating wounds or iatrogenic spread of infection after catheterisation (Alexander et al.,1968; Liston.,1843). The pseudoaneurysms is most likely seen as a result of tonsillitis-induced parapharyngeal abscess, reaching the left ICA adventitia. In our case, ischemia of the carotid artery wall led to its rupture and subsequent development of pseudoaneurysms. We could not exclude a perioperative trauma of ICA during emergency tonsillectomy. Usual bacterial agents causing pseudoaneurysms are *Staphylococcus aureus or Streptococcus pyogenes* (Gralla et al.,2004).

A mycotic carotid pseudoaneurysms most likely present as a growing, pulsatile cervical mass, manifested with dysphagia, odynophagia, and fever. Less frequently, lower cranial nerve palsies, Horner's syndrome or trismus may occur. Severe and life-threatening complications may include a carotid artery rupture, intermittent massive nasopharyngeal haemorrhage, and septic or non-septic embolic events leading to a neurological deficit. The usual interval between the infection and the pseudoaneurysms development is between 2 and 8 weeks. The treatment of carotid artery pseudoaneurysms is complex. The typical management of an infected pseudoaneurysms is twofold: systemic antibiotic administration (predominantly penicillin or clindamycin) and/or surgery, with either a traditional by-pass, or a ligation of ICA (Gralla et al.,2004; Heyd & Yinnon,1994; Jebara et al.,1991; Naik et al.,1995). Endovascular therapy of a non-infected and infected carotid artery pseudoaneurysms has been increasingly used (Gralla et al.,2004; Oishi et al.,2002). With this treatment, the ICA lumen may be better preserved. Several approaches are available.

The novel technique "parent artery occlusion" is achieved by positioning detachable balloons distally and proximally to the lesion (Serbinenko,1974). However, this approach demands preliminary evaluation of the collateral pathways in the circle of Willis. The occlusion test requires the patient to be awake, in order to monitor possible neurological deficits. The inherent risk of the occlusion test includes development of neurological deficits and/or failure to identify a delayed ischemia. Another endovascular approach preserving the carotid artery lumen is a stent or stent-graft implantation with/or without a coil deposition to the pseudoaneurysms. Since the pseudoaneurysms lacks a true arterial wall, the potential risk of the coils compaction and dislocation is always present. A simple stent or a stent-graft implantation is regarded to be the most effective and faster treatment (Glaiberman et al.,2003;Schonholz et al.,2006).

Choice of the endovascular treatment is mainly influenced by the unfavourable deep location of the pseudoaneurysms nearby the skull base, thus making the conventional surgery more risky. We can initially chose between an uncovered bare stent or two overlapping stents, rather than a covered stentgraft, to minimize the amount of foreign material to be inserted and to lessen the risk of the stentgraft thrombosis or infection.

6. Conclusion

Intracranial infectious pseudoaneurysms can occur not only in connection with a heart disease or HIV patients, but they also frequently occur in younger patients with the history of drug abuse or in prematurely born patients. Last but not least, multimodality approach is inevitable in the treatment of ruptured or unruptured infectious pseudoaneurysms. Teamwork brings the largest benefit for the successful future outcome.

In the extracranial area, infectious pseudoaneurysms of ICA have traditionally been treated with a surgical resection of the lesion, in addition to the extended i.v. antibiotic course. Recent advances in interventional radiology, together with the development of new materials, opened up a wide spectrum of new endovascular treatment options. A more radical approach involves a complete occlusion of the affected ICA with detachable balloons. It is also possible to conclude, that intra-arterial stent placement offers less invasive option with preservation of the vessel lumen. The use of either a dense-mash bare stent or a coated stentgraft promises to be a particularly appropriate choice in young individuals presenting with a surgically inaccessible ICA pseudoaneurysms.

Author details

Václav Procházka, Tomáš Jonszta, Daniel Czerný and Jan Krajča
Radiodiagnostic Institute FN Ostrava Poruba, Czech Republic

Michaela Vávrová
Radiodiagnostic department MNOF Ostrava, Czech Republic

Tomáš Hrbáč
Neurosurgery department FN Ostrava Poruba, Czech Republic

7. References

Alexander DW, Leonard Jr, Trail ML: Vascular complications of deep neck abscesses. A report of four cases. Laryngoscope. 78:361-370,1968.

Cloud GC, Rich PM. et Al. : "Serial MRI of a mycotic aneurysm of the cavernous carotid artery." Neuroradiology 45(8): 546-9.,2003.

Cohen J, Rad I: Contemporary management of carotid blowout. Curr Opin Otolaryngol Head Neck Surg. 12: 110-115,2004.

Gawin FH: „Cocaine addiction": Psychology and neurophysiology. Science 251: 1580-1586,1991

Glaiberman CB, Towbin RB, Boal DKB: Giant mycotic aneurysm of the internal carotid artery in a child: Endovascular treatment. Pediatr. Radiol. 33: 211-15,2003.

Gralla J, Brekenfeld C, Schmidli J, Caversaccio M, Do Dai-Do, Schroth G: Internal Carotid Artery Aneurysm with Life-Threatenig Hemorrhages in a Pediatric Patient. J Endovasc Ther. 11:734-738,2004.

Grinspoon L, Bakalar JB: Adverse effects of cocaine: Selected issues. Ann. N Y Acad Sci 362: 125-131,1981.

Heyd J, Yinnon AM: Mycotic aneurysm of the external carotid artery. J Cardiovascular Surg (Torino). 35:329- 331,1994.

Chun JY, Smith W, Halbach Van V, Randal, et Al.: „Current Multimodality Management of Infectious Intracranial aneurysma". Neurosurgery 48 (6): 1203-1214,2001.

Jain K: Mechanism of rupture of intracranial saccular aneurysma. Surgery 54: 347-350, 1963.

Jebara VA, Acar C, Dervanian P, et Al.: Mycotic aneurysms of the carotid arteries – case report and review of the literature. J Vasc Surg. 14:215-219,1991.

Kanaan I, Lasjaunias P et Al.: "The spectrum of intracranial aneurysms in pediatrics." Minim Invasive Neurosurg 38(1): 1-9.,1995.

Lasjaunias P, Ter Brugge KG: Intracranial Aneurysms in Children. Vascular Diseases in Neonates, Infants and Children, Springer-Verlag Berlin Heidelberg: 373-392; 1997.

Lasjaunias P, Wuppalapati S, Alvarez H, Rodesch G, Ozanne A.: Intracranial aneurysms in children aged under 15 years: Review of 59 consecutive children with 75 aneurysms. Childs Nerv Syst.21:437-450,2005.

Lichtenfeld PJ, Rubin DB, Fledman RS: Subarachnoid hemorrhage precipitated bycocaine snorting, Arch Neurol 41:223-224,1984.

Liston R: On a variety of false aneurysms. Br Foreign Med Rev. 15:155-161,1843.

Madden JA, Powers RH: Effect of cocaine and cocaine metabolites on cerebral arteries in vitro. Life Sci 47: 1109- 1114,1990.

Molinari GF, Smith L, Goldstein MN, Satran R: „Pathogenesis of cerebral mycotisaneurysms". Neurology 23: 325-332,1973.

Naik DK, Atkinson NR, et Al.: Mycotic cervical carotid aneurysm . Aust N Z J Surg. 65:620-621,1995.

Nanda A, Vannemereddy P, Polin R, Willis B: Intracranial Aneurysma and Cocaine Abuse: Analysis of Prognostic Indicator [Clinical Studies] Neurosurgery 46 (5): 1063-1069, 2000.

Oishi O, Yoshida K, Oyama M, et Al.: Combination of stenting and coil embolisation for carotid artery pseudoaneurysm causing symptomatic mass effect: Case report. No Schinka Geka-Neurol.Surg 30(4):437-41,2002.

Reisner A, Marshall GS, Bryant K, et Al.: Endovascular occlusion of a carotid artery pseudoaneurysm complicating deep neck space infection in a child. J. Neurosurg. 91: 510–14,1999.

Rodesch G, Noterman J, Thys JP, Flament-Durand J, Hermanus N: Treatment of intracranial mycotic aneurysm: Surgery or not. A case report. Acta Neurochir (Wien) 85:63-68,1987.

Salinger S., Pearlman S J., Hemorrhage from pharyngeal adn peritonsillar abscesses. Arch. Otolaryngol. 1933;18:464-509

Serbinenko FA. Balloon catheterization and occlusion of major cerebral vessels J Neurosurg. 1974 Aug;41(2):125- 45

Schonholz C, Krajcer Z, Carlos Parodi J, et al. Stent-graft treatment of pseudoaneurysms and arteriovenous fistulae in the carotid artery. Vascular.2006 May-Jun;14(3): 123-9

Chapter 17

Saphenous Vein Graft Aneurysms

G. Kang and K. Kang

Additional information is available at the end of the chapter

http://dx.doi.org/10.5772/46035

1. Introduction

Saphenous Vein Grafts were introduced to the technique of coronary artery bypass surgery for the treatment of severe coronary artery stenoses more than 40 years ago (1,2). Saphenous vein graft aneurysm defined as abnormal dilation of the bypassed vein graft remains a rare complication but increases the risk of morbidity and mortality (3,4). Vein graft aneurysms are associated with extensive plaque and atherosclerotic debris and can lead to angina and myocardial infarction both with graft occlusion and distal embolization (3,4,5). Saphenous vein aneurysms can rupture with devastating effects leading to shock or fistula formation and also cause compression of surrounding structures. This can lead to enlarged mediastinum (4), atrial fistulas (3), pulmonary leakage with hemoptysis (3), and repeat coronary artery bypass grafting (4). In my practice, I have reported, a leaking saphenous vein graft aneurysm large enough to compress the right heart chambers causing tamponade physiology (4).

2. Definition and epidemiology

The aneurysms are uncommon, are usually, 1 cm to 14 cm in size and taking the rarity of reporting into account, the aneurysms are seen in less than 1% of coronary bypass patients on follow up (5). Aneurysms are seen at an average age of 59 years and more often in men (5). Saphenous vein graft aneurysms, like the aneurysms elsewhere are defined as vessel dilations of 1.5 times the size of the reference vessel and were first described 7 years after the first Coronary Bypass surgery in 1975 (6).

2.1. Pathophysiology

An aneurysm may be true aneurysm where all the three vessel layers are involved or false where the endothelium or even the media may be disrupted leading to an intramural hematoma or hemorrhage (5). The most common etiology is atherosclerosis but other causes include formation of true or false aneurysms post angioplasty, true aneurysm formation at the site of a venous valve or false aneurysms at the site of suture rupture or false aneurysm from infectious etiology (5). Aneurysms may result from chronic steroid use or unsuspected harvesting of varicose veins (5).

The true aneurysms are fusiform and often in the middle of the graft and the false aneurysms are saccular and often at the origin of the graft but the aneurysms can be seen anywhere (4,5). Inflammatory causes as in aneurysms elsewhere may also be considered but lack any specific anti-inflammatory therapy (7).

2.1.1. Symptoms

True aneurysms are often asymptomatic in about half of the patients that present to medical attention and are discovered incidentally on imaging studies (5). They are seen most often in left anterior descending artery venous bypasses followed by right coronary and circumflex artery bypasses, respectively.

A triad of chest pain, mediastinal enlargement and previous coronary bypass may raise suspicion of a saphenous vein graft aneurysm (4). The symptoms at presentation are usually angina, myocardial infarction, congestive heart failure or variety of symptoms from graft occlusion, embolization, fistula formation or compression of surrounding structures (4,5). False aneurysms are usually symptomatic, however. Only minority of patients with false aneurysms is asymptomatic and the majority of the patients with false aneurysm present with the same symptoms as true aneurysms but the incidence of rupture is higher than with true aneurysms (5). Rupture of the aneurysm into the lung may lead to hemoptysis and into a cardiac chamber can lead to a fistula (8,9,10). Also, compression of left internal mammary artery graft by an aneurysm was recently described (9).

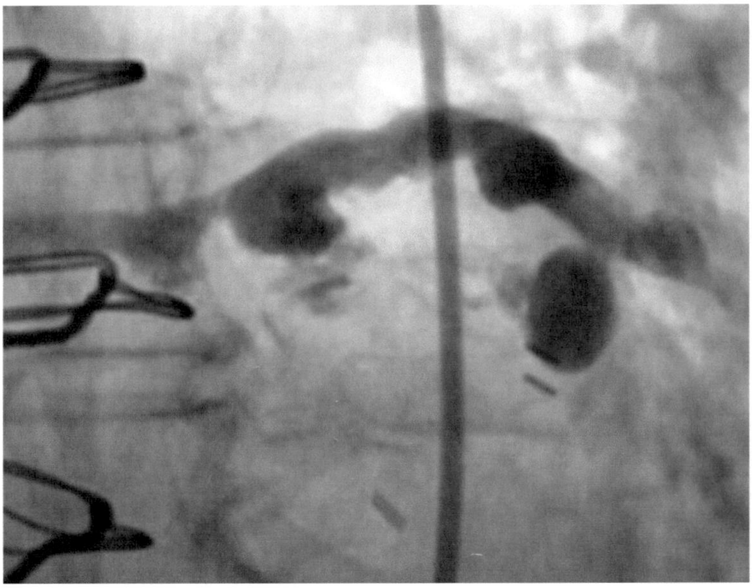

Figure 1. Multiple aneurysms and pseuodaneuyrsms with a narrow neck.

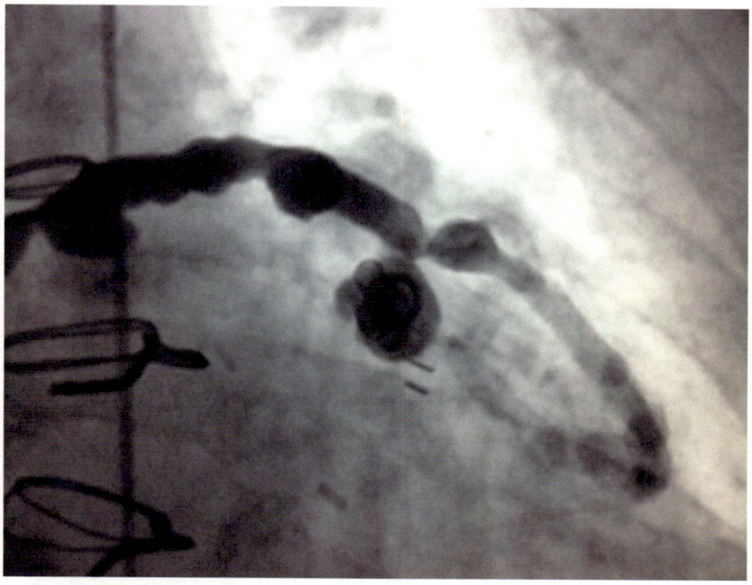

Figure 2. Coil embolization of a large pseudoaneurysm on the patient above.

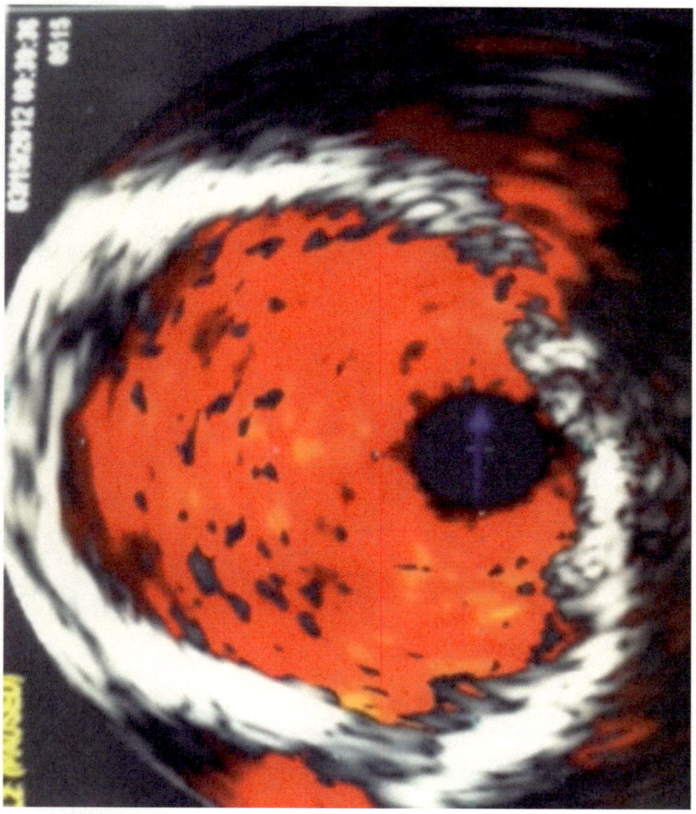

Figure 3. Intravascular ultrasound showing pseudoaneurysm at the 2O'clock position with disrupted endothelium

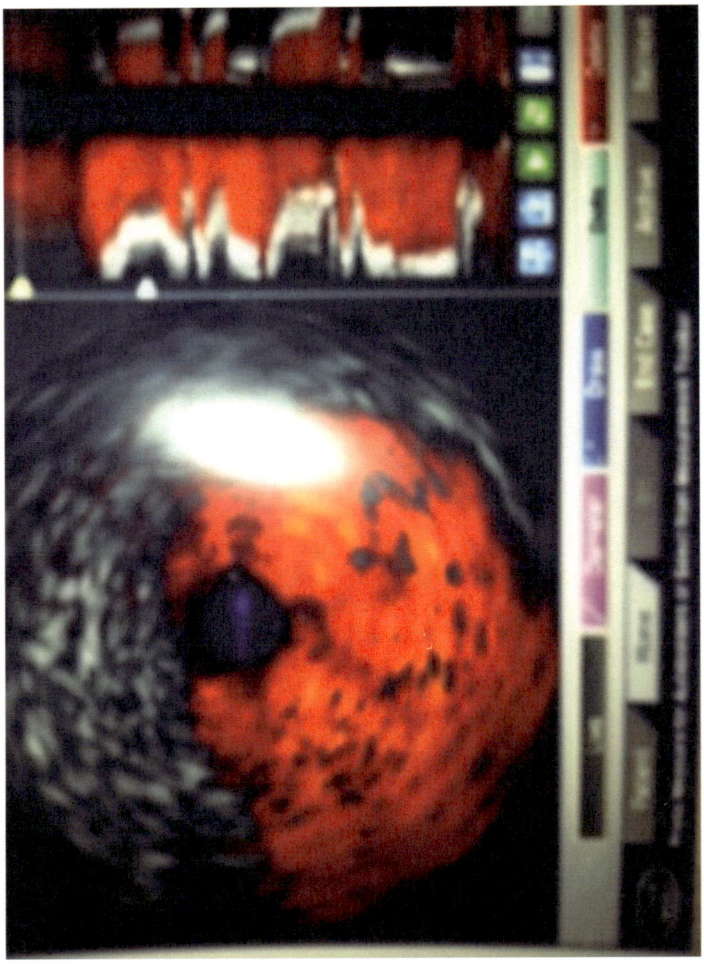

Figure 4. True aneurysm from 4 to 6O'clock position on intravascular ultrasound

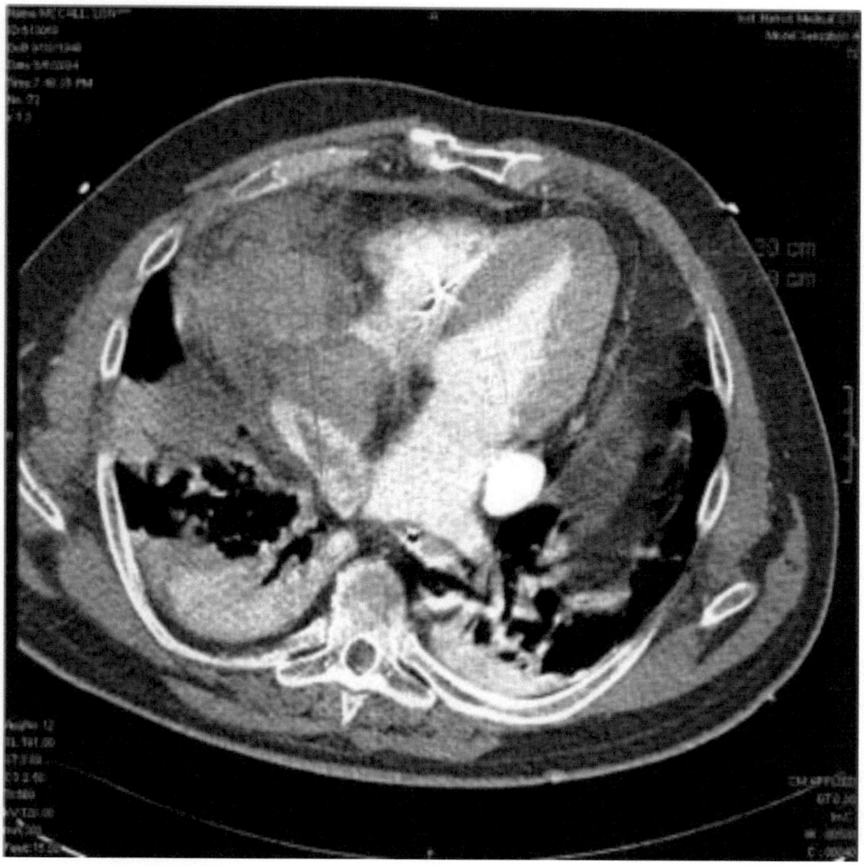

Figure 5. Chest CT scan image of a large leaking aneurysm compressing the right atrium

3. Signs

A variety of signs related to the pathophysiology at the time of presentation may be seen. A pulsatile mass on palpation or ischemia causing a gallop rhythm may be noted. If the rupture of the aneurysm occurs then murmurs related to fistula formation or shock secondary to bleeding or compression may be evident (4,5,8,9,10).

4. Workup

EKG may show ischemia, infarction or tamponade depending on presentation (4). CXRay may show mediastinal enlargement or pleural effusion (4). Diagnostic test of choice is often coronary angiography that is the gold standard before therapeutic decision-making (5). CT or MRI scanning can also accurately define the extent and size of the aneurysm and the associated complications (4). Echocardiography may show a mass as well (4).

5. Conclusion

The average time to diagnosis is 10-20 years post CABG (5) and over that time period, systemic pressures in veins and atherosclerotic disease progression is the most likely cause of aneurysm formation. Medical treatment for atherosclerotic disease is, hence, recommended as primary treatment (4,11). Antiplatelet, cholesterol lowering and anti-hypertensive drugs are standard of care in the treatment (4,11).

The surgical treatment is recommended for large aneurysms but is still controversial as to the size where surgery is necessary (4,11,12). The graft diameter of more than 2 cm is arbitrarily, an indication for surgery (4,5). But, thicker aneurysmal wall or excellent flow through a graft may sway towards medical therapy in borderline cases. Pseudoaneurysms are often treated surgically and distinguished by the narrow neck and ultrasound findings of a disrupted vein graft wall (4,5).

Surgery may involve ligating the aneurysmal graft (4,12,13) and placing a new graft for revascularization (most commonly). Percutaneous techniques are experimental and may include investigational use of stenting and coil embolization or placement of Amplatzer vascular plugs (14). Additionally, covered Jomed stents (Abbott) or even multiple regular stents with prolonged balloon inflation have been tried (15). Other covered stents like Arium iCAST have been tried in our catheterization laboratory. (4,15). In my practice, I have injected platinum coils with expandable hydrogel polymer directly into the pseudoaneurysms with narrow neck or through stent struts for aneurysms with wide neck.

Author details

G. Kang and K. Kang
University of Pittsburgh Medical Center/Hamot Hospital, USA

Acknowledgement

I acknowledge Hamot Hospital and the patients.

6. References

[1] Favaloro RG. Saphenous vein autograft replacement of severe segmental coronary artery occlusion. Operative technique. Ann Thorac Surg 1968;5:334-9.

[2] Favaloro RG. Saphenous vein graft in the surgical treatment of coronary artery disease. Operative technique. J Thorac Cardiovasc Surg 1969;58:178-85.

[3] Williams M.L., Rampersaud E., Wolfe W.G.: A man with saphenous vein graft aneurysms after bypass surgery. Ann Thorac Surg 77. 1815-1817.2004;

[4] Kang G, Shepherd J, Ferraro R, Butler M, Petrella R. Cardiac tamponade caused by a leaking coronary saphenous vein graft aneurysm. Am J Emerg Med. Sep 2007;25(7):858.e1-2.

[5] Wight , Jr. , Jr.J.N., Salem D., Vannan M.A., Pandian N.G., Rozansky M.I., Dohan M.C., Rastegar H.: Asymptomatic large coronary artery saphenous vein bypass graft aneurysm: a case report and review of the literature. Am Heart J 133. 454-460.1997

[6] Riahi M, Vasu CM, Tomatis LA, et al. Aneurysm of saphenous vein bypass graft to coronary artery. J Thorac Cardiovasc Surg. Aug 1975;70(2):358-9.

[7] Hellmann DB, Grand DJ, Freischlag JA. Inflammatory abdominal aortic aneurysm. JAMA 2007;297:395-400

[8] Fares W, Sharifi M, Steele R, Sarhill N, Sopko J, Ramana CV, et al. Superior vena cava syndrome secondary to saphenous venous graft aneurysm with right atrial fistula. Catheter Cardiovasc Interv. Sep 2003;60(1):45-7.

[9] Agarwal SC, Adams PC, Ahmed JM. Aneurysm of saphenous vein graft causing anterior myocardial infarction by possibly compressing left internal mammary artery. Int J Cardiol. May 10 2006;109(2):284-5.

[10] Nishimura Y., Okamura Y., Hiramatsu T., et al: Hemoptysis caused by saphenous vein graft aneurysm late after coronary artery bypass grafting. J Thorac Cardiovasc Surg 129. 1432-1433.2005;

[11] Dieter R.S., Patel A.K., Yandow D., et al: Conservative vs. invasive treatment of aortocoronary saphenous vein graft aneurysms: treatment algorithm based upon a large series. Cardiovasc Surg 11. 507-513.2003;

[12] Rosin MD, Ridley PD, Maxwell PH. Rupture of a pseudoaneurysm of a saphenous vein coronary arterial bypass graft presenting with a superior caval venous obstruction. Int J Cardiol 1989;25:121-3.

[13] Couto WJ, Livesay JJ, Allam A. Off-pump repair of a giant pseudoaneurysm of a distal saphenous vein bypass graft. Ann Thorac Surg. Dec 2005;80(6):2376-8.

[14] Mylonas I, Sakata Y, Salinger MH, Feldman T. Successful closure of a giant true saphenous vein graft aneurysm using the Amplatzer vascular plug. Catheter Cardiovasc Interv. Apr 2006;67(4):611-6

[15] Ho P.C., Leung C.Y.: Treatment of post-stenotic saphenous vein graft aneurysm: special considerations with the polytetrafluoroethylene-covered stent. J Invasive Cardiol 16. 604-605.2004;

Chapter 18

Giant Intracranial Aneurysms – Surgical Treatment, Accessory Techniques and Outcome

Tomasz Szmuda and Pawel Sloniewski

Additional information is available at the end of the chapter

http://dx.doi.org/10.5772/46033

1. Introduction

There are various intracranial aneurysms: saccular, fusiform, dissecting or mycotic. Saccular aneurysms are the most common type and account for up to 98% of all intracranial aneurysms (Yasargil, 1984). If the widest diameter of the aneurysm is equal to or exceeding 25 millimetres (mm), the aneurysm is defined by convention as giant (GIA). The etiology of GIAs is similar to smaller ones (Lemole, 2000), theories about the development of all saccular aneurysms include congenital and acquired artery defects. GIA's and other aneurysms are etiologically divided into "sidewall" and "bifurcation" aneurysms (LeRoux, 2003). In flow-related phenomena, constant enlargement of a small aneurysm in the distal part of the neck results in GIA formation. However, de novo development of GIA has also been described (Barth, 1994). The histology of GIA wall is different from smaller aneurysms: GIAs often lack a muscular layer as well as elastic laminar layers show degeneration. The incidence of intraluminal thrombosis significantly increases with the lumen size of aneurysms; in GIAs this phenomena may occur in approximately 60% of cases (LeRoux, 2003). Krings publication (Krings, 2005) was a breakthrough in large aneurysms formation knowledge; he proved that the GIA development in the internal carotid artery (ICA) and vertebral artery (VA) differ from those in other locations. Repeated subadventitial haemorrhages from vasa vasorum are a predominant factor in GIA aneurysm pathogenesis. Therefore, GIA formation can be considered as a "proliferative disease of the vessel wall induced by extravascular activity". Historically GIA rupture is known as devastating due to higher amount of extravasated blood. In contrast, recent papers indicate that rupture of some smaller aneurysms leads to more extensive SAH. The study ISUIA (Kassell, 1990) proved that the risk of rupture of GIA can reach 40% in five-year follow-up, while treatment of unruptured intracranial aneurysm carries relatively low mortality that does not exceed 2% (Molyneux, 2005). Therefore, treatment is warranted for most patients suffering from GIAs. There are two treatment modalities that can be offered to patients afflicted with GIA pathology: endovascular or surgical. In general endovascular treatment is less invasive and has fewer complications than surgery, and therefore is preferable. Surprisingly, no randomized comparison study of these two methods in GIA treatment have been published. However, the outcome measurement and analysis may be difficult to conduct a trial in GIAs; these aneurysms constitute a heterogeneous group and they are treated using different methods in different institutions. Furthermore, there is not enough observational data in the literature discussing results of treatment and their pertinence to quality of life in patients with GIAs in comparison to smaller ones. Additionally, radiographic results assessed several years post-operatively have not been reported sufficiently. Probably it is due to the unique peculiarity of GIAs as these require extensive comprehension of the treatment strategies to achieve better results. The current study is not only aimed at describing available methods, but to compare the prognosis after treatment of GIAs versus smaller aneurysms. A new neurovascular surgeon should be accustomed to all surgical techniques for GIAs. All of the treatment possibilities, technical issues and their clinical implications are to be learned meticulously and considered preoperatively.

2. Epidemiology and clinical presentation

Approximately 2% to 5% of all intracranial aneurysms are classified as giant. Epidemiological studies have demonstrated increased incidence of GIAs in elderly, most cases present in the fifth to seventh decades of life (Anson, 1995). These lesions are slightly more common in females. In the paediatric population approximately 5 to 10% of all aneurysms exceed 25mm. Up to 40% of GIAs are found in posterior cerebral circulation while 80% to 90% of smaller aneurysms are located in anterior cerebral vasculature. ICA is the predominant localization. In general 40% of GIAs are seen in the carotid artery, 25% in the anterior (ACA) and middle (MCA) cerebral arteries, and 30% per cent in the vertebrobasilar (VB) arteries (Fig. 1).

The ratio of giant aneurysms to all other intracranial aneurysms is six to one in the posterior circulation, which is statistically higher than in anterior circulation. The cause of somewhat different distribution of GIAs from that of smaller aneurysms is unknown. Krings theory about the role of repeated subadventitial haemorrhages in giant VA and ICA aneurysm formation partially explains referral patterns. Above all, adduced aneurysm distribution is only based on clinical publications referring to hospitalized patients, although population based studies have not been performed (Table 1).

	Peerless n=635	Kodama n=1023	Weir n=573	Karavel n=309	Sharma n=181	own series n=128
ICA	34%	**51%**	**39%**	**42%**	**84%**	**61%**
V-B	**56%**	27%	25%	33%	7%	9%
ACA	3%	8%	16%	10%	2%	12%
MCA	16%	13%	12%	15%	7%	18%

Table 1. The distribution of GIAs based on large series studies (Peerless, 1990, as cited in Youmans, 1990; Kodama, 1982; Weir, 1987; Karavel, 1988; Sharma, 2008) and own material.

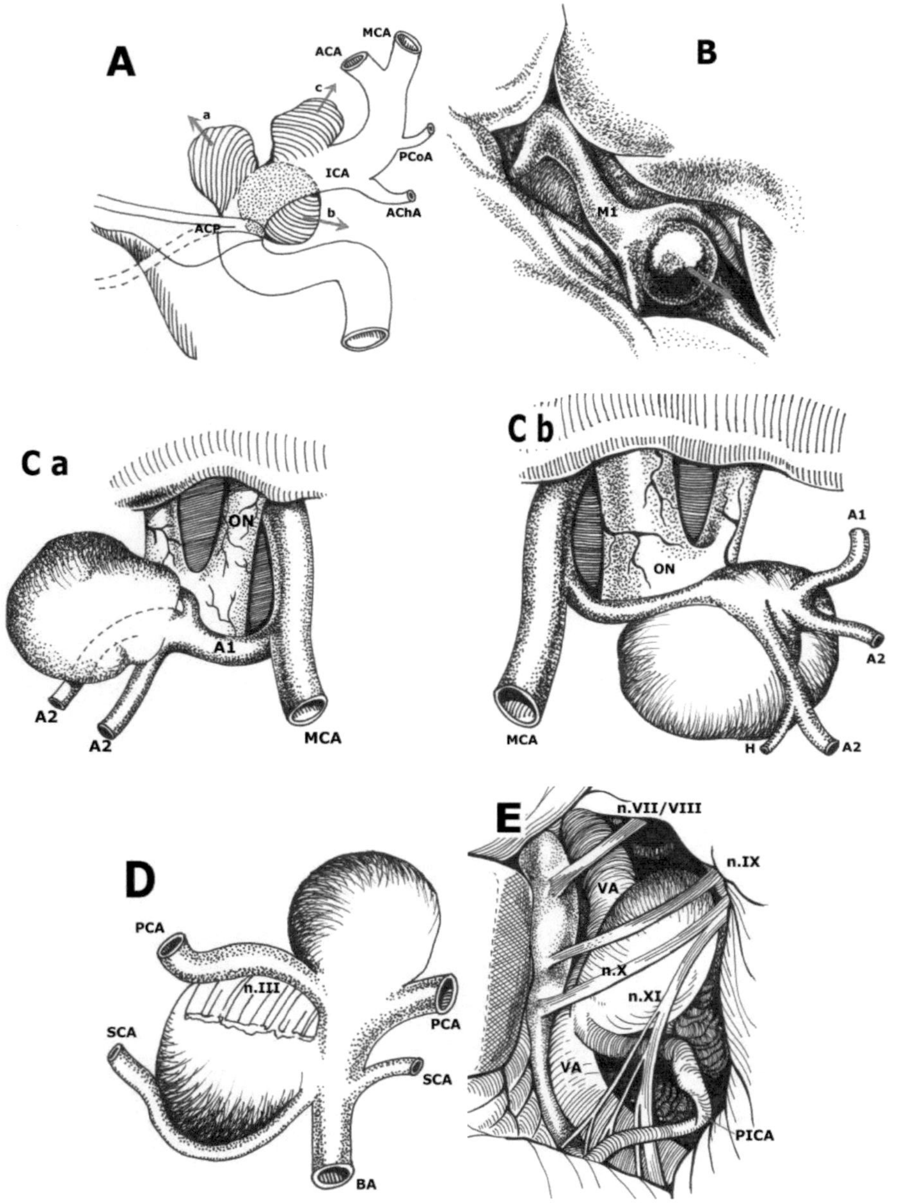

Abbreviations: ACA - anterior cerebral artery; A1-first segment of ACA; A2 - second segment of ACA; ACP - anterior clinoid process; AChA - anterior choroidal artery; H - artery of Heubner; BA - basilar artery; MCA - middle cerebral artery; M1 - first segment of MCA; n.VII/VIII - complex of facial and vestibulocochlear cranial nerves; n.IX - glossopharyngeal cranial nerve; n.X – vagus cranial nerve; n.XI - accessory cranial nerve; ON – optic nerve; PCA - posterior cerebral artery; PCoA - posterior communicating artery; PICA - posterior inferior cerebellar artery; SCA - superior cerebellar artery; VA - vertebral artery;

Figure 1. The location of selected GIAs and their projection. (A) Three variations of ophthalmic segment of ICA aneurysms and their growth projection: a - supraclinoid, b - carotid cave, c - dorsal wall blood blister-like). (B) MCA bifurcation growth direction. (C) ACoA (two variations: a - anterior, b - posterior) (D) BA bifurcation and SCA. (E) PICA.

Both smaller aneurysms and GIAs can present as either mass effect or subarachnoid haemorrhage (SAH). Unruptured smaller aneurysms are rarely symptomatic and therefore are found accidentally in computed tomography (CT) or magnetic resonance imaging (MRI) due to unspecific symptoms or after head trauma. On the contrary, almost two-thirds of GIAs are diagnosed before rupture. The location of the GIA determines its symptoms due to the size and direct contact with neural structures. Coexisting retro-orbital pain, diplopia, ptosis, trigeminal pain and mild headache are characteristic manifestation of GIAs from cavernous portion of the ICA. Visual loss and Horner's syndrome are rare findings even in large or giant aneurysms. The observational study of 20 non-treated cases demonstrated that cranial neuropathies may improve due to compression-induced cranial nerve ischemia resolution (Linskey, 1990).

If the aneurysm erodes surrounding bones massive epistaxis can lead to sudden death before admission. The history of patients with ruptured cavernous GIAs, derived from our own records, confirm that cavernous aneurysms are the last resort diagnosis for chronic haemorrhage from the nose.

Medially directed GIAs of paraclinoid segment and may present visual loss or hypopituitarism (Cawley, 1998). Retro-orbital pain, ophthalmic nerve paresis and headaches are sporadic however clinically relevant. Smaller aneurysms of the paraclinoid segment tend to remain asymptomatic for years. Asymmetrical visual field defects and visual loss are pathognomonic signs of GIAs in the ophthalmic segment of ICA, but are rarely observed in smaller aneurysms. Superior hypophyseal artery aneurysms may expand superomedially remaining ophthalmic aneurysms. Inferomedial aneurysms are called 'carotid cave aneurysms' and if they meet giant classification, produce superior bitemporal hemianopsia or hypopituitarism, generally indicative of pituitary tumours. Supraclinoid segment of ICA include aneurysms at posterior communicating artery (PCoA), anterior choroidal artery (AChA) and ICA bifurcation. Approximately one fourth of all aneurysms arise from ICA at the PCoA origin. Third-nerve palsy is usually complete and is observed in both GIAs and smaller PCoA aneurysms. However, expanding giant PCoA aneurysm may also produce 'thunderclap headaches'. No specific presentation is associated with smaller AChA and ICA bifurcation aneurysms. Nevertheless, GIAs arising from AChA origin may occasionally present third-nerve palsy and GIA's in the ICA bifurcation may cause visual deficits, epilepsy, and dementia, hemiparesis or aphasia. Posterior and anterior ICA wall GIAs are rarely symptomatic before rupture as those lesions usually have friable neck and thin wall. ACoA aneurysms may have different dome projection (Out of place). Mental disturbances, visual deficit, monocular blindness are common in GIAs, however, they are very sporadic symptoms in patients with smaller aneurysm of ACoA origin. Giant basilar artery (BA) bifurcation aneurysms and superior cerebellar artery (SCA) typically cause oculomotor palsy, Weber's syndrome, ataxia, hydrocephalus, gait disturbances or dementia. Other ocular findings observed, including Parinaud's syndrome supranuclear gaze palsy and internuclear ophthalmoplegia. If oriented anteriorly, GIAs in BA bifurcation may mimic sellar lesions by compressing the optic apparatus and causing visual disturbances. Anterior inferior cerebellar artery (AICA), BA trunk, inferior junction of vertebral artery (VA) and posterior inferior cerebellar artery (PICA) GIAs may manifest themselves by hydrocephalus or symptoms referable to brain stem or cranial nerve compression (mimicking cerebellopontine angle tumours). In contrast, smaller aneurysms of the earlier mentioned locations often remain asymptomatic prior to rupture. Unlike ACoA, ICA and posterior circulation aneurysms, GIAs in MCA often reach large sizes before producing pressure-related symptoms. Moreover, focal neurologic deficits before rupture are indicative but not diagnostic in GIAs of MCA; in which, transient ischemic attacks (TIA), epilepsy, dysphasia, hemiparesis and occasionally bruits can be observed. Distally located GIAs, including posterior cerebral artery (PCA), anterior cerebral artery (ACA) and MCA, are diagnosed before rupture by epilepsy or brain stem compression symptoms.

The symptomatology of GIAs in all locations is typically characteristic. On the contrary, most of patients with smaller aneurysms do not present with indicative symptoms, but tend to be diagnosed after experiencing SAH. Based on Laplace's law, tension on the wall is higher in large or giant aneurysms than smaller ones. Drawing from the conclusion of the above law: the rupture of GIA causes a more severe haemorrhage than in smaller aneurysms. That is convincible theory; however, it was contradicted by other observational studies. Some authors (Roos, 2000; Russell, 2003; Taylor, 2004) find in contrast to Laplace's law that rupture of some smaller aneurysms (ACoA and ICA at the PCoA origin) lead to more extensive SAH. Therefore, the size of an aneurysm may not be regarded as a single prognostic factor in patients with SAH due to ruptured GIA. Based on ISUIA study (Kassell, 1990), unruptured GIAs' are related to high annual risk of rupture. Five-year cumulative rupture rates for patients who did not have a history of SAH for aneurysms less than 7 mm, 7-12 mm, 13-24 mm and 25 mm or greater reached 2.5%, 14.5%, 18.4% and 50% respectively. Moreover, the probability of SAH was also higher for BA bifurcation and ICA at the PCoA origin than for other locations. Others proved that the shape of GIA, neck to dome ratio and other factors should be considered in risk of rupture estimation (Patel, 2010). Untreated GIAs have a poor natural history, as the mortality rate can attain 100% within 2 years (Peerless, 1990, as cited in Youmans, 1990). High SAH rate in patients with unruptured GIAs justifies treatment in most cases. The potential consequences of the aneurysm rupture are devastating and usually have a sudden onset. Two-third of all patients after rupture will die or suffer from mental or physical deficits in the near future. Even when treated, unfavourable results usually exceed 30%. The incidence of SAH increases with age as well as related to some genetic diseases.

3. Treatment

Endovascular and surgical techniques are the options considered in treatment of GIAs. Although endovascular treatment has a short history of 50 years, the beginning of surgery for GIAs is dated at 19th century and. Extracranial internal carotid artery (ICA) ligation was the first attempt of excluding GIA from circulatory system in 1885 (Youmans, 1990). In 1911 Harvey Cushing, despite scepticism to abovementioned method, used alloy clip for extracranial ICA ligation. Dandy was a pioneer in aneurysm treatment. In 1936, he ligated ICA proximally and distally to the aneurysm (nowadays called trapping method) and one year later he used Cushing's clip to obliterate the aneurysm neck. Dandy's work diffused a new era of clipping the aneurysms neck. Herbert Olivecrona modified the silver clip by adding winged blades, than Schwartz introduced miniaturized spring forceps as clips. However, Mayfield brought significant innovation by the use of an applicator and various types of detachable stainless steel clips. Followed by Mayfield, whose further development was merely a minor modification on Mayfield's work. Sundt developed Teflon-lined, encircling clip-graft, used for emergent reconstruction of a torn GIA. Sugita created very long clips, which are used for securing GIAs, and developed bayonet applicators and clips. Nowadays the optimized preoperative and intraoperative clip selection seems to play the most important role in correct GIA clipping approaches, as clipping still remains the "gold standard" among microsurgical methods. The features of clips intended for GIAs differ from those used for smaller aneurysms. The blades of standard aneurysm clips are usually longer and some clips (T-bar or J-shaped) are produced specifically for large or giant aneurysms (Fig. 2).

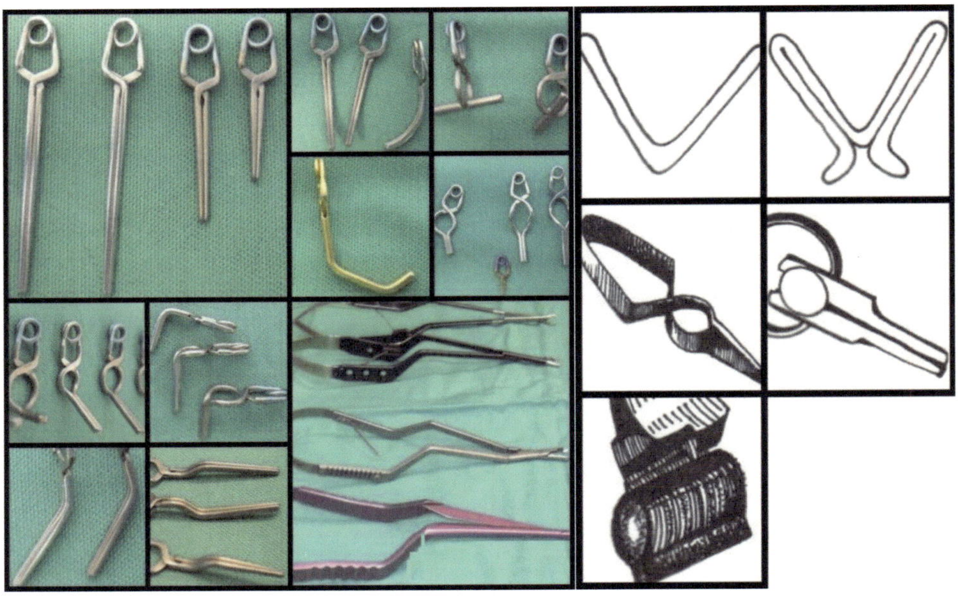

Figure 2. Left combined photo: contemporary permanent clips used for a GIA securing. Clips come in a variety of sizes and curve (straight, fenestrated, curved, bent, angled, bayonet, deflected, J-shaped, T-bar, et cetera). Right graphics: historical clips used in both smaller aneurysms and GIAs.

In the sixties and seventies, an enormous number of surgical approach improvements were observed. Yasargil described pterional craniotomy, which is still a routine approach to most of supratentorial GIAs. Temporary by-pass or hypothermia, bipolar coagulation, floating operating microscope and pharmacological neuroprotection were supportive methods, which led to significant GIA mortality reduction. At the end of 20th century, sweeping improvements of microsurgical techniques, stemming from technological development and microsurgical training, were ceased by the novel endovascular approach. The introduction of Guglielmi Detachable Coils (GDC) in 1991 began the modern era of neurovascular surgery and soon revolutionized aneurysm treatment. Initially GBC devices were approved for aneurysms and patients not amenable for surgery, although they have been used successfully to occlude all types of GIAs in patients with any neurovascular aneurysm condition. However, complete occlusion with only GDC remains insufficient in treatment of GIAs with particularly broad necks, thus balloon-assisted GDC placement or stent intervention was introduced to remedy this problem. For the last decade microsurgical occlusion of GIAs is constantly being displaced, as current endovascular techniques are regarded as having a lower risk for the patient. It is quite unusual in Evidence Based Medicine that rapidly developing endovascular techniques quickly (smoothly doesn't work here) became the standard for securing GIAs, when the neurosurgical discipline has developed a multitude of different approaches and advancements in the treatment of aneurysms. Despite the above dispute, GIAs are the most challenging lesions for both experienced neurosurgeons and experienced neuroradiologists.

Since the first attempt at excluding giant ICA aneurysms from circulatory system in 1885, many surgical occlusion and accessory techniques have been developed and elaborated. Although the introduction of Guglielmi Detachable Coils changed aneurysm treatment, soon limitations of its inability to occlude giant and widenecked aneurysms required further exploration. Constantly developing endovascular techniques are regarded as having lower risks for patients than open surgery and still seem to be unsatisfactory in terms of durability in aneurysm occlusion. The balloon-assisted remodelling and stent-assisted techniques partially solved the problem of neck remnants. Therefore microsurgery and the combination of microsurgical and endovascular method will still be up-to-date for years.

3.1. Treatment considerations

There are two main considerations regarding GIAs:

- Should we treat or observe unruptured GIAs ?
- Should we clip or insert endovascular coils to treat GIAs ?

Since 2003, when the ISUIA study was published, a justification for any treatment for GIA unanimously has been found. Up to 40% risk of rupture was observed in five-year observation. However, Wermer's publication (Wermer, 2007) complicated treatment decision making. As a result of the previously mentioned meta-analysis, the size, site and type of aneurysm should be considered when deciding whether to treat an unruptured aneurysm. Other factors like age, gender and population are also important risk factors of rupture estimation. Those multifactorial results are convincing as the material comprised sixty SAH cases among observed untreated GIAs. Before patient treatment, a pooled analysis of individual data is needed to identify the independent risk of rupture and possible risk of therapy complications. The presence of some factors significantly affects GIAs' treatment and the outcome. The number of people older than 65 years is still growing. Comorbid diseases that are often related to the elderly population include: cardiac disease, hypertension, atherosclerosis, carotid disease and multiple aneurysms. Conservative approaches to GIAs can be applied to older patients with comorbidities, although it is controversial. The risk of surgery in older patients is greater than in younger patients in part because of comorbid disease. Some studies (LeRoux, 2003) suggest that not only old age, but the patient's clinical condition should determine treatment decision. However, no randomized trial has compared treatment with conservative management in elderly patients.

To date, there is no consensus in treatment modality for ruptured, unruptured, and furthermore giant aneurysms. Probably the unique peculiarity of GIAs requires extensive comprehension of the treatment strategies, suggesting that individual approach is preferred. In year 2005, ISAT study (Molyneux, 2005) was a landmark in choosing treatment modality. 2143 patients with ruptured aneurysms took part in the multicentre trial and were randomly assigned to neurosurgical clipping or endovascular coiling. Despite of the fact that rebleeding was lower, one-year survival rate and epilepsy rate was higher in the clipped group. The overall short-term conclusions of ISAT study engendered controversy on several fronts, as the results somewhat favoured endovascular coiling. The awaited long-term follow-up of ISAT patients was published in Lancet in 2009 (Molyneux, 2009). The results confirmed early observations: the risk of death at 5 years was significantly lower in the coiling group than in the clipping group. However, the insight revision of ISAT study revealed basic inconsistencies. The main remark refers to intent-to-treat analysis conception. Only 30% of screened patients with ruptured aneurysms were included to the study and randomized. If we exclude patients who died before treatment, there is the same mortality rate in neurosurgical and endovascular group (Bakker, 2010). However, the main problem is that the results of ISAT study were wrongly adjusted to the unruptured aneurysms by neuroradiologists, though the management and prognosis of ruptured and ruptured aneurysms differ fundamentally. Additionally, the results of above trial are absolutely inconclusive in term of GIAs. There were 155 patients with aneurysms exceeding 11 mm whereas GIAs were not distinguished. The mortality rates in endovascular coiling and microsurgical clipping groups were similar for patients with large aneurysms. The question about the ideal treatment for specific GIA characteristics remained unanswered. Fraser (Fraser, 2011) opposed handling GIAs the same way as other aneurysms, and suggested that case-based aneurysm treatment should be applied for GIAs. Indeed, revising the literature neither retrospective nor prospective randomized trials comparing endovascular and microsurgical approach regarding GIAs' exists. Lack of published comparisons stems from diversity of GIAs as one is amenable to endovascular therapy and another for surgery. Such lesions often demand a combined endovascular and microsurgical approach. The full armamentarium should be available to the cerebrovascular team to facilitate a comprehensive treatment method for these lesions. Maximizing efficacy and minimizing risk should always be a goal of effective approach for GIAs. Tabulated comparisons of these two methods, based on other publications, elaborate the present controversy in GIA treatment (Table 2). Mortality and rehemorrhage rates are similar, but complete occlusion and retreatment rates are higher in endovascular therapy studies. However, the assessment is valid only when meta-analysis would be performed. Listed series rarely exceed a hundred patients, comprises both patients with ruptured and unruptured GIAs and where different therapy strategies were applied in different publications. It seems impossible to provide one and ultimately the best treatment modality or to perform randomized trials for patients suffering from GIAs.

Author	Year of publication	No of patients	Mortality (%)	Retreatment (%)	Rehemorrhage (%)	Complete occlusion (%)
			Endovascular			
Gruber	1999	28	UNK	82	4	61
Sluzewski	2003	29	21	55	7	17
Jahromi	2008	39	29	54	5	36
Shi	2009	9	11	0	0	100
Lylyk	2009	8	UNK	0	0	67
Summary		8-39	11-29	0-82	0-7	17-100
			Neurosurgical			
Lawton	2002	28	14	0	0	100
Jafar	2002	29	3	0	0	100
Hauck	2008	62	15	0	3	90
Sharma	2008	181	9	0	0	90
Sano	2010	109	22	0	0	100
Sughrue	2010	140	13	1	1	84
Sloniewski	2011	75	13	UNK	0	UNK
Summary		28-181	3-22	0-1	1-3	84-100

Abbreviations: UNK – unknown

Table 2. The comparison of treatment results: endovascular versus neurosurgical therapy in GIAs. Data derived from various authors (Gruber, 1999; Sluzewski, 2003; Jahromi, 2008; Shi, 2009; Lylyk, 2009; Lawton, 2002; Jafar, 2002; Hauck, 2008; Sharma, 2008; Sano, 2010; Sughrue, 2010; Szmuda & Sloniewski, 2011).

The current results for the endovascular treatment of GIAs with parent vessel preservation are not encouraging and are not as favourable as those for smaller aneurysms. However, most GIAs are amenable to endovascular coiling alone, balloon-assisted or stent-assisted coil embolization. Vessel reconstruction, especially in fusiform aneurysms, can be achieved by flow diverting stents. Nevertheless endovascular therapy is a treatment of choice in the majority of GIAs in most centres. A continuous development of techniques and devices can supersede surgery of GIAs in the future.

3.2. Microsurgical techniques

Large neck-to-dome ratio and limited surgical access are the main challenging therapeutic characteristics of GIAs. A part of the parent vessel proximally and distally to GIA, associated perforators, adjacent vessels and neural structures should be identified before GIA securing. These actions are imperative to reduce the consequences of intraoperative GIA rupture. Additionally, skull base surgery can cause severe complications which should be considered preoperatively. The aim of every craniotomy or craniectomy is an enhanced exposure achieved by removing additional bone and therefore minimizing cerebral retraction. Aneurysm location dictates the appropriate approach (Fig. 3).

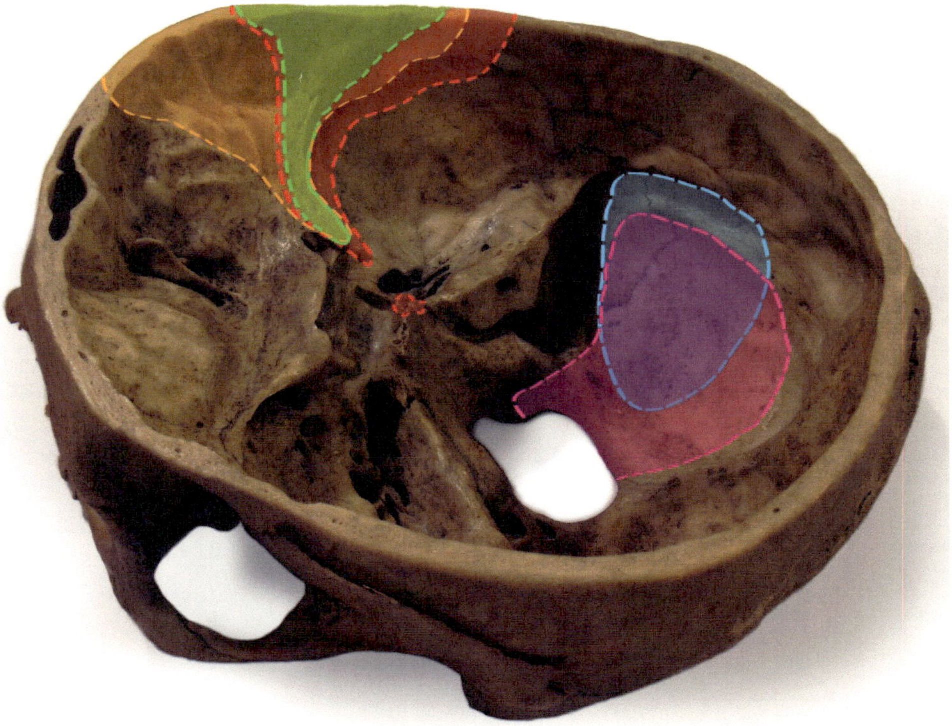

Figure 3. The skull base approaches to GIAs (marked in colours) recommended by authors: orange – orbitozygomatic; green – pterional; red – modification of pterional approach to aneurysms of BA bifurcation; pink – far lateral; blue – retrosigmoid.

Pterional or orbitozygomatic craniotomy is dedicated for most GIAs: ICA, ACoA, MCA and BA bifurcation. Pterional craniotomy is preferred as it is a routine approach in neurosurgery. Additional opening of the superior orbital fissure should always precede dura incisure. Extended exposure for proximal ICA GIAs is reached by extradural or most often intradural anterior clinoid process removal (Fig. 4). This manoeuvre effectively increases the angle of view, although it can rarely cause postoperative cerebrospinal fluid leakage. The anterior clinoid process assessment in preoperative CT is strongly recommended. When deemed necessary, optic strut drilling is performed.

BA bifurcation can also be approached by a modification of pterional approach, which is commonly used in our institution (Krisht, 2005; Sloniewski, 2008). We do not use extent bone by drilling the whole zygomatic arch but we remove only its upper part. The anterior clinoid process is occasionally removed while the lateral part of the orbit and zygomatic notch widening (by drilling its superior aspect) should be performed. These techniques increase the angle of view at about approximately 10° comparing to the classical pterional craniotomy (Sloniewski, 2008). Midbasilar, SCA, AICA, VA and PICA GIAs can be secured by either of petrosal, extended retrosigmoid and far-lateral craniectomies. We always propose the use of limited a far-lateral craniectomy with opening of the foramen magnum and without posterior C1 arch removal. In our opinion the visualization of cerebellar tonsils

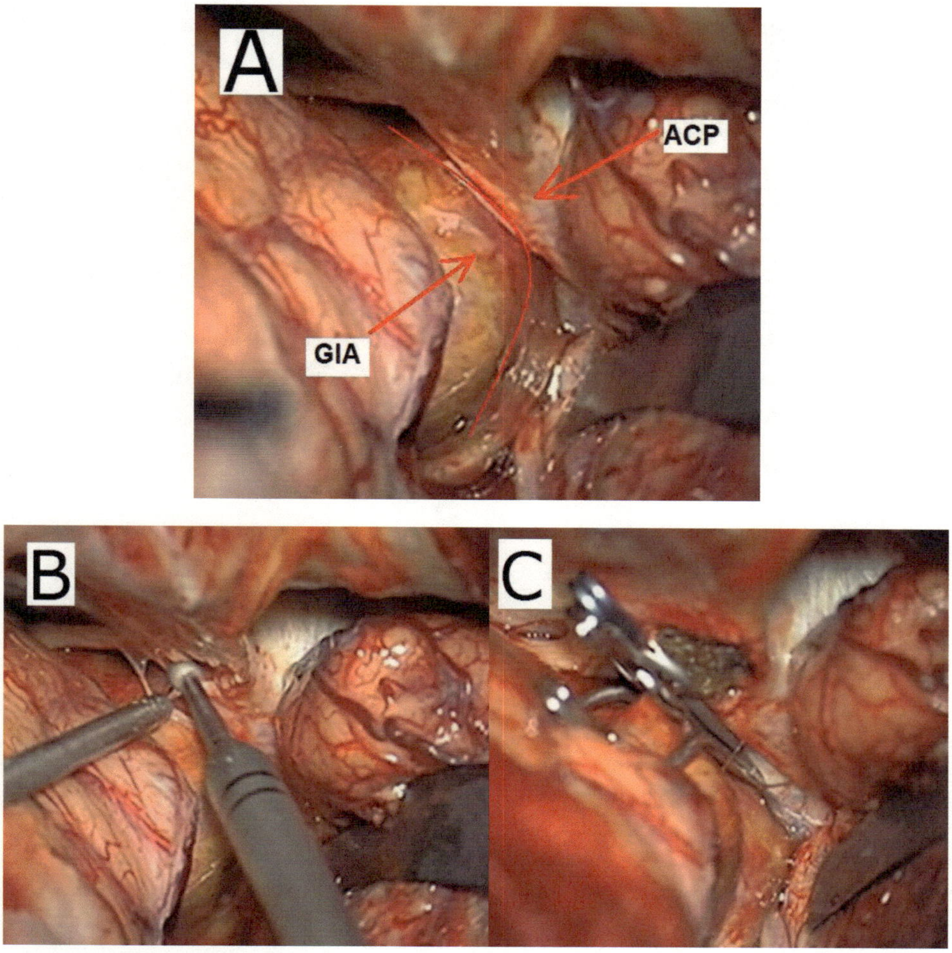

Abbreviations: ACP - anterior clinoid process.

Figure 4. Intradural anterior clinoid process removal. (A) ACP is in direct contact with GIA's neck at ophthalmic ICA origin, what prevents safe clipping. (B) ACP removal by the use of high speed drill with small diamond burr. (C) The hole that remained after ACP removal is filled with wax and haemostatic material (Surgicel®). Drilled ACP gives a space for prudent aneurysm neck clipping.

(via C1 arch osteotomy) is not essential while operating most GIAs. Petrosal or transclival approaches are associated with higher complication rates and therefore discontinued for GIA treatment in our institution. A possible cerebrospinal fluid leakage, meningitis, massive intraoperative bleeding outweigh extended exposure. Retrosigmoid approach is not originally intended for posterior circulation GIAs. This approach can be applied occasionally for some GIAs at the PICA or inferior junction of VA origin when the neck of the aneurysm is located higher than normal. Using a retrosigmoid craniectomy for GIA surgery should be supported by accessory and temporary endovascular balloon occlusion.

A variety of microsurgical occlusion techniques are available for vascular neurosurgeons: aneurysm neck clipping, aneurysmectomy, trapping of parent vessel, wrapping aneurysm dome or extra- to intracranial by-pass. Typically, GIAs with well-defined neck are the most feasible for clipping. Vascular clips and microsurgical skills used in GIAs securing are different from those used in smaller aneurysms. A neurosurgeon should prepare before the surgery and be equipped with a complete selection of aneurysm clips: small and large, straight, angled, bayonet, fenestrated, Sugita and Sundt. One clip usually cannot bring the aneurysm walls together thus several clips or tandem angled fenestrated clips are placed in wide-necked or fusiform aneurysms (Fig. 5). These techniques are used to reconstruct the lumen of the afflicted parent vessel. Aneurysm clips have their limitations, whereas the most important in GIA surgery is weak closing forces. Placing several clips or stacking one on the top of another can prevent clip slippage. Intraluminal thromboses located at the aneurysm's neck, quite often in GIAs, need to be evacuated before definite clipping, which in a sense complicates the procedure.

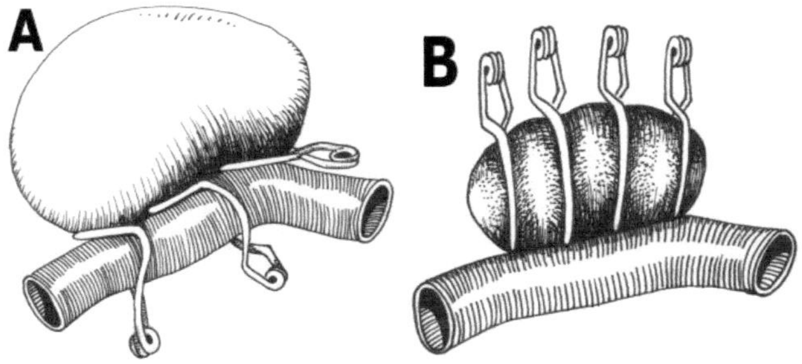

Figure 5. Schematic drawings of clipping techniques used in GIAs: (A) Tandem of fenestrated angled clips. (B) Several straight clips placement.

However, in two different situations - when a clip cannot embrace a GIA's broad neck and a standard clip slips from the aneurysm, we first place a fenestrated clip to form the neck. Then it is easier to stack the second clip, usually a straight or bayonet clip. All of the above microsurgical manoeuvres can lead to aneurysm rupture by puncturing the wall by the tip of a blade. Massive bleeding is a devastating event that results in altered clip positioning, differing from the positioning originally intended. In emergent situations, when other techniques are not feasible, parent artery sacrifice (trapping) can save a patient's life, although is regarded as a complication of aneurysm surgery. Aneurysmectomy, followed by clipping, theoretically resolves the compression of GIA on the neural structures. However, the studies of coiled GIAs revealed that neuropathies were caused by the pulsation of the aneurysm (Gonzalez, 2006). Therefore the aneurysmectomy or thrombosis evacuation may be abandoned. Aneurysm dome incision produces massive bleeding if the aneurysm neck is incompletely clipped.

Wrapping is used as a sole method of securing GIAs or combined with clipping (clip-wrapping technique). The treatment of GIAs should not be aimed at wrapping, although long-term findings based on 63 cases indicated that it is safe and durable method (Deshmukh, 2006). In our opinion, preventing rehaemorrhage from a GIA before further by-pass or coiling is the goal of wrapping. Various materials can be used, including cotton, muscle, gauze, Teflon, adhesives (fibrin glue and sealant) or collagen-impregnated Dacron fabric. We prefer to use cotton because it causes an intermediate inflammatory response (Herrera, 1999). The previous results suggested that wrapping ruptured aneurysms is less effective than clipping in preventing rehaemorrhage or regrowth (Minakawa, 1987; Todd, 1989). The contemporary papers showed that wrapping of unclippable aneurysms (mostly GIAs) may be protective. Furthermore, the risk of complications due to wrapping is low.

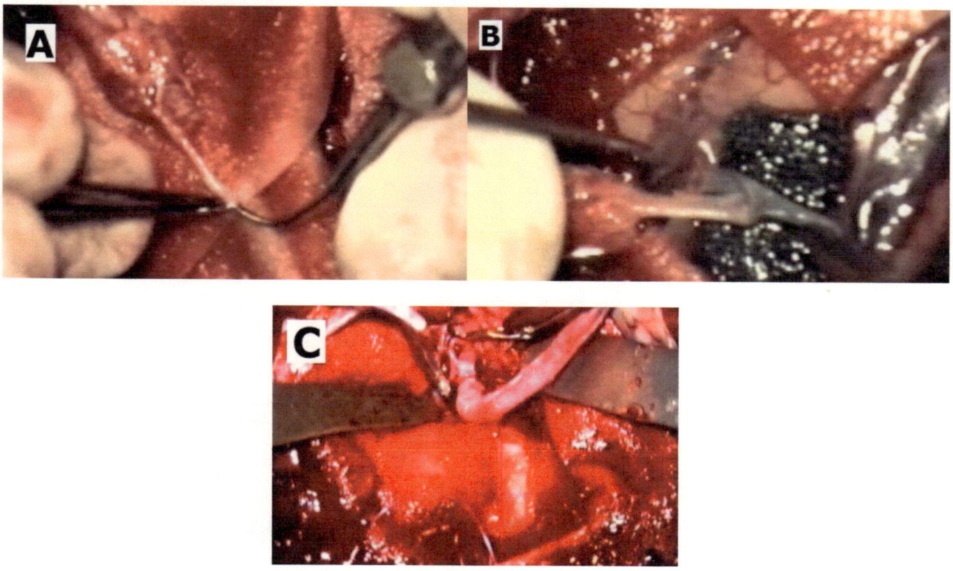

Figure 6. Extracranial to intracranial bypass. (A) Saphenous vein graft filled with saline and heparin. (B) The graft was anastomosed to the M4 segment, as part of an ICA to MCA bypass. (C) Temporary clips are being opened and the vein graft is filled with circulating blood.

Some GIAs' have features that do not permit direct clipping or endovascular obliteration. Incorporation of parent vessels, giant dome, arteriosclerosis or dense calcification of the aneurysm dome and neck, or fusiform shape may prevent successful obliteration. Excluding GIA from the circulation by Hunterian ligation and trapping (parent artery sacrifice) without bypass are not recommended techniques nowadays, as approximately 30% of patients have insufficient collateral flow (Barnett, 1994). The balloon occlusion test (BTO) is useful method for proper qualification of an individual for trapping or extracranial to intracranial bypass surgery with positive predictive value of 98% (vanRooij, 2005). However, BTO has several variations, technical nuances and interpretations (Lesley, 2009). The adjunct of $xenon^{133}$ cerebral blood flow measurement, single-photon-emission in computer tomography and transcranial Doppler ultrasonography increased the sensitivity of BTO (Fraser, 2011). Bypass is an alternative method of securing from further rupture. Since the first superficial temporal artery (STA) to MCA by-pass, the revascularisation methods have significantly developed. Radial artery or saphenous veins are used as a graft material. The anatomic location of a particular GIA dictates the endpoint of the by-pass. VA, petrous segment of ICA or external carotid artery (ECA) to MCA or PCA connections were made by various authors and described (LeRoux, 2003). Contemporarily the ICA to MCA high–flow bypasses are the most common. In addition microvascular skills are required and should be maintained by constant training. When performing bypass surgery, even by skilful neurosurgeons, the temporary occlusion of the proximal major brain artery can result in brain ischemia. To solve the problem of temporary occlusion of the main brain arteries Tulleken developed the Excimer laser-assisted nonocclusive technique (ELANA) (Tulleken, 1995). The above method constructs an anastomosis without the need for temporary occlusion of brain arteries. For other bypasses a balloon occlusion test (BTO) or Xenon computer tomography are useful methods for proper qualification of individuals for extracranial to intracranial bypass surgery or parent artery sacrifice.

3.2. Accessory techniques

In many GIA cases, direct clipping is impossible. Therefore accessory techniques have been refined for years to provide adequate alternatives to patients with such presentations. Temporary occlusion by vessel clipping, endovascular balloon occlusion, temporary extracranial to intracranial by-pass, or retrograde suction decompression comprise some of the safest accessory techniques facilitating microsurgical exclusion of an aneurysm from circulation.

Temporary occlusion is a valuable method, which is used by most neurosurgeons in most clipped GIAs. Safety of this method varies according to the vessel occluded and the respective time of occlusion. To date, there are no time-limits for arterial occlusion. High tolerable occlusion times (without infarction observed in postoperative CT) of 60 minutes for ICA, 35 minutes for MCA and 19 minutes for BA were observed (LeRoux, 2003). Others used sophisticated techniques and proved that even brief episodes of cerebral vessel occlusion produced changes in the brain signals (Jiang, 2009). We use no more than three minutes of arterial occlusion and four to five minutes of reperfusion. However, poor clinical condition of patients with ruptured aneurysms and advanced age are significant risk factors for stroke related to temporary artery occlusion. Intermittent episodes of occlusion and reperfusion are controversial and therefore not recommended. The application of intraoperative monitoring (electroencephalography or somatosensory evoked potentials) during temporary clipping reduces the risk of ischaemic complications, although complicates the whole procedure. Instead of a surgical temporary clip, endovascular balloon introduction may be used for temporary occlusion. The efficacy of both methods is similar. The use of endovascular balloon does not carry surgery-related complications, though both methods of temporary obstruction increase the risk of ischemic deficit by local endothelial cell damage (MacDonald, 1994).

The role of STA to MCA bypass in excluding GIAs is regarded as historical. However, temporary low-flow bypass can be applied in some individuals when a prolonged clipping is regarded preoperatively. On the contrary to temporary occlusion of parent vessels, a circulatory may be superseded by low-flow shunt, which is not limited by time required for GIA securing. Neck clipping of a GIA with accessory temporary occlusion of the parent artery is a superior treatment to accessory by-pass, although it is inevitably associated with the risk of cerebral ischemia. Hongo proposed a 'double insurance bypass' of both the STA and radial artery to different portions of the MCA (Hongo, 2002). The STA is anastomosed to the distal cortical branch of the MCA and is responsible for the blood flow to the distal territory while the radial artery is sutured to M2 or M3 and secures the ICA territory during temporary occlusion of the ICA during clipping a GIA. The results of this safe accessory technique were encouraging (Hongo, 2002; Ishikawa 2005), however, not confirmed by other authors.

Circulatory arrest and deep hypothermia are abandoned in most institutions nowadays. If neurosurgeons were to explore the abovementioned method, remarkable discussion concerning thorough technique learning, potential risk of complication and alternatives would be required. Hypothermia and cardiac arrest are still relatively high-risk procedures related to high rates of mortality and morbidity. The complications include hemodilution, coagulopathies, fibrinolysis, impairment of platelets as well as postoperative haematomas. Circulatory arrest should not exceed 30 minutes because of the increased occurrence of significant hypothermia-induced coagulopathy. Limited time is an additional factor in securing GIAs in cardiac arrest.

Retrograde suction decompression is a simple and effective method used in paraclinoid as well as distal portion of ICA GIAs. A method consists of retrograde suction of blood from closed circulatory resulting in deflation of the aneurysm. Followed by surgical exposure of the ECA, superior thyroid artery is dissected and then catheterised. After temporary clipping of the ECA proximally to an introduced catheter and the ICA distal to the aneurysm, manual syringe suction is performed (Fig. 7). The dome of the aneurysm collapses facilitating the aneurysm neck preparation and its clipping. The drawback of that method is the development of thromboses within the lumen of a GIA, which is relatively common complication. A variety of modifications has been published including novel employment of endovascular embolectomy device for retrograde suction (Hoh, 2007).

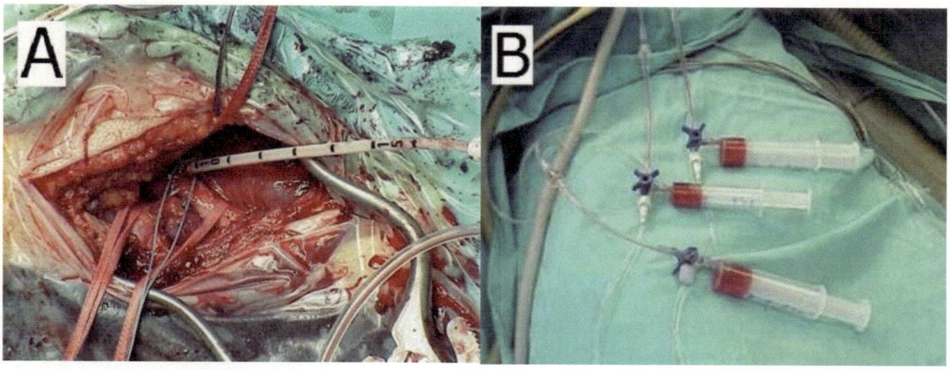

Figure 7. Retrograde suction. (A) The superior thyroid artery is catheterised by means of common central venous catheter. The external carotid artery is temporarily closed at the moment of suction. (B) We use three syringes: two for retrograde suction and one filled with heparin for flushing purposes.

Several monitoring methods test vascular patency and proper aneurysm occlusion: intraoperative fluorescence, Doppler ultrasonography examination or intraoperative angiography. The last one is supposed to be the most beneficial over others, though is invasive and thus related to increased complication rate. A routine use of intraoperative angiography in all operated aneurysms is debatable. In literature, necessary intraoperative angiography was performed in about 6% of cases of altered aneurysm clip position (Klopfenstein, 2004). Some aneurysms, including GIAs, are more succeptable to incomplete clipping and therefore may require intraoperative evaluation with angiography. The authors of retrospective analysis in postoperative angiography following aneurysm clipping concluded that the routine intraoperative angiography is recommended in treatment of GIAs (Kivisaari, 2004). In large and giant aneurysms the incomplete occlusion rate exceeded 50% and these patients required further complementary endovascular therapy or surgical revision.

Intraoperative fluorescence is obtained by the addition of near infrared imaging to surgical microscopes and high resolution videoangiography. When administered intravenously, the dye reacts in plasma in approximately 4 minutes. Then the fluorescence (indocyanine green) is induced by near infrared and recorded by a camera (Snyder, 2011). Intraoperative fluorescence angiography is helpful in performing 'Matas test' during clipping ACoA GIA (Murai, 2011) or ensuring the patency of the parent artery and perforators. However, in 5% of cases the image quality is poor (Raabe, 2005). The limitations of fluorescence angiography refer to GIAs affected by calcifications, thrombosed and those with thick walls (Snyder, 2011).

Colour Doppler and micro-Doppler ultrasonography are reliable and simple methods to verify the correct placement of the clip in aneurysm surgery. Micro-Doppler can detect incomplete exclusion of the aneurysm, stenosis of a parent vessel or occlusion of the parent or adjacent arteries and therefore is used routinely in GIAs. The confirmation of proper blood flow confirmed in ultrasonography allows an addition of another clip to a GIAs neck and afterwards in case of stenosis the clip can be removed. Comparing to other intraoperative vascular patency methods, the cost efficiency of micro-Doppler is favourable (Kapsalski, 2005).

Gruber compared the intraoperative monitoring and vascular imaging methods (Gruber, 2011). He concluded that these methods rather complement than compete. None of them are reliable when used as a single method.

3.4. Complications

Open surgery of GIAs results in more complications than any endovascular securing method (Gobin, 1996; Johnston, 1999). Many of the surgically treated GIAs referencing adverse events are dated prior to the introduction of Guglielmi detachable coils, microsurgery and neuroanaesthesiology development. Issues regarding complication rates of endovascular and surgical methods are indications for performing randomised trials in GIAs.

General and procedure-related adverse events are distinguished. General ones derive from aneurysm rupture, anaesthesia and imperfection of postoperative care.

Procedure	Specific complications of method
Craniotomy	
Pterional	Impaired memory or cognition (due to brain damage), facial nerve paresis, temporal muscle atrophy, cerebrospinal fluid leakage.
ACP removal	GIA or ICA wall damage, cerebrospinal fluid leakage through paranasal sinuses.
Orbitozygomatic	Severe orbital swelling, changes in visual activity, cerebrospinal fluid leakage through paranasal sinuses.
Retrosigmoid	VA injury, cranial nerves deficits, nasal cerebrospinal fluid leakage through mastoid cells, injury of venous sinuses.
Far-lateral	VA injury, cranial nerves deficits, nasal cerebrospinal fluid leakage through mastoid cells, injury of venous sinuses.
Securing methods used in GIAs	
Clipping	Intraoperative aneurysm rupture or cerebral injury, brain swelling due to spatulas use, major vessel stenosis or occlusion, clip slippage, aneurysm residue.
Wrapping	Major vessel stenosis or occlusion, recurrent haemorrhage, vasospasm, arachnoiditis, granuloma in the region of wrapping that can cause cranial nerves neuropathies.
Trapping	Cerebral ischemia in the region of occluded parent artery, thrombotic occlusion of perforators.
By-pass	Cerebral ischemia due to bypass insufficiency, thrombotic occlusion of perforators, heparin-induced haemorrhages.
Accessory techniques	
Temporary vascular occlusion	Cerebral ischemia in the region of temporarily occluded parent artery, endothelial damages.
Retrograde suction	Cerebral ischemia in the region of temporarily occluded parent artery, thrombotic occlusion of arterial branches, endothelial damages.
Deep hypothermia and cardiac arrest	Thrombophlebitis, cardiac arrhythmia, new neurologic deficits occurrence, temperature instability, delayed awakening, coagulopathies, interstitial fluid sequestration.
Temporary bypass	Cerebral ischemia in the region of occluded parent artery, thrombotic occlusion of perforators, heparin-induced haemorrhages.
Intraoperative angiography	Femoral artery thrombosis or pseudoaneurysm, thrombotic occlusion of cerebral arteries, groin hematoma, aortic dissection.
Fluorescence angiography	Possible vasovagal reactions, contraindicated in patients with a history of iodine allergy.
Doppler ultrasonography	None.

Table 3. The characteristic of specific complications related to craniotomies, securing methods and accessory techniques used in GIAs.

The course of treatment following SAH is different than methods used in patients with unruptured GIAs. The consequences of aneurysm rupture include: hypovolemia, hyponatremia, hydrocephalus, cardiac problems, seizures, rebleeding from unsecured aneurysms, symptomatic cerebral ischemia secondary to cerebral vasospasm, coma and death.

However, the main complication of SAH from a neurosurgical point of view is cerebral vasospasm. It is defined as self-limited narrowing of a cerebral vasculature and is observed angiographically with or without clinical manifestation. Angiographic vasospasm refers up to 97% of patients, while neurological signs are observed only in 33% (Dorsch, 1994). Cerebral vasospasm is responsible for about 10% of deaths and 10% of permanent disability after SAH (Dorsch, 1994). These high rates of unfavourable outcomes followed by cerebral vasospasm underestimate the role of postoperative management secondary to SAH and underline the remaining challenges (LeRoux, 2003). Rebleeding from previously secured GIAs occurs rarely in the postoperative period, however, is related to high mortality.

The complications after general anaesthesia in GIAs and smaller aneurysms are similar. Theoretically, the prolonged surgery of GIAs may result in higher rate of adverse events. SAH increases the risk of pulmonary complications, including pneumonia, pulmonary emboli or oedema, adult respiratory distress syndrome (Solenski, 1995) and cardiac arrhythmia (up to 5%). Hypovolemia, hypokalaemia and hypotension generally are iatrogenic consequences of inappropriate management after SAH.

Procedure-related complications are divided into groups of procedures: craniotomy, aneurysm securing and accessory techniques (Table 3). Brain contusion is the most serious, while surgical wound infection is the most common consequence of craniotomy.

Amongst GIA securing methods a bleed from a ruptured neck or dome of the aneurysm without any vascular control is the most dangerous intraoperative failure. All of the accessory techniques are low risk procedures, in contrast to deep hypothermia.

However, the number of complications can differ significantly among authors.

LeRoux indicates that complication rate can reach 100%, depending on accepted criteria applied by investigator (LeRoux, 2003).

4. Outcome

Surgical mortality of GIAs is estimated on average rate at 10% and may range from 4 to 21% (Sharma, 2008). Short-term outcome of ruptured GIAs achieved in a multicentre study was worse than smaller ones (Kassell, 1990). The study from our institution (Szmuda & Sloniewski, 2011) did not coincide with the stereotype of unfavourable treatment results in GIAs. Mortality rate, short and long-term outcome after the operation of giant and smaller ICA aneurysms were similar. Our results proved that size of an aneurysm is not a prognostic factor, but there are other more prominent variables to explore when determining mortality. A thorough multivariate analysis should be a tool used in prognosis evaluation. Moreover, the outcomes of ruptured and unruptured GIAs differ and therefore should be analysed separately. However, the quantification of outcomes in treated aneurysms is an elusive problem. Beyond dispute mortality is the most important endpoint in GIA studies, followed by clinical condition at discharge, functional status, and all aspects with regards to the quality of life several years following the operation. The radiological outcome of secured GIAs should run parallel to both the physical and mental assessment of treated patients. The results of surgery based on older publications do not reflect the current practice in the treatment of GIAs (Sughrue, 2010). The concern about the best treatment method in that group is challenging, whereas evidence based proofs are ambiguous.

Recent studies emphasize economic evaluations. Cost-effective analyses, comparing endovascular and microsurgical methods, should be translated into GIAs.

4.1. Radiological outcome

Postoperative subtracted angiography or occasionally computer tomography angiography after successful by-pass or occlusion of a GIA can reveal initial complications. Cerebral vasospasm, clip slippage or critical stenosis in some cases may result in postoperative management alteration or a second operation. Clip slippage after successful occlusion occurs in 0.2% of cases (Asgari, 2003) due to inadequate closing forces of clips, which are intended for use in smaller aneurysms, are used in the treatment of GIAs. If clip displacement is observed intraoperatively it can be replaced safely once again and additionally strengthen by the positioning of a second forcing clip. Even application of several aneurysm clips may be insufficient. In our series, clip displacement in further control angiography was noted in one patient of 128 operated GIAs (0.8%). The adhesions around complex of clips prevented their safe reposition during the revision (Fig. 8). However, a slipped clip may lead to fatal intracerebral haemorrhage (Wester, 2009).

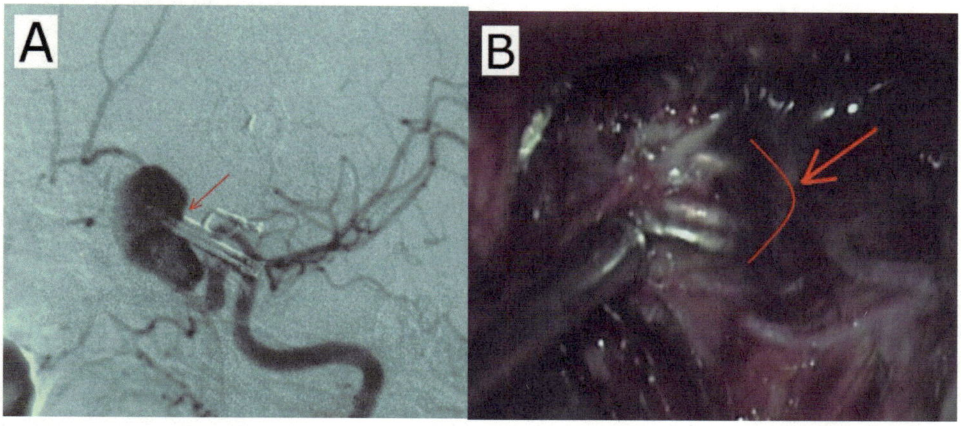

Figure 8. Slipped complex of two straight clips and one fenestrated bayonet clip from ICA GIA. (A) The blades of the fenestrated clip are totally out of the aneurysm's dome. Probably the summary closing force of applied clips proved to be insufficient. (B) Four months after initial surgery the adhesion of the clips located outside the Sylvian fissure, prevented their safe reposition.

The evaluation methods measuring the visual degree of an aneurysm occlusion in postoperative angiography may vary among studies (Gonzalez, 2006). Modified Raymond classification is commonly used following endovascular coiling (Raymond, 1997). The application of the above scale to surgical occlusion assessment is erroneous as a dog-ear remnant is a characteristic finding after coiling. The occlusion of GIAs can be classified using postoperative angiography as incomplete – more than 5% of remaining aneurysm lumen, minimal contrasting aneurysm residue – small neck remnant and as complete – no remnant (Sughrue, 2010). Complete occlusion refers to the majority of clipped GIAs in various studies (see Table 2), although in one study (Kivisaari, 2004) is lower (57%). In our institution postoperative assessment of the duration of occlusion was not assessed in every case, therefore it is impossible to compare our results with other reported works (Szmuda & Sloniewski, 2011). In term of occlusion rate endovascular therapy methods seems to be inferior to surgery; postprocedural incomplete occlusion after coiling can be as low as 17% (Sluzewski, 2003). However, a part of contrasting neck is quite often observed in GIAs (Kivisaari, 2004). Supplementary stent or coil embolization of the aneurysm residue could be offered after angiographic assessment (Fig. 9). The significant limitation of supplementary endovascular therapy is that during the acute phase of subarachnoid haemorrhage stenting is not recommended, due to the need of anticoagulant therapy and should be postponed (Gonzalez, 2006).

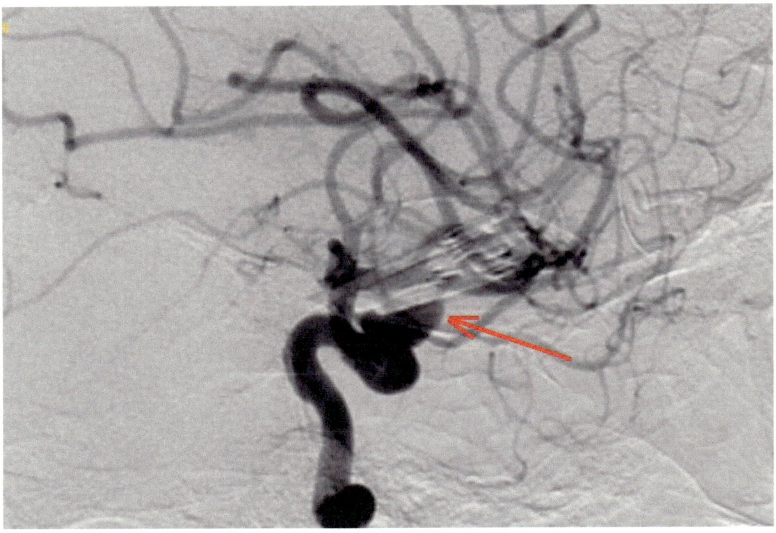

Figure 9. Four long straight clips were applied in unruptured paraclinoid GIA. Residual aneurysm neck was observed in postoperative DSA. The patient required a supplementary coiling of an incompletely occluded GIA.

4.2. Clinical outcome analyzis

We analysed the clinical outcome following treatment of single artery ICA GIAs in our institution from 1997 to 2006. In 2011 two papers concerning our treatment results were published (Szmuda & Sloniewski, 2011, 2011) and one another is in press. ICA saccular aneurysms were assessed; the retrospective analysis of series consisted of 78 GIAs and 250 smaller aneurysms. Both groups comprised ruptured and unruptured aneurysms. All patients suffering from GIAs of ICA origin were offered surgery and all underwent surgical treatment by our senior author (PS). Therefore the analysis reflected a single-surgeon experience measured by means of clinical treatment results. The general outcomes of GIA surgery were published in Acta Neurochirurgica (Szmuda & Sloniewski, 2011). There were no significant differences between GIAs and smaller ICA aneurysms with respect to mortality, unfavourable outcomes rates as well as quality of life. Moreover, the treatment results were similar in separate comparisons of size aneurysm groups among ruptured and unruptured ones. Mortality of presented GIAs' as well as unfavourable outcome rates were comparable to other published works. Postoperative death rate for GIAs depends on group characteristic and ruptured to unruptured aneurysm ratio. Mortality rate may vary from 4 to 21%, with an average of 10% (Sharma, 2008), while in our study was 12.8% (Table 4).

	GIAs (n; %)	**Smaller aneurysms** (n; %)	*p*
All ICA aneurysms	**78**	**250**	
Mortality rate	10; 12.8%	30; 12.0%	*0.84*
Unfavourable short-term outcome rate (GOS score equal or lower than 3)	22; 61.1%	119; 57.8%	*0.26*
Low quality of life rate (total SF-36 score equal or lower than 50)	21; 41.2%	70; 45.1%	*0.62*
Ruptured ICA aneurysms	**36**	**206**	
Mortality rate	6; 16.7%	30; 14.6%	*0.74*
Unfavourable short-term outcome rate (GOS score equal or lower than 3)	14; 38.9%	87; 42.2%	*0.78*
Low quality of life rate (total SF-36 score equal or lower than 50)	6; 27.3%	56; 45.2%	*0.12*
Unruptured ICA aneurysms	**42**	**44**	
Mortality rate	4; 9.5%	0; 0.0%	*0.06*
Unfavourable short-term outcome rate (GOS score equal or lower than 3)	6; 14.3%	3; 6.8%	*0.26*
Low quality of life rate (total SF-36 score equal or lower than 50)	16; 54.8%	15; 48.3%	*0.19*

Table 4. The comparison of general treatment results between giant and smaller ICA aneurysms based on own series (Szmuda & Sloniewski, 2011).

Most of ICA GIAs (n=57; 73%) were clipped; the rest of the aneurysms were excluded from circulation via parent vessel occlusion with extracranial to intracranial bypass (n=15; 19%) or without graft surgery (n=2; 3%). ECA to distal segment (M3 or M4) of MCA bypass was the most common (n=10), while ICA to MCA or low-flow (STA to MCA) bypasses were performed occasionally (n=5). In one individual the aneurysm was wrapped and in three patients a GIA was not secured at all. The operative methods were analysed regarding mortality, short and long term outcome. There were no statistically significant differences observed between these results, although two of three patients that GIA was not secured intraoperatively died and one of two patients after trapping experienced permanent disability. The outcome of these two patients with unsecured GIA from our series is a reflection of a poor natural history of untreated lesions reported by Peerless (Peerless, 1990, as cited in Youmans, 1990). Mortality rates were 68% and 85% in two and five years of follow-up respectively. ICA occlusion due to ruptured GIA without performing by-pass (trapping) is a permissible surgical method in case of intraoperative bleeding. A permanent neurological deficit in patients from our series with occluded ICA is a consequence of both SAH and rescue clipping. In two individuals low-flow bypasses were found to be insufficient as one patient died due to cerebral ischemia. (Table 5)

GIA securing method	**Mortality rate** % (n)	**Unfavourable short-term outcome** (%)	**Unfavourable long-term outcome** (%)
Clipping	10.7% (6/57)	18.0% (9/50)	40.5% (15/37)
High-flow by-pass	10.0% (1/10)	0.0% (0/12)	33.3% (4/12)
Low-flow bypass	20.0% (1/5)	0.0% (0/4)	25.0% (1/4)
Trapping	0.0% (0/2)	50.0% (1/2)	100.0% (1/1)
Wrapping	0.0% (0/1)	0.0% (0/1)	0.0% (0/1)
Not secured	66.6% (2/3)	no FU	no FU

Abbreviations: no FU – no follow-up

Table 5. Characteristic of outcomes in ICA GIAs by treatment methods, derived from own series (Szmuda & Sloniewski, 2011).

A variety of accessory techniques were used in eight cases from the series. Temporary low-flow bypass (n=1), retrograde suction (n=4), temporary balloon occlusion (n=1) and deep hypothermic circulatory arrest (n=2) were undoubtedly beneficial in clipping. Both patients with GIA secured under cardiac arrest survived, did not experience any method-related complication and were discharged home with favourable outcome. However, abovementioned excellent outcome of used hypothermia refer to small group of GIAs at the ICA origin, the complication rate in patients operated on due to other indications was increased. The application of deep hypothermic cardiac arrest is contemporarily limited in our institution to individuals when simultaneous cardiosurgical approach is needed. In our opinion, retrograde suction is a powerful tool in paraclinoid GIAs among accessory techniques. The simplicity and low complication rate are its two main advantages.

In our series the giant size of ICA aneurysms was not related to mortality and short and long-term outcome. However, the analyzis of clinical outcomes in ruptured aneurysms should include other factors directly related to SAH. The summary of various analyses led to the creation of an accepted neurosurgical doctrine, in which, the triad of factors: age, clinical status on admission and vasospasm affect mortality after surgery in ruptured intracranial aneurysms (Salary, 2007; Roos, 2000; Taylor, 2004). Kassell also introduced the size of the aneurysm is an independent factor of a worse outcome (Kassell, 1990). Moreover, an aneurysm occurrence at the posterior circulation resulted in a higher rate of poor treatment results. Concluding from Kassell's study the analysis of factors that might influence the outcome following SAH should comprise the patients with aneurysms derived from a selected artery, for instance ICA. Multivariate analyses of outcome in ruptured ICA aneurysms was published (Szmuda & Sloniewski, 2011). As a result of these analyses various factors appeared significant, although different for mortality and short-term outcome (Fig. 10). Moreover, when mortality and unfavourable short-term outcome were analysed together there were also discrepancies. Clinical state at admission (based on Hunt-Hess scale) and delayed cerebral ischemia (as a resolution of cerebral vasospasm) affected all outcome measurements. SAH intensity (Fisher scale) influenced short-term outcome as well as a combined mortality and unfavourable short-term outcome. However, older age was prevalent in determining clinical state on discharge, although was not related with mortality. Geriatric populations are considered to be more sensitive to surgery due to comorbidities affecting the course of treatment. No significant factors connected with long-term quality of life were found.

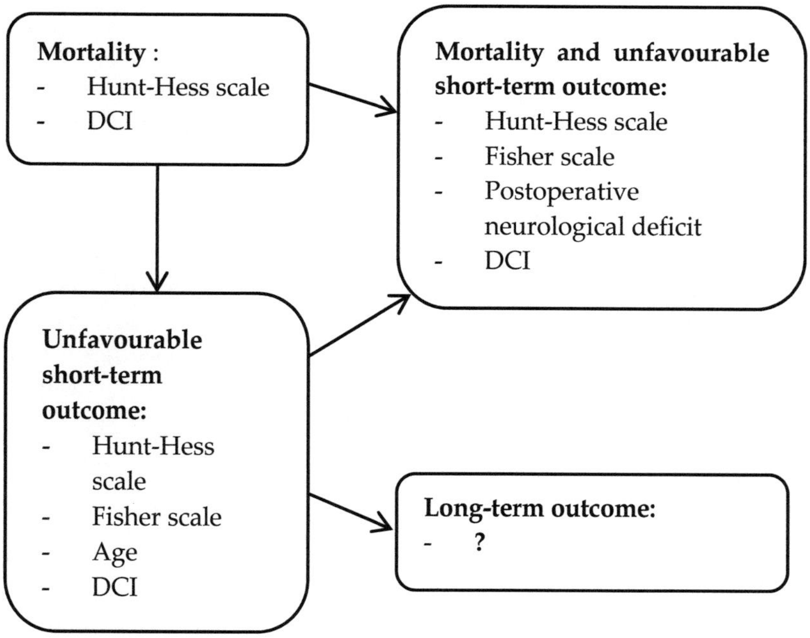

Abbreviations: DCI - delayed cerebral ischemia.

Figure 10. Diagram presenting factors determining mortality, short and long-term outcome in ruptured ICA aneurysms.

Fourth or fifth grade in Hunt-Hess scale found to be dominant factor in determining mortality and unfavourable short-term outcome in ruptured ICA aneurysms based on a statistical tool called receiver operating characteristic (ROC). Followed by poor clinical state, a massive bleed assessed by the Fisher scale, postoperative neurological deficit occurrence and delayed cerebral ischemia were consecutively responsible for worse outcome (Fig.11).

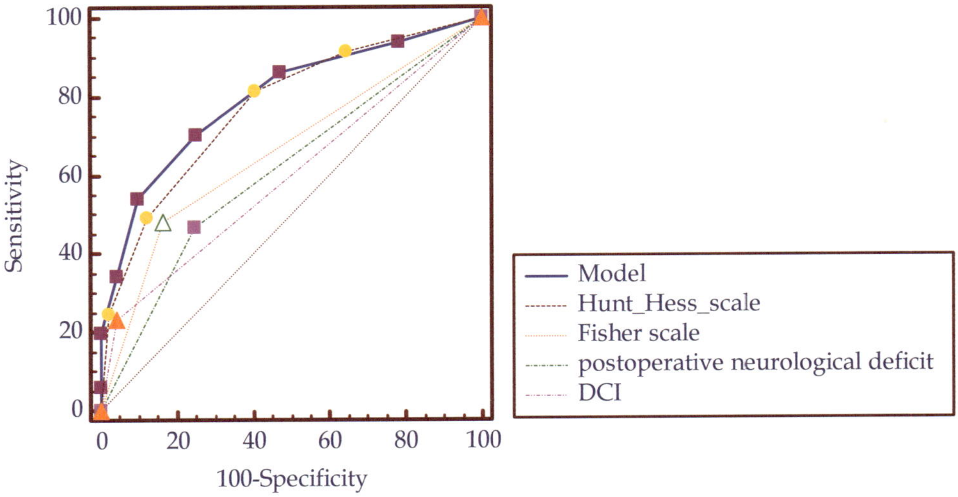

Abbreviations: DCI – delayed cerebral ischemia.

Figure 11. Receiver operating characteristic curve (ROC curve) presenting consecutive factors (according to importance) responsible for combined postoperative mortality and unfavourable short-term outcome in ruptured ICA aneurysms.

Another important issue is how the cost-effectiveness of GIAs therapy compares with smaller aneurysms. The undoubted increased cost of GIA therapy in comparison with smaller aneurysms is related to more complex operative procedures, increased time of surgery and hospital stay. There is a lack of publications regarding such comparisons, however, the economic analysis of unruptured aneurysms proved that treatment is cost-effective if addressed to large aneurysms and GIAs (Johnston & Gress, 1999). These lesions produce symptoms by compressing neural structures and have a high risk of rupture. Therefore a symptomatic patient harbouring unruptured GIA may potentially benefit more quality-adjusted life-years (QALY) (Qureshi, 2007).

5. Evidence-based paradigms for treatment:

GIAs can be secured effectively by neurosurgical or endovascular therapy, though there is a subset of factors (size, morphology, location, segment of artery, related anatomy, comorbidities as well as timing of surgery) which complicate treatment decision. Understanding the ability of variety techniques to the cerebrovascular team facilitates a comprehensive method for treating these lesions, maximizing efficacy and minimizing risk. In 2011 Fraser from Cornell University (New York) created a paradigm for approaching all aneurysms at the institution using currently accessible technology. We reported single-surgeon's experience of ICA GIAs treatment. Based on literature (Fraser, 2011; Cantore, 2008; Kai, 2007, Sharma, 2008), American Society of Anaesthesiologists as well as senior author (PS) reflections, we propose the detailed model of treatment methods to decision making processes in GIAs, also indicating the possible alternatives. However, it should be pointed that a paradigm is a proposal referring to current technology in our institution.

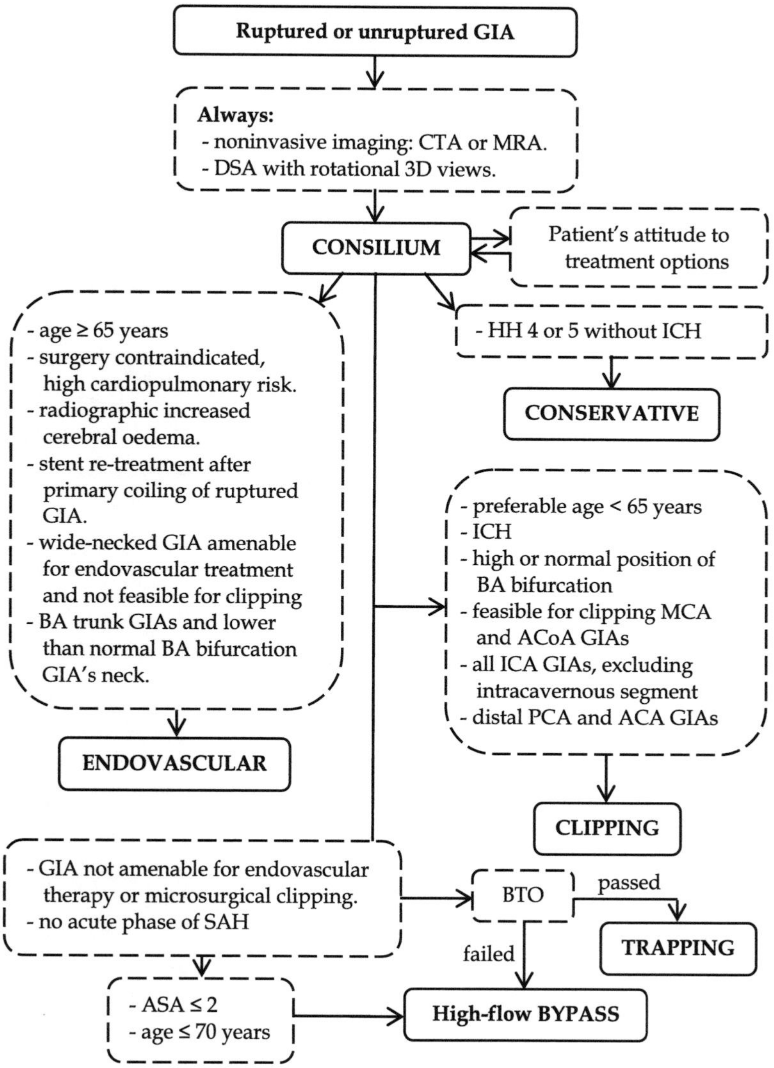

Abbreviations: ASA - American Society of Anaesthesiologists scale; BTO - balloon occlusion test; CTA - computer tomography angiography; HH - Hunt-Hess scale; ICH - intracranial haematoma; MRA - magnetic resonance angiography.

Figure 12. Treatment algorithm for GIAs evaluation and treatment in our institution.

Despite patient's previous radiograms, a meticulous preoperative diagnosis is to be complemented by means of cerebral rotational, three dimensional subtracted angiography (3D DSA) and computer tomography angiography (CTA) or optionally by magnetic resonance angiography (MRA). 3D DSA enables a visualisation of a detailed GIA's anatomical features and originating perforators, though its ability to demonstrate calcification or thrombosis is limited (Hoit, 2006). CTA accomplishes above limitations and moreover shows surrounding bony structures. In posterior fossa or ICA GIAs MRA can visualise adhering neural structures, although is performed occasionally in our institution. Conservative approach is preferred in individuals in fourth or fifth Hunt-Hess grade, excepting those with intracerebral haemorrhage. Conscious and informed patient's attitude to proposed GIA's treatment method is an important factor in making a decision. Endovascular therapy is approached to older individuals with high cardiopulmonary risk and when surgery is contraindicated. For ruptured GIAs an increased radiographic cerebral oedema may prevent direct clipping. Wide-necked GIAs not feasible for clipping should be secured by endovascular methods. GIAs originating at BA trunk or BA bifurcation with the neck located lower than normal are also offered endovascular treatment. A preferable group of patients for direct neck clipping are those younger than 65 years old. All GIAs amenable for clipping in neurosurgeon's opinion should be secured in this manner. In our institution distal PCA or ACA GIAs are excluded from a circulation by clipping technique. However, the most controversy refers to GIAs that are not suitable for both endovascular therapy and microsurgical clipping. In this case an endovascular therapy transforms these lesions into a chronic disease with a relapsing clinical course by further retreatments and repeated risk exposure (Sughrue, 2010). Flow-diverting stents potentially offer a meaningful benefit over surgery, although the outcome has not been sufficiently confirmed. Nonetheless, if endovascular therapy or direct clipping are not amenable bypass or parent artery sacrifice (trapping) is recommended, though bypass is not allowed in acute phase of SAH. Proper qualification to one of above surgical method is validated in balloon occlusion test (BTO). However this test is not meticulous enough, therefore the decision of treatment method can be supplemented by Xenon computer tomography or single-photon emission computed tomography (SPECT). Patients younger than 70 years old with equal or lower than grade II in American Society of Anaesthesiologists scale are qualifying for high-flow bypass without BTO, which is in accordance with contemporary literature (Cantore, 2008).

The contemporary experience with GIAs is limited to retrospective analysis of selected group of ICA GIAs (Szmuda & Sloniewski, 2011). Nonetheless, it demonstrates that experienced neurosurgeon (senior author - PS) can achieve excellent results using a single surgery, definitive and durable therapy.

6. Conclusions/perspectives

General unsatisfactory outcomes of GIAs do not warrant risky microsurgical or endovascular interventions. The more accustomed the neurovascular surgeon is the more difficult is the selection of the appropriate method for securing GIAs. However, in experienced hands the outcomes after treatment of giant and smaller aneurysms do not differ. In elderly populations, the efficacy must be weighed against the natural history of the GIA by considering expected remaining lifetime.

Endovascular embolization competes with open microsurgery in the field of cerebral aneurysms. Prospective and randomized trials (CURES, ATENA and STAT) are intent-to-treat analyses, therefore not dedicated for GIAs. The promising outcomes achieved by endovascular therapy for small aneurysms nevertheless remain unconfirmed for GIAs. Application of these results to GIAs is misleading. To date, the knowledge is based on small published series.

Forced by the completion of both treatment options, continuous development of neither endovascular nor microsurgical methods is being observed. Hopefully for patient's benefit!

Author details

Tomasz Szmuda and Pawel Sloniewski
Neurosurgery Department, Medical University of Gdansk, Poland

Acknowledgement

The authors thank Mrs M.Sc. Aleksandra Prusinowska (Academy of Fine Arts in Gdansk, Poland) for her graphics and the photo presenting approaches and MD Michael Kindrachuk for medical and neurosurgical proofread.

7. References

Anson, JA. (1995). Epidemiology and natural history, In: *Giant Intracranial Aneurysms*, Awad IA, Barrow DL, pp. (23–33), American Association of Neurological Surgeons, Park Ridge.

Asgari, S., Wanke, I., Schoch, B., Stolke, D. (2003). Recurrent hemorrhage after initially complete occlusion of intracranial aneurysms. *Neurosurg Rev*, 26, 4, October 2003, (269–274), 0344-5607.

Bakker, N.A. (2010). International subarachnoid aneurysm trial 2009: Endovascular coiling of ruptured intracranial aneurysms has no significant advantage over neurosurgical clipping. *Neurosurgery*, 66, 5, May 2010, pp. (961-962), 0148-396X.

Barnett, D.W., Barrow, D.L., Joseph, G.J. (1994). Combined extracranial-intracranial bypass and intraoperative balloon occlusion for the treatment of intracavernous and proximal carotid artery aneurysms. *Neurosurgery*, 35, pp. (92–97), 0148-396X.

Barth, A., de Tribolet, N., Barth, A. (1994). Growth of small saccular aneurysms to giant aneurysms: presentation of three cases. *Surgical Neurology*, 41, pp. (277–280), .

Cantore, G., Santoro, A., Guidetti, G., Delfinis, C.P., Colonnese, C., Passacantilli, E. (2008). Surgical treatment of giant intracranial aneurysms: Current viewpoint. *Neurosurgery*, 63, 4., October 2008, pp. (279-289), 0148-396X.

Cawley, C.M., Zipfel, G.J., Day, A.L. (1998). Surgical treatment of paraclinoid and ophthalmic aneurysms. *Neurosurg Clin North Am*, 9, pp. (765-783), .

Deshmukh, V.R., Kakarla, U.K., Figueiredo, E.G., Zabramski, J.M., Spetzler, R.F. (2006). Long-term clinical and angiographic follow-up of unclippable wrapped intracranial aneurysms. *Neurosurgery*, 58, 3, March 2006, pp. (434-442), 0148-396X.

Dorsch, N.W., King, M.T. (1994). A review of cerebral vasospasm in aneurysmal subarachnoid haemorrhage Part I: Incidence and effects. *Journal of Clinical Neuroscience*, 1, 1, January 1994, pp. (19-26), .

Fraser, J.F., Stieg, P.E. (2011) Surgical bypass for intracranial aneurysms: Navigating around a changing paradigm. *World Neurosurgery*, 75, 3-4, March 2011, pp. (414-417), .

Gobin, Y.P., Vinuela, F., Gurian, J.H., et al. (1996). Treatment of large and giant fusiform intracranial aneurysms with Guglielmi detachable coils. *J Neurosurg*, 1996, 84, 1, pp. (55-62), .

Gonzalez, N.R. et al. (2006). Challenges in the endovascular treatment of giant intracranial aneurysms. *Neurosurgery*, 59, 5, November 2006, pp. (S3-113), 0148-396X.

Gruber, A., Killer, M., Bavinzski, G., Richling, B. (1999). Clinical and angiographic results of endosaccular coiling treatment of giant and very large intracranial aneurysms: a 7-year, single-center experience. *Neurosurgery*, 1999, 45, 4, pp. (793-803), 0148-396X.

Gruber, A., Dorfer, C. , Standhardt, H., Bavinzski, G., Knosp, E. (2011). Prospective comparison of intraoperative vascular monitoring technologies during cerebral aneurysm surgery. *Neurosurgery*, 68, 3, March 2011, pp. (657-673), 0148-396X.

Hauck, E.F., Wohlfeld, B., Welch, B.G., White, J.A., Samson, D. (2008). Clipping of very large or giant unruptured intracranial aneurysms in the anterior circulation: an outcome study. *J Neurosurg*, 109, 6, 2008, pp. (1012-1018), .

Herrera, O., Kawamura, S., Yasui, N., Yoshida, Y. (1999). Histological changes in the rat common carotid artery induced by aneurysmal wrapping and coating materials.

Neurol Med Chir (Tokyo), , 39, 1999, pp. (134–139), .

Hoh, D.J., Larsen, D.W., Elder, J.B., Kim, P.E., Giannotta, S.L., Liu, C.Y. (2008). Novel use of an endovascular embolectomy device for retrograde suction decompression-assisted clip ligation of a large paraclinoid aneurysm: technical case report. *Neurosurgery*, 62, 5 Suppl 2, May 2008, pp. (412-413), 0148-396X.

Hoit, D.A., Malek, A.M. (2006). Fusion of three-dimensional calcium rendering with rotational angiography to guide the treatment of a giant intracranial aneurysm: Technical case report. *Neurosurgery*, 58, Suppl 1, February 2006, pp. (173-174), 0148-396X.

Hongo, K. , Horiuchi, T., Nitta, J., Tanaka, Y., Tada, T., Kobayashi, S., Barrow, D.L., Sekhar, L.N., Rak, R., Miyamoto, S., Hashimoto, N., Yamaura, A. (2003). Double-insurance bypass for internal carotid artery aneurysm surgery. *Neurosurgery*, 52, 3, March 2003, pp. (597-602), 0148-396X.

Jafar, J.J., Russell, S.M., Woo, H.H. (2002). Treatment of giant intracranial aneurysms with saphenous vein extracranial-to-intracranial bypass grafting: indications, operative technique, and results in 29 patients. *Neurosurgery*. 51, 1, 2002, pp. (138-144), 0148-396X.

Jahromi, B.S., Mocco, J., Bang, J.A., et al. (2008). Clinical and angiographic outcome after endovascular management of giant intracranial aneurysms. *Neurosurgery*, 63, 4, pp. (662-674), 0148-396X.

Jiang, Y.,Bu, B.,Xu, B.-N.,Sun, Z.-H.,Jiang, J.-L.,Zhou, D.-B.,Yu, X.-G. (2009). Intraoperative neuroelectrophysiological monitoring of cerebral blood supply after parent-artery occlusion during intracranial aneurysm surgery. *Chinese Journal of Cerebrovascular Diseases*, 6, 11, November 2009, pp. (577-580).

Johnston, S.C., Dudley, R.A., Gress, D.R., Ono, L. (1999). Surgical and endovascular treatment of unruptured cerebral aneurysms at university hospitals. *Neurology*, 52, 1999, pp. (1799–1805).

Johnston, S.C., Gress, D.R., Kahn, J.G. (1999). Which unruptured cerebral aneurysms should be treated? A cost-utility analysis. *Neurology*, 1999, 52, pp. (1806–1815).

Kai, Y., Hamada, J., Morioka, M., Yano, S., Mizuno, T., Kuroda, J., Todaka, T., Takeshima, H., Kuratsu, J. (2007). Treatment strategy for giant aneurysms in the cavernous portion of the internal carotid artery. *Surgical Neurology*, 67, 2, February 2007, pp. (148-155).

Kapsalaki, E.Z., Lee, G.P., Robinson III, J.S., Grigorian, A.A., Fountas, K.N. (2008). The role of intraoperative micro-Doppler ultrasound in verifying proper clip placement in intracranial aneurysm surgery. *Journal of Clinical Neuroscience*, 15, 2, February 2008, pp. (153-157).

Kassell, N.F., Torner, J.C., Jane, J.A., Haley, E.C. Jr, Adams, H.P. (1990). The International Cooperative Study on the Timing of Aneurysm Surgery. Part 2. Surgical results. *J Neurosurg*, 73, 1, pp. (37–47).

Keravel, Y. (1988). *Giant Intracranial Aneurysms*, (1ed), Springer-Verlag, 3540181318, Berlin.

Kivisaari, R.P., Porras, M., Ohman, J., Siironen, J., Ishii, K., Hernesniemi, J. (2004). Routine cerebral angiography after surgery for saccular aneurysms: Is it worth it? *Neurosurgery*, 55, 5, November 2004, pp. (1015-1022), 0148-396X.

Klopfenstein, J.D., Spetzler, R.F., Kim, L.J., Feiz-Erfan, I., Han, P.P., Zabramski, J.M., Porter, R.W., Albuquerque, F.C., McDougall, C.G., Fiorella, D.J. (2004). Comparison of routine and selective use of intraoperative angiography during aneurysm surgery: A prospective assessment. *Journal of Neurosurgery*, 100, 2, February 2004, pp. (230-235), .

Kodama, N., Suzuki., J. (1982). Surgical treatment of giant aneurysms. *Neurosurg Rev*, 5, 1982, pp. (155), .

Krings, T., Piske, R.L., Lasjaunias, P.L. (2005). Intracranial arterial aneurysm vasculopathies: targeting the outer vessel wall. *Neuroradiology*, 47, pp. (931–937).

Krisht, A.F., Kadri, P.A.S. (2005). Surgical clipping of complex basilar apex aneurysms: A strategy for successful outcome using the pretemporal transzygomatic transcavernous approach. *Neurosurgery*, 56, 4 Suppl., April 2005, pp. (261-272), 0148-396X.

Lawton, M.T. (2002). Basilar apex aneurysms: surgical results and perspectives from an initial experience. *Neurosurgery*, 50, 1, 2002, pp. (1-8), 0148-396X.

Lemole, G.M., Henn, J., Spetzler, R.F., Riina, H.A. (2000). Surgical management of giant aneurysms. *Operative Techniques inNeurosurgery*, 3, 4, 2000, pp. (239-254), .

LeRoux, PD. (2003). *Management of Cerebral Aneurysms*, (1ed), W.B. Saunders, 0721687547, Pennsylvania.

Lesley, W.S., Rangaswamy, R. (2009). Balloon test occlusion and endosurgical parent artery sacrifice for the evaluation and management of complex intracranial aneurysmal disease. *Journal of NeuroInterventional Surgery*, 1, 2, December 2009, pp. (112-120).

Linskey, M.E., Sekhar, L.N., Hirsch Jr., W., Yonas, H., Horton, J.A. (1990). Aneurysms of the intracavernous carotid artery: Clinical presentation, radiographic features, and pathogenesis. *Neurosurgery*, 26, 1, 1990, pp. (71-79), 0148-396X.

Lshikawa, T., Kamiyama, H., Kobayashi, N., Tanikawa, R., Takizawa, K., Kazumata, K. Experience from "double-insurance bypass." Surgical results and additional techniques to achieve complex aneurysm surgery in a safer manner. *Surgical Neurology*, 63, 5, May 2005, pp. (485-490).

Lylyk, P., Miranda, C., Ceratto, R., et al. (2009). Curative endovascular reconstruction of cerebral aneurysms with the pipeline embolization device: the Buenos Aires experience. *Neurosurgery*, 64, 4, 2009, pp. (632-642), 0148-396X.

MacDonald, J.D., Gyorke, A., Jacobs, J.M., Mohammad, S.F., Sunderland, P.M., Reichman, M.V., Mayberg, M.R., Selman, W.R. (1994). Acute phase vascular endothelial injury: A comparison of temporary arterial occlusion using an endovascular occlusive balloon catheter versus a temporary aneurysm clip in a pig model. *Neurosurgery*, 34, 5, 1994, pp. (876-881), 0148-396X.

Minakawa, T., Koike, T., Fujii, Y., Ishii, R., Tanaka, R., Arai, H. (1987). Long term results of ruptured aneurysms treated by coating. *Neurosurgery*, 21, 1987, pp. (660–663), 0148-396X.

Molyneux, A., Kerr, R., Stratton, I., et al. (2005). International Subarachnoid Aneurysm Trial (ISAT) of neurosurgical clipping versus endovascular coiling in 2143 patients with ruptured intracranial aneurysms: A randomised trial. *Lancet*, 366, 2005, pp. (809-817).

Molyneux, A.J., Kerr, R.S., Birks, J., Ramzi, N., Yarnold, J., Sneade, M., Rischmiller, J. (2009). Risk of recurrent subarachnoid haemorrhage, death, or dependence and standardised mortality ratios after clipping or coiling of an intracranial aneurysm in the International Subarachnoid Aneurysm Trial (ISAT): long-term follow-up. *The Lancet Neurology*, 8, 5, May 2009, pp. (427-433).

Murai, Y., Adachi, K., Takagi, R., Koketsu, K., Matano, F., Teramoto, A. (2011). Intraoperative Matas test using microscope-integrated intraoperative indocyanine green videoangiography with temporary unilateral occlusion of the A1 segment of the anterior cerebral artery. *World Neurosurg*, 76, 477, 2011, pp. (E7-477.E10).

Patel, U. (2010). The development of a calculator to predict the risk of rupture of unruptured intracranial aneurysms@neurisk. *World Neurosurgery*, 73, 4, April 2010, pp. (231-233).

Qureshi, A.I., Janardhan, V., Hanel, R.A., Lanzino. Comparison of endovascular and surgical treatments for intracranial aneurysms: an evidence-based review. *Lancet Neurology*, 6, 9, September 2007, pp. (816-825).

Raabe, A., Nakaji, P., Beck, J., Kim, L.J., Hsu, F.P., Kamerman, J.D., Seifert, V., Spetzler, R.F. (2005). Prospective evaluation of surgical microscope-integrated intraoperative nearinfrared indocyanine green videoangiography during aneurysm surgery. *J Neurosurg*, 103, 2005, pp. (982-989).

Raymond, J, Roy, D. (1997). Safety and efficacy of endovascular treatment of acutely ruptured aneurysms. *Neurosurgery*, 41, 1997, pp. (1235-1246), 0148-396X.

Roos, E.J., Rinkel, G.J., Velthuis, B.K., et al. (2000). The relation between aneurysm size and outcome in patients with subarachnoid hemorrhage. *Neurology*, 54, 2000, pp. (2334-2336).

Russell, S.M., Lin, K., Hahn, S.A., et al. (2003). Smaller cerebral aneurysms producing more extensive subarachnoid hemorrhage following rupture: a radiological investigation and discussion of theoretical determinants. *J Neurosurg*, 99, 2003, pp. (248-253).

Salary, M., Quigley, M.R., Wilberger, J.E. (2007). Relation among aneurysm size, amount of subarachnoid blood, and clinical outcome. *J Neurosurg*, 107, 2007, pp. (13-17).

Sano, H. (2010). Treatment of complex intracranial aneurysms of anterior circulation using multiple clips. *Acta Neurochir Suppl*, 107, 2010, pp. (27-31).

Sharma, B.S., Gupta, A., Ahmad, F.U., Suri, A., Mehta, V.S. (2008). Surgical management of giant intracranial aneurysms. *Clin Neurol Neurosurg*, 110, 7, 2008, pp. (674–681).

Shi, Z.S., Ziegler, J., Duckwiler, G.R., et al. (2009). Management of giant middle cerebral artery aneurysms with incorporated branches: partial endovascular coiling or combined extracranial-intracranial bypass—a team approach. *Neurosurgery*, 65, 6 Suppl., 2009, pp. (121-129).

Sloniewski, P., Dzierzanowski, J., Szmuda, T. (2008). Modyfikacja dojscia pterionalnego do patologii dolu miedzykonarowego – technika, morfometria i wyniki leczenia. *Neurol Neurochir Pol*, 42, 2 Suppl., 2008, pp. (160–168).

Sluzewski, M., Menovsky, T., van Rooij, W.J., Wijnalda, D. (2003). Coiling of very large or giant cerebral aneurysms: long-term clinical and serial angiographic results.

Am J Neuroradiol, 24, 2, 2003, pp. (257-262).

Snyder, L.A., Spetzler, R.F. (2011). Current indications for indocyanine green angiography. *World Neurosurgery*, 76, 5, November 2011, pp. (405-406).

Solenski, N.J., Haley Jr., E.C., Kassell, N.F., Kongable, G., Germanson, T., Truskowski, L., Torner, J.C., Spetzler, R.F., Selman, W.R., Warf, B., Barnett, G.H., Solomon, R.A., Friedman, A.H., Campbell, R.L., Horner, T., Nauta, H.J., Heros, R.C., Muizelaar, J.P., Mohr, G., et al. (1995). Medical complications of aneurysmal subarachnoid hemorrhage: A report of the multicenter, cooperative aneurysm study. *Critical Care Medicine*, 23, 6, 1995, pp. (1007-1017).

Sughrue, M.E., Saloner, D., Rayz, V.L., Lawton, M.T. (2011). Giant intracranial aneurysms: Evolution of management in a contemporary surgical series. *Neurosurgery*, 69, 6, December 2011, pp. (1261-1270), 0148-396X.

Szmuda, T., Sloniewski, P. (2011). Early and long-term outcome of surgically treated giant internal carotid artery aneurysms—comparison with smaller aneurysms. *Acta Neurochir*, 153, 2011, pp. (1611–1619).

Szmuda, T., Sloniewski, P., Dzierzanowski, J., Rut, M. (2011). Predictors of postoperative mortality in ruptured aneurysms of internal carotid artery. *Neurologia i Neurochirurgia Polska,*; 45, 6, 2011, pp. (543-555).

Taylor, C.L., Steele, D., Kopitnik, T.A., Jr, et al. (2004). Outcome after subarachnoid hemorrhage from a very small aneurysm: a case control series. *J Neurosurg*, 100, 2004, pp. (623-625).

Todd, N.V., Tocher, J.L., Jones, P.A., Miller, J.D. (1989). Outcome following aneurysm wrapping: A 10-year follow-up review of clipped and wrapped aneurysms. *J Neurosurg*, 70, 1989, pp. (841–846).

Tulleken, C.A., Verdaasdonk, R.M. (1995). First clinical experience with Excimer assisted high flow bypass surgery of the brain. *Acta Neurochir (Wien)*, 134, 1995, pp. (66–70).

van Rooij, W.J., Sluzewski, M., Slob, M.J., Rinkel, G.J. (2005). Predictive value of angiographic testing for tolerance to therapeutic occlusion of the carotid artery. *Am J Neuroradiol*, 26, 2005, 175-178.

Weir, B. (1987). *Aneurysms Affecting the Nervous System*, (1ed), Williams & Wilkins, 0683089250, Baltimore.

Wermer, M.J.H., Van Der Schaaf, I.C., Algra, A., Rinkel, G.J.E. (2007). Risk of rupture of unruptured intracranial aneurysms in relation to patient and aneurysm characteristics: An updated meta-analysis. *Stroke*, 38, 4, April 2007, pp. (1404-1410).

Wester, K. (2009). Lessons learned by personal failures in aneurysm surgery: what went wrong, and why? *Acta Neurochir*, 151, 2009, pp. (1013–1024).

Yasargil, MG. (1984). *Microneurosurgery vol 2*, (1ed), Georg Thieme Verlag Stuttgart, 9783136449011, New York.

Youmans, JR. (1990). *Neurological Surgery*, (3ed), W.B. Saunders, 0721696554, Philadelphia.

Chapter 19

The Critical Care Management of Aneurysmal Subarachnoid Hemorrhage

Vishal N. Patel and Owen B. Samuels

Additional information is available at the end of the chapter

http://dx.doi.org/10.5772/48474

1. Introduction

Aneurysmal subarachnoid hemorrhage (SAH) is a neurosurgical emergency that results from the rupture of an aneurysm in the subarachnoid space (see figure 1). SAH carries a high mortality rate, estimated at 45%; additionally, a significant amount of patients are left with impaired neurologic function [1]. The critical care management of SAH requires an appreciation of both neurologic and general critical care principles; it is best thought of as a systemic multi-organ disease.

1.1. Epidemiology & morbidity

The clinical burden of aneurysmal SAH is immense. Case fatality approaches 50%, and approximately 1 in 8 patients die prior to reaching the hospital [2]. Of those that survive, nearly 50% will have significant functional impairment [3]. Aneurysmal SAH accounts for approximately 85% of all non-traumatic SAH. Approximately 30,000 Americans are affected annually [1]. The incidence of aneurysmal SAH ranges from 6-21/100,000 patient years [4].

1.2. Risk factors

Risk factors for development of aneurysmal SAH can be categorized as modifiable and non-modifiable. Modifiable risk factors include cocaine abuse, hypertension, and cigarette smoking [4]. It is estimated that cigarette use increases the risk of aneurysmal SAH by a factor of 3.7-3.9 [5]. Non-modifiable risk factors include sex, ethnicity, family history, and collagen-vascular diseases. The female:male ratio for aneurysmal SAH is approximately 2:1 [6]. The incidence of aneurysmal SAH is higher amongst people of Finnish and Japanese descent; and the incidence of aneurysmal SAH is almost three times greater in Finland than other parts of the world [4]. The incidence of intracranial aneurysms is higher in patients with collagen vascular diseases, such as Marfan's Syndrome, Ehlor's-Danlos Disease, Neurofibromatosis Type 1, and Autosomal dominant polycystic kidney disease [7].

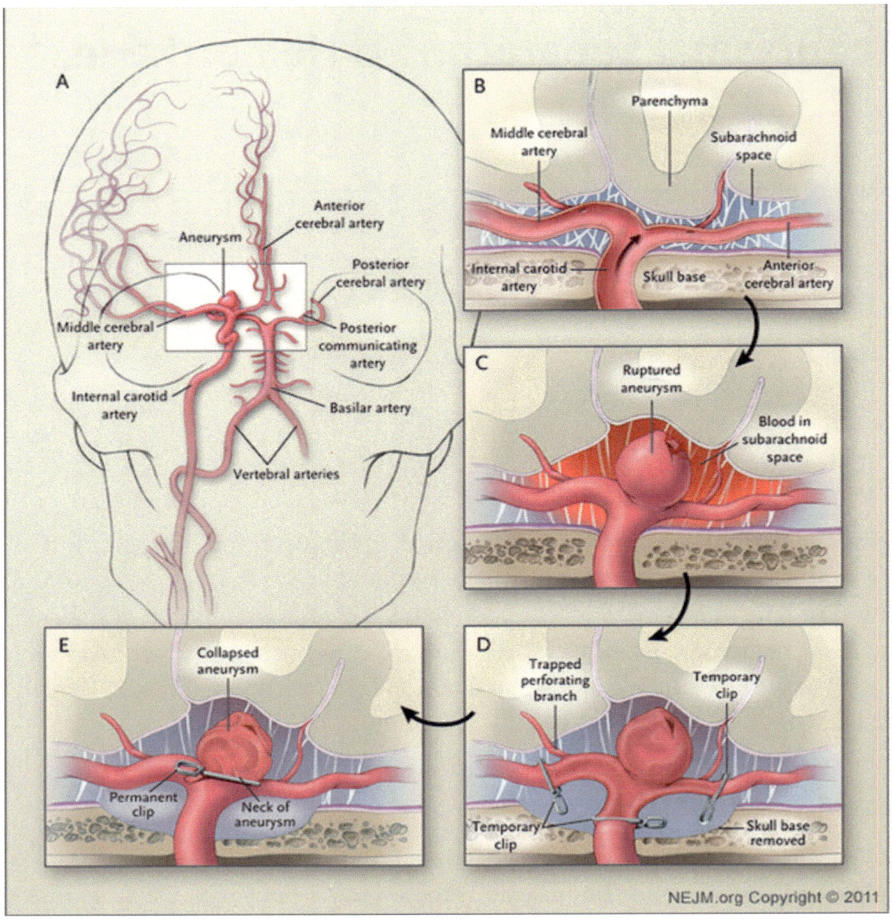

Borrowed with permission: Ellegala D, Day A. (2005) Ruptured Cerebral Aneurysms. New England Journal of Medicine. 352: 121-124

Figure 1. The arterial blood supply to the brain is located primarily in the subarachnoid space (Panel B). Aneurysm formation occurs in the subarachnoid space (Panel C), which must be surgically accessed to provide definitive treatment of the aneurysm (Panel E).

2. Diagnosis

2.1. Clinical presentation

The classic presentation of a patient with aneurysmal SAH is thunderclap headache, often described as the "worst headache of my life." It is generally abrupt in onset and reaches maximal intensity instantly. However, this classic description is seen in only 50% of patients presenting with aneurysmal SAH [8]. Conversely, in those patients prospectively screened for acute severe headache, only 6-17% were demonstrated to have SAH [9,10]. Common features at presentation can include seizure, loss of consciousness, and nausea and emesis preceding onset of headache [9]. The concept of 'sentinel headache' remains controversial; it is thought to be related to changes in the wall of the aneurysm versus a microbleed. A sentinel headache generally presents as a severe headache lasting greater than an hour, but diagnostic evaluation does not lead to the confirmation of SAH. These patients are at higher risk for early re-bleeding and aneurysmal SAH. The estimated relative odds ratio is 2.5-3.8 increase in early re-bleeding in patients who present initially with a sentinel headache [11].

2.2. Physical examination

Patients with aneurysmal SAH can have a variety of examination findings at presentation. These may range from a headache without focal neurologic deficits to being comatose. Most commonly, patients may have a depressed level of consciousness or confusional state. Cranial nerve palsies are also frequently seen as a direct result of an aneurysm; though cranial nerve 6 palsy may be a sign of elevated intracranial pressure. Focal weakness is also noted in a small percentage of patients. Fundoscopic examination may reveal subhyaloid hemorrhages and papilledema. Clinical correlation with outcome is best defined by the Hunt & Hess grading scale (see Table 1) [12].

2.3. Neuro-imaging

In addition to clinical presentation, the vast majority of SAH is diagnosed with correlating neuro-imaging. Non-contrast Head CT is the preferred modality of choice for the initial evaluation. Retrospective analysis has reported a sensitivity of 91-100% [13]. The sensitivity of non-contrast head CT diminishes as time elapses from the time of onset. It is best during the first 24 hours and diminishes to 85% at 5 days and subsequently to 50% at 1 week [14]. False negatives may occur in patients with anemia and is dependent upon the experience of the reading neuroradiologist [15]. MRI offers a higher sensitivity to detect SAH in patients presenting outside of first 48 hours after onset; however MRI is not readily available at most institutions and some patients may not be suitable for MRI. The FLAIR (fluid attenuated inversion recovery) and GRE (gradient echo) sequences are the most reliable method for detection of SAH in MRI [16].

Detection of aneurysms is best with catheter digital subtraction angiography, which remains the gold standard. In our practice, we perform a CT angiogram at admission, which carries a 85-98% sensitivity in comparison to catheter angiography. On average, 10-20% of patients with non-traumatic SAH will have a non-diagnostic catheter angiogram [17]. Practice varies in terms of repeat angiography; our current practice is to repeat an angiogram between 10-14 days.

2.4. Lumbar puncture

Cerebro-spinal fluid (CSF) analysis remains an essential aid in diagnosis in CT-Negative patients presenting with acute onset of severe thunderclap headache. Lumbar puncture should ideally occur 6-12 hours after onset of symptoms to optimize sensitivity. Lysis of red cells and the formation of oxyhemoglobin and bilirubin produce xanthochromia, ideally detected visually by inspection and confirmed by spectophotometry. CSF can remain positive for up to 7 days following ictus [18].

2.5. Classification

Various classifications exist for SAH. These range from clinical grading systems to radiographic scales. The most commonly used scales are Hunt & Hess, and World Federation of Neurological Surgeons (WFNS) scales [19]. (See Table 1)

Grade	Hunt & Hess	WFNS	Survival
1	Asymptomatic or minimal headache and slight nuchal rigidity	GCS 15, no motor deficit	70%
2	Moderate to severe headache, nuchal rigidity, no neurology deficit other than cranial nerve palsy	GCS 13-14, no motor deficit	60%
3	Drowsy, confusion, or mild focal deficit	GCS 13-14, motor deficit	50%
4	Stupor, moderate to severe hemiparesis, possibly early decerebrate rigidity and vegetative disturbances	GCS 7-12 with or without motor deficit	20%
5	Deep coma, decerebrate rigidity, moribund appearance	GCS 3-6 with or without motor deficit	10%

Adapted from - Rosen et al. (2005) Subarachnoid Hemorrhage Grading Scales: A Systemic Review. Neurocrit Care. 2: 110-118.

Table 1. Clinical grading scales for aneurysmal SAH and percent survival correlated with Hunt & Hess.

2.6. Differential diagnosis

Not all non-traumatic SAH is necessarily aneurysmal; however all non-traumatic SAH is treated as aneurysmal unless it is evident from clinical history or radiographic imaging that it is low risk. Most commonly, angiographic negative SAH is secondary to perimesencephalic hemorrhages. These compromise 10% of all SAH and two-thirds of non-traumatic SAH with negative angiograms. Blood is generally located ventral to brainstem in the prepontine and perimesencephalic cisterns. Generally, intraventricular hemorrhage (IVH) is rare. The average patient with perimesencephalic SAH is above the age of 50 and has less severe deficits. Rebleeding and vasospasm are infrequent in these patients [17].

Most SAH is in fact traumatic; however a collaborating history is not always obtained. Of those patients that have non-traumatic, non-aneurysmal SAH, intradural dissection is a concern; this is typically of the vertebral artery. Rupture of arteriovenous malformations (AVM) can occasionally extravasate blood into the cisternal space. Additionally, Arteriovenous Dural fistulas, mycotic aneurysms, pituitary apoplexy, and moya moya disease should remain on the differential, though there is generally additional history to suggest these. Cerebral vasculitis should remain a diagnosis of exclusion in patients with unexplained subarachnoid hemorrhage. The pattern of SAH on neuroimaging directs further work up. A non-classic pattern of cisternal hemorrhage suggests perimesencephalic or AVM related SAH. Blood present in the cortical sulci is generally thought to be traumatic, though can be associated with AVM rupture and vasculitis [17].

3. Management

The critical care management of aneurysmal SAH can be thought of as three distinct phases: Immediate management (prior to securing the culprit aneurysm), entrapment of the aneurysm, and post entrapment management. Technical aspects and surgical management in entrapment of the aneurysm are described elsewhere [20, 21]. In this chapter we focus primarily on critical care management of aneurysmal SAH and potential complications.

3.1. Immediate management

The major risk of fatality following aneurysmal SAH occurs within the first 24 hours and is related to the risk of re-rupture of the aneurysm. Rebleeding occurs primarily within the first 8 hours and is present in 9-17% of patients within the first 72 hours [22]. Rebleeding carries a significant mortality rate – up to 50% [17]. Therefore, prevention of rebleeding is key in management.

Management in the 1980's of aneurysmal SAH incorporated the use of antifibrinolytics to diminish the risk of rebleeding. In these patients, antifibrinolytics were continued for weeks at a time. However, this practice was subsequently abandoned when further studies suggested that though rebleeding was diminished, complications of delayed cerebral ischemia, primarily vasospasm, increased and there was little difference in outcomes [23].

Recently, there has been renewed interest in the use of short-term (12-48 hours) antifibrinolytic therapy. Because complications of delayed cerebral ischemia and vasospasm generally occur after day 3, and the greatest risk of re-rupture is within the first 48 hours, a short duration of antifibrinolytic therapy may improve outcomes. A significant reduction in the rate of rebleeding, 11% to 2.5% has been observed in patients treated with an early short course of the antifibrinolytic tranexamic acid [24]. However, no study to date has been powered adequately to assess clinical outcome benefit with early short duration antifibrinolytic therapy. One study, however, has shown an increase in the rate of DVT's associated with the use antifibrinolytic therapy [25]. The Neurocritical Care Society's consensus statement on management of SAH recommends considering an initial early short course of an antifibrinolytic with early definitive treatment of the aneurysm [26]. Our current practice is to utilize antifibrinolytic therapy as early surgery/intervention is being arranged.

No clear hemodynamic goals have been defined in patients with aneurysmal SAH prior to entrapment of the aneurysm. Practice varies from center to center with the general consensus that elevated blood pressure raises the concern for early rebleeding. Early studies reported that induced hypertension and hypervolemia were associated with aneurysmal rebleeding and hemorrhagic transformation; however, further studies have failed to demonstrate this link. The consensus statement from the Neurocritical Care Society observed that modest hypertension (SBP <160mmHg, MAP < 110mmHg) was not associated with rebleeding [26].

Hydrocephalus is a frequent complication of aneurysmal SAH and is seen in 15-30% of SAH patients. The clinical impact of hydrocephalus is variable. Patients may be asymptomatic to obtunded. CSF diversion thru ventriculostomy generally resolves hydrocephalus and often times, a marked improvement is noted in level of consciousness [1]. Our clinical practice is to place ventriculostomies in all Hunt and Hess Grade 3 or higher aneurysmal SAH.

3.2. Securing the aneurysm

The key treatment of aneurysmal SAH is securing or trapping the aneurysm, thereby reducing the probability of rebleeding. Patients who have early surgery, within the first 72 hours, had an overall mortality rate equivalent to patients with delayed surgery (days 11-32); however, those with early surgery had significantly better clinical recovery [27]. The general consensus is that aneurysms should be secured within the first 24-48 hours following rupture The technical aspects and surgical management in entrapment of the aneurysm are beyond the scope of this chapter and are described elsewhere [20, 21]

3.3. Post entrapment management

The majority of the length of stay for aneurysmal SAH patients occurs post-surgical trapping. It is during this time that patients remain at high risk for neurologic deterioration secondary to vasospasm, delayed cerebral ischemia, seizures, hyponatremia, and other complications.

Management during this period relies on close serial neurologic assessment, and prompt management of complications.

Traditionally, patients with aneurysmal SAH have been treated with triple H therapy – consisting of hypervolemia, hemodilution, and hypertension. As our understanding of aneurysmal SAH advances, this strategy has changed significantly.

3.3.1. Volume status

Monitoring volume status in critically ill patients can be challenging, but remains essential to optimizing medical care. Patients with aneurysmal SAH frequently develop hypovolemia and hyponatremia as a consequence of cerebral salt wasting syndrome. Retrospective studies demonstrate an increase in ischemia and worse outcomes in patients with hypovolemia [28].

Fluid balance does not necessarily reflect intravascular volume [29]. Some have advocated CVP while others rely on PAC to optimize volume status. CVP appears to be unreliable as an indicator of volume status and the use of routine PAC is cumbersome and the risks outweigh the benefits [30, 31]. Few have shifted to beside ultrasound and distensibility of the inferior vena cava [32]. However, none of these measures of intravascular volume have proven reliable. A combination of both invasive and non-invasive monitoring in conjunction with other clinical indicators of volume status provide the best guide for targeting therapy [26].

Induced hypervolemia has been investigated in two prospective randomized trials – no benefit was found in vasospasm or clinical outcome [33, 34]. Therefore, our clinical practice is to target euvolemia. Preferred volume of choice is isotonic crystalloid [26]. Mineralocorticoid supplementation with fludrocortisone has demonstrated the reduction in need of intravenous fluids needed to maintain euvolemia [35].

3.3.2. *Prophylactic measures*

3.3.2.1. *Nimodipine*

Calcium antagonists have been studied as agents to reduce the incidence of vasospasm associated with aneurysmal SAH. To date, nimodipine, a member of the dihydropyridine family of calcium antagonists, has been the only medication shown to have significant improvement in clinical outcome in patients with aneurysmal SAH [37]. Typical dosing is 60mg every 4 hours orally and is continued for 21 days. Treatment with nimodipine led to a relative risk reduction of 24% for poor outcome [37].

3.3.2.2. *Magnesium*

Magnesium has attracted study in patients with aneurysmal SAH as it is a non-competitive calcium antagonist with important vascular and potential neuroprotective effects [38]. Dosing and optimal magnesium levels are not well agreed upon; however, hypomagnesemia is related to a worse outcome. Studies have yielded conflicting results. The largest trial to date did not demonstrate any outcome difference between those targeted with hypermagnesemia [39]. A second Phase III study, MASH-II, is currently underway. Our current practice is to target Magnesium levels between 2.0 and 3.0 mg/dL, and to avoid hypomagnesemia pending results of MASH-II [26].

3.3.2.3. *Statins*

The many beneficial effects of statins have made them targets for consideration as prophylactic agents in aneurysmal SAH patients. Clinical trials have, however, not demonstrated a consistent beneficial effect. A meta-analysis suggested that there may be a reduction in delayed cerebral ischemic (DCI) with statins, however, patients in these studies had a higher rate of DCI than typically reported elsewhere [40]. Another meta-analysis of 4 randomized trials showed no benefit with statin prophylaxis in Trans-Cranial Doppler (TCD) detected vasospasm, functional outcome, or mortality [41].

Though no studies have directly addressed continuing or withdrawing statins in patients with aneurysmal SAH, there is data from patients with ischemic stroke and myocardial infarction that suggests acute statin withdrawal can worsen outcome [42, 43]. Until further data is available from clinical trials, the consensus is not to initiate treatment with a statin; however, one should be continued if it has been prescribed prior to aneurysmal SAH [26].

3.3.2.4. Seizure

Seizures may occur with aneurysmal rupture; patients may also develop chronic epilepsy following aneurysmal SAH. The incidence of seizures during the acute phase of aneurysmal SAH varies: studies estimate a range between 8-30% [1]. Other estimates are more conservative ranging between 1-7% at the time of rupture [21]. Continuous EEG monitoring in patients with poor grade SAH demonstrated a 10-20% prevalence of non-convulsive seizures [44]. Risk factors for developing seizures include age > 65 years, thick subarachnoid clot, rupture of a middle cerebral artery aneurysm, and intraparenchymal hemorrhage [45].

Prophylactic treatment of seizures has been commonplace; however, recent studies have investigated the benefit and risks involved [26]. Prophylactic use with phenytoin has been demonstrated to lead to worse outcomes [46]. Shorter duration prophylaxis has been advocated and a 3-7 day course of prophylaxis is general practice. Other anti-epileptic agents have been investigated and levetiracetam has been shown to be equally efficacious in reducing early seizures as well as improved functional recovery in comparison to those patients treated with phenytoin [47]. The current recommendation is to consider using short-term (3-7 days) of agents other than phenytoin, such as levetiracetam, for seizure prophylaxis. For patients with poor grade SAH with unexplained neurologic deterioration, continuous EEG monitoring is recommended [26].

3.3.2.5. DVT

Aneurysmal SAH induces a prothrombotic condition that can lead to an increase in deep venous thrombosis (DVT), and pulmonary embolism (PE). Incidence of DVT varies between 1.5-1.8%, with poor grade SAH having a higher incidence [48].

Conventionally, sequential compression devices (SCDs), unfractionated heparin, and low-molecular weight heparin have been used. One meta-analysis showed all were similarly effective in preventing DVT, but there was a trend towards higher rates of hemorrhage (intracerebral and non-cerebral) in those with low molecular weight heparins [49]. Timing of initiation is controversial, but generally, it is felt safe to assume pharmacologic prophylaxis after 24 hours from onset. Similarly, pharmacologic prophylaxis should be held 24 hours before and after intracranial procedures [26].

3.3.2.6. Glycemic control

Hyperglycemia is often diagnosed in patients with SAH; numerous studies have associated admission hyperglycemia with poor clinical grade and outcome [50]. The optimal range of glycemic control in patients with aneurysmal SAH is unknown. One study has shown improved outcomes with tight glycemic control: 80-140mg/dL, achieved thru insulin infusion [51]. However, when tightened to 80-110mg/dL, outcomes were worse secondary to episodic hypoglycemia and vasospasm [52]. Extrapolating data from other critically ill populations suggests that patients on insulin infusions are more likely to develop hypoglycemia [53]. Microdialysis studies have shown cerebral glucose levels to decrease, even without systemic hypoglycemia [54]. Based on the available data, hypoglycemia should be avoided and system glycemic control should target < 200mg/dL [26].

3.3.2.7. *Pyrexia*

Fever is very common in patients with SAH; studies report between 41-72% of patients with aneurysmal SAH will have fever. Fever is independently associated with poor outcome in retrospective studies of SAH [55]. As such, aggressive work up of fever is obligatory to look for underlying infection, drug reaction, or thrombosis. No clinical trial has prospectively examined induced normothermia and outcome; however, given the increased morbidity with fever, it is prudent to manage pyrexia [56]. Strategies to decrease fever include medications such acetaminophen, and NSAIDs. More aggressive devices include cooling blankets, and intravascular temperature modulation devices. The deleterious effects of aggressive cooling can include shivering and should be monitored for and aggressively combated [26].

3.3.2.8. *Anemia*

Anemia develops in over 50% of patients with Aneurysmal SAH and Hemoglobin concentrations decrease to less than 11g/dL in more than 80% of patients [57]. Because under normal circumstances when cerebral oxygen delivery demands metabolic demand, these levels are well tolerated. However, patients with aneurysmal SAH are at risk for developing vasospasm and DCI; their metabolic needs may not be met.

The optimal target hemoglobin in this patient population is not known. Retrospective studies have demonstrated that higher hemoglobin concentrations were associated with good functional outcomes [58]. PET imaging studies show an improvement in delivery of cerebral oxygen when hemoglobin is improved from 8g/dL to 10g/dL thru red cell transfusion [59]. However, evidence from broader based critically ill patients suggest that there is lower mortality in patients with a restrictive transfusion strategy [60].

Current guidelines suggest minimizing blood loss from blood drawing, as well as consideration of packed red cells to maintain hemoglobin concentrations between 8-10g/dL. Patients with DCI are the most likely to benefit from this higher transfusion strategy [26].

3.3.3. *Complications of aneurysmal subarachnoid hemorrhage*

Direct neurologic complications include cerebral vasospasm and delayed cerebral ischemia. Acute hydrocephalus and a diminished threshold for seizures have been discussed previously. Systemic complications of aneurysmal SAH include cardiac, pulmonary, and electrolyte abnormalities (see Figure 2). Fever, anemia, hyperglycemia are also common and have been discussed previously.

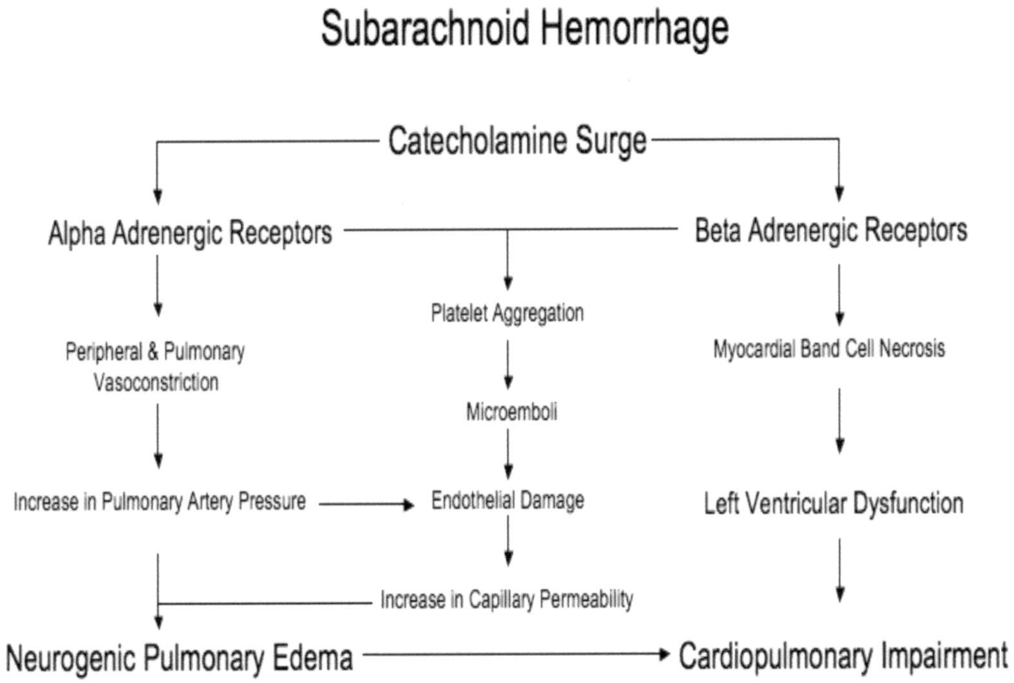

Adapted from – Coppadoro A, Citerio G (2011) Subarachnoid Hemorrhage: An Update for the Intensivist. Minerva Anestesiologica. 77: 74-84.

Figure 2. Cardio-pulmonary complications of aneurysmal SAH are related to the surge in catecholamines.

3.3.3.1. Cardiac complications

Cardiac complications following aneurysmal SAH are frequent and range from hemodynamic instability to cardiac arrhythmias to myocardial injury and heart failure. Given the high prevalence of cardiac complications, all patients with aneurysmal SAH should have an ECG, cardiac enzymes, and echocardiogram on admission.

ECG abnormalities most commonly seen following aneurysmal SAH are ST segment alterations, prominent U waves, QT-prolongation and other conduction abnormalities. Older age, hyperglycemia, and longer length of state are associated with atrial fibrillation and atrial flutter [61].

Troponin I is elevated on admission in 20-34% of patients with aneurysmal SAH. Studies have suggested that elevated troponin I is an independent risk factor for severe disability and death at hospital discharge. Higher grade SAH, IVH, and loss of consciousness at ictus have all been associated with elevated troponin I [62].

Acute heart failure and myocardial injury are most commonly seen in higher-grade SAH patients; the most severe form is neurogenic stunned myocardium. The surge of catecholamine release associated with SAH is thought to be responsible for neurogenic stunned myocardium, however the exact mechanism remains poorly understood. The classic pathologic findings are myocardial contraction band necrosis. Presentation includes transient lactic acidosis, cardiogenic shock, pulmonary edema, widespread T wave inversions, and reversible wall motion abnormalities [63]. One prospective study revealed a 18% (35% in Grade III-V) prevalence of wall motion abnormalities on echocardiogram in patients with aneurysmal SAH [64]. Takotsubo cardiac myopathy, also known as apical ballooning syndrome, is a subset of stunned myocardial injury seen most commonly in post-menopausal women and is associated with pulmonary edema and prolonged mechanical ventilation [65].

3.3.3.2. Pulmonary complications

Pulmonary complications are frequent (22%) and include impairment in gas exchange, pneumonia (20%), pulmonary edema (14%), and pulmonary embolism (0.3) [61]. These represent common manifestations of pulmonary disease in general critical care patients. Patients with aneurysmal SAH are however prone to develop aspiration pneumonias given a higher frequency of impaired consciousness. Thus, vigilant aggressive pulmonary toilet and aspiration precautions are important.

Neurogenic pulmonary edema (NPE) is associated with various neurologic insults, including SAH, seizures, and traumatic brain injury. It is thought to be a result of massive sympathetic discharge and catecholamine release at ictus, resulting in vasoconstriction and an increase in MAP with subsequent shift of intravascular volume to a lower-resistance pulmonary bed. The role of cardiac dysfunction in association aneurysmal SAH also contributes to pulmonary edema in these patients. NPE is associated with poor outcomes and is seen in patients with higher grade SAH. These patients are challenging to manage. Maintaining euvolemia in SAH patients decreases the risk of vasospasm; and it is well accepted that hypovolemia increases risk of vasospasm. Thus, cautious use of diuretic therapy is indicated when oxygenation and/or hemodynamic instability as a result of heart failure develop [66].

3.3.3.3. Hyponatremia

Hyponatremia is prevalent in up to 57% of patients with aneurysmal SAH [67]. It is the most commonly encountered electrolyte abnormality in NeuroScience ICU's. Severe hyponatremia is associated with seizures, and worsening of cerebral edema. In patients with aneurysmal SAH, hyponatremia is associated with increasing risk of vasospasm, likely secondary to its association with hypovolemia [68].

Hyponatremia in the setting of aneurysmal SAH can either be caused by Cerebral salt wasting (CSW) or the Syndrome of Inappropriate Antidiuresis (also known as Syndrome of Inappropriate Antidiuretic Hormone – SIADH). The proportion of patients with CSW versus SIADH as the cause of hyponatremia in aneurysmal SAH varies depending on the study, but CSW is more likely. Distinguishing CSW and SIADH is of clinical importance as the management is different, and can adversely affect outcomes in patients with aneurysmal SAH [68].

CSW is a result of natriuresis: loss of sodium resulting in loss of free water leading to hyponatremia; it is thus a hypovolemic hyponatremia. SIADH results from inappropriate anti-diuresis and is thus a euvolemic hyponatremia. Distinguishing the two is often difficult. Generally, patients with SIADH have decreased urine output in comparison to CSW. Urine osmolality is generally lower to normal in patients with CSW and high in patients with SIADH. Urine sodium levels are elevated in both. However, these are not always reliable; volume status, if determined reliably, is likely the most accurate method for distinguishing CSW from SIADH [69].

The mechanism of CSW is not completely understood. It is thought to result from interference of sympathetic input to the kidney and from elevated circulating natriuretic factors seen after cerebral injury [68].

CSW in patients with aneurysmal SAH are treated with Na supplementation and restoration of volume. This is achieved thru the use of salt tablets and hypertonic saline solutions. Mineralocorticoid supplementation is useful to increase Na and volume; typically, fludrocortisone is used. Therapy is targeted to maintain Na >135 [68].

More recently, the vasopressin receptor antagonist conivaptan has become available. It may cause an increase in diuresis and lead to a negative fluid balance. Though originally intended for the treatment of SIADH, it has been used cautiously in the hyponatremic patient with aneurysmal SAH [70].

3.3.3.4. Systemic Inflammatory Response (SIRS)

The catecholamine release associated with aneurysmal subarachnoid hemorrhage along with pro-inflammatory cytokines can lead to SIRS. The presence of SIRS criteria on admission (body temperature, heart rate, respiratory rate, and white blood cell count) in patients with aneurysmal SAH is a significant independent predictor of vasospasm and hydrocephalus. It is also associated with a higher mortality and morbidity rate [71].

3.3.3.5. Vasospasm and delayed cerebral ischemia

Vasospasm refers to the narrowing and vasoconstriction of cerebral arteries following aneurysmal SAH; it is prevalent in 70% of patients with aneurysmal SAH. Delayed cerebral ischemia refers specifically to the clinical and neurologic deterioration, often related to severe cerebral vasospasm, and occurs in 20-30% of patients with aneurysmal SAH.

The best predictor of cerebral vasospasm is thickness of cisternal clot and intraventricular hemorrhage, as seen on CT scan [72]. The Fisher and modified Fisher grading scales are used to predict expected risk of vasospasm (see table 2) [73].

Cerebral vasospasm typically starts after post-bleed day 3 and can extend thru 21 days, though most cases resolve within 14 days. The generation of microemboli, cortical spreading ischemia, and microcirculatory spasm are thought to add to DCI [74, 75]. (See Figure 3)

Grade	Fisher Scale	Percent with Symptomatic Vasospasm	Modified Fisher Scale	Percent with Symptomatic Vasospasm
1	Focal Thin	21%	Focal or Diffuse Thin SAH, no IVH	24%
2	Diffuse Thin SAH	25%	Focal or Diffuse Thin SAH, with IVH	33%
3	Thick SAH Present	37%	Thick SAH Present, no IVH	33%
4	Focal or Diffuse thin SAH with significant ICH or IVH	31%	Thick SAH Present, with IVH	40%

Adapted from – Frontera et al. (2006) Prediction of Symptomatic Vasospasm After Subarachnoid Hemorrhage: The Modified Fisher Scale. Neurosurgery. 58: 21-26

Table 2. Fisher and Modified Fisher grading scales for aneurysmal SAH with percentage of patients within grade with symptomatic vasospasm.

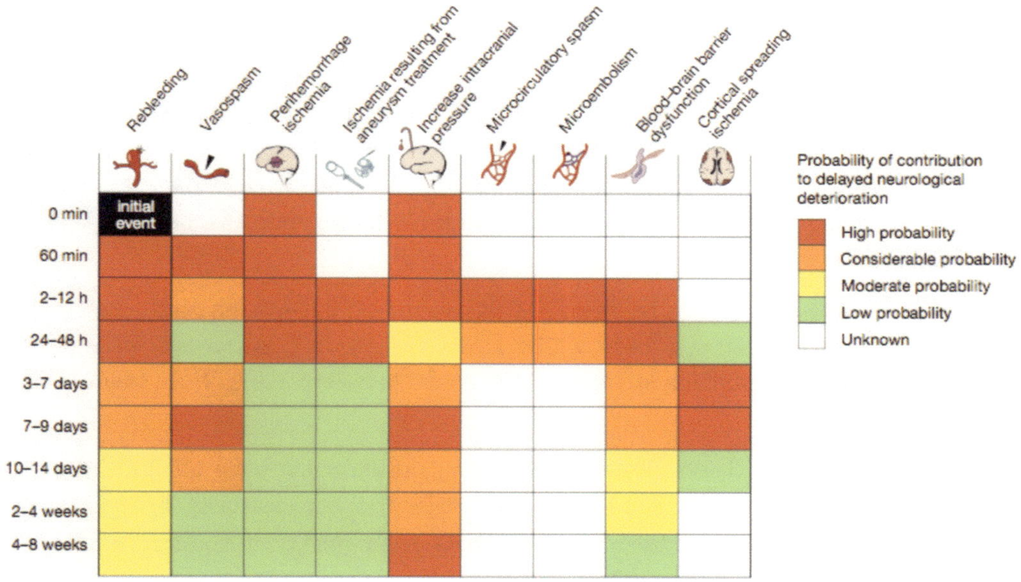

Borrowed with permission: MacDonald R et al. (2007) Cerebral Vasospasm After Subarachnoid Hemorrhage: The Emerging Revolution. Nature Clinical Practice Neurology. 3: 256-263.

Figure 3. Complications and risk against time in aneurysmal SAH

Cerebral vasospasm is the highest contributing factor to morbidity in patients with aneurysmal SAH. Cerebral vasospasm may have evolved as a protective measure to prevent re-rupture of a cerebral aneurysm; however, its diffuse cerebral effects are deleterious and add significant morbidity to aneurysmal SAH. Vasospasm is thought to occur secondary to blood product degradation in the subarachnoid space. Deoxy-hemoglobin and oxy-hemoglobin decrease perivascular nitric oxide and increase endothelin-1 respectively. The net result is a pathologic prolongation of calcium in smooth muscle, leading to an increase in spasm, apoptosis, and vascular remodeling [75].

Monitoring for vasospasm is of great value in the management of aneurysmal SAH. TCD, CT Angiography with perfusion imaging, and conventional digital subtraction angiography are options for monitoring for cerebral vasospasm.

The advantages of TCD are its noninvasive low risk profile; however it's sensitivity is variable and dependent on the skill of the ultrasonographer. Many patients have poor trans-cranial windows, making monitoring with TCD's difficult, if not impossible. Mean flow velocities are typically utilized for detection of vasospasm. Using a mean fellow velocities less than 120cm/s has a 94% negative predictive value for cerebral vasospasm. Mean flow velocities greater than 130cm/s have been proposed as the threshold for mild-moderate vasospasm; this carries a 73% sensitivity and 100% specificity for detecting vasospasm. Mean flow velocities greater than 200cm/s reliably predict moderate to severe angiographic vasospasm. The Lindegaard ratio compares intracranial MCA mean flow velocity to extracranial ICA mean flow velocity; the advantage of a ratio is to distinguish hyperemic states from vasospasm. Ratios greater 4 are suggestive of vasospasm; a ratio greater than 6 reliably predicts cerebral vasospasm [76].

CT angiography has a 87-95% percent sensitivity for angiographic vasospasm, but carries a high negative predictive value approaching 99%. However, CT angiography and perfusion are cumbersome and may pose additional risk to the patient secondary to iodinated contrast. CT angiography with perfusion may be a surveillance option for patients who have poor TCD windows [26].

Non-interventional strategies to combat cerebral vasospasm include the traditional triple H model. Augmenting MAP has been utilized to decrease DCI associated with cerebral vasospasm [74]. Our practice utilizes MAP goals between 110-140 to treat cerebral vasospasm.

Few centers have utilized intrathecal calcium antagonists. Some have utilized intrathecal nicardapine with success in decreasing flow velocities as measured by TCD's [77]. Multicenter randomized trials utilizing have yet to be completed demonstrating efficacy.

The trigger for intervention varies between centers. Many centers choose an aggressive intervention including endovascular delivery of local intra-arterial verapamil (and other calcium antagonists) that have an immediate effect with resulting local vasodilatation. Specific management of interventional management of vasospasm associated with aneurysmal SAH are described in more detail elsewhere [78]. The current gold standard for refractory cerebral vasospasm includes angioplasty in conjunction with intra-arterial delivery of calcium channel antagonists [26].

4. System based practice

Most patients with aneurysmal SAH are treated at small volume centers seeing fewer than 18 cases per year. Mortality is substantially greater at small volume centers compared to larger high volume referral centers [79]. Moreover, studies suggest that the utilization of a dedicated neurocritical care team is associated with improvement in hospital discharge disposition in patients with aneurysmal SAH [80].

5. Conclusion

Aneurysmal SAH is a complex critical illness with multisystem complications that requires the close attention of a dedicated neurocritical care team. Mortality and morbidity are high; the likelihood of a good outcome depends on presentation grade and careful and diligent management of complications.

Author details

Vishal N. Patel
Emory University School of Medicine,Marcus Stroke & NeuroScience Critical Care Center, Grady Memorial Hospital, Atlanta, GA

Owen B. Samuels
Emory University School of Medicine, Division of Neurointensive Care, Emory University Hospital, Neuroscience Critical Care and Stroke Units, Atlanta, GA

6. References

[1] Wendell L, Levin J. (2010) How Should Aneurysmal Subarachnoid Hemorrhage Be Managed. In: Deutschman C, Neligan P, editors. Evidence-Based Practice of Critical Care. Philadelphia: Saunders. pp 414-421.
[2] van Gijn et al. (2007) Subarachnoid Haemorrhage. Lancet. 369: 306-318.
[3] Suarez et al (2006) Aneurysmal Subarachnoid Hemorrhage. N Engl J Med. 354: 387-396.
[4] Linn et al. (1996) Incidence of Subarachnoid Hemorrhage: Role of Region, Year, and Rate of Compute Tomography: A Meta-Analysis. Stroke. 27: 625-629.
[5] Bell B, Symon L. (1979) Smoking and Subarachnoid Haemorrhage. BMJ. 1: 577-578.
[6] Kongable G et al. (1996) Gender-Related Differences in Aneurysmal Subarachnoid Hemorrhage. J Neurosurg. 84: 43-48.
[7] Schievink. (1997) Intracranial Aneurysms. N Engl J Med. 336: 28-40.

[8] Linn et al. (1998) Headache Characteristics in Subarachnoid Hemorrhage and Benign Thunderclap Headache. J Neuro Neurosurg Psychiatry. 65: 791-793.

[9] Linn et al (1994) Prospective Study of Sentinel Headache in Aneurysmal Subarachnoid Haemorrhage. Lancet. 344: 590-593.

[10] Morgenstern et al. (1998) Worst Headache and Subarachnoid Hemorrhage: Prospective, Modern Computed Tomography and Spinal Fluid Analysis. Annals of Emergency Medicine. 32: 297-304.

[11] Beck J et al. (2006) Sentinel Headache and Risk of Rebleeding After Aneurysmal Subarachnoid Hemorrhage. Stroke. 37: 2733-2737.

[12] Hunt E, Hess R (1968). Surgical Risk as Related to Time of Intervention in the Repair of Intracranial Aneurysms. J Neurosurg. 28: 14-20.

[13] Byyny et al. (2008) Sensitivity of Noncontrast Cranial Computed Tomography for the Emergency Department Diagnosis of Subarachnoid Hemorrhage. Annals of Emergency Medicine. 51: 697-703.

[14] van Gijn et al (1982) The Time Course of Aneurysmal Haemorrhage on Computed Tomograms. Neuroradiology. 23: 153-156.

[15] Edlow et al. (2000) Avoiding the Pitfalls in the Diagnosis of Subarachnoid Hemorrhage. N Engl J Med. 342: 29-36.

[16] Mitchell P et al. (2001) Detection of Subarachnoid Hemorrhage with Magnetic Resonance Imaging. J Neurol Neurosurg Psychiatry. 70: 205-211.

[17] van Gijn et al. (2001). Subarachnoid Haemorrhage: Diagnosis, Causes, and Management. Brain. 124: 249-278.

[18] Irani, D (2008) Cerebrospinal Fluid in Clinical Practice. Philadelphia: Sauders. 317p.

[19] Rosen et al. (2005) Subarachnoid Hemorrhage Grading Scales: A Systemic Review. Neurocrit Care. 2: 110-118.

[20] Lawton M (2011) Seven Aneurysms. New York: Thieme Medical Publishing, 224p.

[21] Molyneux et al. (2005) International Subarachnoid Aneurysm Trial (ISAT) of Neurosurgical Clipping Versus Endovascular Coiling in 2143 Patients with Ruptured Intracranial Aneurysms: A Randomized Comparison of Effects on Survival, Dependency, Seizures, Rebleeding, Subgroups, and Aneurysm Occlusion. Lancet. 366: 809-817.

[22] Starke et al. (2011) Rebleeding After Aneurysmal Subarachnoid Hemorrhage. Neurocrit Care. 15: 241-246.

[23] Roos et al (2003) Antifibrinolytic Therapy for Aneurysmal Subarachnoid Hemorrhage. Cochrane Database of Systemic Reviews. 2: CD001245

[24] Hillman et al. (2002) Immediate Administration of Tranexamic Acid and Reduced Incidence of Early Rebleeding After Aneurysmal Subarachnoid Hemorrhage: A Prospective Randomized Study. J Neurosurg. 97: 771-778.

[25] Starke et al. (2008) Impact of a Protocol for Acute Antifibrinolytic Therapy on Aneurysm Rebleeding after Subarachnoid Hemorrhage. Stroke. 39: 2617-2621.

[26] Diringer et al. (2011) Critical Care Management of Patients Following Aneurysmal Subarachnoid Hemorrhage: Recommendations from the Neurocritical Care Society's Multidisciplinary Consensus Conference. Neurocrit Care. 15: 211-240.

[27] Haley E, Kassell N, and Torner J (1992) The International Cooperative Study on the Timing of Aneurysm Surgery: The North American Experience. Stroke. 23: 205-214.

[28] Wijdecks et al. (1985) Volume Depletion and Natriuresis in Patients with Ruptured Intracranial Aneurysms: Is Fluid Restriction Harmful? Ann Neurol. 17: 137-140.

[29] Hoff et al. (2008) Fluid Balance and Blood Volume Measurement After Aneurysmal Subarachnoid Hemorrhage. Neurocrit Care. 8: 391-397.

[30] Hoff et al (2009) Blood Volume Measurement to Guide Fluid Therapy After Aneurysmal Subarachnoid Hemorrhage: A Prospective Controlled Study. Stroke. 40: 2575-2577.

[31] Mutoh et al. (2009) Performance of Bedside Transpulmonary Thermodilution Monitoring for Goal Directed Hemodynamic Management after Subarachnoid Hemorrhage. Stroke. 40: 2368-2374.

[32] Moretti R, Pizzi B (2010) Inferior Vena Cava Distensibility as a Predictor of Fluid Responsiveness in Patients with Subarachnoid Hemorrhage. Neurorcit Care. 13: 3-9.

[33] Lennihan et al. (2000) Effect of Hypervolemic Therapy on Cerebral Blood Flow After Subarachnoid Hemorrhage: A Randomized Controlled Trial. Stroke. 31: 381-338.

[34] Egge et al. (20001) Prophylactic Hyperdynamic Postoperative Fluid Therapy After Aneurysmal Subarachnoid Hemorrhage: A Clinical, Prospective, Randomized Controlled Study. Neurosurgery. 49: 593-605.

[35] Woo M, Kale-Pradhan P (1997) Fludrocortisone in the Treatment of Subarachnoid Hemorrhage Induced Hyponatremia. Ann Pharmacother. 31: 637-639.

[36] Allen et al. (1983) Cerebral Arterial Spasm – A Controlled Trial of Nimodipine in Patients with Subarachnoid Hemorrhage. N Engl J Med. 308: 619-624

[37] Felgin et al. (1998) Calcium Antagonists in Patients with Aneurysmal Subarachnoid Hemorrhage: A Systematic Review. Neurology. 50: 876-883.

[38] Taccone F (2010) Vasodilatation and Neuroprotection: The Magnesium Saga in Subarachnoid Hemorrhage. Crit Care Med. 38: 1382-1384.

[39] Wong et al. (2010) Intravenous Magnesium Sulphate for Aneurysmal Subarachnoid Hemorrhage (IMASH): A Randomized, Double-Blinded, Placebo-Controlled, Multicenter Phase III Trial. Stroke. 41: 921-926.

[40] Kramer A, Fletcher J (2009) Statins in the Management of Patients with Aneurysmal Subarachnoid Hemorrhage: A Systematic Review and Meta-Analysis. Neurocrit Care. 12: 285-296.

[41] Vergouwen et al. (2009) Effect of Statin Treatment on Vasospasm, Delayed Cerebral Ischemia, and Functional Outcome in Patients with Aneurysmal Subarachnoid Hemorrhage: A Systematic Review and Meta-Analysis Update. Stroke. 41: e47-52.

[42] Blanco et al. (2007) Statin Treatment Withdrawal in Ischemic Stroke: A Controlled Randomized Study. Neurology. 69: 904-910.

[43] Heeschen et al. (2002) Withdrawal of Statins Increases Event Rates in Patients with Acute Coronary Syndromes. Circulation. 105: 1446-1452.

[44] Little et al (2007) Nonconvulsive Status Epilepticus in Patients Suffering Spontaneous Subarachnoid Hemorrhage. J Neurosurg. 106: 805-811.

[45] Choi et al. (2009) Seizures and Epilepsy Following Aneurysmal Subarachnoid Hemorrhage: Incidence and Risk Factors. J Korean Neurosurg Soc. 46: 93-98.

[46] Naidech et al. (2005) Phenytoin Exposure is Associated with Functional and Cognitive Disability after Subarachnoid Hemorrhage. Stroke. 36: 583-587.

[47] Szaflarski et al (20010). Prospective, Randomized, Single-Blinded Comparative Trial of Intravenous Levetiracetam Versus Phenytoin for Seizure Prophylaxis. Neurocrit Care. 12: 165-172.

[48] Ray W et al. (2009) Incidence of Deep Venous Thrombosis After Subarachnoid Hemorrhage. J Neurosurg. 110: 1010-1014.

[49] Collen J et al. (2008) Prevention of Venous Thromboembolism in Neurosurgery: A Meta-Analysis. Chest. 134: 237-249.

[50] Kruyt N et al. (2009) Hyperglycemia and clinical Outcome in Aneurysmal Subarachnoid Hemorrhage: A Meta-Analysis. Stroke. 40: e424-430.

[51] Pasternk J et al. (2008) Hyperglycemia in Patients Undergoing Cerebral Aneurysm Surgery: Its Association with Long-Term Gross Neurologic and Neuropsychological Function. Mayo Clin Proc. 83: 406-417.

[52] Naidech A et al. (2010) Moderate Hypoglycemia is Associated with Vasospasm, Cerebral Infarction, and 3-Month Disability after Subarachnoid Hemorrhage. Neurocrit Care. 12: 181-187.

[53] Finfer S et al. (2009) Intensive Versus Conventional Glucose Control in Critically Ill Patients. N Engl J Med. 360: 1283-1297.

[54] Schlenk F et al. (2008) Insulin-Related Decrease in Cerebral Glucose Despite Normoglycemia in Aneurysmal Subarachnoid Hemorrhage. Crit Care. 12: R9.

[55] Fernandez A et al. (2007) Fever after Subarachnoid Hemorrhage: Risk Factors and Impact on Outcome. Neurology. 68: 1013-1019.

[56] Aiyagari V, Diringer, M. (2007) Fever Control and its Impact on Outcomes: What is the Evidence? J Neurol Sci. 261: 39-46.

[57] Kramer A et al. (2009) Relationship Between Hemoglobin Concentrations and Outcomes Across Subgroups of Patients with Aneurysmal Subarachnoid Hemorrhage. Neurocrit Care. 10: 157-165.

[58] Naidech A et al. (2007) Higher Hemoglobin is Associated with Improved Outcome after Subarachnoid Hemorrhage. Crit Care Med. 35: 2383-2389.

[59] Dhar R et al. (2009) Red Blood Cell Transfusion Increases Cerebral Oxygen Delivery in Anemic Patients with Subarachnoid Hemorrhage. Stroke. 40: 3039-3044.

[60] Hebert P et al. (1999) A Multicenter, Randomized, Controlled Clinical Trial of Transfusion Requirements in Critical Care. Transfusion Requirements in Critical Care Investigators, Canadian Critical Care Trials Group. N Engl J Med. 340: 409-417.

[61] Wartenberg K, Mayer S. (2010) Medical Complications After Subarachnoid Hemorrhage. Neurosurg Clin N Am. 21: 325-338.

[62] Naidech et al. (2005) Cardiac Troponin Elevation, Cardiovascular Morbidity, and Outcome After Subarachnoid Hemorrhage. Circulation. 112: 2851-

[63] Mayer S et al. (1994) Cardiac Injury Associated with Neurogenic Pulmonary Edema Following Subarachnoid Hemorrhage. Neurology. 44: 815-820.

[64] Kothavale A et al. (2006) Predictors of Left Ventricular Regional Wall Motion Abnormalities After Subarachnoid Hemorrhage. Neurocrit Care. 4: 199-205.

[65] Lee V et al. (2006) Tako-Tsubo Cardiomyopathy in Aneurysmal Subarachnoid Hemorrhage: an Underappreciated Ventricular Dysfunction. J Neurosurg. 105: 264-270.

[66] Friedman J et al. (2003) Pulmonary Complications of Aneurysmal Subarachnoid Hemorrhage. Neurosurgery. 52: 1025-1031.

[67] Sherlock M et al. (2006) The Incidence and Pathophysiology of Hyponatremia After Subarachnoid Hemorrhage. Clin Endocrinol. 64: 250-254.

[68] Yee et al. (2010) Cerebral Salt Wasting: Pathophysiology, Diagnosis, and Treatment. Neurosurg Clin N Am. 21: 339-352.

[69] Palmer B. (2000) Hyponatraemia in a Neurosurgical Patient: Syndrome of Inappropriate Antidiuretic Hormone secretion versus Cerebral Salt Wasting. Nephrol Dial Transplant. 15: 262-268.

[70] Wright W et al. (2009) Conivaptan for Hyponatremia in the Neurocritical Care Unit. Neurocrit Care. 1: 6-13.

[71] Yoshimoto et al. (2000) Acute Systemic Inflammatory Response Syndrome in Subarachnoid Hemorrhage. Stroke. 32: 1989-1993.

[72] Classen et al. (2001) Effect of Cisternal and Ventricular Blood on Risk of Delayed Cerebral Ischemia After Subarachnoid Hemorrhage: the Fischer Scale revisited. Stroke. 32: 2012-2020.

[73] Frontera et al. (2006) Prediction of Symptomatic Vasospasm After Subarachnoid Hemorrhage: The Modified Fisher Scale. 58: 21-26

[74] Lazaridis C, Naval N. (2010) Risk Factors and Medical Management of Vasospasm After Subarachnoid Hemorrhage. Neurosurg Clin N Am. 21: 353-364.

[75] MacDonald R et al. (2007) Cerebral Vasospasm After Subarachnoid Hemorrhage: The Emerging Revolution. Nature Clinical Practice Neurology. 3: 256-263.

[76] Marshall S et al. (2010) The Role of Transcranial Doppler Ultrasonography in the Diagnosis and Management of Vasospasm After Aneurysmal Subarachnoid Hemorrhage. Neurosurg Clin N Am. 21: 291-303.

[77] Ehtisham A et al. (2009) Use of Intrathecal Nicardapine for Aneurysmal Subarachnoid Hemorrhage-Induced Vasospasm. South Med J. 102: 150-153.

[78] McGuinness B, Gandhi D. (2010) Endovascular Management of Cerebral Vasospasm. Neurosurg Clin N Am. 21: 281-290.

[79] Cowan et al. (2003) Outcomes After Cerebral Aneurysm Clip Occlusion in the United States: the Need for Evidence-Based Hospital Referral. J Neurosurg. 99: 947-952.

[80] Samuels O et al. (2011) Impact of a Dedicated Neurocritical Care Team in Treating Patients with Aneurysmal Subarachnoid Hemorrhage. Neurocrit Care. 14: 334-340.

Section 4

Special Case

Chapter 20

False Aneurysms

Igor Banzić, Lazar Davidović, Oliver Radmili,
Igor Končar, Nikola Ilić and Miroslav Marković

Additional information is available at the end of the chapter

http://dx.doi.org/10.5772/48656

1. Introduction

Although great strides have been made in vascular and endovascular surgery in last decade, still remains challenge to resolve problems with false aneurysm or pseudoaneurysm. This problem is especially connected to sites that are managing vascular patients mostly with open surgical treatment.

2. Definition

All aneurysms can be classified by location, size, shape and etiology. However, there is always significant confusion about what a false aneurysm or pseudoaneurysm is. True aneurysm presents with all three layers of arterial wall. Pseudoaneurysm or false aneurysm occurs as result of blood flow outside the normal layers of the arterial wall. Basically blood is going through the hole in the wall of artery into contained space outside. That blood is compressed by surrounding tissue so it finally reenters the artery during the cardiac cycle. Repeating this process, false aneurysm (outside the artery) begins to grow.

False aneurysm could be caused by trauma, infections, iatrogenic or every kind of conditions that could promote focal weakness within the arterial wall.

3. False traumatic aneurysms (FTA)

The management of FTA of arteries has a long history. One of the earliest texts known, the Ebers Papyrus (2000 BC), contains a description of FTA of the peripheral arteries [1]. During the second century AD; Antyllus treated FTA by applying a ligature above and below the lesion, incising the aneurysmal sac, and extracting the clot. In 1873 Pick provided an interesting and detailed account on his management of an FTA of a large femoral artery by digital compression, which had an unsatisfactory final result [1]. The first reported FTA repair was by Matas in 1888. He operated on a young male patient with a large FTA of the brachial artery that had developed after multiple gunshots [2]. After ligation of the main proximal and distal arteries, he opened the aneurysm sac and sutured all collaterals with back-bleeding. Fifteen years later, Matas described this procedure as a reconstructive endoaneurysmorrhaphy [3]. Vojislav Soubbotich, a Serbian surgeon treated 60 FTA and 17 traumatic arteriovenosum fistulas (TAVF) during the Balkan wars between 1912 and 1913. He performed some of the reconstructive procedures in 32 cases [4]. Rich published an interesting article titled, "Matas Soubottich Connection." He said that Soubbotich's technique and results had been outrun 40 years later, during the Korean conflict [5].

4. Incidence

It is difficult to determine the true incidence of FTA. Some series combine iatrogenic with traumatic lesions. During World War II Elkin and Shumacker noted that there were 558 (22.58%) FTA and TAVF among the total 2471 vascular injuries [6]. According to Hughes and Jahnke's data, 215 cases of TAVF and FTA were described during the Korean conflict [7]. The largest series of surgically treated combat-related vascular injuries of about 1000 cases was published by Rich after the Vietnam war. They included 558 (incidence 55.8%) TAVF and FTA [8]. The first large civilian series of traumatic AVF and false aneurysms were published by Pattman et al. in 1964 [9], and Hewitt et al. in 1973 [10]. The incidence of TAVF and FTA was 2.3% (6/256) in the first study and 6.8% (14/206) in the second. According to experience of Davidović et al, is not that low. The incidence of TAVF and FTA, which included 140 cases, was 17.85%, and in civilian study with 273 cases it was 21.24% [11].

The most frequent cause of penetrating wounds during wars, as under civilian conditions, are bullets (figure 1) and fragments from various exploding devices (figure 2). In civilian experience, FTA and TAVF result from stab wounds as well [12]. FTA can also be caused by secondary damage, followed by pathologic moving of a bone fracture after penetrating and blunt trauma. In Davidović et al study, most of the FTA (superficial femoral 23.4% and popliteal 19.15%) were found at vessels near long bones (figure 3 and 4) [13]. Blunt trauma without associated bone fracture can also result in FTA and [14-16] (figure 5).

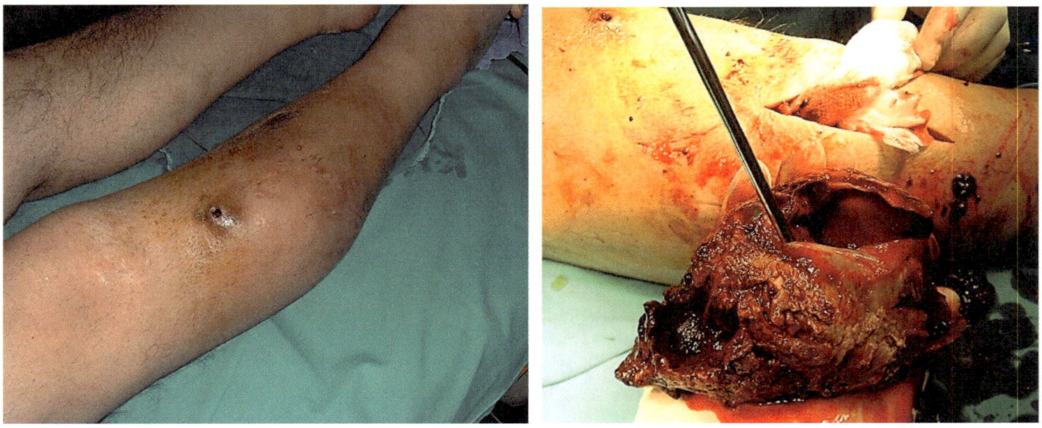

Figure 1. FTA after gun-shut injury

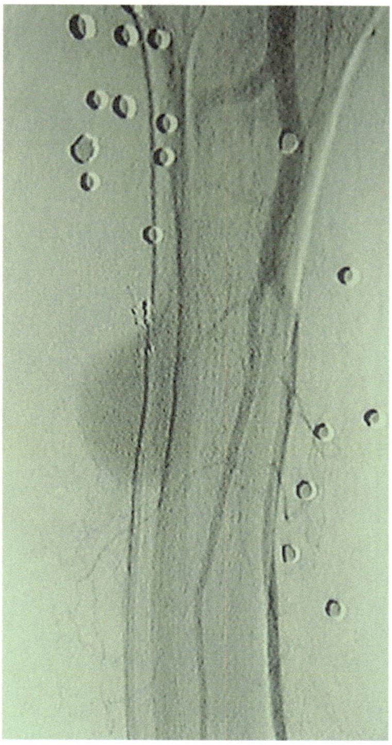

Figure 2. FTA and multifragments in right limb

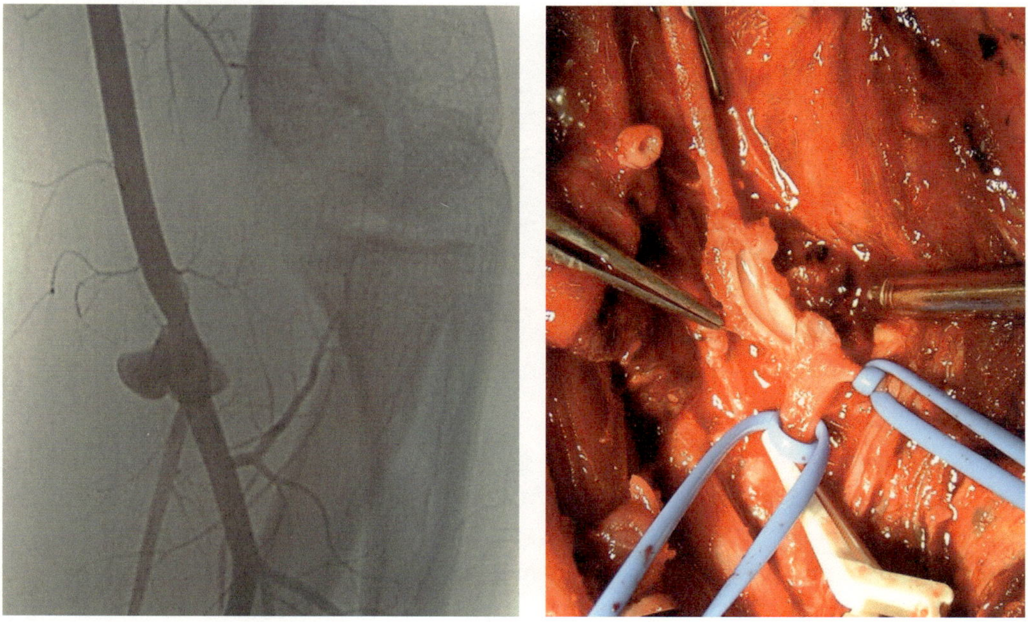

Figure 3. False traumatic aneurysm of the left-side brachial artery developed after a stab injury, which was accidental, job-related, and self- inflicted. a Angiography. b Intraoperatively, a laceration is apparent on the front wall of the brachial artery

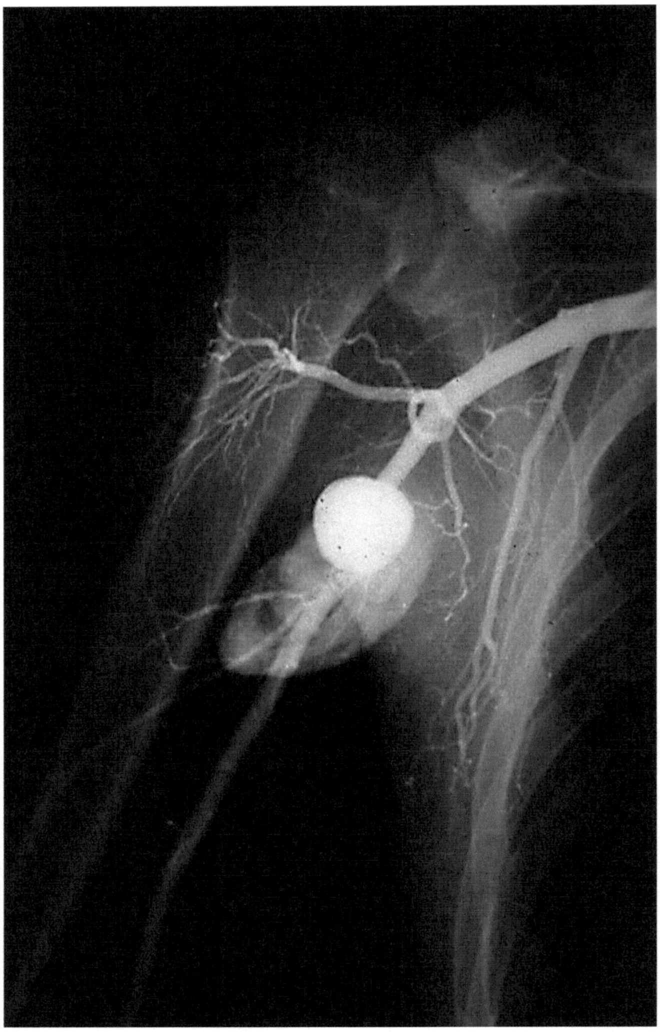

Figure 4. False traumatic aneurysm of the right-side axillary artery developed as the result of a gunshot injury

Lesions of the intrathoracic segment of the supraaortic branches can be often fatal. Formation of an FTA is not uncommon [17,18]. In 1968, Vollmar and Krumhaar described two such cases among 200 FTA, while Beall et al [19], Rich et al. [5], and Davidović et al [13] found only one such case (figure 6). In the most important war studies published between 1946 and 1975, all carotid arteries (common, external, internal) were involved in 3.8–20.5% of cases [6-8,20]. The incidence of all carotid arteries (common, external, internal) being involved, according to two of the most important civilian studies published during the same period, was 14.3–18% [10,12,13,21] (figure 6, 7 and 8).

In all of these studies FTA were mainly associated with lower extremity vessel (46.0–69.46%).[6-13, 20]

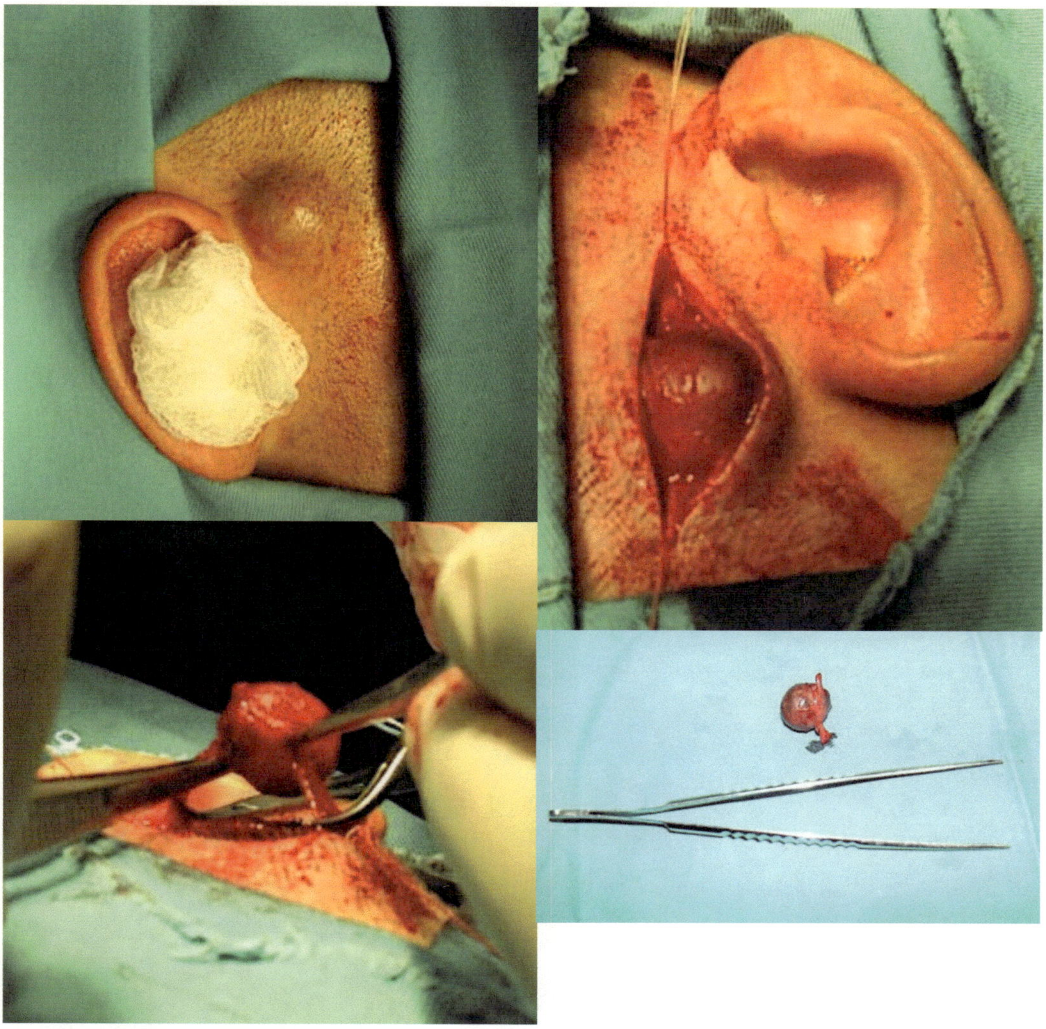

Figure 5. FTAof temporal artery after blunt injury

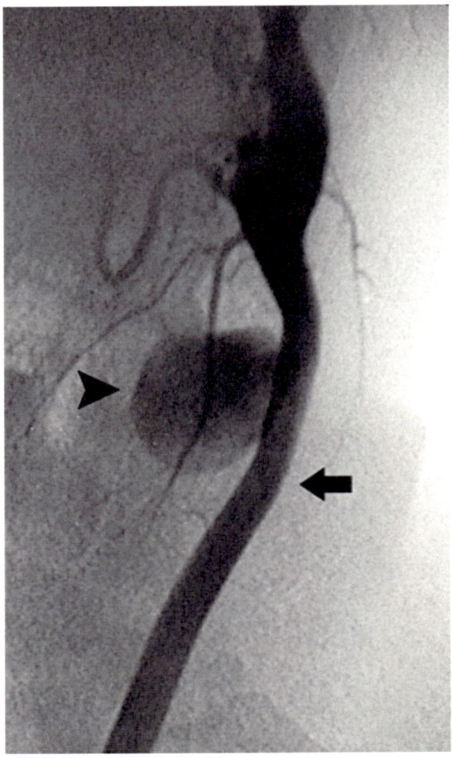

Figure 6. False traumatic aneurysm (arrowhead) of the left common carotid artery (arrow) developed after blunt trauma

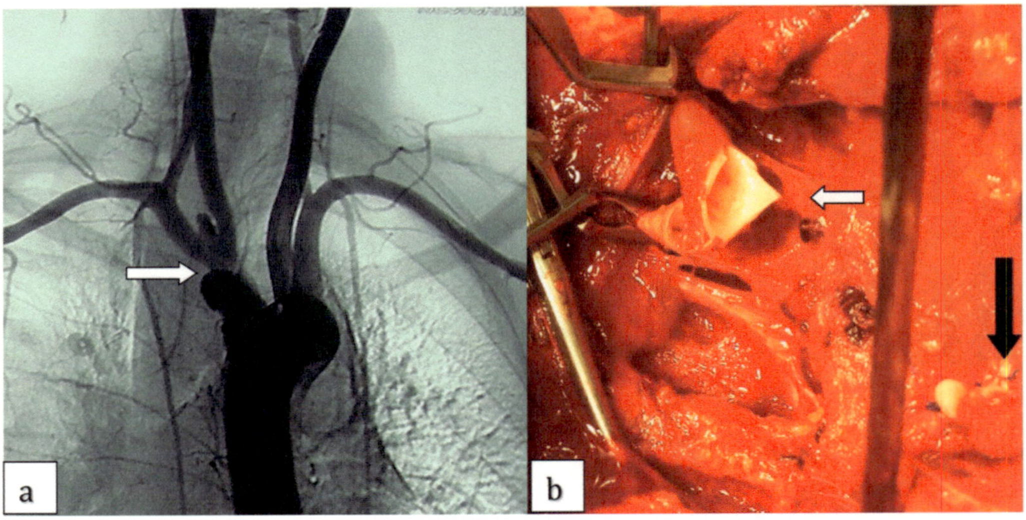

Figure 7. a Angiography reveals a false traumatic innominate artery aneurysm (arrow) that developed after chest blunt trauma during a car accident. b Note the right common carotid artery (white arrow) and the closed proximal end of the innominate artery (black arrow)

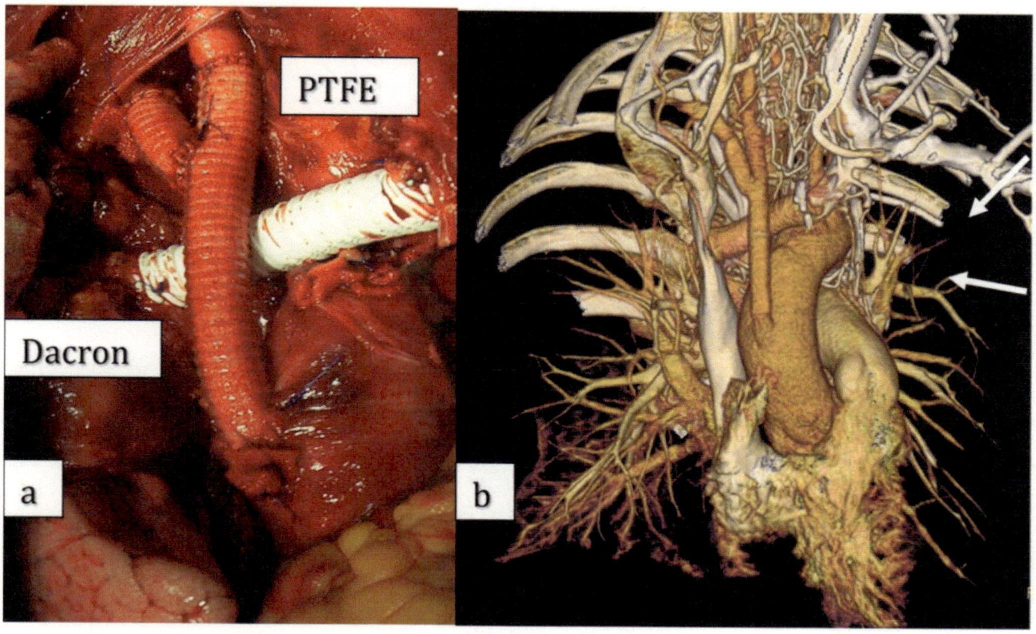

Figure 8. a Dacron bypass graft from the ascending aorta to the right common carotid and right subclavian artery. An 8-mm ringed polytetrafluoroethylene (PTFE) graft has been used to repair the injured left brachiocephalic vein. b MSCT performed 1 month later showed that both Dacron and PTFE grafts are patent

5. Diagnostic

The diagnosis of FTA is not difficult when the "hard signs" are present [22-24]. The problem is finding a way to recognize these signs and avoid failing to recognize FTA when the clinical picture is not typical [25]. Angiography has still very important roll as method of diagnostic, appropriate surgical approach as well as the type of vascular repair. Sophisticated diagnostic procedures, such as computed tomography, are extremely useful in cases of complex FTA.

6. Natural history and treatment

Natural history of FTA could be distal embolization (figure 9), rupture (figure 10), neurogenic compression or venous (figure 11) and cardiac failure. These lesions require prompt treatment. The treatment is relatively simple if the interval between injury and operation is not long [8,14,25-31]. Primary arterial repair without grafting is usually not feasible in late-presenting cases owing to the chronic nature of the FTA and the presence of fibrosis and inflammation. In the case of a small aneurysm, resection and primary end-to-end repair can be the safest alternative, although some advocate graft interposition [32]. The material of choice for repair is autologous saphenous vein [8,26,28-32]. The use of synthetic grafts is not recommended during the early phase because of infection. Synthetic grafts should be used only for a chronic FTA that involves large arteries (e.g., common femoral, subclavian).

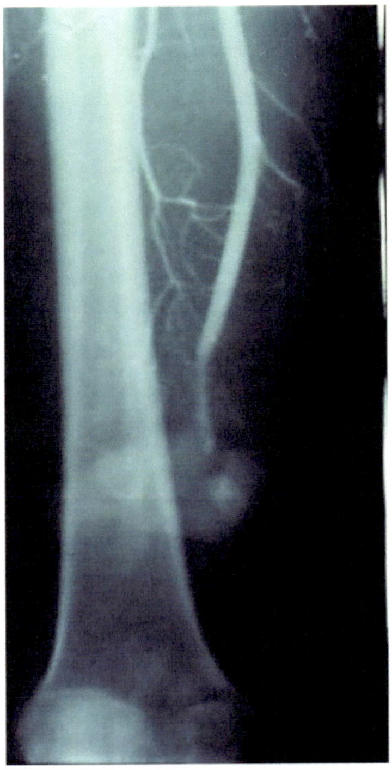

Figure 9. Embolization FAA and severe right foot ischemia after femoropopliteal reconstruction

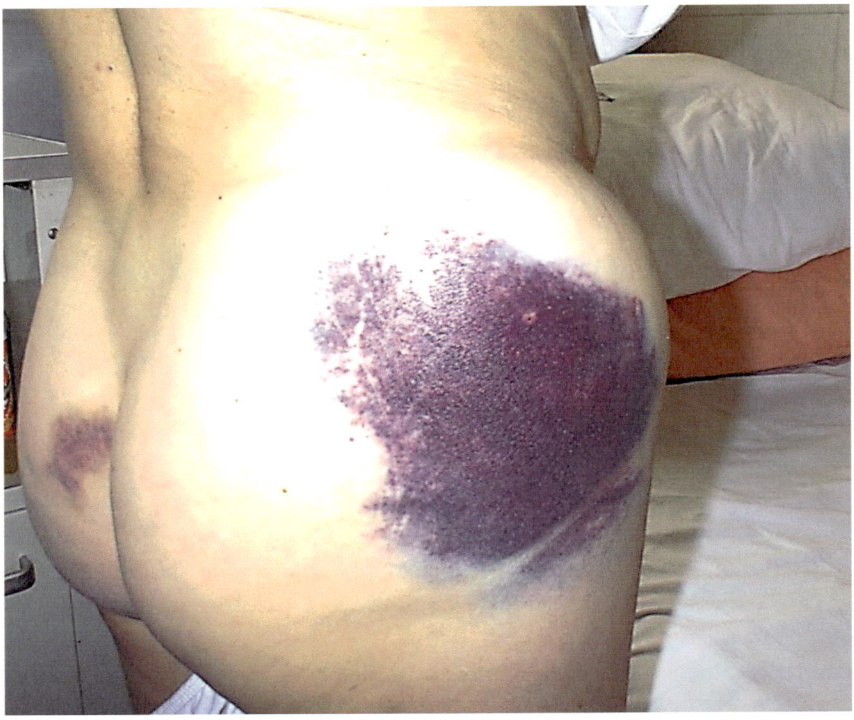

Figure 10. Rare case of ruptured FTA after blunt injury in right gluteal reg.

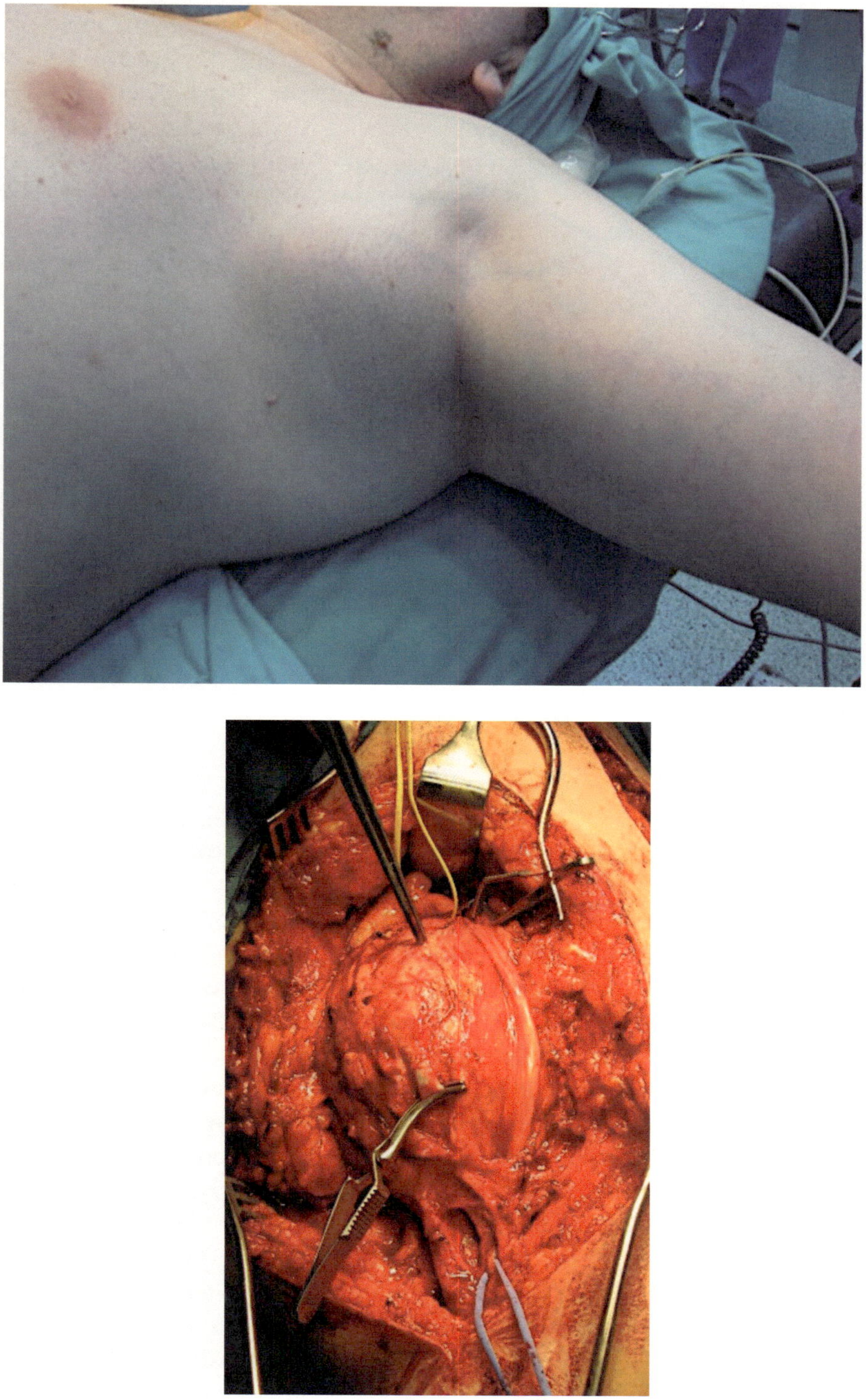

Figure 11. FTA of left axillar artery; neurogenic and venous compression

According to some, endovascular procedures can be important in the management of critically injured patients, as well as those with chronic FTA [33-43]. Endovascular repair of a peripheral FTA seems attractive because it theoretically results in less morbidity and shorter hospitalization [33]. However, this experience is still limited, especially in young patients. There is also skepticism regarding the use of stents in the popliteal artery. The reason is the mobility of the knee joint. Because of their history of numerous complications, FTAs require prompt treatment. The treatment is simpler if there is not an extended interval between the injury and the operation. Endovascular repair is mostly indicated in locations where a surgical approach is not easily attained.

7. False anastomotic aneurysms (FAA)

Most common false aneurysm belongs to group of anastomotic aneurysms and they present clinical challenges in detection, evaluation, and treatment. The incidence is approximately between 1.4% and 4% [44]. Claytor and associates, in 1956, reported the first case of anastomotic aneurysm in a patient after prosthetic aortic graft placement [45].

In 1978, Wesolowski outlined these common causes of FAA [46]:

1. Suture material
2. Prosthesis defects in manufacture
3. Arterial changes
4. Other factors

Although silk was used as a suture material for anastomosis (prior to 1967), the most frequent cause of FAA was breaking of the suture material [47-54]. Introduction of synthetic polyfilament suture materials has significantly decreased this cause. Also, the prosthesis defects in manufacture have long ceased to be the cause of the FAA. A whole range of arterial wall changes could lead to the formation of an FAA: infection arterial degeneration, aseptic necrosis of the suture line, extensive endarterectomy, and large "patch" or anastomosis, according to the Laplace rule [53-63]. A mechanical stress in the anastomotic area was the most important cause from the group of "other" factors. Movements in the hip area creating this kind of stress are recognized as the reason for the most frequent occurrence of FAA in the inguinal area after aortobifemoral reconstruction [49,55,62,64,65]. Growth of tissue created between the graft and the inguinal ligament prevents the graft from "sliding" over the ligament when a hip movement is performed [49]. For this reason, the FAA often develops after aortofemoral reconstruction but rarely develops after axillofemoral, femorofemoral, or femoropopliteal reconstruction. Szilagyi and colleagues believed this is the reason for the FAAs that manifest later [53]. In his discussion of the Stoney and Albo study [47], Baker suggested that anastomosis in the femoral region must be covered by a mobilized sartorius muscle to decrease stress. Mechanical stress caused by insufficient graft length [50] or configuration of end-to-side anastomosis [47,56,66] and the mechanical stress caused by an extensive mismatch, occurring if the prosthesis is too rigid, are also described. With every pulse wave, the anastomotic part of the artery is dilated at least 10% more than the prosthesis. Given that this difference increases with the size of mismatch, the least resistant structures (suture material, artery, prosthesis) could be broken [57,67-70]. These pathogenic mechanisms are more likely to happen on an end-to-side than on an end-to-end anastomosis [66-71]. At first sight, it is normal to expect that FAAs develop more often after the reconstructive procedures performed owing to aneurysmal and not occlusive diseases. In other words, it could be expected that aneurysmal degeneration can enhance FAA development. However, there are not many studies on that.

There are some systemic factors which are thought to contribute to anastamotic aneurysm formation: smoking, hypertension, hyperlipidemia, anticoagulation, systemic vasculitides and generalized arterial weakness [72,73].

8. Incidence

According to the literature, FAAs most often develop in the inguinal area [74-78]. They can develop after the aortofemoral or infrainguinal bypass (figure 13, 14 and 15). They develop in 14 to 44% of inguinal anastomoses [57,63,68,79], although the cumulative risk in clinically significant FAAs is probably less than 10% [80-84]. Inguinal FAA development is clearly a matter of time for the risk increases with the age of the patient and the graft. The literature cites the following frequency of FAA after the aortofemoral bypass operation: 0.4% [85], 1.4% [86], 2% [87], 3.2% [88], 3.3% [89], 3.9% after 17 years of monitoring [53], 4% [90], 4.7% [91], 7% [92], 3.88% [93], and 4.3 [94]%. Cintora and colleagues stated that the FAA incidence in the aortobifemoral position is 4% if a Dacron graft is used and just 1% if a PTFE graft is used, all types taken into account [95]. If the publishing dates are analyzed, the number of FAAs was larger at an early age owing to the poorer quality of the prosthesis and suture material. Data in table 1. show changes in interval of inguinal FAA development through time [96].

Period	*Time Interval (mo)*
Before 1975	36–48 [53,100]
1976–1980	37–73 [52,70,78,88]
1981–1990	72–92 [49,83,99]
After 1990	111 [99]

Table 1. Time Intervals of the Appearance of False Anastomotic Aneurysm

The main reason for this is the improvement in surgical technique and better quality of prosthetic and suture material. Also, it takes longer for the other etiopathogenetic factors, with the exception of the infections, to develop. Some literature data cite the fact that partial section of the inguinal ligament and enlargement of the tunnel in which the prosthesis lies, combined with free omental wrapping of the entire suture line, decrease the incidence of FAA [80].

Aortic FAAs are rare [77,97-99], and with the total number of operations in mind, their incidence of occurrence ranges from 2 to 10% [68-71]. They are believed to be more frequent after emergency procedures. Also, they are much more frequent after end-to-side than after end-to-end anastomosis [77] (figure 16) Owing to the development of surgical procedures, the occurrence of aortic FAAs has decreased to less than 1% [99]. With the lack of symptoms, it is difficult to diagnose aortic FAA. They are often detected during the evaluation of other abdominal diseases and conditions. Sometimes patients can notice the existence of a pulsatile abdominal mass, back pain, or weight loss [97,98]. Unfortunately, many aortic FAAs present only with acute expansion, rupture, gastrointestinal bleeding, infection, or distal embolism [94,95,97]. They are, in that manner, similar to abdominal aortic aneurysms.

The incidence of anastomotic aneurysm after carotid endarterectomy (with or without patch angioplasty) is approximately 0.3% [100]. They are most commonly associated with prosthetic infection [101].

9. Natural history and treatment

The disease development course of FAA, as well as that of any other aneurysm in general, can be complicated by a rupture (figure 12), compression, thrombosis, neurogenic compression and distal embolism [53,59,77,78,102,104,105]. Demarche and colleagues describe their experience with 142 femoral anastomotic aneurysms [106]. 64% were presented as an asymptomatic pulsatile mass, 19% presented with acute limb ischemia, 9% presented as a painful groin mass, 7% presented with acute hemorrhage, two patients (1%) presented with distal microemboli and limb edema. Infection was presented in 7% of all anastomotic aneurysms. Other series report similar presentations [107-109].

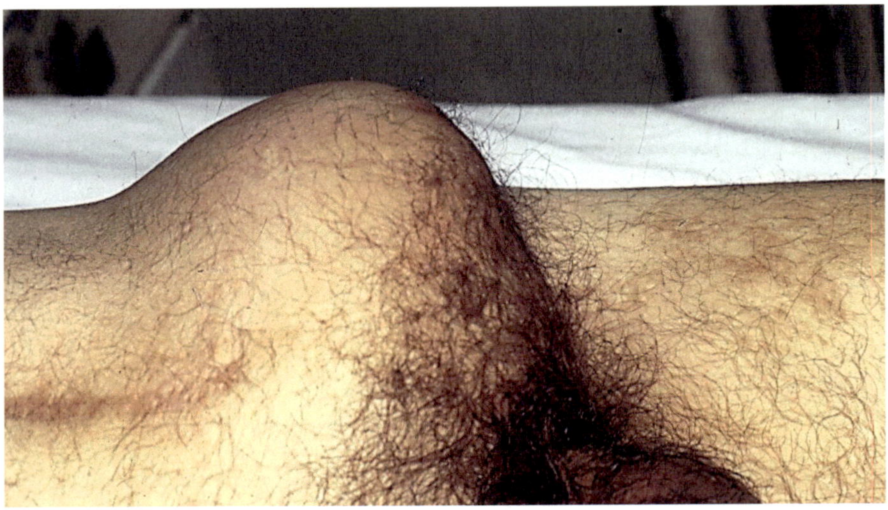

Figure 12. Ruptured FAA in left groin

Sometimes it is very difficult to prove that infection is the cause of an FAA. Keeping in mind that an intraoperative culture and blood culture can often have a false-negative result, the surgeon has to rely on intraoperative findings. Perigraft infiltration or fluid and the absence of graft incorporation in the surrounding tissue could be the only signs of graft infection. Laboratory parameters such as CRP level and white blood cell count can help us make a decision. In cases characterized by the absence of infection, there is a choice in FAA treatment between the methods of complete or partial resection and graft interposition or bypass procedure [58,92,94,96,105]. In case of an infection as the cause of the FAA, only two treatment options are considered: "in situ" repair with a homoarterial graft and EAR [67,110]. Incidence of infection as a cause of FAA can be an underestimation considering the existence of low-virulence pathogens and false-negative intraoperative culture examinations. On the other hand, Edwards and colleagues found in their 45-month follow-up study that only 5.5% had FAA as a symptom of late graft infection [63]. Reinfection after 30 postoperative days appeared in one patient (4.8%).

Other than standard surgical approach, there have been cases in the literature recently in which FAA was treated by an endovascular placed graft [111]. Using this method in cases of FAA in the groin, problems can be caused by kinking and thrombosis of the implanted stent graft. It is hoped that very soon technology development will resolve this problem and provide a fast, safe, and less invasive procedure with better results. Several authors have published recent series on successful endovascular treatment of anastomotic aneurysms (table 2).

Series	Year	Number of Patients	Location	Technique	Adjunctive Procedure	Infected	Results (%)				Mean Follow-up (mo)
							Technical Success	Major Compli-cations	30-Day Mortality	Patency	
Yuan et al.[112]	1997	12	A/I	Covered stent	No	No	100	17	0	100%	16
Curti et al.[113]	2001	11	I	Covered stent	No	Yes	100	0	0	100%	28
Magnan et al.[114]	2003	10	A	Covered stent	Yes	No	100	10	0	90%	17.7
Faries et al.[115]	2003	33	A/I	Covered stent	Yes	No	100	11	0	—	—
Gawenda et al.[116]	2003	10	A/I	Covered stent	Yes	No	100	0	10	100%	—
van Herwaarden et al.[117]	2004	8	A/I	Covered stent	No	No	100	20	0	88%	12
Derom and Nout[118]	2005	7	F	Covered stent	No	No	100	0	0	100%	18.6
Mitchell et al.[119]	2007	10	A/I	Covered stent	Yes	No	100	10	0	—	—
Di Tommaso et al.[120]	2007	6	A	Covered stent	Yes	No	100	0	0	100%	26.1
Lagana et al.[121]	2007	30	A/I	Covered stent	Yes	No	100	0	3	91%	19.7
Piffaretti et al.[122]	2007	22	A/I	Covered stent	Yes	No	100	5	0	96%	16
Sachdev [123]	2007	65	A/I	Covered stent	Yes	Yes	98	9	3.80	94%	18.1

A, aortic; F, femoral; I, iliac.

Table 2. (Taken from Rutherford's Vascular Surgery, 7th ed. -- *Endovascular Management of Anastomotic Aneurysms)*

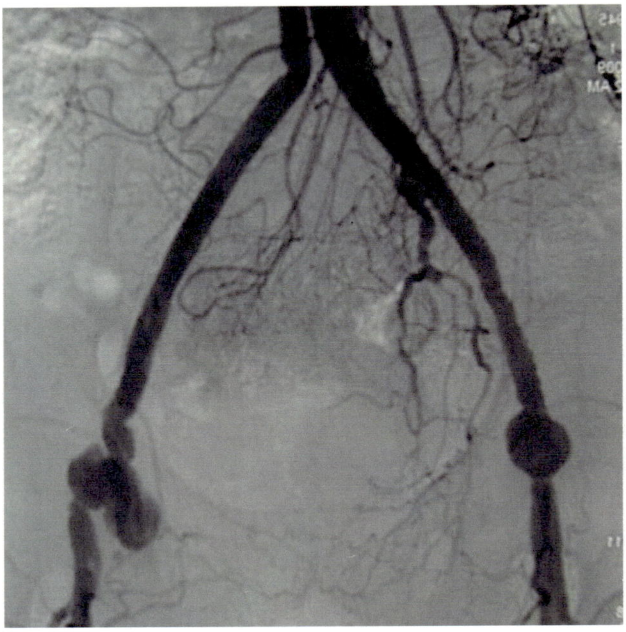

Figure 13. Angiography; False anastomotic aneurysms in both groins

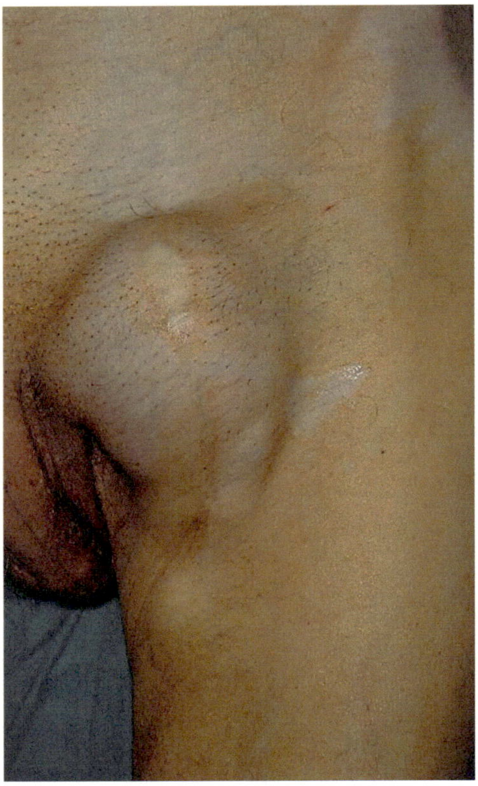

Figure 14. FAA in left groin after femoropopliteal reconstruction

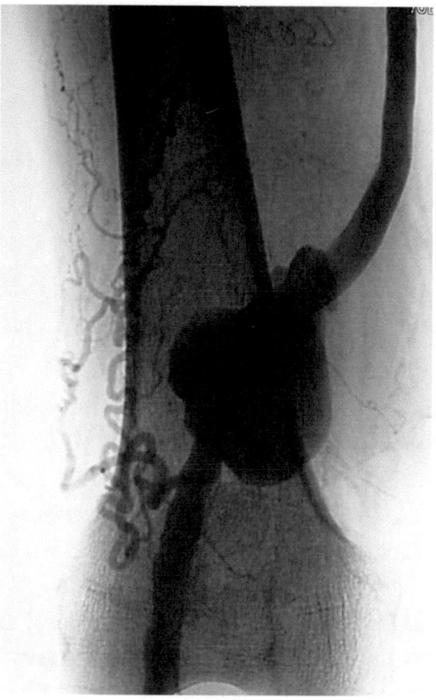

Figure 15. FAA in distal anastomosis after femoropopliteal reconstruction

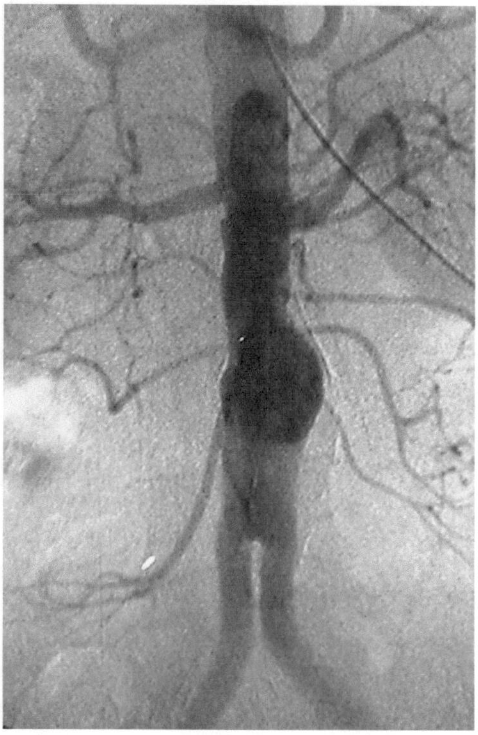

Figure 16. FAA after aortobifemoral reconstruction with end to side proximal anastomosis

Author details

Igor Banzića, Lazar Davidovića, Oliver Radmilia,
Igor Končara, Nikola Ilić and Miroslav Marković
Clinic for Vascular and Endovascular Surgery, Clinical Center of Serbia, Belgrade, Serbia
Medical Faculty, University of Belgrade, Serbia

10. References

[1] Schwartz AM (1958) The historical development of methods of hemostasis. Surgery 44:604
[2] Matas R (1888) Traumatic aneurysm of left brachial artery. Med News 53:462
[3] Matas R (1909) Aneurysms. In: Keen WW, Da Costa JC (eds) Surgery: its principles and practice, vol 5. Saunders, Philadelphia, pp 266–268
[4] Soubbotich V (1913) Military experiences of traumatic aneurysms. Lancet 2:720–721
[5] Rich NM, Clagett GP, Salander JM et al (1983) The Matas/ Soubbotitch connection. Surgery 93:17–19
[6] Elkin DC, Schumacker HB Jr (1955) Arterial aneurysms and arteriovenous fistula: general considerations. In: Elkin DC, De Bakey ME (eds) Surgery in World War II. Vascular surgery. Office of the Surgeon General, Department of the Army, Washington, DC, pp 149–180
[7] Hughes CW, Jahnke EJ Jr (1958) The surgery of traumatic arteriovenous fistulas and aneurysms: a five year follow up study of 215 lesions. Ann Surg 148:790–797
[8] Rich NM, Hobson RW, Collins GJ Jr (1975) Traumatic arterio- venous fistulas and false aneurysms: a review of 558 lesions. Surgery 78:817–828
[9] Pattman RD, Poulos E, Shires GT (1964) The management of civilian arterial injuries. Surg Gynecol Obstet 118:725–738
[10] Hewitt RL, Smith AD, Drapanas T (1973) Acute traumatic arteriovenous fistulas. J Trauma 13:901–906
[11] Davidovic LB, Cinara IS, Ille T et al (2005) Civil and war peripheral arterial trauma: review of risk factors associated with limb loss. Vascular 13:141–147
[12] Roobs JV, Carrim AA, Kadwa AM et al (1994) Traumatic arte- riovenous fistula: experience with 202 patients. Br J Surg 81:1296
[13] Davidovic LB, Banzić I, Rich N, Dragaš M, Cvetkovic SD, Dimic A. False traumatic aneurysms and arteriovenous fistulas: retrospective analysis. World J Surg. 2011 Jun;35(6):1378-86.
[14] Megalopoulos A, Siminas S, Trelopoulos G (2007) Traumatic pseudo aneurysm of the popliteal artery after blunt trauma: case report and a review of the literature. Vasc Endovasc Surg 1:499–504 17.
[15] Gillespie DL, Cantelmo NL (1991) Traumatic popliteal artery pseudo aneurysms: case report and review of the literature. J Trauma 31:412–415 18.
[16] Rosenbloom MS, Fellows BA (1989) Chronic pseudo aneurysm of the popliteal artery after blunt trauma. J Vasc Surg 10:187–189

[17] Matas R (1902) Traumatic arteriovenous aneurysms of the subclavian vessels, with an analytical study of fifteen reported cases, including one operated upon. JAMA 38:103 20.

[18] Gallen J, Wiss DA, Cantelmo N et al (1984) Traumatic pseudo-aneurysm of the axillary artery: report of three cases and literature review. J Trauma 24:350–354

[19] Beall AC Jr, Harrington OB, Crawford ES et al (1963) Surgical management of traumatic arteriovenous aneurysms. Am J Surg 106:610–618

[20] Vollmar J, Krumhaar D (1968) Surgical experience with 200 traumatic arteriovenous fistulae. In: Hiertonn T, Rybeck B (eds) Traumatic arterial lesions. Forsvarets Forskningsanstalt, Stockholm

[21] Yetkin U, Gurbuz A (2003) Investigation of post-traumatic pseudo aneurysm of the brachial artery and its surgical treatment. Tex Heart Inst J 30:293–297

[22] Woodlark JD, Reddy DS, Robs JV (2003) Delayed presentation of traumatic popliteal artery pseudo aneurysms: a review of seven cases. Eur J Vasc Endovasc Surg 23:255–25930.

[23] Pritchard DA, Malonez JD, Barnhorst DA et al (1977) Traumatic popliteal arteriovenous fistula: diagnostic methods and surgical management. Arch Surg 112:849–85231.

[24] La ̈dermann A, Stern R, Bettschart V et al (2008) Delayed post- traumatic pseudoaneurysm of the anterior tibial artery mimicking a malignant tumor. Orthopedics 31:500

[25] Davidovic L, Lotina S, Vojnovic B et al (1997) Post-traumatic AV fistulas and pseudoaneurysms. J Cardiovasc Surg 38:645–651

[26] Linder F (1985) Acquired arterio-venous fistulas: report of 223 operated cases. Ann Chir Gynaecol 74:1 27.

[27] Hegarty MM, Angorn IB, Gollogly J et al (1975) Traumatic arterio-venous fistulae. Injury 7:20

[28] Treiman L, Cohen L, Gaspard J et al (1971) Early repair of acute arteriovenous fistulas. Arch Surg 102:559–561

[29] Kollmeyer R, Hunt L, Ellman A et al (1981) Acute and chronic traumatic arteriovenous fistulae in civilians. Arch Surg 116: 697–702

[30] Folley J, Allen V, Janes M (1956) Surgical treatment of acquired arteriovenous fistulas. Am J Surg 91:611

[31] Losev RZ, IuA Burov, Alimov VK et al (1994) The treatment of posttraumatic and true arterial aneurysms of the extremities. Vestn Khir Im I Grek 153:43–47

[32] Darbari A, Tandon S, Chandra G et al (2006) Post-traumatic peripheral arterial pseudo aneurysms: our experience. Indian J Thorac Cardiovasc Surg 22:182–187

[33] Marin ML, Veith FJ, Panetta TF et al (1994) Transluminally placed endovascular stented graft repair for arterial trauma. J Vasc Surg 20:466–472

[34] Dorros G, Joseph G (1995) Closure of a popliteal arteriovenous fistula using an autologous vein-covered Palmaz stent. J Endo- vasc Surg 2:177–181

[35] Uflacker R, Elliot BM (1996) Percutaneous endoluminal stent- graft repair of an old traumatic femoral arteriovenous fistula. Cardiovasc Interv Radiol 19:120

[36] Criado E, Marston WA, Ligush J et al (1997) Endovascular repair of peripheral aneurysms, pseudoaneurysms, and arteriovenous fístulas.AnnVascSurg11:256–263

[37] Manns RA, Duffield RG (1997) Case report: intravascular stenting across a false aneurysm of the popliteal artery. Clin Radiol 52:151–153

[38] Reber PU, Patel AG, Do DD et al (1999) Surgical implications of failed endovascular therapy for posttraumatic femoral arteriovenous fistula repair. J Trauma 46:352

[39] Coldwell DM, Novak Z, Ryu RK et al (2000) Treatment of posttraumatic internal carotid arterial pseudoaneurysms with endovascular stents. J Trauma 48:470–472

[40] Redekop G, Marotta T, Weill A (2001) Treatment of traumatic aneurysms and arteriovenous fistulas of the skull base by using endovascular stents. J Neurosurg 95:412–419

[41] Assali AR, Sdringola S, Moustapha A et al (2001) Endovascular repair of traumatic pseudoaneurysm by uncovered self-expand- able stenting with or without transstent coiling of the aneurysm cavity. Catheter Cardiovasc Interv 53:253–258

[42] Ramsay DW, McAuliffe W (2003) Traumatic pseudoaneurysm and high flow arteriovenous fistula involving internal jugular vein and common carotid artery: treatment with covered stent and embolization. Australas Radiol 47:177–180

[43] Self ML, Mangram A, Jefferson H et al (2004) Percutaneous stent-graft repair of a traumatic common carotid-internal jugular fistula and pseudoaneurysm in a patient with cervical spine fractures. J Trauma 57:1331–1334

[44] Goldstone J: Anastamotic aneurysms. In:Bernard VM., Towne JB, ed. Complications in Vascular Surgery, St Luis, MO: Quality Medical Publishing; 1991.

[45] Birch L, Cardwell ES, Claytor H, et al: Suture-line rupture of a nylon aortic bifurcation graft into small bowel. AMA Arch Surg 1954;73:947

[46] Wesolovski AS. A plea for early recognition of late vascular prosthetic failure. Surgery 1978;84:575–6.

[47] Stoney RJ, Albo EJ. False aneurysms occurring after arterial grafting operations. Am J Surg 1965;110:153–61.

[48] Moore WS, Hall AD. Late suture failure in the pathogenesis of anastomotic false aneurysms. Ann Surg 1970;172:1064–8.

[49] Read RC, Thompson BW. Uninfected anastomotic false aneurysms following arterial reconstruction with prosthetic grafts. J Cardiovasc Surg 1975;16:558–61.

[50] Kim GE, Imparato AM, Nathan I, Riles TS. Dilatation of synthetic grafts and junctional aneurysms. Arch Surg 1979;114:1296–303.

[51] Sawyers JL, Jacobs JK, Sutton JP. Peripheral anastomotic aneurysms. Arch Surg 1967;95:802–9.

[52] Gaylis H. Pathogenesis of anastomotic aneurysms. Surgery 1981;90: 509–15.

[53] Szilagyi DE, Smith RF, Elliot JP, et al. Anastomotic aneurysms after vascular reconstruction: problems of incidence, etiology and treatment. Surgery 1975;78:800–16.

[54] Markovic DM, Davidović LB, Kostić DM, Maksimović ZL, Kuzmanović IB, Koncar IB, Cvetkovic DM. False anastomotic aneurysms. Vascular. 2007 May-Jun;15(3):141-8.

[55] Watanabe T, Kusaba A, Kuma H, et al. Failure of Dacron arterial prostheses caused by structual defect. J Cardiovasc Surg 1983;24: 95–100.

[56] Clark ET, Gewertz BL. Pseudoaneurysms. In: Rutherford RB, editor. Vascular surgery, 4th ed. Philadelphia: W.B. Saunders; 1995. p. 1153–61.

[57] Gutman H, Zelinovski A, Reiss R. Ruptured anastomotic pseudo- aneurysms after prosthetic vascular graft bypass procedures. J Med Sci 1984;20:613–7.

[58] Broyn T, Christensen O, Fossdal E, et al. Early complications with a new bovine arterial graft (Solcograft-P). Acta Chir Scand 1986; 152:263–6.

[59] Seabrook GR, Schmitt DD, Bandyk DF, et al. Anastomotic femoral pseudoaneurysm: an investigation of occult infection as an etiologic factor. J Vasc Surg 1990;11:629–34.

[60] Merrill EW, Salzam EW. Properties of material affecting the behavior of blood and their surfaces. In: Sawyer PN, Kaplitt MJ, editors. Vascular graft. New York: Appleton Century Crofts; 1978. p. 119–29.

[61] Nunn DB, Freeman MH, Hudgins L. Postoperative alterations in size of Dacron aortic grafts: an ultrasonic evaluation. Ann Surg 1979;189:741–5.

[62] Dubost C, Allary M, Olconomos N. Resection of an aneurysm of the abdominal aorta. Reestablishment of the continuity by a preserved human arterial graft with result after five months. Arch Surg 1952;64:405–8.

[63] Edwards MJ, Richardson JD, Klamer TW. Management of aortic prosthetic infections. Am J Surg 1988;155:327–30.

[64] Orringer MD, Rutherford RB, Skiner DB. An unusual complication of axillary femoral arterial bypass. Surgery 1972;72:769–71.

[65] Dardik H, Ibrahim IM, Jarah M, et al. Synchronous aortofemoral or iliofemoral bypass with revascularization of the lower extremity. Surg Gynecol Obstet 1979;149:676–80.

[66] Dadgar L, Downs AR, Deng X, et al. Longitudinal forces acting at side-to-end and end-to-side anastomoses when a knitted polyester arterial prosthesis is implanted in the dog. J Invest Surg 1995;8: 163–78.

[67] Paasche RE, Kinly CE, Dolan FG, et al. Consideration of suture line stresses in the selection of synthetic grafts for implantation. J Biomech 1973;6:253–9.

[68] Sieswerda C, Skotnicki SH, Barentz JO, Heystraten FMJ. Anastomotic aneurysms—an underdiagnosed complication after aorto-iliac reconstructions. Eur J Vasc Surg 1989;3:233–8.

[69] McCann RL, Schwartz LB, Georgiade GS. Management of aortic graft complications. Ann Surg 1993;217:729–34.

[70] Bastounis E, Georgopoulos S, Maltezos C, Balas P. The validity of current vascular imaging methods in the evaluation of aortic anastomotic aneurysms developing after abdominal aortic aneurysm repair. Ann Vasc Surg 1996;10:537–45.

[71] Berger K, Sauvage LR. Late fiber deterioration in Dacron arterial grafts. Ann Surg 1981;193:477–91.

[72] Alpagut U, Ugurlucan M, Daytoglu E: Major arterial involvement and review of Behýet's disease. *Ann Vasc Surg* 2007; 21:232.

[73] Oderich GS, Panneton JM, Bower TC, et al: The spectrum, management and clinical outcome of Ehlers-Danlos syndrome type IV: a 30-year experience. *J Vasc Surg* 2005; 42:98.

[74] Wandschneider D, Bull PH, Denck A. Anastomotic aneurysms— an unsoluble problem. Eur J Vasc Surg 1988;2:115–9.

[75] Knox GW. Aneurysm occuring in a femoral arterial Dacron prosthesis five and a half years after insertion. Ann Surg 1962;156: 827–30.

[76] Giordanengo F, Pizzocari P, Rampoldi V, et al. Femoral non-infected anastomotic pseudoaneurysm. Clinical contribution. Minerva Chir 1992;1547:823–9.

[77] Guinet C, Buy JN, Ghossain MA, et al. Aortic anastomotic pseudoaneurysms: US, CT, MR, and angiography. J Comput Assist Tomogr 1992;16:128–8.

[78] Waibel P. False aneurysm after reconstruction for peripheral arterial occlusive disease. Observations over 15 to 25 years. Vasa 1994;23:43–51.

[79] Shwartz LB, Clark ET, Gewertz BL. Anastomotic and other pseudoaneurysms. In: Rutherford RB, editor. Vascular surgery. 5th ed. Philadelphia: W.B. Saunders; 2000. p. 752–63.

[80] Courbier R, Ferdani M, Jausseran JM, et al. The role of omentropexy in the prevention of femoral anastomotic aneurysm. J Cardiovasc Surg 1992;33:149–53.

[81] Melliere D, Becquemin JP, Cervantes-Monteil F, et al. Recurrent femoral anastomotic false aneurysms: is long term repair possible? Cardiovasc Surg 1996;4:480–2.

[82] Millili JJ, Lanes JS, Nemir P. A study of anastomotic aneurysms following aortofemoral prosthetic bypass. Ann Surg 1980;192:69–73

[83] Ernst CB, Elliott JP Jr, Ryan CJ, et al. Recurrent femoral anastomotic aneurysms: a 30-year experience. Ann Surg 1988; 201:401–9.

[84] Ernst CB. Anastomotic aneurysm. In: Ernst CB, Stanley JC, editors. Current therapy in vascular surgery. St. Louis: Mosby-Year Book; 1995. p. 415–9.

[85] Poulias GE, Polemis L, Skoutas B, et al. Bilateral aorto-femoral bypass in the presence of aorto-iliac occlusive disease and factors determining result. J Cardiovasc Surg 1985;26:257–37.

[86] Brewster DC, Darling DC. Optimal methods of aortoiliac reconstruction. Surgery 1978;84:739–47.

[87] Malone JM, Moore WS, Goldstone J. Life expectancy following aortofemoral arterial grafting. Surgery 1977;81:551–5.

[88] Nevelsteen A, Wouters L, Suy R. Long-term patency of the aortofemoral Dacron graft. A graft limb related study on a 25 year period. J Cardiovasc Surg 1991;32:174–80.

[89] Gomes MR, Bernatz PE, Jurgens JL. Influence of clinical factors on results. Arch Surg 1967;95:387–94.

[90] Martinez BD, Hertzer NR, Beven EG. Influence of distal arterial occlusive disease on prognosis following aortobifemoral bypass. Surgery 1973;74:519–23.

[91] Crawford ES, Bomberger RA, Glaeser DH, et al. Aortoiliac occlusive disease: factors influencing survival and function following reconstructive operation over a twenty-five year period. Surgery 1981;90:1055–67.

[92] Crawford ES, Manning LG, Kelly TF. "Redo" surgery after operations for aneurysm and occlusion of the abdominal aorta. Surgery 1977;81:41–52.

[93] Davidovic´ L. Comparison between bifurcated Dacron and PTFE grafts in aortobifemoral position [dissertation]. Belgrade: University of Belgrade School of Medicine; 1995.

[94] Levi N, Schroeder TV. Anastomotic femoral aneurysms: is an increase in interval between primary operation and aneurysms formation related to a change in incidence? Panminerva Med 1998; 40:210–3.

[95] Cintora I, Paero DE, Canon JA. A clinical survey of aortobifemoral bypass using two inherently different graft types. Ann Surg 1988; 208:625–30.

[96] Levi N, Schroeder TV. Anastomotic femoral aneurysms: increase in interval between primary operation and aneurysm formation. Eur J Vasc Endovasc Surg 1996;11:207–9.

[97] Gautier C, Borie H, Lagneau P. Aortic false aneurysms after prosthetic reconstruction of the infrarenal aorta. Ann Vasc Surg 1992;6:413–7.

[98] Chen FZ, Xu X, Fu WG, Wu ZG. Anastomotic false aneurysm following abdominal aortic aneurysmectomy and prosthetic grafting. Chin Med J (Engl) 1994;107:832–5.

[99] De Monti M, Ghilardi G, Sgroi G, Scorzo R. Proximal anastomotic pseudoaneurysms. Minerva Cardioangiol 1995;43:127–34.

[100] Branch Jr CL, Davis Jr CH: False aneurysm complicating carotid endarterectomy. *Neurosurgery* 1986; 19:421.

[101] Borazjani BH, Wilson SE, Fujitani RM, et al: Postoperative complications of carotid patching: pseudoaneurysm and infection. *Ann Vasc Surg* 2003; 17:156.

[102] DeBakey ME, Crawford ES, Morris GC, Cooley LA. Patch graft angioplasty in vascular surgery. J Cardiovasc Surg 1963;3: 106–41.

[103] Satiani B, Karmers M, Evans NE. Anastomotic arterial aneurysms. Ann Surg 1980;192:674–82.

[104] Tridico F, Zan S, Panier Suffat P, et al. Femoral anastomotic pseudoaneurysms. The etiopathogenetic hypotheses and the therapy. Minerva Chir 1992;47:37–40.

[105] Morbidelli A, Caron R, Caldana G, et al. Bilateral thrombosis of a femoral pseudoaneurysm. Minerva Chir 1995;50:1013–8.

[106] Demarche M, Waltregny D, van Damme H, et al: Femoral anastomotic aneurysms: pathogenic factors, clinical presentations and treatment. A study of 142 cases. *Cardiovasc Surg* 1999; 7:315.

[107] Schellack J, Salam A, Abouzeid MA, et al: Femoral anastomotic aneurysms: a continuing challenge. *J Vasc Surg* 1987; 6:308.

[108] Youkey JR, Clagett GP, Rich NM, et al: Femoral anastomotic false aneurysms: an 11-year experience analyzed with a case control study. *Ann Surg* 1984; 199:703.

[109] Argifoglio G, Costantini A, Lorenzi G, et al: Femoral noninfected anastomotic aneurysms.. *J Cardiovasc Surg* 1990; 31:453.

[110] Mulder EJ, van Bockel JH, Maas J, et al. Morbidity and mortality of reconstructive surgery of noninfected false aneurysms detected long after aortic prosthetic reconstruction. Arch Surg 1998;133:45–9.

[111] Dorros G, Jaff MR, Parikh A, et al. In vivo crushing of an aortic stent enables endovascular repair of a large infrarenal aortic pseudoaneurysm. J Endovasc Surg 1998;5:359–64.

[112] Yuan JG, Marin ML, Veith FJ, et al: Endovascular grafts for noninfected aortoiliac anastomotic aneurysms. *J Vasc Surg* 1997; 26:210.

[113] Curti T, Stella A, Rossi C, et al: Endovascular repair as first-choice treatment for anastomotic and true iliac aneurysms. *J Endovasc Ther* 2001; 8:139.

[114] Magnan PE, Albertini JN, Bartoli JM, et al: Endovascular treatment of anastomotic false aneurysms of the abdominal aorta. *Ann Vasc Surg* 2003; 17:365.

[115] Faries PL, Won J, Morrissey NJ, et al: Endovascular treatment of failed prior abdominal aortic aneurysm repair. *Ann Vasc Surg* 2003; 17:43.

[116] Gawenda M, Zaehringer M, Brunkwall J: Open versus endovascular repair of para-anastomotic aneurysms in patients who were morphological candidates for endovascular treatment. *J Endovasc Ther* 2003; 10:745.

[117] Van Herwaarden JA, Waasdorp EJ, Bendermacher BLW, et al: Endovascular repair of paraanastomotic aneurysms after previous open aortic prosthetic reconstruction. *Ann Vasc Surg* 2004; 18:280.

[118] Derom A, Nout E: Treatment of femoral pseudoaneurysms with endograft in high-risk patients. *Eur J Vasc Endovasc Surg* 2005; 30:644.

[119] Mitchell JH, Dougherty KG, Strickman NE, et al. Endovascular repair of paraanastomotic aneurysms after aortic reconstruction. *Tex Heart Inst J*. 2007;34:148-153.

[120] Di Tommaso L, Monaco M, Piscione F, et al. Endovascular stent grafts as a safe secondary option for para-anastomotic abdominal aortic aneurysm. *Eur J Vasc Endovasc Surg*. 2007;33:91-93.

[121] Lagana D, Carrafiello G, Mangini M, et al: Endovascular treatment of anastomotic pseudoaneurysms after aorto-iliac surgical reconstruction. *Cardiovasc Intervent Radiol* 2007; 30:1185.

[122] Piffaretti G, Tozzi M, Lomazzi C, et al: Endovascular treatment for para-anastomotic abdominal aortic and iliac aneurysms following aortic surgery.. *J Cardiovasc Surg* 2007; 48:711.

[123] Sachdev U, Baril DT, Morrissey NJ, et al. Endovascular repair of para-anastomotic aortic aneurysms. *J Vasc Surg*. 2007;46:636.

Chapter 21

Marfan Syndrome – Advances in Diagnosis and Management

Miguel Angel Ramirez-Marrero, Beatriz Perez-Villardon,
Ricardo Vivancos-Delgado and Manuel de Mora-Martin

Additional information is available at the end of the chapter

http://dx.doi.org/10.5772/48482

1. Introduction

Cardiovascular disease is the leading cause of death in most Western societies and it is increasing steadily in many developing countries. Aortic diseases constitute an emerging share of the burden. New diagnostic imaging modalities, longer life expectancy in general, longer exposure to elevated blood pressure, and the proliferation of modern non-invasive imaging modalities have all contributed to the growing awareness of acute and chronic aortic syndromes. Despite recent progress in recognition of both the epidemiological problem, diagnostic and therapeutic advances, the cardiology community and the medical community in general are far from comfortable in understanding the spectrum of aortic syndromes and defining an optimal pathway to manage aortic diseases.

Aortic aneurysms and dissections are the main disorders that can affect this artery in the thoracic cavity. Thoracic aortic aneurysms are usually asymptomatic, a silent disease, and they may not be diagnosed until a serious complication appears, such as acute aortic dissection or rupture. Those complications have a high morbidity and mortality, and entail a considerable healthcare expenditure. Prophylactic aortic surgery is being applied to prevent these potentially catastrophic aortic complications. It is very important to correctly identify patients at high risk, by establishing periodic monitoring and follow-up with imaging tests to determine the size of the aorta and the rate of aortic growth.

There have been identified many genetic syndromes that may predispose to the development of thoracic aortic aneurysms and type A aortic dissections. The most important is the Marfan syndrome, as almost all patients with this syndrome will develop an ascending aortic aneurysm throughout his life.

2. Body

The Marfan syndrome (MFS) is an autosomal dominantly inherited disorder of connective tissue with multisystem involvement. It is caused by mutations in the *FBN1* gene on chromosome 15, which encodes a glycoprotein called fibrillin-1, a component of the extracellular matrix. Over 1700 mutations have been identified in the fibrillin-1 gene associated with MFS, other genes related with the disease have been discovered and other disease-related genes with phenotypes very similar to this clinical syndrome (which need a thorough differential diagnosis) have been also identified. Because connective tissue is found throughout the body, MS can affect many body systems, including the ocular, cardiovascular, skeletal, and pulmonary Systems, as well as the skin and dura mater. The most serious signs and symptoms associated with MS involve the cardiovascular system; the cardiac complications, particularly aortic dilatation, dissection and rupture and involvement of the aortic and mitral valves, lead to a greatly reduced life expectancy.

2.1. Diagnostic criteria for Marfan´s syndrome

The MFS was described by the first time in 1896 by Antoine-Bernard Marfan, and it was not until 1995 that it was included in the connective tissue diseases classification. In 1986 a group of experts established a set of clinical criteria for the diagnosis of MFS (Berlin nosology). Later, in 1996 [1], it suffered a modification, known as Ghent's nosology (table 1), in order to avoid the overdiagnosis and to facilitate the differentiation with other similar syndromes. These criteria have been used throughout the world for the diagnosis of the SM, with a high specificity, as mutations in the gene FBN1 had been detected in up to 97 % of the patients who assemble these criteria [2]. Nevertheless, it presents some limitations, such as not consider the dependence on the age for some clinical manifestations, preventing the diagnosis in children, or to include not specific clinical manifestations, or with a poorly established diagnostic value. These facts may involve the overdiagnosis of MFS in patients with ectopia lentis or mitral valve prolapse syndrome; or on the contrary they may restrict the diagnosis in patients with ectopia lentis and aortic dilatation without sufficient skeletal manifestations.

Organ / System	Requirements for the classification of major criteria	Requirements for the affectation of organs/systems
Skeletal	At least four of the following ones: 1. *Pectus carinatum* 2. *Pectus excavatum* that needs surgery 3. Reduced upper segment / lower segment ratio, or increased armspan / height 4. Thumb and wrist´s signs 5. Curvature of the spine (20◦) o	At least two findings for major criteria, or one of those and two of the following minor criteria: 1. Moderate severity pectus excavatum 2. Articular hypermobility 3. Marked arch palate, or dental agglomeration

	espondilolistesis 6. Reduced elbow extension (<170◦) 7. Medial displacement of the internal ankle causing plain flat feet 8. Protrucio acetabulae	4. Typical facial appearance (dolichocephaly, malar hypoplasia, retrognathia, downward slanting palpebral fissures, enophthalmos)
Ocular	Ectopia lentis	Al least two of the following minor criteria: 1. Flattened cornea 2. Increase of the axial lenght of the eyeball 3. Miosis reduced by iris of ciliary muscle hipoplasy
Cardiovascular	Al least one of the following ones: 1. Ascending aortic dilatation, with or without regurgitation, concerning Valsalva sinus 2. Ascending aortic dissection	At least one of the following minor criteria: 1. Mitral valve prolapse, with or without regurgitation 2. Pulmonary artery dilatation, in absence of estenosis or other cause in adults < 40 years 3. Mitral ring calcification in adults < 40 years 4. Aortic dilatation or dissection
Pulmonary	None	At least one of the following minor criteria: 1. Spontaneous pneumothorax 2. Apical bullous
Coverings	None	At least one of the following minor criteria: 1. Skin striae not associated with marked weight changes, pregnancy or repeated stress 2. Recurrent of iincisional hernia
Dura mater	Lumbosacral dural ectasia	None
For the diagnosis of Marfan´s syndrome in patients without family history of the disease, there must be involved two organs / systems that assemble major criteria, and at least the affectation of a third organ / system. In patients with positive family history of this sybndrome, it is needed a major criteria, with information that suggest the affectation of a second system.		

Table 1. Diagnostic criteria of Ghent´s nosology

In order to solve the limitations of Ghent's nosology, it has been proposed a review of this. A group of international experts in the diagnosis and the management of MFS summoned in Brussels by the National Marfan Foundation, published recently *"The revised Ghent nosology"* [3], based on the review of wide cohorts of patients, experts opinion and the available literature about the application of the classic criteria, the differential diagnosis of the MS and the solidity and limitations of the genetic study.

Among the most importants changes, a major value is granted for two cardinal findings of the MFS, the aneurysm/dissection of the root of the aorta and the ectopia lentis, being sufficient the combination of both to establish the diagnosis. The rest of ocular and cardiovascular manifestations, as well as the findings of other organs/systems, contribute to a systemic score that facilitates the diagnosis when the aortic disease is present but not the ectopia lentis (table 2).

A more relevant role is assigned to the genetic study of the gene FBN1 and other related genes (TGFBR1 and TGFBR2). Some of the less specific manifestations lose importance in the diagnostic evaluation.

The new criteria emphasize the need of diagnostic considerations and additional tests if patients assemble sufficient criteria for MS but show unexpected findings, especially because of the possibility of an alternative specific diagnosis. It is emphasized specially in Sphrintzen-Goldberg and of Loeys-Dietz syndromes, and in the vascular form of Ehlers-Danlos's syndrome.

The new diagnostic criteria have been defined for a sporadic index patients, or for a patient with positive family history (table 3).

- **In absence of any family history**, the diagnosis can be established in the following cases:

1. The presence of aortic root dilatation or dissection (Z score ≥2, adjusted to age and body surface area) and ectopia lentis establish the diagnosis, independently of the presence of other systemic findings, except when these are indicative of other genetic syndromes of aortic aneurysm, as Sphrintzen-Goldberg and of Loeys-Dietz syndromes, and the vascular form of Ehlers-Danlos's syndrome
2. The presence of dilatation or dissection (Z-score ≥2) and the identification of a mutation of the FBN1 gene is sufficient to establish the diagnosis of the MS.
3. In presence of dilatation or dissection (Z-score ≥2) without ectopia lentis and ignorance of mutations of the FBN1 gene, diagnosis can be established when sufficient systemic findings exist (≥ 7 points); in this case, there must be excluded the possibility of other genetic aortic aneurisma syndromes.
4. In presence of ectopia lentis without aortic dilatation / dissection, the identification of mutations of the FBN1 gene associated with aortic disease allows the diagnosis of the MS.

Wrist AND thumb sign: 3 (wrist OR thumb sign: 1)
Pectus carinatum deformity: 2 (*pectus excavatum* o chest asymmetry: 1)
Hindfoot deformity: 2 (plain flat foot: 1)
Pneumothorax: 2
Dural ectasia: 2
Protrusio acetabulae: 2
Reduced upper segment/lower segment and increased armspan/height: 1
Scoliosis of thoracolumbar kyphosis: 1
Reduced elbow extension 1
3 of 5 facial features: 1 (dolichocephaly, enophthalmos, downward slanting palpebral fissures, malar hypoplasia, retrognathia)
Skin striae: 1
Myopia >3 diopters: 1
Mitral valve prolapse: 1
Maximum total 20 points; *score* ≥7 indicates systemic affectation.

Table 2. Systemic findings score

- **In the presence of family history**, the diagnosis can be established in the presence of ectopia lentis plus a systemic score ≥ 7 points, or the presence of aortic dilatation (Z ≥2 in adults ≥20 years, or Z ≥3 in individuals <20 years).

In absence of family history for Marfan´s syndrome
1. Ao (Z ≥2) and EL = MFS[a]
2. Ao (Z ≥2) and FBN1 mutation = SMF
3. Ao (Z ≥2) and systemic *score* (≥7 points) = SMF[a]
4. EL and FBN1 mutation identified in individuals with aortic aneurysm = SMF
• EL with or withour systemic score, without FBN1 mutation, or with FBN1 mutation not related to aortic aneurysm/dissection = ELS
• Ao (Z ≥2) and systemic score (≥5 points) without EL = MASS
• PVM and Ao (Z <2) and systemic *score* (<5 points) without EL = SPVM
In the presence of family history
5. EL and FH of MFS = MFS
6. Systemic score ≥7 points and FH of MFS = SMFa
7. Ao (Z ≥2 in > 20 years, Z ≥3 in < 20 years) and FH of MFS = MFS[a]
Ao: aortic diameter in Valsalva sinus (indicated by Z-score) or dissection; FBN1 mutation: mutation in fibrillin 1 gene; EL: ectopia lentis; MASS: phenotype with myopia, mitral valve prolapse, bordering expansion of aortic root (Z<2), skin striae and skeletal findings; PVM: mitral valve prolapse; ELS: ectopia lentis syndrome; MFS: Marfan´s syndrome; VMPS: mitral valve prolapse syndrome; Z: Z-score.
[a] Warning: reject Shprintzen-Goldberg, Loeys-Dietz o vascular type Ehlers-Danlos syndromes, study of TGFBR1/2, COL3A1 mutations, and collagen biochemistry.

Table 3. The revised Ghent nosology for the Marfan Syndrome

In addition, there are considered two new situations in patients younger than 20-year-old. The first of them, the **"unspecific disorder of the connective tissue"** for the cases with insufficient systemic findings (<7 points) and/or bordering dimensions of the aortic root (Z <3), without mutation of the FBN1 gene. The second one, the **"MFS potential"** for the sporadic or family history cases with mutation of the FBN1 gene and aortic dimensions with Z<3 score.

In adults, three alternatives categories are defined: ecopia lentis syndrome (ELS), mitral valve prolapse syndrome (MVPS) and the phenotype MASS.

Finally, the experts' panel recognizes the difficulty for establishing MFS's diagnosis in certain patients due to the overlapping phenotype of diverse entities.

2.2. Hereditary syndromes related to thoracic aorta aneurysms

The thoracic aortic aneurysms (TAA) are a relatively frequent entity, being responsible for approximately 15,000 annual deaths in USA. Up to 20 % of the patients with TAA, a genetic substratum is detected [4].

The familial TAA are classified in syndromics (they appear with phenotypics manifestations to other levels) and non syndromics (they appear as an isolated manifestation but with family aggregation, suggesting a genetic substratum).

The MFS is the most important entity inside the familial syndromics TAA. It is necessary to establish the differential diagnosis between this one and others mixed connective tissue diseases with clinical manifestations and similar phenotypics features. The majority of these diseases (table 4) are monogenics and with a dominant autosomal inheritance.

Familial Syndromic Thoracic Aortic Aneurysm Syndromes	**Non fibrilinopathies** **Loeys-Dietz's syndrome** **Type IV Ehler-Danlos's syndrome** **Turner's syndrome** **Beals's syndrome** **Noonan's syndrome** **Alagille's syndrome** **Autosomal dominant polycystic kidney disease** **Fibrinilopathies** **Shprintzen-Goldberg's syndrome** **Weill-Marchesani's syndrome** **MASS phenotype**
Familial Non Syndromic Thoracic Aortic Aneurysm Syndromes	TAAD1, TAAD2, TAAD3, TAAD4, TAAD5, FAA1 and TAAD associated to ductus arterial persistent Bicuspid aortic valve

Table 4. Differential diagnosis of Marfan's syndrome

Among the genetic syndromes that can be accompanied of TAA, we can emphasize:

MAAS phenotype (mitral valve, aorta, skin, skeletal)

It is included inside the fibrilinopathies group, that is to say, diseases results from mutations in the FBN1 gene. It is characterized by the presence of myopathy, mitral valve prolapse, aortic dilatation (slight and not progressive) and alterations of the cutaneous and musculoskeletal system. At least two systems must be affected.

Loeys-Dietz's syndrome

Autosomal dominant genetic syndrome caused by mutations in the genes encoding transforming growth factor β1 (TGFBR1) or 2 (TGFBR2). Two phenotypic variants can be currently distinguished (table 5).

The aortic aneurysms are very frequent, appearing in 98 % of the cases, at early ages, and they are characterized by a high risk of dissection and / or rupture, even with diameters <5 cm. Up to 53 % of the patients may develop aneurysms in other locations. In general way, it is accepted that those patients with more severe craniofacial manifestations present the most aggressive vascular disease.

Patients with this syndrome are recommended to realize a complete imaging study to evaluate the aorta in the moment of the diagnosis and every 6 months, to check the growth rate of the TAA. An annual craniothoracoabdominal magnetic resonance must be fullfilled for the detection of systemics vascular aneurysms.

	Type I Loeys-Dietz syndrome	**Type II Loeys-Dietz syndrome**
Phenotype	Hypertelorism Craniosynostosis Cleft palate or bifid uvula Arterial tortuosity and aneurysms/dissections	Without other craniofacial anomalies, except bifid uvula Similar to type IV Ehlers-Danlos's syndrome
Mutated genes	TGFBR1 and TGFBR2	TGFBR1 and TGFBR2
Prevalence	Unknown	Unknown
Prognosis	37 years of median survival Average age of death at 26 years	37 years of median survival Average age of death at 26 years

Table 5. Variants of Loeys-Dietz's syndrome

The surgical repair of the TAA in patients with Loeys-Dietz's syndrome must be realized when the internal diameter overcomes 4,2 cm for transesophageal echocardiogram or the external diameter is major than 4,5 cm in a computerized tomography or magnetic resonance.

Ehlers-Danlos's syndrome vascular type or type IV Ehlers-Danlon´s syndrome

It is caused by mutations in the genes encoding the collagenous type 3 (COL3A1) with an autosomal dominant inheritance. It is characterized by vascular and visceral external fragility, which can lead to vascular and visceral spontaneous breaks or with minimal traumatisms. The cutaneous or articular hyperlaxity is less marked that in other subtypes. The majority of the deaths are due to vascular breaks.

It is recommended to carry out non invasive imaging tests because of the high risk of vascular break. It is unknown the usefulness of the aortic surgery in the repair of the not complicated TAA. In case of dissection or rupture, the urgent surgery is indicated, with specially attention to the vascular anastomosis because of the trend to the hemorrhage, vascular fragility and the difficulties in the tissue regeneration capacitiy in this syndrome.

Turner's syndrome

It is a chromosomal abnormality in which the monosomy X is the most common (cariotipe 45, X0). The patients affected with Turner's syndrome present characteristic physical abnormalities such as short stature, webbed necks and sterility. There can be associated differents cardiovascular manifestations, as the coarctation of aorta, early ischemic cardiopathy, bicuspid aortic valve and TAA (up to 40 % of the cases). The incidence of aortic dissection in these patients is greater compared with the healthy population, six-times increased risk, with a median age of presentation of 31 years.

It is recommended to realize an initial imaging test to reject bicuspid aortic valve, coarctation of aorta and / or TAA. If the test is normal and there is no risk factors for aortic dissection it is enough to do an imaging test every 5-10 years. In the opposite case, annual controls are advised. Inthose patients with Turner´s syndrome who are planning the get pregnancy, an imaging test must be realized to determine the risk of aortic dissection.

Autosomal dominant polycystic kidney disease

Disease caused by a mutation in the genes PKD1 and PKD2. Its more frequent complication are the hemorrhages subaracnoideas due to the rupture of cerebral aneurysms. It is also associated with an increase in TAA and type-A aortic dissections.

Beals's syndrome or congenital contractural arachnodactyly

It is an autosomal dominantly inherited connective tissue disorder caused by a mutation in FBN2 gene. Although the clinical features can be similar to Marfan syndrome, multiple joint contractures (especially elbow, knee and finger joints), arachnodactyly, severe kyphoscoliosis, abnormal pinnae, muscular hypoplasia and crumpled ears in the absence of significant aortic root dilatation are characteristic of Beals syndrome and rarely found in Marfan syndrome.

Responsible gene	Familiar Non syndromic TAA	%	Aortic dissection
Unknown gene Locus 5q13-14 Gene that codifies for the proteins versican, trombospondina 4 and protein related to the cartilage	TAAD1		
TGFBR2 Gene that codifies the receptor of the transforming growth factor β2 Mutation in arginina 460, locus 3p24-25	TAAD2 The same gene mutated in the syndrome Loeys-Dietz	5 %	Risk of aortic dissection with diameter <5 cm Recommendations similar to those for Loeys-Dietz's syndrome
MYH11 Heavy chain of the 11-βmiosina, specific for smooth muscle cells. Located in the chromosome 16p	TAAD-persistent arterious ductus	1 %	Risk of aortic dissection with diameter ≤4,5 cm
ACTA2 Gene that codifies for the region alfa2 of the actina of the aortic smooth muscle. Locus 10q22-24	TAAD4	15 %	Risk of type A aortic dissection with diameter <5,0 cm and at early ages of life Risk of type B aortic dissection with < 21 years old
TGFBR1 Gene that codifies the receptor of the transforming growth factor β1 Locus 9q33-34	TAAD5 The same gene mutated in Loeys-Dietz's syndrome and Furlong's syndrome		
FAA1 Locus 11q23-24	FAA1		
FBN1 Gene that codifies the fibrilina 1 Locus 15q21.1 It can present mosaicism in somatic and germinate cells	The same gene mutated in Shprintzen-Goldberg's syndrome, Weill-Marchesani's syndrome and the phenotype MASS (fibrilinopathies)		

Table 6. Familial non syndromic thoracic aortic aneurysm syndromes (*see text*)

The majority of the familial TAA and aortic dissections are produced in patients who cannot be fitted in any of the syndromes described before. The studies of family aggregation suggest that between 11 and 19 % of the patients with TAA or dissections present a first degree relative with this antecedent.

In general, the presentation of aoritc complications (rupture and/or dissection) in patients with familial non syndromics TAA occur at earlier ages in comparison with the sporadic aneurysms (median age of 56,8 years opposite to 64,3 years), though without reaching the precociousness of the syndromics TAA. The aortic dilatation can concern both the tubular portion of the ascending aorta and sinus of Valsalva. The age of appearance and the growth rate are very changeable, event inside the components of a same family.

From a genetic point of view, the familial non syndromic TAA are very heterogeneous, having been located up to 7 different loci, that can explain only 20% of the cases: TAAD1, TAAD2, TAAD3, TAAD4, TAAD5, FAA1 and TAAD-partner to persistent arterial ductus (table 6). The way of inheritance is autosomal dominant with incomplete penetrance, minor in the female sex.

In patients with familial non syndromic TAA it is necessary to realize an individualized genetic advine to the relatives. It is necessary to realize a genetic analysis to the first degree relatives in case of a known mutation in the index case. In the first degree relatives with a negative genetic study, it is recommended an unique imaging test to reject aortic pathology. In case of presenting any of the genetic mutations described mutations, periodic reviews must be made every 2 years approximately.

2.3. Genetics of Marfan's syndrome

Marfan syndrome results from mutations in the fibrillin-1 (FBN1) gene located on chromosome 15q21.1 and, occasionally, by mutations in *TGFβR1* or *TGFβR2* genes (transforming growth factor-β receptor 1 and 2) located on chromosome 9 and on chromosome 3p24.2-p25, respectively [5]. More than 500 fibrillin gene mutations have been identified. Almost all of these mutations are unique to an affected individual or family. Different fibrillin mutations are responsible for genetic heterogeneity. Phenotypic variability in the presence of the same fibrillin mutation suggests the importance of other, yet-to-be-identified factors that affect the phenotype.

Fibrillin-1 (FBN1) gene

The fibrillin-1 gene consists of 65 exones and it is located in the chromosome 15q-21.1. It encodes for the glycoprotein fibrillin, which is a major building block of microfibrils that constitute the structural components of the suspensory ligament of the lens and serve as substrates for elastina in the aorta and other connective tissues.

The FBN1 gene is characterized for having several rich sequences in cysteine, comparable to the factor of epidermal growth (EGF). 47 exones codify a complete domain EGF and 43 of these include the sequence consensus for the union to the calcium *Asp/Asn-x-Asp/Asn-*

Glu/Gln-xm-Asp/Asn-xn-Tyr/Phe* (where x represents any amino acid, * it represents possible beta-hydroxylation of this residue and "m" y "n" represent a variable number of residues). Each of the EGF-similar contains six residues highly preserved of cysteine that form three disulfide bonds between C1 and C3, between C2 and C4 and between C5 and C6, resulting in a structure of βeta strand what is involved in the union to the calcium. Calcium plays a very important role in the stability of the domain and awards a major resistance to the proteolytic degradation.

Nowadays, several strategies can be used in the genetic study of the FBN1 gene, being the reference the direct sequentiation of the exones and the border intron regions. Another method is the high-performance denaturing liquid chromatography liquid, with later confirmation for direct sequentiation. When a mutation is not identified and there is a high clinical suspicion of the presence of the disease, there can be looked big deletion/duplication, impossible to detect for the previous methods, using MLPA (multiplex ligation-dependent probe amplification). Finally, the analysis of genetic linkage can be used to determine if an individual has inherited an allele of the FBN1 gene that is associated with the syndrome in several members of the family, nevertheless its cost and efficiency are limited compared by the sequencing technique.

In order to consider the identified mutation as responsible, the following criteria must be evaluated:

1. If the mutation has been described before, familial consegregation must be demonstrated, that is to say, that in a family with MFS, the ones with the mutation must be affected and those without the mutation must be healthy.
2. If the mutation has not been described before, it is necessary to consider the following premises:
   a. Certain mutations have a high probability of being pathogenic:
      - *Nonsense mutation*, that creates a premature stop codon
      - Insertion/deletion that concerns a number of bases that is not multiple of three, and consistently alters the reading, usually creating a premature stop codon
      - Mutation that affects the *splicing* of the sequence of reference or that alters to level of the cDNA/mRNA ("splice site mutations"); mechanism that forms a part of the mRNA maturation consisting of the elimination of the introns so that a codificant and without interruptions sequence is obtained, and it can be translated into protein.
      - *Missense* mutation that creates or replaces cysteine
      - *Missense* mutation that concerns a preserved residue of the consensus EGF sequence.
   b. The mutation must concern a preserved residue in the evolution. It is considered that the amino acids that have not suffered changes along the evolutionary scale are important for the function of the same one.
   c. For the demonstration of the pathogenic of a mutation, bioninformatic models can be used so that they can predict if the change that induces the mutation can carry deleterious effects or not in the protein.

d. The familial consegregation must be demonstrated if possible, and the absence of the mutation in at least 40 chromosomes of the same etnia, that is to say, at least in 200 subjects.
e. The pathogenicity is high probably in the identified mutations by genetic linkage.

The sensibility to find a mutation in a patient with MFS is high, varying between 76 and 93% in recent studies. It depends on several factors, as the age, the familial history or the method used for the genetic study.

Marfan syndrome is known as an autosomal dominant connective tissue disorder. Hereby, the risk that a son of an affected father has the disease is 50%. Approximately, 75% of the patients with MFS has one of his parents affected, and only in 25% the affected one presents a de novo mutation.

The penetration of the mutations in FBN1 is in general high, being considered to be near to 100%. It has been communicated exceptional cases of incomplete penetration. It is necessary to consider that many of the manifestations appear with the age.

Those patients with severe and progressive forms of the disease (called "The neonatal Marfan Syndrome") usually have mutations in the central part of the gene, between exons 24 and 32 of FBN1. Affected individuals are generally diagnosed at birth or shortly thereafter. Congestive heart failure associated with mitral and tricuspid regurgitation is the main cause of death, whereas aortic diseection is uncommon; survival beyond 24 months is rare. As a general rule, the mutations that produce insertions or deletions with change or displacement of the frame of reading or *splice site mutations*, are usually associated to severer forms of the disease. The patients with mutations that alter the terminal-C-propeptide procesate have been related to predominantly skeletal affectations of the disease. It is evident that it is necessary to compile information about the clinical consequences and the phenotype associated with different mutations, since mutations with the same mechanism can have very different clinical consequences, as it is demonstrated in other genetic pathologies.

The diagnosis of the MFS can be realized without needing a genetic study. Nevertheless, it has a great importance in the following suppositions:

1. It is of great relevancy in patients who do not fulfill clinical criteria, especially in patients with ectopia lentis and patients with cardiovascular suggestive features combined with skeletal findings or in sporadic cases in young subjects.
2. It is very useful in relatives of affected patients, especially children, to know if they have inherited the mutation of their parents and so they will need periodic controls.
3. It must be realized in patients in whom the genetic diagnosis can influence their way of life, as in high competitive sports, for the initiation of the treatment or programming of clinical follow-up.
4. It can be useful for prenatal diagnosis, analyzing DNA extracted from foetal cells obtained of the chorionic villus between 10 and 12 weeks′ gestation. It might be done whenever a causal mutation had been identified in the relative, with pathogenicity

clearly demonstrated, and avoiding the pollution by mother DNA of the studied sample, in the cases in which the mother is affected.

5. In the preimplantational diagnosis in in-vitro fertilization treatments. The use for the prenatal and preimplantational diagnosis is controversial in many countries, with ethical and legal aspects that must be have in mind.

Transforming growth factor-β receptor 1 and 2 (TGFBR 1 and 2)

There have been found mutations in these genes in some of the MFS diagnosed patients or thos with MFS's suspicion. These patients present a more aggressive form of the vascular disease, with dissections and ruptures at earlier ages and with smaller diameters. Initially they were identified by MFS's type 2, leaving the type 1 for mutations in the FBN1 gene. Later, these patients with marfanoid phenotype, aggressive vascular disease and other morphologic features (hyperterolism, bifid uvula, ...) were grouped in Loeys-Dietz's syndrome. Thus, we can find it with both nomenclatures.

2.4. Use of biomarkers in Marfan's syndrome

According to the definition of the National Intitutes of Health, a biomarker is "a characteristic that can be quantified and evaluated in an objective way as an indicator of normal biological processes, pathogenic processes or pharmacological answers to a therapeutic intervention" [6]. The employment of biomarkers facilitates the identification of patients at risk, and they are usually molecules that can be identified by a blood analysis.

Nowadays we don't have many specific bibliography about circulatory biomarkers for the thoracic aortic aneurysm. The not circulatory biomarker that is in use with more frequency is the diameter of the aneurysm.

Below we will detail the biomarkers that could have importance in the clinical management of the thoracic aortic aneurysms, as in Marfan syndrome:

D-dimer

It has been demonstrated that the concentrations of D-dimer allow to detect the Stanford type A acute aortic dissection. The concentration of the D-dimer obtained during the hospital admission is correlated by the survival of these patients. Thus, elevations in the concentration of D-dimer in patients who come to Emergency Room for thoracic pain it should be realized a tomography computerized to reject acute aortic dissection as well as acute pulmonary embolism.

Cellular biomarkers

There have been identified two types of cells that are associated with the evolution of an aneurysm, the CD 28 T-lymphocytes and the natural citolytic lymphocytes or natural killer. It has been demonstrated in studies the presence of population of natural killer lymphocytes in greater number in patients with abdominal aortic aneurysm compared with healthy subjects. The CD 28 T-lymphocytes appear in diverse inflammatory disorders, and express in a more frequent form with the age. It has been observed in patients with aneurysms greater quantity of this cellular type in peripheral blood compared to healthy controls. In addition, on a contradictory way, highest rates are found in patients with smaller aneurysms in comparison with patients with big aneurysms, appearing the hypothesis about the intervention of Cd 28 T-lymphocytes in the genesis of the aneurysms.

Biomarkers in plasma and serum

Several circulating biomarkers have been identified with the aneurysms, in relation to their appearance, diameter or expansion. These can be classify in inflammation biomarkers, indicators of tissue turnover, and others as homocysteine, serum amyloid A, osteopontin, osteoprotegerin and the concentrations of plasmin / antiplasmin complex.

Inflammation biomarkers have been the more widely studied. At present, the formation of the aortic aneurysm is understood as an inflammatory process. Many studies relate diverse inflammatory cytokines (interleukin-1, interleukin-6, tumor necrosis factor-α, interferon γ and cold-reactive proteins) to the formation, expansion or rupture of the aneurysm. Its disadvantage is the lack of specificity, being able to rise their concentrations in other inflammatory processes, reason why their clinical utility as aortic aneurysm biomarker is limited.

Special mention is deserved to the matrix metallooproteinases (MMPs). Their main function is the degradation of the extracelular matrix. The MMPs are active in many pathological processes, either in trivial ones as periodontitis or others more serious as heart failure. In experimental models with animals, there has been demonstrated that MMP's inhibition, by genetic deletion directed or by pharmacological intervention, determines a minor progression of the abdominal aortic aneurysms. In patients with abdominal aortic aneurysm, the circulating concentrations of MMP-9 presented a direct correlation with the concentrations of MMP-9 in the aortic wall. It has been observed an increase in the concentration of MMP-1 and MMP-9 in the thoracic aortic walls with aneurysms or dissections in comparison with healthy controls. It has also been observed an increase of the quotient MMP-9/TIMP-1 (tissue inhibitor of metalloproteinases-1), favoring the proteolysis of the aortic wall. Other studies have documented a correlation of MMP's activity, especially MMP-9, with the genesis and evolution of the thoracic aortic aneurysms.

Molecular biomarkers

It has been studied the RNA of circulating leukocytes and there have been identified characteristics of expression that relate to the appearance of thoracic aneurysms, with an accuracy up to 78%. In the same line, there has been identified a hyperexpression of certain genes in patients with thoracic and abdominal aortic aneurysms. Among these genes, we must emphasize those who codify the intracellular adhesion molecule-1, v-yes-1 oncogene, mitogen activated protein kinase and the MMP-9.

In short, it does not exist a perfect biomaker for a pathological process. In case of the thoracic aortic aneurysms, the best described biomarker and with wide diffusion in the clinical practice is the diameter of the same one. Big advances have been achieved in circulating biomarkers, though further study is required to be able to generalize it to the daily clinical practice.

2.5. Diagnosis of the aortic affectation in the MFS

In a summarized form, the management of the aortic pathology in the MFS is based on the clinical study and imaging techniques to detect and to quantify the progression of the aortic expansion [7].

The initial clinical evaluation of every patient with MFS's suspicion must include anamnesis and a complete clinical examination. The diagnosis of certainty can be reached in almost 90% of the cases through the Ghent´s nosology, being able to be completed by the genetic study as we have described before. To complete the information about diagnostic criteria (table 1) we will carry out an imaging test that allows to evaluate the ascending aorta and the cardiac valves.

The transthoracic echocardiogram (TTE) represents the main technique for the diagnosis of the cardiovascular affectation in the initial evaluation of patients with MFS, allowing to explore the aortic root, the proximal ascending aorta and the aortic arch. The maximum diameters of the aortic annulus, Valsalva sinus, sinotubular junction and of the ascending aorta must be measured perpendicularly to the longitudinal axis of the aorta. The obtained information will be compared in nomogramas with the expected values according to the age, the sex and the corporal surface. The severity of the aortic affectation relates to the degree and the extension of the dilatation, being most important when it spreads from the root over the ascending aorta up to the aortic arch. The second TTE will be carried out at 6 months of the diagnosis to determine the speed of growth. If the diameter remains stable, the ultrasonic study can be realized anually, but if accelerated expansion is detected or when it comes closer to 45mm, the evaluation will have to be more frequent (table 7).

In spite of the fact that the transthoracic echocardiogram is the most used technique to monitor the size of the aortic root, its precision depends on the operator. The computerized tomography (CT) or the magnetic resonance (MRI) are more precise and must be used if the echocardiogram does not give a suitable image of the aorta. It is advisable to know that the echocardiographic measures, being realized between internal edges, can be up to 4mm lower than the obtained ones with MRI or CT, in which the thickness of the wall joins.

Anamnesis, physical examination, echocardiogram: **At the beginning and at the 6 months[a]** **Later: every year, if the growth rate is stable and without complications[a]**
CT or MRI: If there is aortic dilatation or dissection. After the surgery, before the discharge, at 6 months, and then anually.
The evaluation will be more frequent as the aortic root approaches 45mm or if it is registered an accelerated rate of growth (> 5 mm / year)
a Class I recommendation, level of evidence C. b It is consider of utility to correct the aortic diameters in accordance with the age and the corporal size (class IIa, level of evidence C).

Table 7. Cardiovascular follow-up in Marfan's syndrome

2.6. Pharmacological treatment in the prevention of the cardiovascular complications of the MFS

The pharmacological treatment in the prevention of the cardiovascular pathology in patients with MFS is based on the employment of β-adrenergic blocking agents and renin-angiotensin system antagonists [8].

Beta blockers

Many studies have demonstrated that the employment of betablockers can slow down the aortic rate expansion and delay the moment of appearance of the aortic complications of the MFS, as the aortic regurgitation, the aortic dissection, the need of surgery, the congestive heart failure or the death, specially if they are use in the initial phases of the disease, as they can reduce the hemodynamic stress of the thoracic aorta wall.

These benefits are in all the groups of age, being more important in patients with not severe aortic dilatation.

Nowadays the clinical guidelines recommend the employment of betablockers at the right dose in all patients with MFS who tolerate them, independently from the degree of aortic dilatation.

Given that the aortic growth rate changes along the life, presenting a prepuberal peak, it is recommended the beginning of the treatment with betablockers in the infancy, and to support it forever, even in patients who have received aortic prophylactic surgery.

The effects of the pharmacological treatment must have a periodic review to assure an optimal management of the cardiac frequency and the arterial pressure of the patient (table 8).

Betablockers	**Use always in MFS, except in cases of intolerance[a]** **Atenolol: more used (long half-life and cardioselective)** **Dose: to title up to CF at rest <60 lpm and <100 lpm in exercise, if the AP allows it.** **To monitor the efficiency and the doses in periodic visits**
Calcium channel blockers	Verapamil: second line treatment in patients who do not tolerate betablockers
ACE inhibitors	Associated to betablockers when additional treatment is needed to control the AP, specially those with chronic dissection
AT1R-II	AT1 blockers (losartan) *associated to betablockers;* in small not randomized studies, major efficiency in delaying the aortic rate growth[b]. AT1 blockers, *associated to betablockers;* alternative use to ACEi when additional medication is needed for AP's control
	a Class I recommendation, level of evidence B. b Class IIa recommendation, level of evidence B.

Table 8. Pharmacological treatment in the MFS

Renin-angiotensin-aldosterone system antagonists

The influence of the renin-angiotensin-aldosterone system in the aortic wall degeneration of the MFS seems to be increasingly important. The angiotensin II (ATII) stimulates the expression of metalloproteases and promotes the apoptosis of the smooth muscle cells in the aortic wall. The experimental models have demonstrated that the deficiency of *FBN1* increases the TGF-β active, causing the detention of the cellular differentiation cicle, an increase of the apoptosis and deposit of extracelular matrix. The employment of renin-angiotensin system antagonists by means of angiotensin-converting-enzyme inhibitors (ECAs) or with angiotensin II receptor antagonists (ARAII), produces beneficial effects at different levels. The ECAs contribute, apart from the control of the AP, to the decrease of the inflexibility of the aortic wall. The selective block of the type 1 receptor (AT1) of the angiotensin II might reduce the deleterious effects of the TGF-β, independently of the effects on the control of the AP. Though in animal models, losartan has demonstrated to stop and even to revert MFS manifestations, including the aortic aneurysm and its complications, we are waiting for the results of controlled clinical trials in human beings that are in process.

It is important to insist that the medical treatment, based fundamentally on betablockers, which is possible to associate to the renin-angiotensin system block, gets delaying the aortic expansion, but no medicament, up to the moment, has demonstrated either to avoid the development of aortic dissection or to avoid the need for surgery in human beings.

Physical activity

To reduce the hemodynamic stress in the MFS, the restriction of the physical activity complements the pharmacological therapy. The intense isometric exercise is contraindicated due to the marked increases in the peripheral AP and the stress of the proximal aortic wall. Also competitive sports, contact sports and those that with marked changes in the atmospheric pressure are contraindicated, to prevent the arterial traumatism and the pneumothorax. Since the dynamic exercise is associated with minor aortic stress, for the decrease of the peripheral vascular resistance and of the diastolic AP, in patients without high risk, the practice of aerobic activity of moderate intensity is considered to be sure (table 9).

2.7. Prophylactic surgery of the proximal aorta

In the MFS, the prophylactic surgery of the aortic root and the ascending aorta is recommended, because of the high mortality of the emergency aortic replacement and because both, the type A aortic dissection and the aortic rupture, are the complications with major impact in the survival. Though technically more complex, the aortic valve conservation techniques, remodeling or reimplantation, are usually the ones preferred than the valvulated tubes, whenever they offer good results.

Provided that the dissection and mortality risk are proportional to the size of the proximal aorta, the guidelines recommend elective surgery in adults when the *external* diameter is ≥50mm. The surgery also must be considered in patients with diameter <50mm if they present additional risk factors: rapid growth of the aortic diameter (> 5mm/year), familial history of aortic dissection or rupture, or the presence of significant aortic regurgitation (table 10).

With regard to the *timing* of the elective surgery, some considerations must be done. According to the value of the threshold of the diameter, a more or less important proportion of patients will present complications without reaching this value or will surrender unjustibiably to the surgical risk of an elective procedure still being removed from complications. It turns out important to incorporate another information, as the growth rate, and indexing the diameters by body surface. The corporal surface, used in many nomograms on having contemplated the weight, can artificially modify the surgical risk. The current trend is to correct according to the stature, in order that in subjects of minor stature, specially women, but at risk of complication, surgery could be indicated even if their diameters were more near to 45 that to 50mm. In the clinical practice, the surgical indication starts beeing considered when the aorta is expanded (≥2 deviations over the average, Z-score≥2) or when its diameter comes closer to 45mm (before if the stature is lower than 170cm). The surgical results are determinant to indicate prophylactic surgery, preferably preserving the valve and with very low mortality, necessarily lower than 5%.

In *children and teenagers* with MFS, the establishment of a relation with the diameter of the aorta is more difficult than in adults, since the complications are infrequent before 12 years of age. The elective aortic surgery in this population, up to 18 years, is recommended when the aortic diameter exceeds 50mm, when there is a rapid aortic growth (> 10mm/year), when aortic regurgitation appears, or when there is simultaneous affectation of the mitral valve. As for the *timing,* it is necessary to weigh the risk of dissection and the delay of the surgical moment to avoid prosthetic *mismatch,* since the children will continue growing. The paediatric nomograms have been re-calculated to improve their correspondence with those of adults. The normalization for sex, age and corporal surface seems to be suitable, though it will be necessary to define better which is the dilatation of risk in which the benefits of the prophylactic surgery unequivocally overcome the risks.

Type of patient	Recommendation
Every patient with SM: Any degree of aortic root dilatation	To avoid contact sports of contact and those with risk of corporal impact
Low risk: all the following ones: Without aortic root dilatation: • Adults, root <40 mm • Children and teenagers: root Z-score <2 Mitral regurgitation less that moderated Without familial history of dissection or sudden death	Static and dynamic activity of low and moderate intensity[a]
Risk: any of the following ones: Aortic root dilatation • Adults, root ≥40 mm • Children and teenagers: root Z-score ≥2 Moderate or severe mitral regurgitation Previous surgery of aortic root Chronic dissection Familial history of dissection or sudden death	Alone advisable dynamic activity of low intensity

Treatment with betablokers is considered to be a standard for all patients.
a Maximum heart rate during activity <100 lpm (adults) and up to 110 lpm (children) with betablockers.
b If there is usual sport practice, it is suitable to follow-up the growth rate of the aortic root by a transthoracic echocardiogram each six months.
The presence of significant aortic regurgitation with aortic root dilatation makes inadvisable any type of sports practice.

Table 9. Recommendations for the physical activity in Marfan's syndrome

In what concerns the aspects of the *surgical techniques*, the Bono and Bentall procedure has been considered the *gold standard* for the treatment of these patients. It consists in replacing the root and the aortic valve with a composite graft by a dacron vascular graft (rectum or with morphology that imitates to Valsalva's sinus) and a prosthetic valve; the coronary arteries have to be reimplanted into the vascular graft. Diverse technical variations (inclusion vs interposition, *button technique,* Cabrol modification or Svensson) have emerged over the years trying to reduce the early complications (bleeding, coronary occlusion) and the late ones (anastomotic pseudoaneurysms) of the same one, being the most used nowadays the Bono-Bentall by interposition with anastomosis of the coronary arteries in tablets *(button technique).* In young patients, mechanical prosthetic valves are the most used, whereas in those of major age or with contraindications for anticoagulation, biological valves are usually used.

Class I recommendations, level of evidence C
External diameter of proximal aorta ≥ 50 mm
External diameter <50mm with any of the following risk factors:
• **Familial history of dissection or aortic rupture**
• **Rapid progression of the aortic diameter (> 5 mm/year)**
• **Significant aortic regurgitation (moderate or major)**
Class IIa recommendations, level of evidence C
In women with MFS who wish to get pregnancy, it looks reasonable the aortic root and ascending aorta replacement when the diameter is > 40 mm
Aortic surgery will be recommended when the quotient of the proximal aortic maximum area (in cm2) divided by the stature in meters is superior to 10, since the smallest patients and up to 15% of the MFS patients have aortic dissection with diameters <50 mm

Table 10. Criteria for the elective surgery of the aorta proximal in adults with MFS

The immediate and long-term results of this technique are very good, and the rates of the long-term survival are similar to those of the general population. Nevertheless, the results deteriorate considerably when the surgery is realized in an emergent form in the context of an aortic dissection. The long-term morbidity of these patients is in relation with the fact of being carriers of a valve prosthesis. This is the reason why in the last years some techniques have emerged to try to preserve the native aortic valve, which is re-implanted to the dacron vascular graft. They are the valve preserving techniques or *valve-sparing*, basically with two variants, the *reimplantation technique* or David procedure and the *remodeling technique* or Yacoub's surgery. In both cases, the aortic root is cut just above the aortic valve annulus and the coronary ostia; the diseased portion of aorta is removed and a collagen-coated polyester graft is used. In the modified David procedure, the sutures are placed just below the aortic valve, around the left ventricular outflow tract, and these sutures are then tied around a Hegar´s dilator to shape the bottom portion of the aort graft similar to a natural aortic root. Next, the valve is resuspendided within the graft, the aortic valve may be repaired or remodeled, and small holes are produced in the aorta graft for the coronary ostia, which are re-attached through the small holes.

In the Yacoub technique, the graft of dacron stands out imitating Valsalva's bosoms and the graft is sutured to the remnants of aortic fabric that stay close to the insertion of the veils.

David's technique is the one that more followers has inside the surgical community since theoretically it stabilizes better the valvular ring, though there are surgeons who praise the use of Yacoub's technique associated with maneuvers of stabilization to annul (anuloplastias with suture or with external rings), since this skill preserves better the functionality of the aortic root.

Those valve sparing methods can be realized either if the aortic valve is competent in the moment of the intervention or whenit is not, though in the latter case, specially if the regurgitación is very ancient, it maybe not possible to preserve the valve. This owes to the intense elongation that the leaflets can present, with very thin and friable tissue even with big fenestrations, on having been submitted to a great mechanical tension for a long time.

The immediate results of these procedures are similar to those of Bentall's surgery, though they are technically challenging, so they are used only in reference centres [9]. The long-term results also are excellent, remaining the patients free of significant degrees of aortic valve regurgitation and reoperation greater to 90% at 10 years [10].

Given these good long-term results, in many centers the valve sparing surgeries have turned into the new *gold standard* for the patients with Marfan syndrome.

2.8. Elective surgery of the descending aorta

Though the elective surgery of the descending aorta is nowadays a safe procedure, the risk of paraplegia is still present (that should be lower than 5%) depending on the group experience, on the extension of the aortic segment to be replaced and on the spinal cord protection. Since the operative risk increases in the emergency cases (dissection or rupture), and given the limitation for the use of stents in these patients, it is recommended the prophylactic replacement of the aortic segment when the diameter is > 55mm (class I recommendation, level of evidence C).

2.9. Treatment of the acute aortic complications

The treatment of the acute aortic complications in patients with MFS includes the management of the type A and B ascending aortic dissection (table 11).

Type A ascending aortic dissection

Given that the unpredictable nature of the aortic dissection in the MFS, it is necessary to educate the patients on the symptoms of the acute aortic dissection. As in the general population, the type A aortic dissection in the MFS is a emergency surgery emergency in which there must be replaced the sinus and the sufficient extension of the ascending aorta.

Type B descending aortic dissection

The type B aortic dissection represents approximately 10% of the acute aortic dissections in the MFS. Like in other patients, the medical management is initially recommended, except complications or lack of response, in which case, the surgery must be considered. The routine accomplishment of CT or MRI is recommended if the descending aorta is large or if it has been dissected after the repair of a type A dissection. In the type B chronic aortic dissection it is recommended the open surgery when, in the absence of high comorbidity, the aorta diameter is >55mm.

Type A ascending aortic dissection	**Emergency surgery**[a]
Type B descending aortic dissection	Initial management: medial treatment[a]
Type B acute aortic diseection	Surgery indicated if[b]: • Mesenteric ischaemia, limbs or branches of the abdominal aorta • Progression of the dissection • Accelerated rate of the aortic diameter • Inability to control the symptoms (pain...) or PA
Type B chronic aortic dissection	In the absence of a elevated comorbidity, open surgery if the diameter > 55 mm[a]
Endovascular therapy	The stents of the descending aorta are not indicated in patients with MFS, except in those cases with conditions prohibiting the conventional open surgery

a Class I recommendation, level of evidence B.
b Later management: betablockers, additional medication if it is necessary for the control of the arterial pressure, and follow-up with MRI or CT according to the symptoms, the diameter and the aortic growth rate.

Table 11. Treatment of the aortic complications in Marfan's syndrome

2.10. Therapy endovascular with stents

Though the experience with endoprosthesis in the type B acute or chronic aortic dissection in the MFS is limited, it has been observed that in spite of the correct implantation of the stent, with total thrombosis of the false light, the aorta continues expanding. This is the reason for which it is not recommended to use aortic stents in the MFS, except high risk for the conventional surgery. The pseudoaneurysms after aortic replacement can be an exception when it is possible to fix to the previous graft the stent to seal the point of entry of the false aneurysm as an alternative to the surgical reintervention (table 12).

Before discharge postsurgery	**CT or RMI[a]: complete aorta**
At 6 months	CT or RMI: to value diameters • Stable: annual • Progression: every 6 months
Anually	Throughout life, except unstabilization
Appearance of complications	CT or RMI at 1,3, 6 and 12 months If later stable: annual

Class IIa recommendation, level of evidence C.

a The aorta must be valued in its entirety, not only the ascending portion, since a great proportion (almost a third) of the aortic events that compromise the distal aorta happen during the follow-up of these patients.

Table 12. Follow-up after aortic surgery in Marfan's syndrome

2.11. Recommendations after the aortic intervention in the MFS

After the aortic repair, the grafts, relatively rigid, transmit tension towards contiguous territories, as the coronary arteries, the aortic arch and principal trunks, and the descending aorta, predisposing to the late development of aneurysms and dissection. These patients must support the treatment with betablockers and they must be followed by means of imaging techniques throughout life, restricting the irradiation for CT when possible (table 12).

2.12. Surgery of the valvular mitral prolapse in the SM

The mitral and tricuspid affectations constitute the most frequents cardiac finding in the MFS, though the tricuspid rarely has repercussion. The alterations of the mitral connective tissue carry to the growth in a myxoid aspect, with high content of air in its interior, though the histology and the morphology of the mitral valve in patients with MFS are different from the classic myxoid valve disease. In the MFS the leaflets, though thicker than normal, they are longer and thinner than the mixoides ones and with minor celularity.

Patients with MFS present more frequently affectation of both leaflets or the anterior one, which, together with the laxity of the valvular tissue, makes more frequent the prevalency of mitral prolapse in patients with MFS compared with the healthy population (50-80% opposite to 2,4%). In these patients the prolapse can produce moderate mitral regurgitation or major up to 25 % of the cases. It is also typical the trend to the early calcification of the mitral ring, which constitutes a minor diagnostic criteria.

In the most serious forms of the MFS, which begin in the first years of life, the mitral affectation can cause cardiac heart failure and pulmonary hypertension, with very unfavorable surgical results in younger than 2 years old, being an important reason for mortality in children with MFS. In teenagers and adults the surgical repair of the severe mitral severe regurgitation is associated with a high events free survival.

The mitral isolated surgery is infrequent, and in the majority of the occasions we carry out combined conservative procedures on the aorta and the mitral valves to avoid the anticoagulation therapy.

The extensive calcification of the mitral ring is the main contraindication for the mitral repair in the MFS. It is important to insist that not repair severe mitral regurgitation, concerns adversely the aortic hemodynamic stress and the ventricular function in the MFS.

In a similar way to the case of the aortic valve, the classic method used in patients with severe mitral regurgitation is the valve replacement, usually with mechanical prosthesis. Nevertheless, and given the high morbidity that these can produce over the years because of the thromboembolic and infectious events, the conservative mitral valve techniques are the gold standard of the mitral surgery, with long-term results similar to the ones obtained in patients without Marfan's syndrome.

Before this type of valves, the surgeon must use the whole available technical equipment and devices, being in an extensively use the PTFE's neocordae, and always associating annuloplasty rings, preferably rigidly or semi rigid. In occasions, it is used the double orifice technique, described by Alfieri, less demanding technically, though the anatomical repair methods are the ones preferred.

The immediate and long-term results are very good, with events free survival and reintervention free survival of 95 % at 10 years, specially when the early surgery is indicated.

2.13. Other cardiovascular manifestations of the SM

The expansion of the trunk of the pulmonary artery is less frequent than the aortic one, and rarely it causes dissection. In the MFS it is possible to have alterations in the atrioventricular conduction and in the ventricular repolarization (long QT, ST alterations and U waves), that might be associated with ventricular arrhythmias, but it is not clear if these changes are secondary to a primary myocardiopathie or to ventricular dilatation owed to the evolved regurgitations.

3. Conclusion

The diagnosis of Marfan syndrome is inevitably complex, due to the high variability of presentation of affected individuals, the dependence of the age in many clinical manifestations, the absence of gold standards diagnostic tests, and the wide differential diagnosis. The new Marfan syndrome diagnostic criteria are intended to facilitate a correct and early identification by professionals and improve the prognosis of these patients.

In last decades there have been significant changes in the prognosis of the Marfan syndrome. Cardiovascular management of these patients is based on three pillars aimed to increase hope and quality of life: stratification of risk, medical treatment and prophylactic aortic surgery.

Imaging techniques contribute to establish the risk of these patients and select better cases and the most appropriate time for the indication of elective surgery.

All patients should be treated early, at least with beta-blockers. Meanwhile, it will continue to evaluate new therapies aimed at stopping or even reversing the pathological changes associated with the disease.

More and more patients with Marfan syndrome will achieve more advanced stages of life, and this will mean new challenges. It will be tested the acquired knowledge and teamwork from specialized multidisciplinary units will be essential.

Author details

Miguel Angel Ramirez-Marrero*, Beatriz Perez-Villardon,
Ricardo Vivancos-Delgado and Manuel de Mora-Martin
Cardiology Department, Regional University Hospital Carlos Haya, Malaga, Spain

4. References

[1] De Paepe A, Deveraux RB, Dietz HC, Hennekam RC, Pyeritz RE (1996) Revised diagnostic criteria for the Marfan syndrome. Am J Med Genet. 62: 417-426.

[2] Loeys B, Nuytinck L, Belvaux I, De Bie S, De Paepe A (2001) Genotype and phenotype analysis of 171 patients referred for molecular study of the fibrilin-1 gene FBN1 because of suspected Marfan syndrome. Arch Intern Med. 161: 2447-2454

[3] Loeys BL, Dietz HC, Braverman AC, et al (2010) The revised Ghent nosology for the Marfan syndrome. J Med Genet. 47: 476-485.

[4] Cañadas V, Vilacosta I, Bruna I, Fuster V (2010) Marfan syndrome. Part 1: pathophysiology and diagnosis. Nat Rev Cardiol. 7: 256-265.

[5] Arslan-Kirchner M, Arbustini E, Boileau C, et al (2010) Clinical utility gene card for: Marfan syndrome type 1 and related phenotypes [FBN1]. Eur J Hum Genet. 18, doi: 10.1038/ejhg.2010.42.

[6] Botta DM (2010) Biomarcadores para el diagnóstico de aneurisma de la aorta torácica: pros. In Elefteriades JA editor. Controversias en enfermedades de la aorta. Barcelona: Elsevier Inc. pp. 17-22.

* Corresponding Author

[7] Hiratzka LF, Bakris GL, Beckman JA, et al (2010) Guidelines for the Diagnosis and Management of Patients With Thoracic Aortic Disease: Executive Summary. Circulation. 121: 1544-1579.

[8] Cañadas V, Vilacosta I, Bruna I, Fuster V (2010) Marfan syndrome. Part 2: Treatment and management of patients. Nat Rev Cardiol. 7: 266-276.

[9] Forteza A, de Diego J, Centeno J, et al (2010) Aortic valve-sparing in 37 patients with Marfan syndrome: midterm results with David operation. Ann Thorac Surg. 89:93-96.

[10] Cameron D, Alejo D, Patel N, et al (2009) Aortic root replacement in 372 Marfan patients: evolution and operative repair over 30 years. Ann Thorac Surg. 87:1344-1350.

Chapter 22

Vascular Access for Hemodialysis

Ivica Maleta, Božidar Vujičić, Iva Mesaroš Devčić and Sanjin Rački

Additional information is available at the end of the chapter

http://dx.doi.org/10.5772/48787

1. Introduction

Patients with acute kidney failure (AKF) and chronic kidney failure (CKF) require an appropriate vascular access for hemodialysis [1]. Vascular access is needed to allow blood flow through an extracorporeal circulation system with a blood pump connected to a hemodialysis monitor driving the blood through a dialysis filter (dialysator). Satisfactory levels of blood flow range between 300 and 400 mL/min.

The need for vascular access in patients with kidney failure may be temporary or permanent [2].

2. Temporary hemodialysis vascular access

Temporary hemodialysis access is required in patients scheduled to start hemodialysis treatment in several days to six months. It is mostly needed in patients with AKF of various etiology [3]. For that purpose, a hemodialysis catheter is introduced percutaneously into one of the large central veins (the internal jugular, subclavian or femoral veins) under local anesthesia. Catheters are made of different materials (polyurethane, silicon, and so on). Single-lumen catheters are used less often than double-lumen catheters of different lengths (usually 15 to 24 cm, rarely of other lengths – shorter are for pediatric use, and longer for permanent use) and 11.5-14 F in diameter. They are available in two configurations - straight and curved. A catheter is introduced after the puncture of an appropriate vein performed either in a "blinded" fashion or under ultrasound control [4]. Before the venipuncture, ultrasound should be used to visualize the relative anatomic position of the internal jugular vein and common carotid artery and determine the possible direction of puncture angle and depth in order to avoid the unwanted puncture of the common carotid artery (Figure 1).

After the catheter placement, a control chest x-ray is recommended to confirm the correct position of the catheter and exclude possible complications (Figure 2).

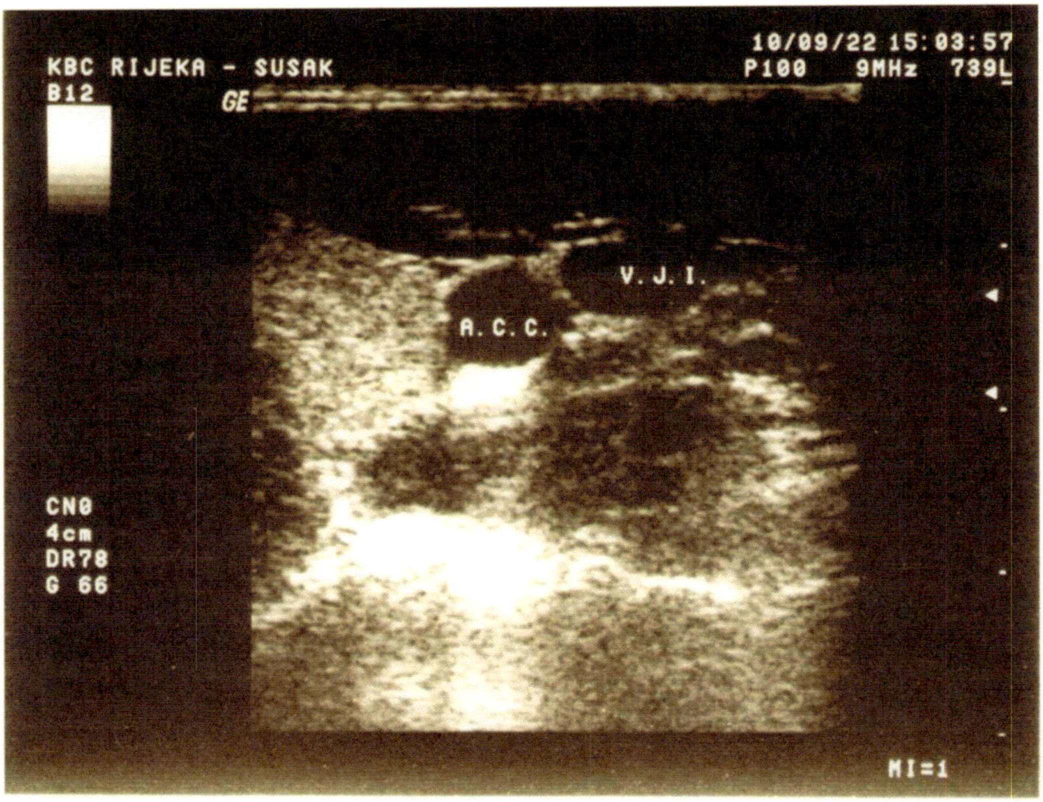

Source: Archive of the Department of Nephrology and Dialysis, University Hospital Rijeka

Figure 1. Ultrasonographic assesment in the B-mode of the internal jugular vein (V.J.I) and common carotid artery (A.C.C.).

Temporary vascular access for hemodialysis is sometimes indicated in patients with CKF stage 5, or end-stage kidney disease (ESKD), who are on regular dialysis, in cases of inadequate function of arteriovenous fistula (AV) or AV graft due to stenosis or thrombosis, and in new hemodialysis patients in whom AV fistula has not been created in a timely manner [5].

3. Permanent hemodialysis vascular access

Permanent vascular access is usually required in patients with CKF stage 4 because of permanent HD treatment [6]. For permanent vascular access, AV shunt (out of clinical use), AV fistula, AF graft or tunneled or non-tunneled hemodialysis catheters may be used. During the pre-dialysis preparation or pre-dialysis education program, the patients should be informed about possible ESKG treatment options, which include HD, peritoneal dialysis (PD), and kidney transplantation.

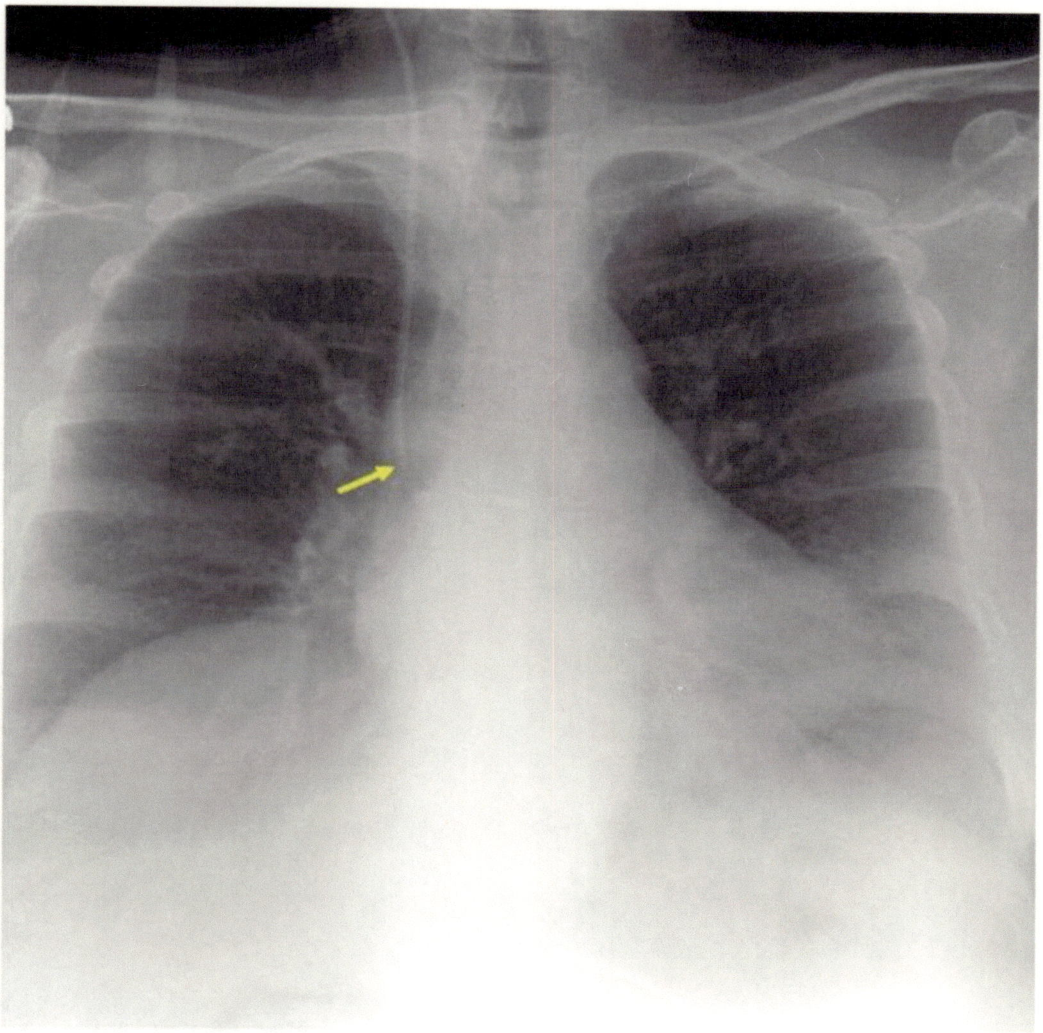

Source: Archive of the Department of Nephrology and Dialysis, University Hospital Rijeka

Figure 2. Chest radiogram showing correct position of the jugular cateter in the right atrium.

3.1. Arteriovenous shunt

External AV shunt belongs to history. It was used between 1960 and 1965, before the first AV fistula was created (Kenneth C. Apple), that is, radiocephalic (Brescia–Cimino 1966) (Figure 3).

3.2. Arteriovenous fistula

In patients on chronic hemodialysis, vascular access should be created in a timely fashion. Native AV fistula is the gold standard and the most frequently used type of vascular access in these patients [2]. After examining the patient in CKF stage 4 (GFR 30-15 mL/min/1.73 m^2), a

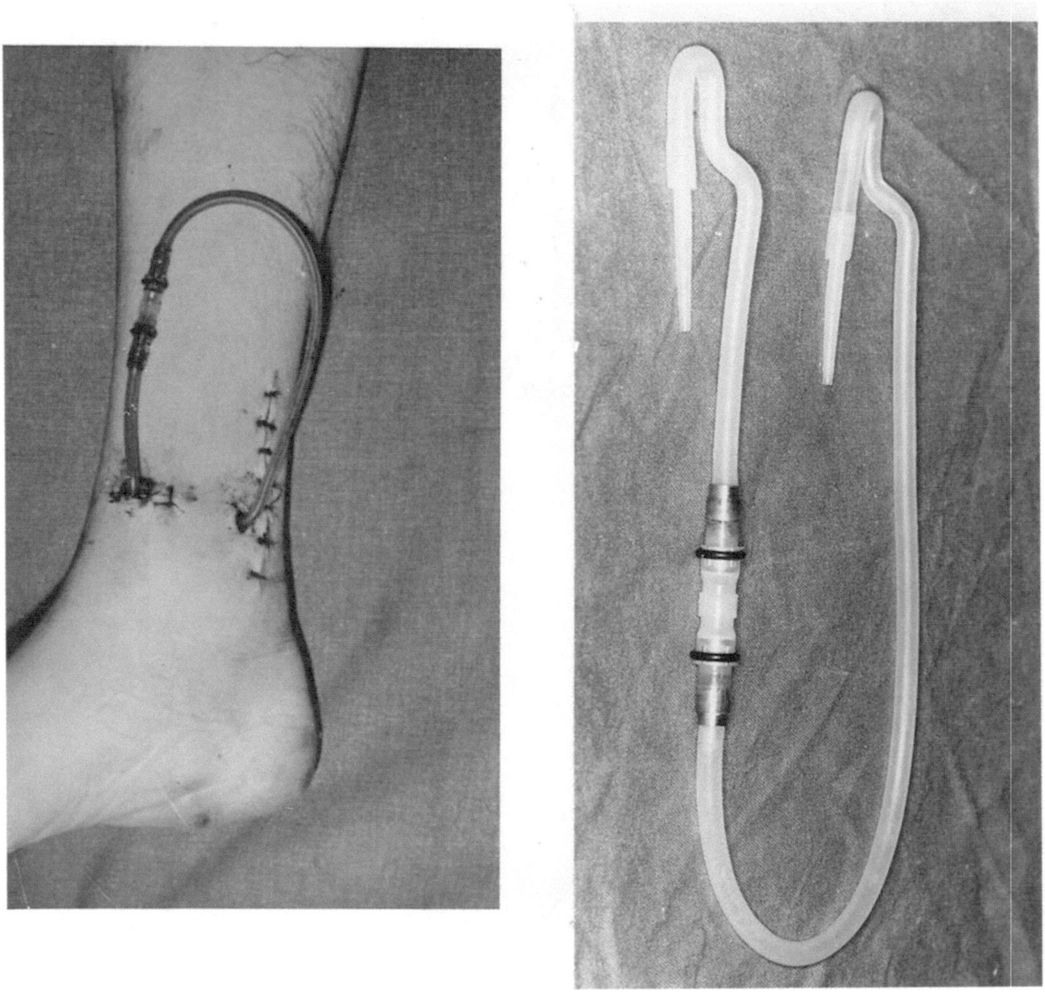

Source: Archive of the Department of Nephrology and Dialysis, University Hospital Rijeka

Figure 3. Quinton-Scribner AV sunt

vascular surgeon makes an assessment of the patient's vascular system in order to plan for the AV fistula construction. In case of progressive kidney failure and/or diabetes mellitus, AV fistula should be created earlier [7]. Before choosing the type of vascular access, peripheral blood vessels (arteries and veins) should be evaluated by clinical examination and ultrasound. If diameters and walls of the blood vessels are satisfactory, AV fistula may be created. It is usually done on the non-dominant arm between the radial artery and cephalic vein as distally as possible. AV fistula is a surgically created subcutaneous anastomosis between an artery and a vein (Figure 4) and it matures by venous dilatation and arterialisation of the vein.

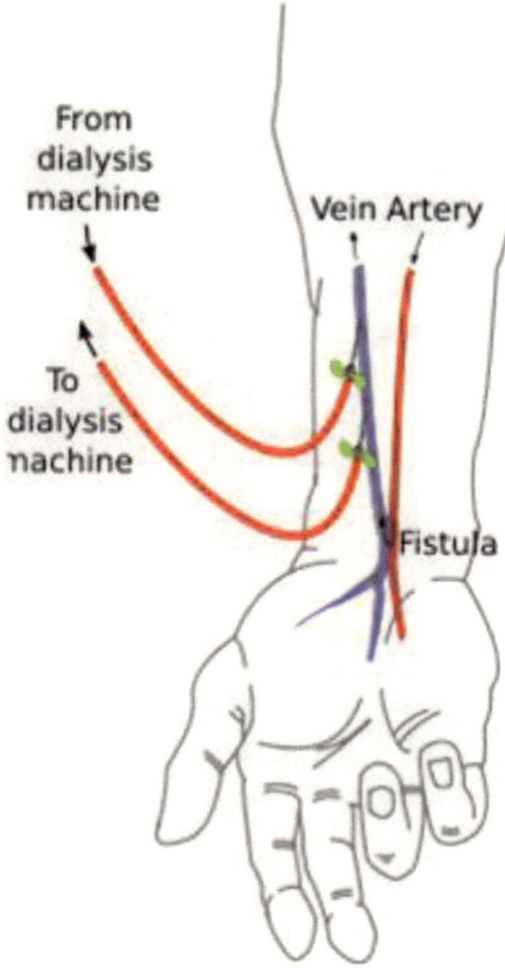

Figure 4. Typical arterivenous fistula (Brescia-Cimino)

The AV anastomosis redirects arterial blood flow into the vein, which then becomes dilated due to new hemodynamic conditions. Over time, the lumen of the vein widens, the venous blood flow increases, and the vein becomes suitable for puncture and hemodialysis usually after three to five weeks [8].

There two most common types of anastomosis. One is "side-to-side" (a standard anastomosis described by Brescia), where an artery and its neighboring vein are cut longitudinally and sewn or stapled together [9]. This type of anastomosis may lead to the venous hyperemia of the arm (Figure 5).

The other is "end-vein to side-artery" anastomosis, where the cephalic vein is completely severed, its distal part toward the hand is ligated, and the proximal part is sewn to the side of the relevant artery (Figure 6).

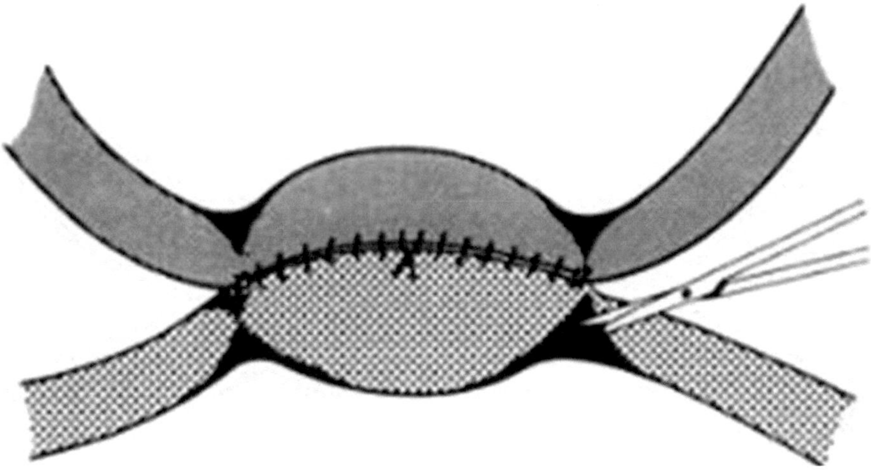

Figure 5. "Side to side" anastomosis of the AV fistula

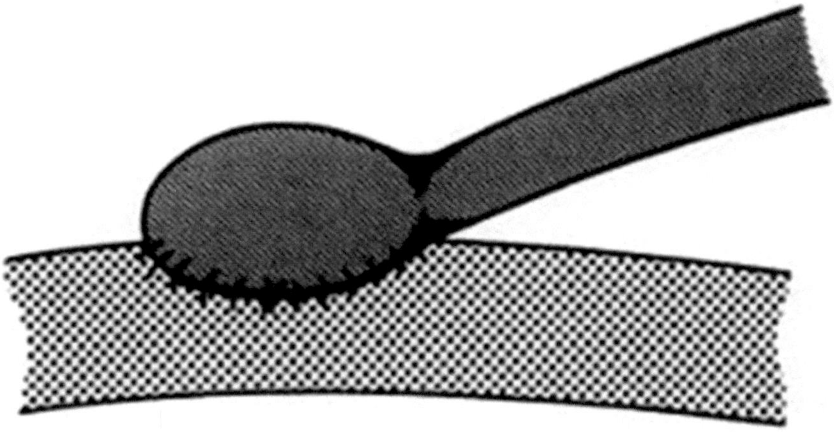

Figure 6. "End to side" anastomosis of the AV fistula

If AV fistula cannot be created at the usual site, i.e., the wrist, it may be created proximally in the middle part of the forearm or cubital fossa. The fistula may also be created between the ulnar artery and the basilic vein.

3.3. AV fistula complications

3.3.1. Thrombosis

AV fistula thrombosis is characterized by a complete cessation of blood flow through the venous part of the AF fistula proximal to the AV anastomosis due to a thrombus, which may develop in any part of the vein (from the anastomosis to the confluence of the subclavian vein into the superior vena cava). Thrombosis may be diagnosed by a standard physical examination. The characteristic sign is the absence of the typical thrill of the fistula on palpation. In some cases, the thrombus in the vein may be palpable. Arterial pulsations may be noticed distal and the absence of blood flow in the empty vein proximal to the site of thrombosis. No AV fistula bruit can be heard with a stethoscope. The findings may be confirmed by ultrasound, i.e. the thrombus may be visualized and measured by B mode ultrasound, and the absence of the circulation proximal to the thrombosis site may be confirmed by Doppler [10].

Thrombosis is the most serious complication leading to the loss of function of the fistula. It is treated surgically by thrombectomy or via endovascular route.

3.3.2. Stenosis

Stenosis is the most frequent complication. It is caused by the luminal narrowing of the vein. Although it may develop in any part of the vein, it is usually found close to the AV anastomosis.

Stenosis leads to AV fistula malfunction characterized by a reduced blood flow through the arterial segment of the fistula in 50% of the cases. Reduced and inadequate blood flow through the AV fistula is registered by the blood pump, which results in inadequate dialysis doses [11]. Stenosis may be suspected if blood flow through a particular segment of the vein

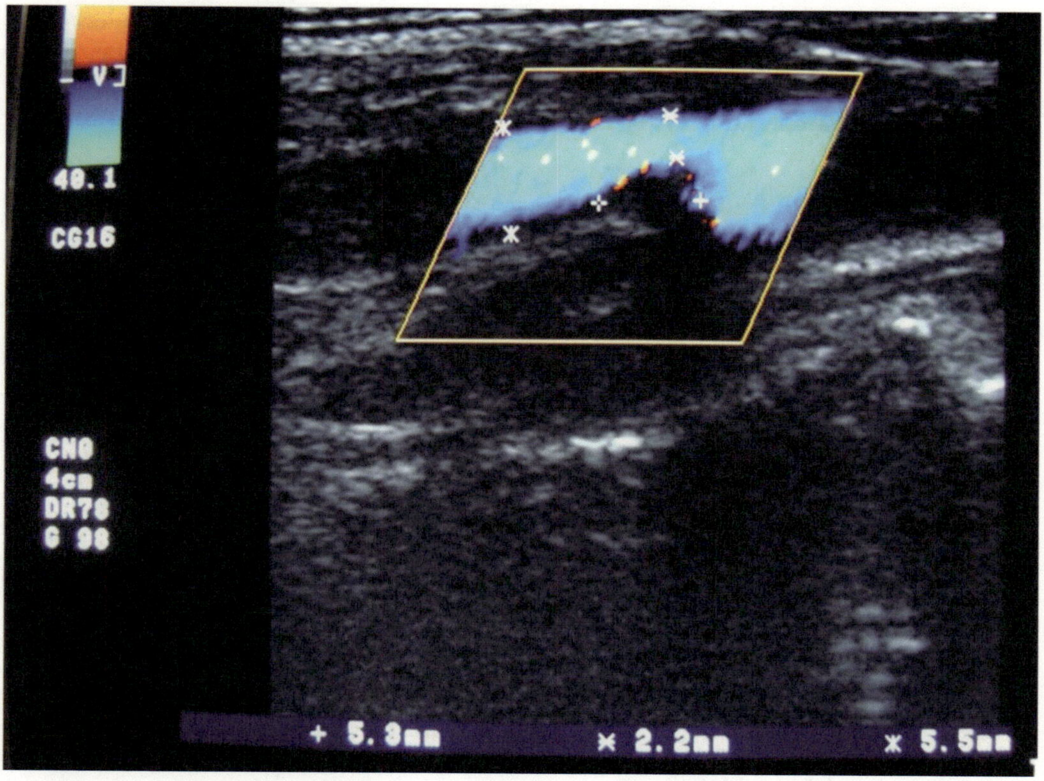

Source: Archive of the Department of Nephrology and Dialysis, University Hospital Rijeka

Figure 7. Stenosos of the AV fistula as shown using ultrasonography in the B-mode with Doppler visualisation of the missing blood flow on the stenosis site.

is reduced. Frequently, a high-pitched bruit can be heard on auscultation. The diagnosis may be confirmed by ultrasound and phlebography. Priority should be given to B mode ultrasound and Doppler sonography, because these are non-invasive techniques that can precisely determine the location and degree of stenosis (Figure 7).

These methods may be used to determine the length of stenosis and measure the diameter of the vein distal and proximal to the stenotic site. In addition, Doppler can detect higher blood flow velocity at the stenotic site [12]. Depending on the findings, a new anastomosis may be created proximal to the stenosis or a stent may be placed at the site of stenosis by a percutaneous intervention. If stenosis develops in the large veins of the neck (usually the subclavian vein), it leads to the edema of the entire arm and pronounced collateral venous blood flow through the subcutaneous veins. HD is complicated by high percentage of blood recirculation, difficult puncture of the vessel, and high venous resistance. The diagnosis of subclavian stenosis is made on the basis of physical and phlebographic findings; ultrasound may not produce reliable results. This complication is managed by percutaneous dilatation and stenting [13].

3.3.3. Aneurysm

Aneurysm is defined as a localized dilation of the vein, usually proximal to the site of stenosis where the pressure on the vessel wall is increased due to blood turbulence and results in the aneurysmal widening of the vein [14]. Turbulent blood flow in aneurysmal dilatation often leads to AV fistula thrombosis. Aneurysms are diagnosed by inspection, palpation, and ultrasound (Figure 8).

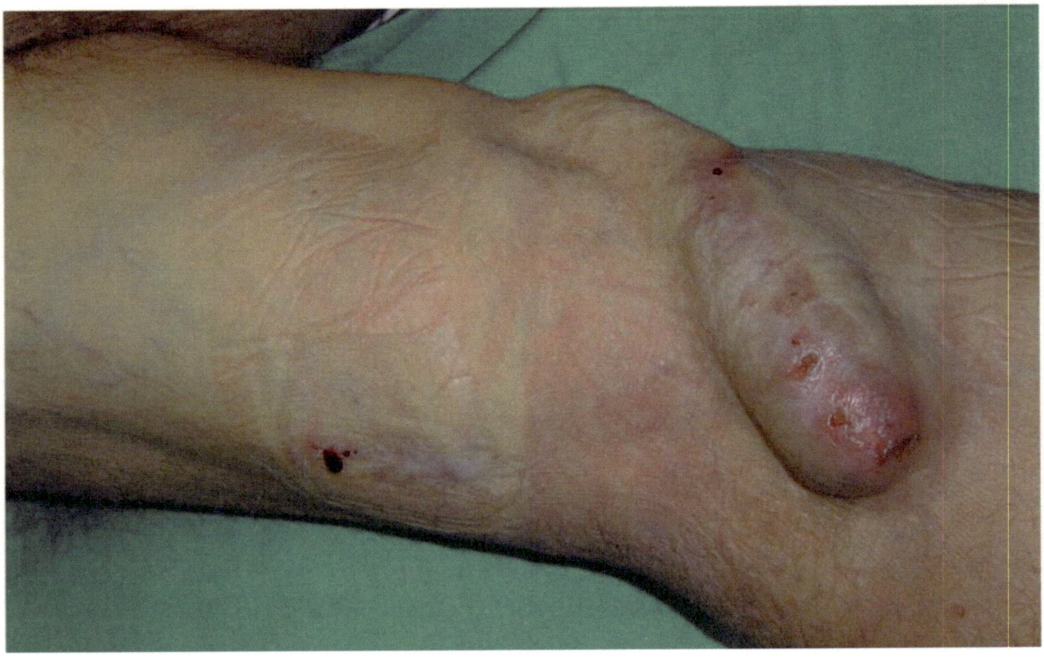

Source: Archive of the Department of Nephrology and Dialysis, University Hospital Rijeka

Figure 8. Aneurismatic enlargment of the AV fistula.

3.3.4. *Pseudoaneurysm*

As opposed to aneurysm, pseudoaneurysm does not contain vessel wall. It expands into the surrounding soft tissue after the destruction of the vessel wall, usually after a careless puncture of the artery or graft. Pseudoaneurysms more often develop as complications of synthetic AV grafts than native fistulas and are diagnosed by ultrasound.

3.3.5. *Hematoma*

Hematoma most often develops between the venipuncture site and the skin due to inadequate and short compression of the venipuncture site after a dialysis session. It may cause external compression of a segment of a blood vessel and create stenosis. Hematoma is diagnosed by inspection and ultrasound examination (Figure 9).

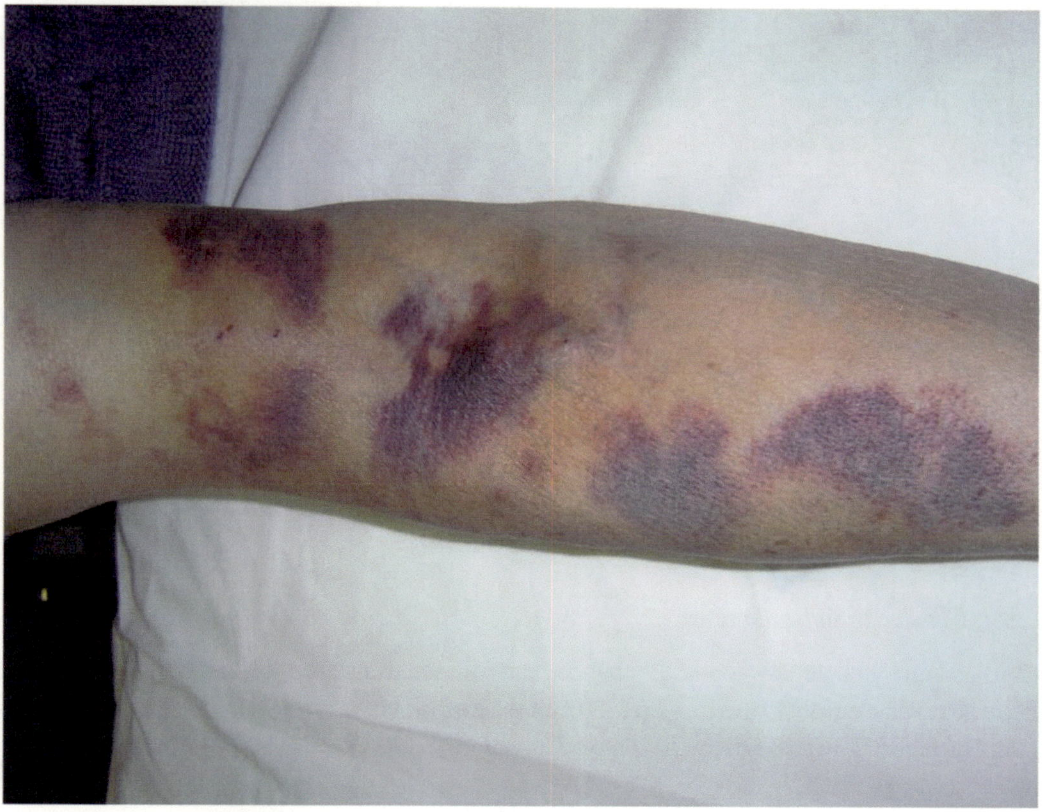

Source: Archive of the Department of Nephrology and Dialysis, University Hospital Rijeka

Figure 9. Hematom on the puncture sites of the AV fistula.

3.3.6. *Peripheral ischemia*

Since blood flow from the radial artery to the palmar arch and fingers is decreased after the creation of an AV fistula, vascular access "steal syndrome" may develop, resulting in ischemia of the fingers. The thumb, index finger, and middle finger, which are supplied by the radial artery, are most often affected. The syndrome develops mostly in patients with diabetes mellitus and changes on the peripheral arteries (intimal hyperplasia, fibrosis, calcifying plaques, stenoses) due to diabetic angiopathy and reduced peripheral arterial circulation. Therefore, antecubital AV fistulae should be avoided in patients with diabetes mellitus [15]. Patients often complain of cold fingers and pain and they may develop trophic changes on the acral parts, including gangrene (Figure 10).

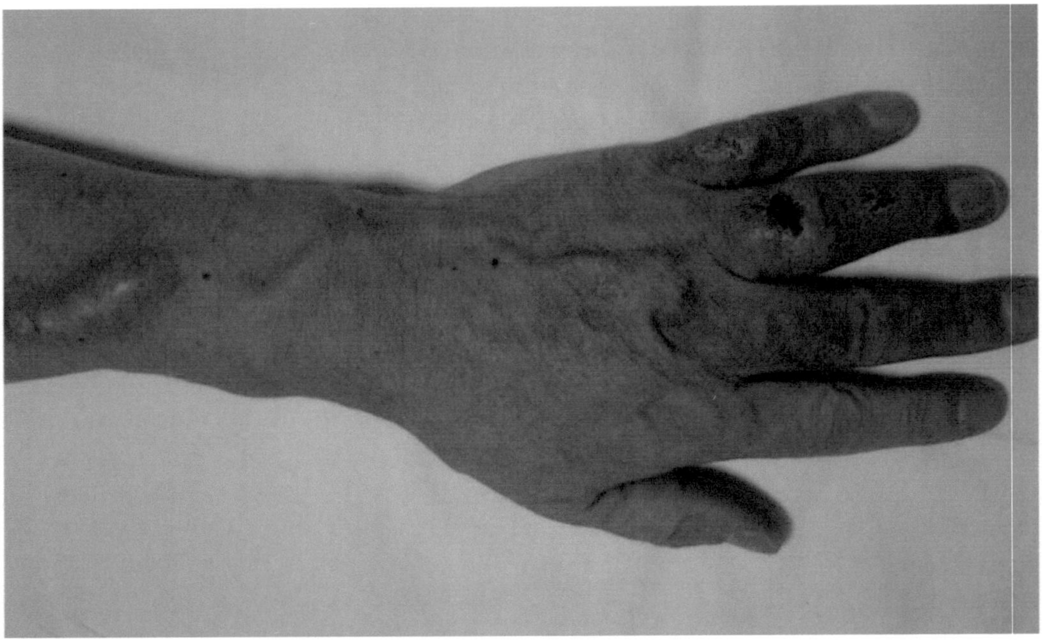

Source: Archive of the Department of Nephrology and Dialysis, University Hospital Rijeka

Figure 10. Pereipheral ishemia caused by "steal syndrome" as a consequence of the insufficient blood flow in the distal part of the arm after AV fistula anastomosis.

3.3.7. Cardiac complications

Cardiac patients may develop additional cardiac complications after the creation of AF fistula, because cardiac output is increased (20–50% of the cardiac volume flows through an AV fistula) [16]. The blood flow through the AV fistula, depending on its location, is 600 - 2000 mL/min.

3.3.8. Infection

Infections most often occur after a non-sterile puncture of AV fistula and are characterized by redness and edema of the skin over the fistula. Due to the inflammatory changes, the blood vessel was may be weakened and rupture, especially if the changes affect the aneurysm.

These complications are treated medically with antibiotics or surgically in case of imminent rupture (Figure 11) [17].

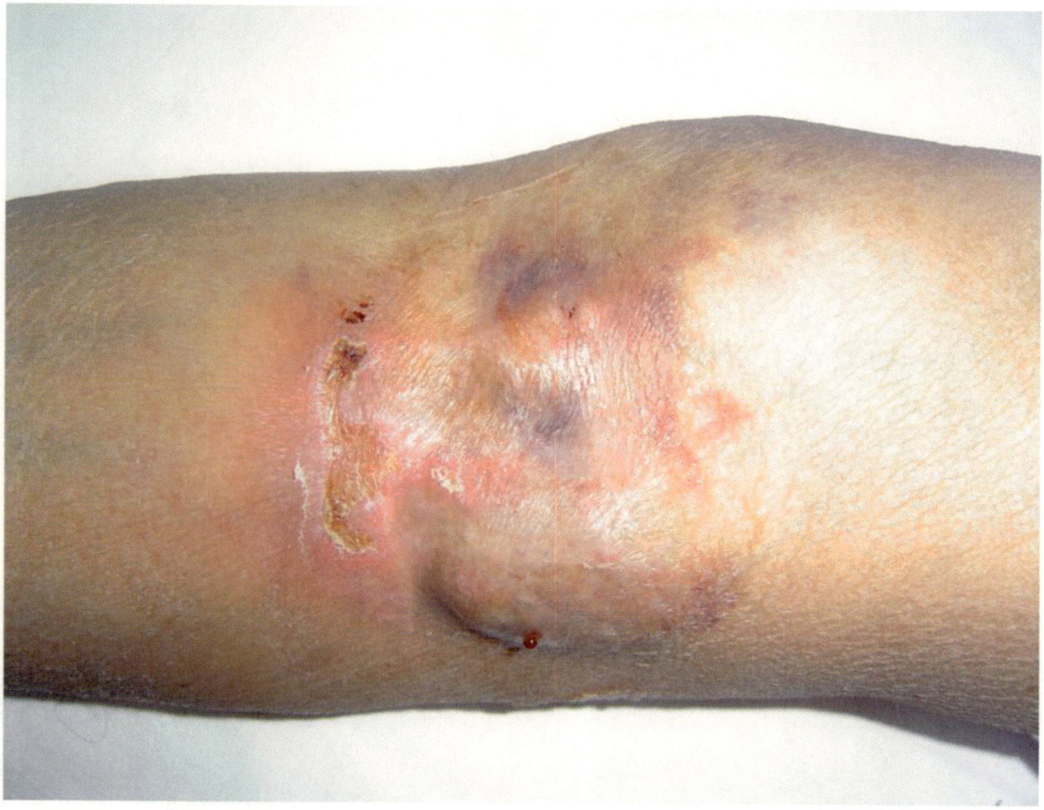

Source: Archive of the Department of Nephrology and Dialysis, University Hospital Rijeka

Figure 11. Infection of the AV fistula. Serotic extravasation is present on the puncture site. Crusta formations are sign of the active inflammatory process.

3.4. Arteriovenous graft

If native AV fistula cannot be created due to inadequate blood vessels (poorly developed veins or arterial insufficiency), a synthetic blood vessel may be implanted between the artery and the vein. Such an implanted vessel is called AV graft. A graft is made of biocompatible material, such as polyesther (Dacron), expanded polytetrafluoroethylene (Goretex) or polyurethane (Vectra), in order to avoid allergic reactions, thrombosis, and infection. It is implanted subcutaneously to be available for puncture, mostly on the upper arm between the brachial artery and axillary vein and less often on the forearm or thigh (Figure 12) [20].

3.4.1. Complications

AV graft complications are similar to those described for native AV fistulas and include thrombosis, stenosis, pseudoaneurysm, and infections and are managed in a similar way.

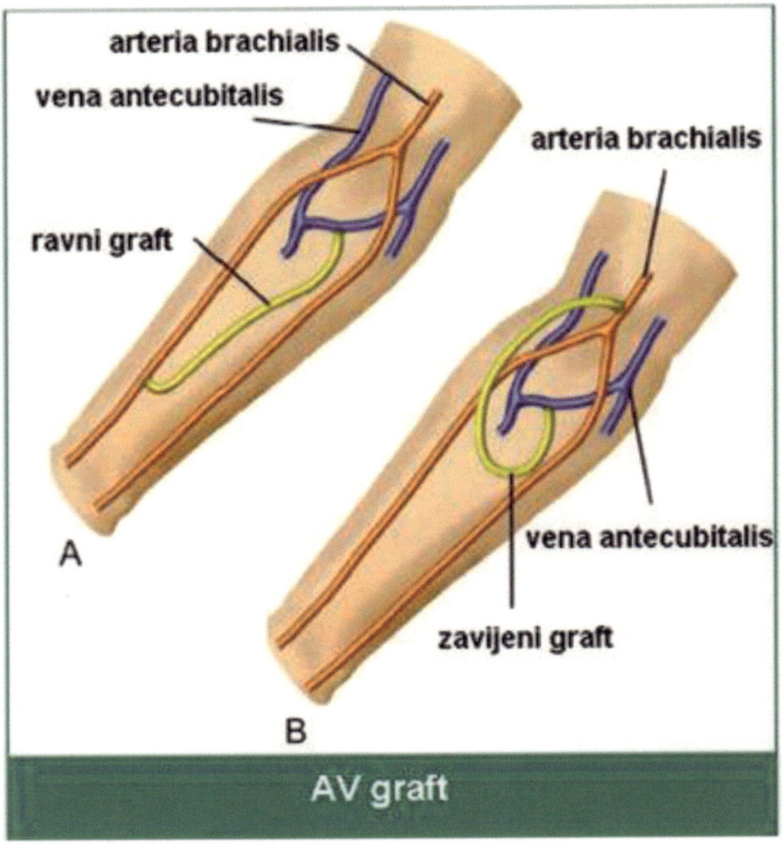

Figure 12. Schematic view of the arteriovenous graft

3.5. Tunneled central venous catheters

In some elderly patients with chronic heart failure syndrome and inadequate peripheral blood vessels, it is not possible to create an AV fistula or implant a synthetic AV graft. Therefore, a permanent tunneled central venous catheter (CVC) with a subcutaneous synthetic cuff is often implanted in these patients [19]. Connective tissue grows into the cuff and anchors the catheter in place, at the same time reducing the possibility of infection (Figure 13).

This approach is used in the treatment of 10–15% patients in the chronic HD program. The patients should be informed about the tunneled CVC-associated complications, which are more frequent than those associated with AV fistulas or AV grafts (thrombosis, bacteremia, sepsis). Double-lumen catheters are introduced through large veins (the internal jugular, subclavian or femoral veins) and connected via tubing with the blood pump, which ensures a sufficient blood flow (300 to 400 mL/min) and is controlled via an HD monitor. The most desirable site for tunneled CVC placement is the right internal jugular vein. Alternative sites include the external jugular vein, subclavian vein, femoral vein, and inferior vena cava. If the vascular access is temporary, it should not be placed on the same side of the body where

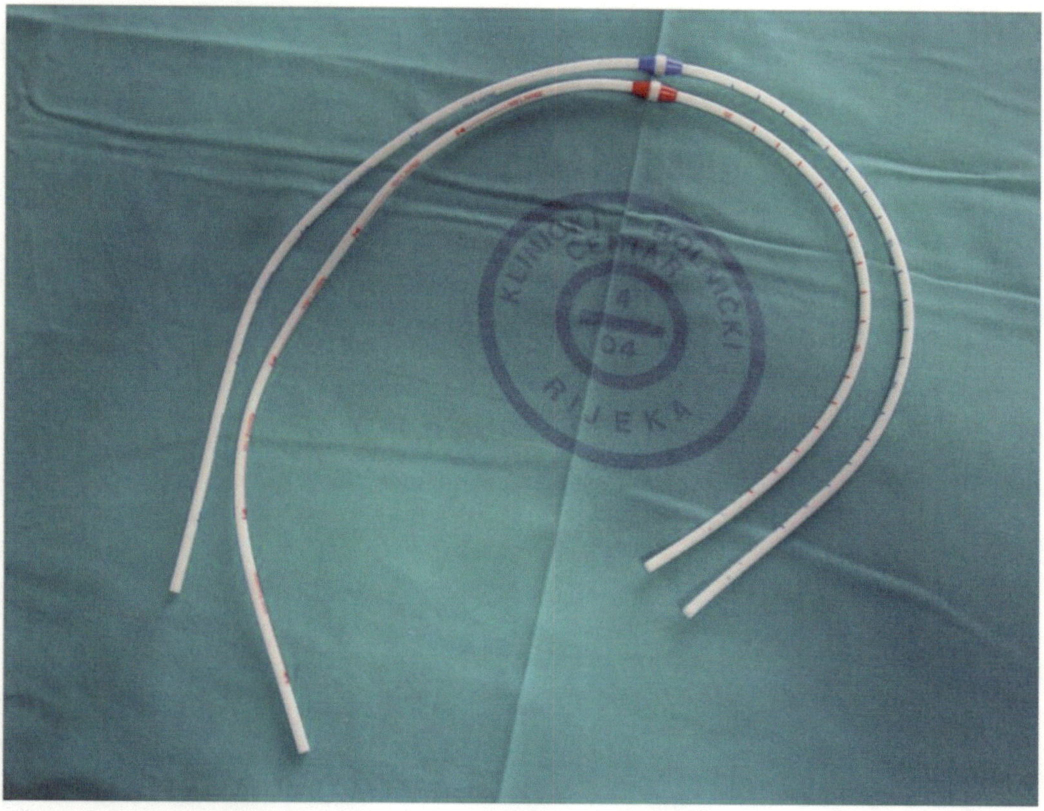

Source: Archive of the Department of Nephrology and Dialysis, University Hospital Rijeka

Figure 13. Tunneled catheter for hemodialysis, Tesio model. Two separate lumen are suitable for better blood flow and less recirculation.

the creation of fistula is planned. The subclavian vein should be used only if jugular access is not possible. The catheter is inserted using the modified Seldinger technique under ultrasound control. The jugular access is located superior and lateral to the sternal end of the clavicle. After a successful placement, the position of tunneled CVC should be confirmed by x-ray. There are several advantages of tunneled CVC. It may be used immediately after placement, it does not require venipuncture (lower risk of heparin-associated bleeding), and possible thrombotic complications at the access site are easier to manage. Disadvantages of a tunneled CVC include lower blood flow through the dialyzer, possible complications during catheter placement, higher risk of infection, stenosis of the subclavian vein, and cosmetic problems [2].

3.5.1. Complications

Complications related to tunneled hemodialysis catheters may be early and late. Early complications are usually mild, such as hematoma at the puncture site, puncture of the common carotid artery, inadequate catheter position (most often due to stenosis of the bachiocephalic vein), hoarseness, and paresthesia of the limb on the puncture side due to anesthetic infiltration to the innervating area of the recurrent nerve and brachiocephalic nerve plexus. More severe complications include pneumothorax, hemothorax, and hemopericardium with an imminent cardiac tamponade. Late complications include thrombosis, infection (usually in the subcutaneous tunnel) resulting in bacteremia and, in severe cases, sepsa (Figure 14) [20].

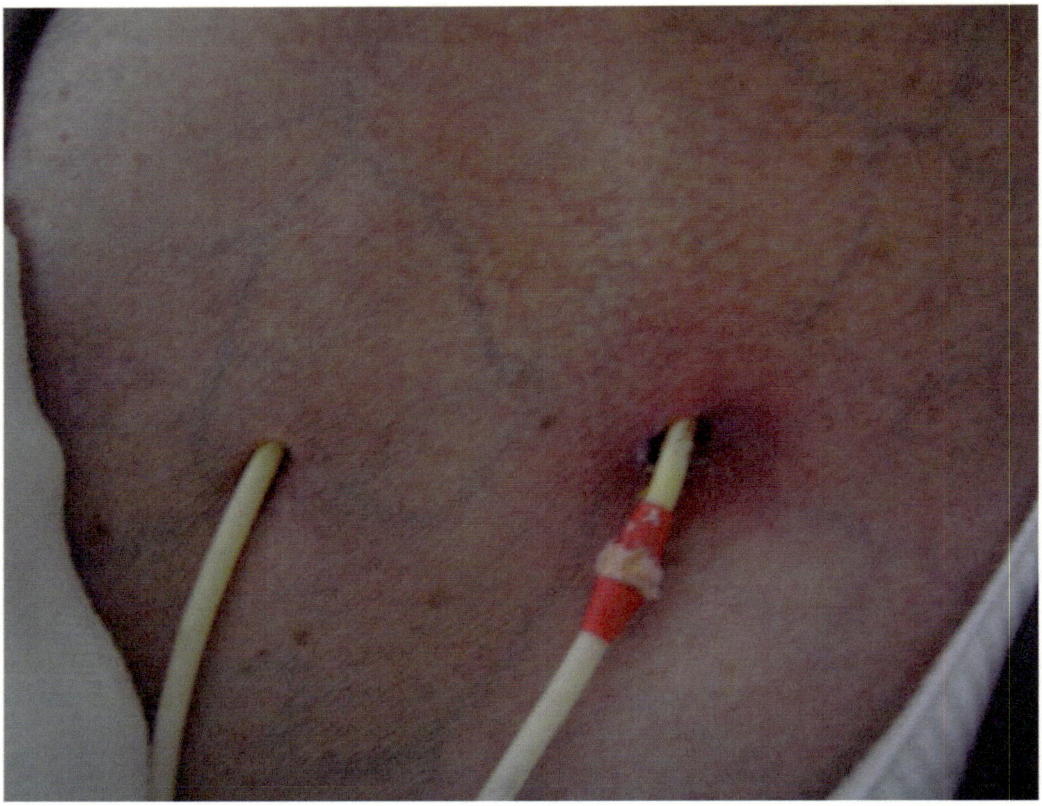

Source: Archive of the Department of Nephrology and Dialysis, University Hospital Rijeka

Figure 14. Infection of the exit-site of the catheter lumen. Complete protrusion of the cuff.

3.5.2. Thrombosis

Thrombosis leads to inadequate blood flow through the catheter. It is a relatively frequent complication in dialysis patients with intravenous catheters. Reduced blood flow reduces the delivered dialysis dose. Tunneled catheters normally have a blood flow rate of >300 mL/min. If the blood flow rate is lower, incomplete obstruction caused by endoluminal fibrin deposits may be suspected. In case of complete obstruction, dialysis is not possible; therefore, the non-functional catheter should be replaced by a new one via new subcutaneous tunnel [21].

Fibrinolytic agents (urokinase, tissue plasminogen activator – tPA) may be administered over 3-6 hours. In case of incomplete obstruction, instillation of antithrombotic solutions (standard heparin, low-molecular-weight heparin, sodium citrate) into the lumen of the catheter is recommended [22, 23].

Sodium nitrate has recently been used more often than standard heparin for the prevention of hemodialysis catheter infection and thrombosis. As a polysaccharide, heparin attracts microbes and contributes to the development of biofilm on catheter surfaces. If it enters the systemic circulation, it increases the risk of bleeding. Sodium citrate prevents possible infection by "binding" calcium needed for bacterial growth and prevents the formation of thrombus by blocking calcium. If it enters the systemic circulation, it has no systemic effect because it is rapidly metabolized in the liver and muscle tissue to neutral bicarbonates. The observed adverse reactions (occurring in approximately 10% of the patients) are transitory and include metallic taste and numbness in the fingers and toes while the lumen of the catheter is being filled with the solution. These reactions may be avoided it the volume of the administered solution is tapered in 0.1 ml decrements in each subsequent dialysis session until the symptoms resolve. The concentrations of sodium citrate that are in use include 23%, 30% i 46.7% solutions [24, 25].

3.5.3. *Infection*

Catheter-associated infections are the most frequent cause of illness in patients with this type of vascular access. Diagnosis is not difficult to make. It is based on increased body temperature and pain and redness around the catheter exit site or subcutaneous tunnel often accompanied by discharge. The diagnosis of silent endoluminal contamination is more difficult to make, especially if the external signs of inflammation are absent. It that case, positive hemoculture or positive bacterial culture from intraluminal thrombus helps the diagnosis.

The most common causative agents (80%) include Gram-positive bacteria (Staphylococcus epidermidis, Staphyloccus aureus), whereas Gram-negative bacteria and fungi (Enterococcus, Escherichia coli, Pseudomonas, Candida species) are less common (20%). Specific blood markers (leukocytosis, increased C-reactive protein, increased procalcitonin) may help in the diagnosis of catheter-associated bacterial infection [26].

Management of known catheter-associated infection

a. In case of the catheter exit site or tunnel infection with negative hemoculture, toilet of the exit or tunnel should be performed. Exit swabs should be taken for microbiological analysis and a two-week antibiogram-based antibiotic therapy should be administered. Since Gram-positive bacteria are the causative agents in 80% of the cases, treatment with antibiotics to which Gram-positive bacteria are susceptible may be introduced immediately and maintained until the microbiological results become available.
b. In case of positive hemoculture without any clinical signs of the catheter exit site or tunnel infection, it is advisable to replace the catheter and introduce antibiotic prophylaxis based on the microbial susceptibility test results over the next 4 weeks.
c. In case of the catheter exit site or tunnel infection and positive hemoculture, the catheter should be immediately removed and antimicrobial treatment should be administered over the next 4 weeks to decrease the risk of catheter-associated sepsis and possible

development of metastatic infection, such as endocarditis, osteomyelitis, and vertebral abscess, which may sometimes develop even after the catheter has been removed

3.5.4. *Infection prevention*

Strict hygienic measures during dialysis sessions, the use of sodium citrate solution for the maintenance of the catheter patency between dialysis sessions due to its antithrombotic and antiseptic characteristics, and preventive application of protective antimicrobial ointment on the skin around the catheter exit site will reduce the risk of bacteremia [28].

4. Conclusion

Adequate patient preparation for hemodialysis includes AV fistula construction in time. AV fistula is the most appropriate type of vascular access for hemodialysis with less complication in comparison to other vascular access types. Use of endovenous catheters is sometimes needed, but should be limited only for emergency or in the patients with exhausted vessels for AV fistula or AV graft construction.

Author details

Ivica Maleta, Božidar Vujičić* and Sanjin Rački
Department of Nephrology and Dialysis, University Hospital Rijeka, Rijeka, Croatia

Iva Mesaroš Devčić
Polyclinic for Hemodialysis "Fresenius Medical Care", Delnice, Croatia

5. References

[1] Ortega T, Ortega F, Diaz-Corte C, Rebollo P, Ma Baltar J, Alvarez-Grande J (2005) The timely construction of arteriovenous fistula: a key to reducing morbidity and mortality and to improving cost management. Nephrol. dial. transplant. 20:598-603.

[2] NKF-K/DOQUI Clinical Practice Qudelines for Vascular Access: Update (2000) Am j. kidney dis. 37:137-181.

[3] Weijmer MA, ter Wee PM (2004) Temporary Vascular Access for Hemodialysis reatment. In: Ronco C, Levin NW, editors. Hemodialysis Vascular Access and Peritoneal Dialysis Access. Contrib. nephrol. Basel: Karger. pp. 94-111.

[4] Ash SR (2002) The evolution and function of central venous catethers for dialysis. Semin.dial. 14:416-424.

[5] Mickley V (2002) Central venous catheters: Many questions, few answers. Nephrol. dial. transplant.17:1368-1373.

[6] Pisoni LR (2002) Vascular Access use and outcomes: Results from DOPPS. Contrib. nephrol. 137:13-19.

---

* Corresponding Author

[7] Ryner HC, Pisoni RL, Gillespie BW (2003) Creation, cannulation and survival of arteriovenous fistulae: data from DOPPS. Kidney int. 63:323.

[8] Brunori G, Ravani P, Mandolfo S, Imbasciati E, Malberti F, Cancarini G (2005) Fistula maturation: doesn't time matter at all? Nephrol. dial. transplant. 20:684-687.

[9] Corpataux JM, Haesler E, Silacci P, Ris HB, Hayoz D (2002) Low-pressure enviroment and remodelling of the forearm vein in Brescia-Cimino vascular access. Neprol. dial. transplant. 17:1057-1062.

[10] Schwab SJ, Raymond JR, Saeed M, Newman GE, Dennis PA, Bollinger RR (1989) Prevention of hemodialysis fistula thrombosis. Early detection of venous stenoses. Kidney int. 36:707-711.

[11] Schwab SJ, Oliver MJ, Suhocki P, McCann R (2001) Hemodialysis arteriovenous access: Detection of stenosis and response to treatment by vascular access blood flow. Kidney int. 59:358-362.

[12] Bay WH, Henry ML, Lazarus JM, Lew NL, Ling J, Lowrie EG (1998) Predicting hemodialysis access failure with color flow Doppler ultrasound. Am. j. nephrol. 18:296-304.

[13] Turmel-Rodrigues L, Pengloan J, Rodrigue H, Brillet G, Lataste A, Pierre D et al. (2000) Treatment of failed native arteriovenous fistulae for hemodialysisi by interventional radiology. Kidney int. 57:1124-1140.

[14] Kronung G (1984) Plastic deformation of Cimino fistula by repeated puncture. Dial. transplant 13:635-638.

[15] Miles AM (2000) Upper limb ischaemia after vascular access surgery. Diferential diagnosis and management. Semin. dial. 13:312-315.

[16] Foley RN (2003) Clinical epidemiology of cardiac disease in dialysis patients: Left ventricular hyperthrophy, ischaemic heart disease, and cardiac failure. Semin. dial. 16:111-117.

[17] Dhingra RK, Young EW, Hulbert-Shearon TE, Leavey SF, Port FK (2001) Type of vascular access and mortality in U.S. hemodialysisi patients. Kidney int. 60:1443-1451.

[18] Miller PE, Carlton D, Deierhoi MH, Redden DT, Allon M (2000) Natural history of arteriovenous grafts in hemodialysis patients. Am. j. kidney dis. 36:68-74.

[19] O'Dwyer H, Fotheringham T, O'Kelly P, Doyle S, Haslam P, McGrath F et al. (2005) A prospective comparison of two types of tunneled hemodialysis catheters: The Ash Split versus Perm Cath. Cardiovascular intervent. radiol. 28:23-29.

[20] Capdevila JA, Planes AM, Palomar M, Gasser I, Almirante B, Pahissa A et al. (1992) Value of differential quantitative blood cultures in the diagnosis of catheter related sepsis. Eur j. clin. microbiol. infect. dis. 11:403-407.

[21] McCann M, Moore ZE (2010) Interventions for preventing infectious complications in haemodialysis patients with central venous catheters. Cochrane database syst. rev. 20;(1):CD006894

[22] Rockall AG, Harris A, Wetton CW, Taube D, Gedroyc W, Al-Kutoubi MA (1997) Stripping of failing haemodialysis catheters using the Ampltaz gooseneck snare. Clin. radiol. 52: 616–620.

[23] Merport M, Murphy TP, Egglin TK, Dubel GJ (2000) Fibrin sheath stripping versus catheter exchange for the treatment of failed tunneled hemodialysis catheters: randomized clinical trial. J. vasc. interv. radiol. 11: 1115–1120.

[24] Ash SA, Mankus RA, Sutton M (2000) Concentrated Sodium Citrate (23%) for Catheter Lock. Hemodialysis int. 4: 22-31.

[25] Wijmer MC, Debets-Ossenkopp YJ, Van de Vondervoort FJ, Ter Wee PM (2002) Superior antimicrobial activity of trisodium citrate over heparin for catheter locking. Nephrol. dial. transplant. 17:2189-2195.

[26] Tordoir J, Canaud B, Haage P, Konner K, Basci A, Fouque D et al. (2007) EBPG on Vascular Access. Nephrol. dial. Transplant. 22: 88-117.

Chapter 23

Atrial Septal Aneurysm

Soh Hosoba, Tohru Asai and Tomoaki Suzuki

Additional information is available at the end of the chapter

http://dx.doi.org/10.5772/48407

1. Introduction

ASA is a rare entity incidentally diagnosed during conventional transthoracic echocardiography (TTE). It is defined as the presence of redundant and mobile interatrial septal tissue extending to at least 15 mm during the cardiorespiratory cycle. The incidence of ASA has been reported at about 2% in patients undergoing TTE [1]. Patent foramen ovale (PFO) and ASA have been cited as potential risk factors for cryptogenic stroke. For example, ASA was observed in 7.9% of patients with a history of possible embolic stroke. Most patients with previous cerebral ischemic events and ASA also have an interatrial shunt, usually via PFO. Interatrial shunt has been reported in 56-78% of patients with ASA [2]. To our knowledge, there have been few reports of surgical intervention in ASA, for which the surgical indications are not yet defined. We describe herein two cases of surgical repair of giant ASA.

2. Case report 1

A 59-year-old Asian female referred to our surgical team was admitted to our hospital for investigation of ASA after complaining of frequent palpitations starting eight years previously. ASA had been confirmed two years earlier in an examination for palpitation, to which the patient was very sensitive, making frequent visits to the emergency department. The arrhythmia consisted of paroxysmal atrial fibrillation (AF), which was refractory to antiarrhythmic medication. The medication did not include any anticoagulant or antiplatelet agents. Physical examination was normal. Auscultation detected no murmurs, rubs, or gallops, but a split S1 was noted. Laboratory data on admission were within normal limits except for slightly elevated liver enzyme, possibly due to chronic hepatitis C. Initial EKG showed no abnormality. Chest radiograph demonstrated a cardiothoracic ratio of 0.50 and no remarkable findings. TTE revealed a giant ASA with mobility into the right atrium and nearly prolapsing into the tricuspid orifice (Figure 1). It also showed a mildly dilated right ventricle with no valvular dysfunction. Right ventricular systolic pressure was calculated to be 43 mm Hg. Chest computed tomography (CT) with contrast dye showed 47×22 mm of protruding tissue at the site of the atrial septum. Transesophageal echocardiogram demonstrated PFO at a site close to the superior vena cava and ascending aorta. In view of the enlarged right ventricle and paroxysmal AF, in addition to the high risk of stroke, surgical repair was recommended and performed.

The surgical approach was through medial sternotomy. Cardiopulmonary bypass was established and bilateral pulmonary vein isolation was performed with a bipolar radiofrequency device. Right atriotomy was then carried out. The aneurysm lay next to the fossa ovalis, enabling detection of PFO (Figure 2). The aneurysm in the interatrial septum was removed, a right atrium maze procedure was performed, and the defect was closed with a 4-0 polypropylene running suture.

The patient tolerated surgery very well and had an uneventful postoperative recovery without occasional paroxysmal AF. A postoperative MRI was performed, but no shunt flow was detected. TTE showed the same result. The patient was discharged uneventfully after surgery and remains symptom-free and in good health at two years postoperatively.

Macroscopically, the mass consisted of a thin protrusion of the atrial septum. The histological results from the septum showed a degenerative cardiac muscle with fibrosis. There was no evidence of atherosclerosis, specific inflammation, or tumorous lesion.

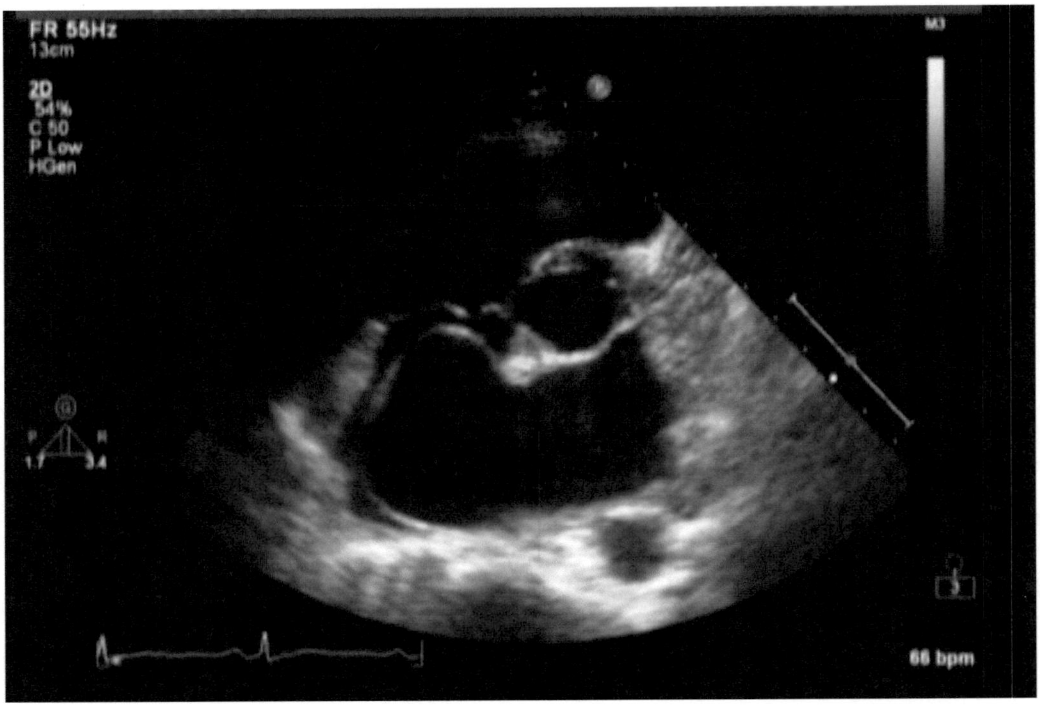

Figure 1. Giant atrial septal aneurysm (47×23 mm) with mobility into the right atrium nearly prolapsing into the tricuspid orifice

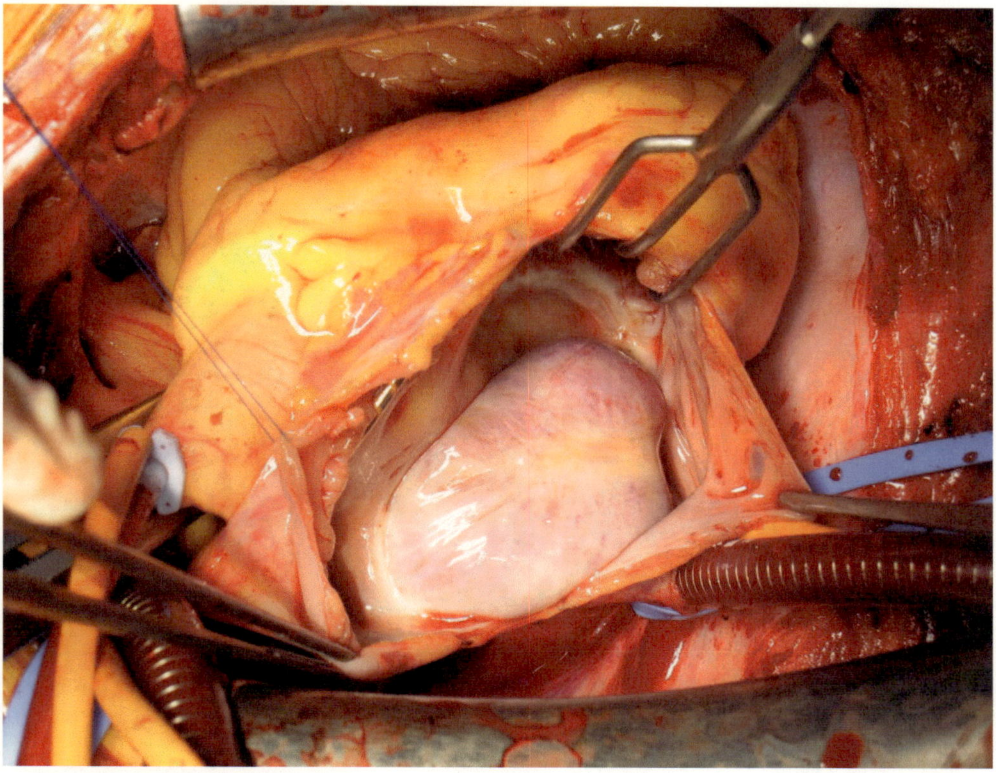

Figure 2. Intraoperative picture showing 50×25 mm of protruding tissue at the site of the atrial septum

3. Case report 2

A 37-year-old Asian woman with a 10-month history of general malaise and dyspnea was referred to our division. The patient had been well until a month earlier, when she began to have episodes of chest oppression. Transthoracic echocardiography showed almost normal wall motion without valvular dysfunction apart from the unusual feature of atrial septal defect (ASD) (Figure 3). It showed the atrial septum extending into right atrium and multidirectional right to left shunt flow using the color Doppler image. The ejection fraction was 64% and the shunt ratio was 50% (Qp/Qs=2.0). The patient was referred to our surgical team as a case of ASD.

The patient underwent an ASD closure. Following medial sternotomy, cardiopulmonary bypass was established. Right atriotomy was then carried out. The defect appeared to resemble ASD secundum, but protruded as seen in ASA had two large cribriform holes and numerous small pinholes (Figure 4). The aneurysm in the interatrial septum was removed and the defect was closed with a 4-0 polypropylene running suture.

The patient tolerated surgery very well and had an uneventful postoperative recovery without symptoms. The patient was discharged uneventfully after surgery and remains symptom-free and in good health at 12 months postoperatively.

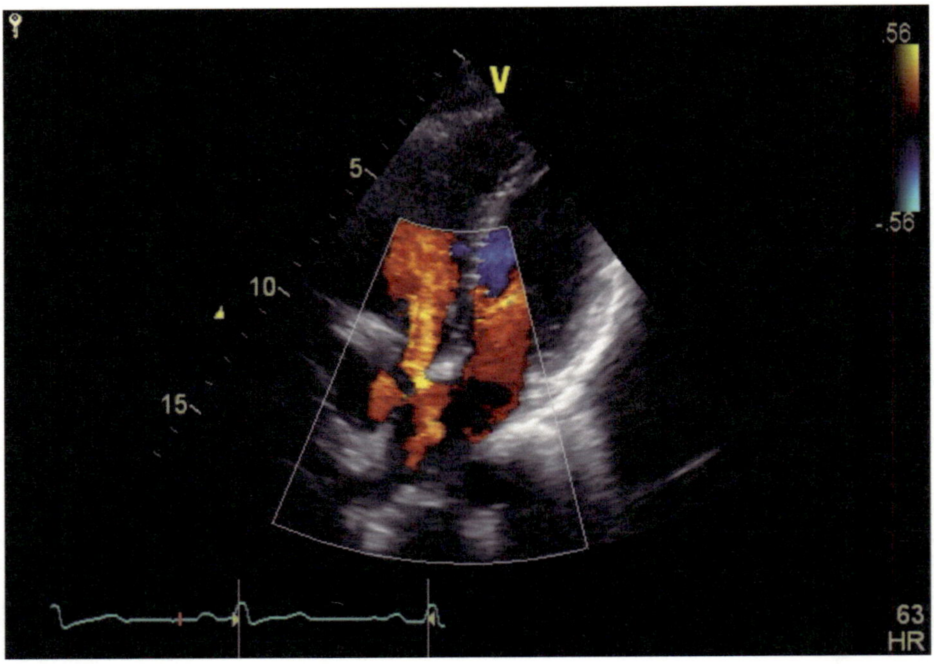

Figure 3. Echocardiography showing shunt flow through atrial septal defect. The multiple direction of the flow suggested the presence of a number of holes in the atrial septum.

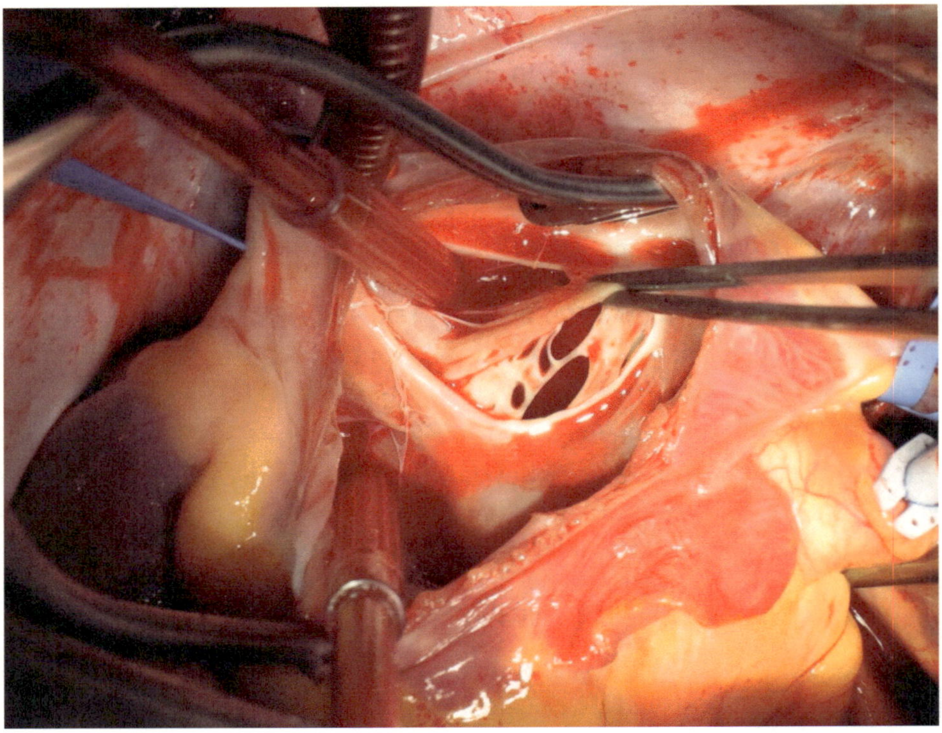

Figure 4. Figure 4. Atrial septum with numerous small pinholes and cribriform atrial septal defect

4. Discussion

The incidence of ASA has been found to be higher after a cerebral ischemic event in patients evaluated with transesophageal echocardiogram. A meta-analysis of case-control studies found that the presence of a PFO, ASA, or both was significantly associated with ischemic stroke in subjects less than 55 years of age [2, 3]. It is reported from PFO-ASA study that the presence of PFO together with ASA is a significant predictor of recurrent stroke [4]. Aggressive therapy such as warfarin or surgical repair may be the best option in such patients, but this question needs to be assessed in randomized clinical trials. The 2004 American Academy of Neurology practice parameter concluded that the combination of PFO and ASA increases the risk of subsequent stroke in medically treated patients below age 55 compared with other cryptogenic stroke patients without atrial abnormalities. It also concluded that there is insufficient evidence to evaluate the efficacy of surgical or endovascular closure [5].

The pathological mechanisms that lead to the development of ASA have not yet been clarified. To explain the association between ASA and cryptogenic stroke, two mechanisms have been proposed. Because of the frequency of intraatrial shunt, paradoxical embolism may occur. In patients with ASA without intracardiac shunt, it has been hypothesized that direct thrombi form within the aneurysm or as a result of atrial fibrillation, causing embolism [6].

Surgery is seldom performed for ASA patients. Shinohara and colleagues reported on a three-year follow-up of ASA [7], while Aoyagi and colleagues reported on a case of ASA and stenotic mitral valve [8]. In these two cases ASA was successfully removed and the atrial septum repaired with a pericardial patch. The reports concluded that surgery may be considered as an alternative therapy for patients with atrial arrhythmia and ASA.

The present cases occurred in patients without history of stroke, but who had numerous strong predictors of cryptogenic stroke, including ASA, PFO, ASD, and AF. The right ventricle was mildly dilated and right ventricular pressure mildly elevated in one case. Although the indications for surgical treatment of ASA and PFO remain undetermined, we considered that the symptoms were unlikely to resolve and that surgical intervention was the only curative treatment available. We reported in the above on cases of ASA. We believe surgical repair should be considered for giant ASA to reduce the future risk of cerebral embolism or heart failure.

Author details

Soh Hosoba*, Tohru Asai and Tomoaki Suzuki
Division of Cardiovascular Surgery,
Department of Surgery, Shiga University of Medical Science, Otsu, Japan

* Correspondig Author

5. References

[1] Hanley, PC, Tajik, AJ, Hynes, JK, Edwards, WD, Reeder, GS, Hagler, DJ, Seward, JB (1985) Diagnosis and classification of atrial septal aneurysm by two-dimensional echocardiography: report of 80 consecutive cases. J Am Coll Cardiol; 6:1370-1382.

[2] Agmon, Y, Khandheria, BK, Meissner, I, Gentile, F, Whisnant, JP, Sicks, JD, O'Fallon, WM, Covalt, JL, Wiebers, DO, Seward, JB (1999) Frequency of atrial septal aneurysms in patients with cerebral ischemic events. Circulation 99:1942-1944

[3] Overell, JR, Bone, I, Lees, KR (2000) Interatrial septal abnormalities and stroke: a meta-analysis of case-control studies. Neurology 55:1172-1179.

[4] Mas, JL, Arquizan, C, Lamy, C, Zuber, M, Cabanes, L, Derumeaux, G, Coste, J (2001) Patent Foramen Ovale and Atrial Septal Aneurysm Study Group. Recurrent cerebrovascular events associated with patent foramen ovale, atrial septal aneurysm, or both. N Engl J Med 345:1740-1746.

[5] Messe, SR, Silverman, IE, Kizer, JR, Homma, S, Zahn, C, Gronseth, G, Kasner, SE (2004) Quality Standards Subcommittee of the American Academy of Neurology. Practice parameter: recurrent stroke with patent foramen ovale and atrial septal aneurysm: report of the Quality Standards Subcommittee of the American Academy of Neurology. Neurology 62:1042-1050.

[6] Schneider, B, Hanrath, P, Vogel, P, Meinertz, T (1990) Improved morphologic characterization of atrial septal aneurysm by transesophageal echocardiography: relation to cerebrovascular events. J Am Coll Cardiol. 16:1000-1009.

[7] Shinohara, T, Kimura, T, Yoshizu, H, Ohsuzu, F (2001) Three-year follow-up of an atrial septal aneurysm. Ann Thorac Surg. 71:1672-1673.

[8] Aoyagi, S, Kosuga, T, Fukunaga, S, Ueda, T (2009) Atrial septal aneurysm associated with mitral valve disease. Ann Thorac Surg. 88:1024.